Quality and Cost in Neurological Surgery

VOLUME 10: CONCEPTS IN NEUROSURGERY

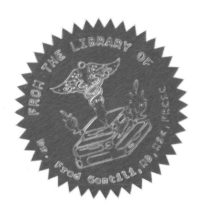

Quality and Cost in Neurological Surgery

VOLUME 10: CONCEPTS IN NEUROSURGERY

EDITORS

Mark E. Linskey, M.D.

Associate Professor of Neurological Surgery
Department of Neurosurgery
University of Arkansas for Medical Sciences
Little Rock, Arkansas

Michael J. Rutigliano, M.D., MBA

Assistant Professor of Neurological Surgery
Department of Neurological Surgery
University of Pittsburgh School of Medicine
Pittsburgh, Pennsylvania

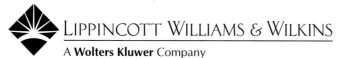

LIPPINCOTT WILLIAMS & WILKINS
A **Wolters Kluwer** Company
Philadelphia · Baltimore · New York · London
Buenos Aires · Hong Kong · Sydney · Tokyo

Copyright © 2001
THE CONGRESS OF NEUROLOGICAL SURGEONS

Accurate indications, adverse reactions, and dosage schedules for drugs are provided in this
book, but it is possible that they may change. The reader is urged to review the package
information data of the manufacturers of the medications mentioned.

Printed in the United States of America
(ISBN 0-781-732603)

01 02 03 04
1 2 3 4 5 6 7 8

Foreword

In the final volume under our series editorship, we have asked Mark Linskey to address the fundamental questions in the delivery of neurosurgical services: "how do we maintain and improve the quality of care?" and "how do we do so at a reasonable cost?" He has assembled a formidable team of experts to meet the challenge.

The answers are not obvious, the methods are frequently unfamiliar but the rigor and intensity of work required is familiar to neurosurgeons. What is important, and what we hope the neurosurgical community will gain from this publication, is that these issues, more than those of science or technology, will determine the role of neurological surgery in the 21st century. Those who pay for health care will increasingly demand high quality service at reasonable cost. It will be their definitions of "quality" and "reasonable" that will affect us. On the other hand, we have immense capability to influence their understanding, and therefore the way they define the terms. It is one of our most important tasks, if we are to thrive as a profession in American society, to be sure that the public definitions of "quality" and "reasonable cost" are informed by the knowledge of the real impact of neurologic disease, the true value of treatment and the belief that we are committed to providing our patients care of the highest quality in the most cost-effective way.

Dr. Linskey and his team provide an outline. The work is left to all of us.

Stephen J. Haines, M.D.
Charleston, SC

Paul B. Nelson, M.D.
Indianapolis, IN

Preface

The leadership, management, business, and accounting components of Neurosurgery practice do not have the popular allure of the sexier and more fashionable surgical tenchique, new technology, and scientific components. When we were first approached to take on the task of producing a monograph on "Quality & Cost in Neurological Surgery", we were both skeptical as to the level of genuine interest present in the Neurosurgical community at large. We feared that the very large amount of effort invested to produce a worthwhile monograph of this subject would be wasted due to generalized apathy toward the subjects and inability to entice Neurosurgeons to even read the work. However, as we thought further on the subject, we realized that the topic was too important to let these fears squash development at the point of conception. Even if we only reached a few seminal individuals, or produced a work that could serve as a reference for future study as the Neurosurgery climate evolved and matured, we would be performing a worthwhile service.

At one time we were together side-by-side as residents-in-training at the University of Pittsburgh. However, we took markedly different paths from that point onward. Dr. Rutigliano had strong interests in the business aspects of Neurosurgical practice and healthcare policy. He recognized that traditional Neurosurgical residency training was inadequate to prepare him for advanced academic work in these areas. Fortunately, he was able to convince a visionary department chairman, Dr. Peter Jannetta, of the academic value of allowing him to pursue and complete a M.B.A. during his research years within his residency. He is now on the staff at the University of Pittsburgh in charge of clinical practices for surrounding community hospitals affiliated with the main university hospital. As such, he spans the gap between an academic university neurosurgeon and a private practice community neurosurgeon. His academic publications on cost-effectiveness and other business aspects of Neurosurgery are well known and help fill out the content of this monograph.

Dr. Linskey started active duty with the United States Navy shortly after residency to pay back a scholarship commitment, and found himself thrust, at a precocious age, into a position of leadership, managerial, and fiscal responsibility—directing a department of five neurosurgeons at one of the Navy's largest military hospitals. In order to optimize his function in this new role, he studied to become a Quality Advisor for his hospital department through the Naval Leadership Training Unit (NTLU) at the Marine Corps Amphibious Base in Coronado, CA. The NTLU was in charge of training west coast and Pacific theatre Naval and Marine Corps officers in Total Quality Leadership (TQL) (the Navy's version of Total Quality Management). Individual intensive, full-time, two-week courses toward Quality Advisor certification included: Fundamental of TQL, Team Skills and Concepts, Systems Approach to Process Improvement, and Methods of Managing Quality. Dr. Linskey has since left active duty and is currently an academic neurosurgeon at the University of Arkansas. He has relied heavily on his military leadership experience and total quality training in producing and editing this monograph.

Currently, the number of individuals within our own Neurosurgical community with training and experience in quality management and advanced business assessments at the healthcare policy level are too few to allow thorough presentation of all relevant topics. As a result, we have had to also draw on authors outside of our Neurosurgical community in order to provide a complete and comprehensive treatment of the subject. Within this monograph, you will find experts from other surgical disciplines, from private consulting firms, from the military, from insurance companies, from the Joint Commission on Accreditation of Health Care Organizations, and from other non-health science university academic departments. Authors include physicians in academic settings, physicians in private practice settings, physicians in military healthcare settings, physician-executives from the insurance industry, physicians working as full time business consultants, Deans of medical schools, as well as Ph.D.'s, M.B.A.'s, and R.N.'s. We believe that the broad base of expertise thus represented will not only serve to strengthen the "hybrid vigor" of the monograph, but also serves to present a diverse viewpoint with regard to the issues of quality, and health care cost.

The monograph is divided into two separate parts. Dr. Linskey edits the first part on "Quality". The second part on "Cost", is edited by Dr. Rutigliano. Given the large amount of business and quality management jargon involved in the publication, a comprehensive glossary of terminology is provided at the end of the monograph to assist the reader as they make their way through each chapter. Chapter 14 includes lists of quality-related journals, web sites, software, and outside consulting firms, as well as an extensive general, and healthcare-related quality bibliography. A short "Editor's Comment" is included at the beginning of each chapter to help orient the reader to the specific relevance of each chapter to the overall goal of each of the two portions of the monograph.

We both recognized that we were poorly prepared by traditional Neurosurgery residency training to assume our later roles. Success as a Neurosurgeon often thrusts us into positions such as senior partner, Division or Department Head, Program Director, or officer in a Neurosurgical organization, where we are expected to succeed as leaders, managers, and businessmen. Unfortunately, those qualities that led us to become successful individual neurosurgeons do not ensure success in these additional roles. Most neurosurgical training programs only familiarize us with the concepts and tools necessary to successfully discharge these new responsibilities. This monograph is intended to serve as a resource for those individuals who find themselves in positions of leadership and/or business responsibility, as well as all Neurosurgeons who have an interest in these subjects, or aspire to these positions.

Contributors

SERIES EDITORS

Stephen J. Haines, M.D., F.A.C.S.
Chairman
Department of Neurosurgery
Medical College of South Carolina
Charleston, South Carolina

Paul B. Nelson, M.D.
Professor and Chairman of Neurological
  Surgery
Indiana University School of Medicine
Indianapolis, Indiana

VOLUME EDITORS

Mark E. Linskey, M.D.
Associate Professor of Neurological Surgery
Department of Neurosurgery
University of Arkansas for Medical Science
Little Rock, Arkansas

Michael J. Rutigliano, M.D., MBA
Assistant Professor of Neurological Surgery
Department of Neurological Surgery
University of Pittsburgh School of Medicine
Pittsburgh, Pennsylvania

John F. Alksne, M.D.
San Diego Health Sciences
University of California
San Diego, California

Peter McLaren Black, M.D., Ph.D.
Neurosurgical Services
Brigham & Women's Hospital and Children's
   Hospital
Boston, Massachusetts

Barbara I. Braun, Ph.D.
Associate Director for Health ServiceResearch
Joint Commission on Accreditation of
   HealthcareOrganizations
Oakbrook Terrace, Illinois

Ken Brodeur, Ph.D.
Director for Technical Support
Office of Continuous Improvement
Naval Medical Center
San Diego, California

Alex M. Chehansky
Intern
Office of Continuous Improvement
Naval Medical Center
San Diego, California

Stephen L. David, M.B.A.
President
SkyMark Corporation
Pittsburgh, Pennsylvania

Aaron Fausz, Ph.D.
Strategic Improvement Consultant
Executive Learning
Brentwood, Tennessee

Donald E. Fetterolf, M.D., MBA
Clinical Assistant Professor of Medicine
University of Pittsburgh School of Medicine;
Medical Director
Healthcare Informatics and Research
Highmark, Inc.
Pittsburgh, Pennsylvania

Robert E. Florin, M.D., FACS
Clinical Professor of Neurosurgery
Department of Neurosurgery
University of Southern California School of
   Medicine
Los Angeles, California

Peter C. Gersten, M.D., M.P.H.
Clinical Instructor
Department of Neurological Surgery
University of Pittsburgh Medical Center
Pittsburgh, Pennsylvania

Andrew Glass, M.D.
Health Services Commission of Oregon,
Kaiser Permanente
Portland, Oregon

Linda S. Hanold, MHSA
Director of Performance Measurement
Joint Commission on Accreditation of
   HealthcareOrganizations
Oakbrook Terrace, Illinois

Robert E. Harbaugh, M.D., FACS
Professor of Surgery (Neurosurgery)
Director of Cerebrovascular Surgery
Dartmouth Hitchcock Medical Center
Lebanon, New Hampshire

Julianne R. Howell, Ph.D.
San Diego Health Sciences
University of California
San Diego, California

Terry Howell, Ph.D.
President and CEO
Executive Learning
Brentwood, Tennessee

Eric J. Hummel, Ph.D.
Vice President, Meeting the Challenge Group
Oriel
Madison, Wisconsin

Yuhchang Hwang, Ph.D.
Associate Professor
School of Accountancy and Information
   Management
College of Business
Arizona State University
Tempe, Arizona

Steven F. Isenberg, M.D.
Indianapolis, Indiana

Joseph T. King, Jr., M.D., MSCE
Assistant Professor of Neurological Surgery
   and Medicine
Department of Neurological Surgery
University of Pittsburgh
Pittsburgh, Pennsylvania

Alison J. Kirby, Ph.D.
Associate Professor
School of Management
Boston University
Boston, Massachusetts

Richard G. Koss, MA
Associate Director for Research and
    Development
Joint Commission on Accreditation of
    HealthcareOrganizations
Oakbrook Terrace, Illinois

Mark E. Linskey, M.D.
Associate Professor of Neurological Surgery
Department of Neurosurgery
University of Arkansas for Medical Science
Little Rock, Arkansas

Jerod M. Loeb, Ph.D.
Vice President for Research and Performance
    Measurement
Joint Commission on Accreditation of
    HealthcareOrganizations
Oakbrook Terrace, Illinois

Mary B. McLaughlin, R.N., MBA
Project Specialist, Quality Management
Albany Medical Center
Albany, New York

William Mitchell, M.D.
Resident
Department of Neurosurgery
Jefferson Medical College
Philadelphia, Pennsylvania

Michael J. O'Leary, M.D.
Chief, Division of Neurotology/Skull Base
    Surgery
Otolaryngology Department
Naval Medical Center
San Diego, California

Charles A. Peck, M.D., FACP
Arthur Andersen LLP
Atlanta, Georgia

Gregory J. Przybylski, M.D.
Associate Professor of Neurosurgery
Northwestern University
Chicago, Illinois

Pam Rosato-Lange, R.N.
Department of Neurological Surgery
University of Pittsburgh
Pittsburgh, Pennsylvania

Michael J. Rutigliano, M.D., MBA
Assistant Professor of Neurological Surgery
Department of Neurological Surgery
University of Pittsburgh School of Medicine
Pittsburgh, Pennsylvania

Barbara J. Streibel, Ph.D.
Consultant Manager, Intellectual Capital
    Development
Oriel
Madison, Wisconsin

Mark E. Toso, CPA
TriNet Healthcare Consultants
Chelmsford, Massachusetts

Kristen Upchurch, M.D.
Neurosurgical Services
Brigham & Women's Hospital and Children's
    Hospital
Boston, Massachusetts

John B. Waldman, M.D., FACS
Division of Neurosurgery
Albany Medical College
Albany, New York

**Beverly C. Walters, M.D., M.Sc.,
    FRCSC, FACS**
Chief of Neurosurgery
The Miriam Hospital
Providence, Rhode Island

Contents

PART I

Quality in Neurological Surgery

The Total Quality Movement: A Paradigm Shift in Leadership and Management Philosophy for Neurological Surgery and Health Care in General

MARK E. LINSKEY, M.D.

> EDITOR'S NOTE: Introducing a concept so new to most neurosurgeons means introducing a great deal of new terminology. To limit the confusion caused by this new quality jargon, a glossary of terminology has been provided at the end of this volume. The reader is encouraged to consult this glossary while reading the first 14 chapters of this monograph, until the new terminology becomes clear.
>
> "People work in the system. Management creates the system."
>
> —W. Edwards Deming

Total quality is an approach to assessing a production or service organization that has profound implications on the way these organizations conduct business and manage themselves. The concepts and principles of total quality are equally applicable to both small (three to six employees) organizations and giant multinational corporations. For most health professionals, including neurosurgeons, the total quality approach represents a true "paradigm shift" (4), which is both exciting and frightening at the same time.

There are many reasons for individual neurosurgeons, neurosurgical group practices, academic neurosurgical divisions and departments, and national and international neurosurgical organizations to take an active interest in learning about and applying total quality management (TQM) within their organizations. The most compelling reason is that it is the single most effective and cost-efficient means yet devised of ensuring predictable excellence for the future, ensuring an optimal level of morale and productivity within an organization, and ensuring that the organization maintains its market share and stays in business. Furthermore, as TQM continues to make inroads in industries that purchase health care for their employees, in the managed care industry, in the health insurance industry, and in hospital administration, neurosurgical organizations that can continually demonstrate stable quality data and an organizationwide total quality approach will enjoy a significant competitive advantage over their peers for the business of these organizations. Lastly, because regulatory and governmental agencies such as the Joint Commission for Accreditation of Health Care Organizations, the Health Care Financing Administration, the Veterans Administration health care system, and the Department of Defense military treatment facility systems have made corporate strategic planning and multidisciplinary continuous process improvement mandatory, neurosurgical organizations face mandatory involvement. Why not be prepared and reap the benefits?

HISTORICAL BACKGROUND

The total quality movement has its origins firmly rooted in the United States manufacturing industry before World War II. Its beginnings can be traced to Walter A. Shewhart, a statistician at Bell Laboratories in New York. Shewhart was the father of *statistical process control* (sometimes referred to as *statistical quality control*) (67). He developed techniques to define the limits of random variation in any production task so that any points outside those limits could be studied, and the causes discovered. He also applied the scientific method to acquiring process knowledge by developing the plan-do-check-act (PDCA) cycle (discussed later in the chapter). Statistical process control exploded on the United States industrial scene during World War II, when the concept was applied to wartime material and agricultural production with impressive success. Shewhart was recruited by the United States Department of Agriculture, and it was as a member of this organization that he met and profoundly influenced William Edwards Deming, a Ph.D. physicist who trained at Yale and who had worked at Western Electric's Hawthorne plant in Chicago before the war.

After the war, the Unites States had little, if any, competition in the world markets for manufactured goods. In this environment, quality control techniques came to be considered time-consuming and, ultimately, unnecessary for business success. As the perceived need for statistical process control faded, statistical process control disappeared from the American scene. As Dr. Deming once said, by 1949 "there was nothing—not even smoke" (75). Still, the demonstrated power of statistical process control techniques had a lasting influence on at least three individuals: W. Edwards Deming, Joseph M. Juran, and Philip B. Crosby (31, 50, 69). They each used statistical process control as a core concept in much more extensive and comprehensive theories of quality that addressed all levels of management, not just production processes. Each went on to publish extensively their quality management theories (8–17, 19–22, 39–47, 59), and to establish prominent private quality consulting firms or training institutes. Of the three, Deming has arguably emerged as the most influential, not because his theories of total quality were immediately recognized for their inherent value in the United States, but because of eventual recognition in the United States and

elsewhere of the overwhelming success of the application of his theories in Japan (1, 30, 32, 33, 51, 52, 57, 63–65, 71–73, 75, 76, 81).

In the United States, Deming was better known as an expert in statistical sampling techniques (18), and in 1947 he was invited to Japan to help the Supreme Command of the Allied Powers prepare for the 1951 Japanese census. Once there, he interacted freely with Japanese statisticians. Soon his theories and reputation made their way to the newly formed Union of Japanese Scientists and Engineers, which had been organized by Japanese industry to assist in accelerating their country's economic and industrial reconstruction. The Union of Japanese Scientists and Engineers invited Deming to speak to them in June 1950. A meeting quickly followed this invitation with the 21 presidents of Japan's leading industries in July 1950. Japanese industry never looked back. Deming's total quality philosophy lit a fire in Japan that, within 4 years, led them to economic independence and soon empowered them to lead the world in steel, automobile, electronics, and high-technology manufacturing. Japanese industrial leaders did more than take TQM to heart. Many people, including Akoa (2), Kaizen (48), Ishikawa (36, 37), and Taguchi (35, 60), made their own seminal contributions to advancing and improving the philosophy.

Deming, was "rediscovered" in the United States after the airing of an NBC whitepaper entitled "If Japan can . . . Why can't we?" (56) in June 1980. Since then, the TQM concept has spread like wildfire, and literally hundreds of United States corporations have started their own total quality programs based on Deming's theories. Although initially this concept influenced industrial manufacturing primarily, TQM soon began to make inroads in service industries including the hotel and restaurant franchise, and health care industries.

THE EVOLUTION OF AMERICAN MANAGEMENT

TQM can be thought of as the most recent generation in the progressive evolution of American management (23). During the first generation, leaders "managed by doing." Organizations were small, and the most efficient management style was simply to "do it yourself." In neurosurgery, this management style can still be found in the setting of many solo private practices. Master craftsmen directing their apprentices characterized the second generation. This management style is still represented in neurosurgery in residency training programs, as well as in some solo private practices and many small to medium-size group private practices (in which the apprentices are often office managers, nurse practitioners, and/or physician assistants).

The third generation managed by results (sometimes called managing by objective). This is the most prevalent management style in use in the United States today. In this paradigm, there is a formal and systematic hierarchy of control and accountability within the organization. Management operates through establishment of short-term objectives or goals and the assessment of success in achieving these goals, as well as the exercise of established organizational controls (i.e., formal written policies or "by-laws"). This management style is represented in neurosurgery by university neurosurgical divisions and departments, many large neurosurgical or multispecialty group private practices, most national and international neurosurgical organizations, and most hospitals. TQM represents evolution to a fourth generation of management in which the focus is on management by method. Alternative terms (and their acronyms) for TQM that are in common use include:

- Total quality control (TQC)
- Total quality leadership (TQL)
- Total quality
- Quality function deployment (QFD)
- Continuous quality improvement (CQI)
- Continuous process improvement (CPI)
- Continuous performance improvement
- Continuous improvement

Examples of successful implementation of this management style in neurosurgery are still few in number, and some of them are described in this monograph.

Although management by results demands better results from the *current system* within an organization, TQM provides the methods to study and improve processes continually to achieve better results by *improving the system* (38). The key elements entailed in the quality approach of management by method are:

- Customer focus (internal as well as external)
- Dedication to quality and continuous improvement
- A systems view of the organization
- Committed organizational leadership emphasizing unity and constancy of purpose
- Measurement and analysis of significant processes to identify improvement opportunities
- Cross-functional teamwork to achieve optimal results
- Employee development through education and training
- Open communication

The key differences in the organizational roles of management, supervisors, and employees between management by results and management by method philosophies are illustrated in *Figure 1.1*.

TQM does not succeed overnight. Implementation requires patience, the unswerving commitment and participation of organizational leadership, and a planned program of employee training and education. Ultimately the cultural transformation of the organization does not occur or become self-sustaining until a "critical mass" of people with the necessary position, knowledge, and power within the organization understand the concepts and accept responsibility for the transformation.

Previous Health Care "Quality" Initiatives, *or* What TQM Is Not

In the early and mid 1980s, hospital corporations and individual hospital administrations responded to managed care market pressures by creating a new internal administrative monitoring and regulatory department called *utilization review* (UR). The purpose of UR was to limit hospital financial losses by ensuring that inpatients were not kept in the hospital longer than the number of days that the institution would be reimbursed for their particular medical condition. Reviewers were usually middle- and senior-level nurses who had moved out of the clinical care arena into hospital administrative roles. We are all familiar with the notebook-carrying UR nurse carefully examining our patients' charts (but never examining the patients), and leaving either notes or stickers on the chart cover, requesting further documentation of need for additional hospitalization. The unspoken implication was, of course, that in the absence of extenuating medical circumstances, the physi-

ORGANIZATIONAL ROLES

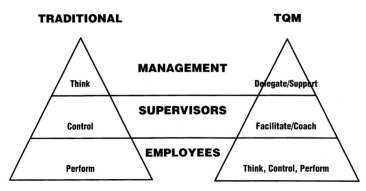

Figure 1.1   A comparison of the differing roles of management, supervisors, and employees in a traditional organization and a total quality organization.

cian should discharge the patient from the hospital regardless of whether the physician judged this to be appropriate.

At about the same time, hospital corporations and individual hospital administrations responded to the pressures of excessive malpractice litigation and insurance costs by establishing *risk management* offices. Initial risk management efforts were based on the belief that many malpractice lawsuits could by avoided altogether if management intervened immediately after an adverse therapeutic outcome by providing additional support services and demonstrating appropriate levels of care and concern. During these initial efforts, risk management relied mostly on physicians to report when adverse events or outcomes occurred, and then worked with them to assist the patients and their families. However, this effort soon evolved into a more active and impersonal institutional surveillance and monitoring system in which specific "red flags" or purported "sentinel events" were specified that automatically triggered risk management investigation. The reporting mechanism was taken out of the hands of the physicians and made a mandatory responsibility of the clinical nursing staff. Each sentinel event report generated required a written response, in way of explanation, from the involved physician. Although this approach did little to aid physicians in improving their health care delivery, this practice did succeed in alienating physicians from their clinical nursing support and wasting valuable time by creating large amounts of additional

paperwork that was required to comply with hospital regulations. Both of these changes were "cost driven" rather than "quality driven."

In the mid to late 1980s, many hospital corporations and individual hospital administrations combined their new UR and risk management services into one department with the new title of *quality assurance* (QA). In some respects, this was an attempt to put a positive "spin" on the UR and risk management programs by converting the older names, which included negative expressions (*review* and *risk*), to a new, positive, and optimistic name. Physicians were not fooled. The same practices of targeting physicians for what were usually process deficiencies, undermining the cooperative team relationship between physicians and their clinical nursing support, and annoying physicians with non-value-added additional paperwork were still in place.

The choice of QA as a name was quite unfortunate. Physicians understandably often have a very negative visceral reaction to the mention of QA, and at first glance quality improvement and quality management are often confused with QA, even though they embody completely different philosophical approaches. This confusion is often compounded by the frequent hospital practice of entrusting their organizational attempts at instituting TQM (i.e., quality improvement or performance improvement) to the same department previously responsible for QA. In many cases, the only real change perceived by physicians is a change in the name on the door of the QA department and a corresponding change in the titles of the personnel within.

Other than "quality" assurance programs, the other management approach most frequently and erroneously confused with TQM is "management by democracy" or "leadership by committee." This confusion is most often expressed by leaders who possess an autocratic leadership style and confuse the quality emphasis on cross-functional teams and consensus building with abdication of leadership responsibilities and leadership vision. As this monograph demonstrates, consensus has nothing to do with majority rule. Winning a vote is not the same as achieving consensus. Furthermore, strong leadership and clear leadership vision are major priorities in TQM because they are the most essential prerequisites for TQM implementation success—establishing the proper priorities and direction for TQM efforts, and avoiding suboptimization within an organization.

The Chain Reaction, the Deming Approach to Quality Management, and Basic Quality Conceptual Definitions

A fundamental principle in Deming's total quality philosophy is the concept of the chain reaction (*Fig. 1.2*) (75). The chain reaction begins with an organizational focus on customers as the agents that define the quality of your products or services. As you improve product or service quality in the eyes of your customers, your costs decrease because of less rework, fewer mistakes, fewer delays, and better use of equipment, time, and materials. As your costs decrease, productivity improves. As productivity

and quality improve while price decreases, you capture a larger market share, stay in business, and provide more jobs. It is the ongoing empiric demonstration that the chain reaction really works, coupled with leadership constancy of purpose that sustains an organization's quality management program once organizational critical mass is achieved.

Simply defined (23–25), TQM is the application of quantitative methods and the knowledge of people to assess and improve:

1. The materials and services supplied to the organization
2. All significant processes within the organization
3. Meeting the current and future needs of the end user

Deming's quality management approach is made up of three key elements—the *system of profound knowledge*, the *fourteen points,* and the *PDCA cycle* aided by *process improvement tools*—and it can be viewed as a triangle (*Fig. 1.3*). Each of these three elements is discussed sequentially in detail, but to understand and appreciate their importance and interrelationships, one must understand the basic concepts of operational definitions, customers, suppliers, processes, stakeholders, data-driven management decisions, and teamwork as they apply to TQM.

Operational Definitions

In the opinion of Deming, there was probably nothing more important or more neglected in management than proper *operational definitions.* To Deming, an operational definition consists of three components:

1. A *criterion* to be applied to an object or service
2. A defined *test* for compliance of the object or service with the agreed-on criterion
3. A *decision rule* for interpreting the test results to adjudicate whether the object or service is in compliance with the agreed-on criterion

An operational definition gives communicable meaning to a concept by specifying how the concept is measured and applied within a given set of circumstances. The operational definition of the same term changes, depending on the application and the circumstances. However, the terms will always mean the same thing to every-

DEMING'S CHAIN REACTION

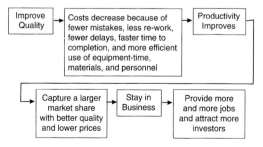

Figure 1.2 W. Edward Deming's chain reaction, which is used to explain how improving quality actually leads to lower costs and becomes a force for organizational growth and development.

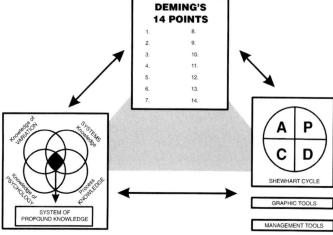

Figure 1.3   Deming's TQM philosophy is composed of three equally important entities that can be thought of in terms of a triangle. The first is his 14 points. The second is the system of profound knowledge that emerges from an understanding of knowledge of variation, knowledge of systems, process knowledge, and knowledge of psychology. The third entity is the practical quality weapons including the PDCA cycle, graphic tools, and quality management tools.

one involved in their formulation, both today and tomorrow (23, 27).

Delineation of specifications is not enough for an operational definition because an explanation of the means for determining compliance with specifications needs to be included as well. Good operational definitions eliminate many unnecessary disagreements and misunderstandings between departments and divisions within an organization. More importantly, good operational definitions eliminate unnecessary misunderstandings between suppliers and customers because the definitions are mutually agreed on between suppliers and customers in advance.

For example, patients may express that timely service is a desirable quality characteristic. An agreed-on operational definition might be that timely service means that patients receive an office appointment within 7 working days of receipt of the written or telephone referral at the neurosurgical clinic, based on the date of the appointment subtracted from the date of referral telephone call or date of fax transmission of the written referral. Then again, a managed care organization contracting for neurosurgical services might express that a low wound infection rate for simple lumbar discectomy is a desirable quality characteristic. An agreed-on operational

definition might be that a low wound infection rate means that less than 2% of patients undergoing simple lumbar discectomy exhibit wound redness, swelling, or drainage associated with an elevated erythrocyte sedimentation rate, white blood cell count, or fever by postoperative day 7.

Customers

In quality management terms, a *customer* is a person or group who receives or uses the output of a process (also known as *end users; Fig. 1.4*). Customers may be internal customers or external customers. An *internal customer* is an individual or group within the producing organization who receives or uses output from a previous stage of a process to contribute to the production of the final product or service. An *external customer* is an individual or group outside the producing organization who receives or uses output from the organizational process. In neurosurgery, examples of internal customers include other clinical services within the hospital that rely on neurosurgery for clinical support, an affiliated medical school, or an affiliated residency training program. Examples of external customers include our patients and their families, referring health care providers, managed

UNIVERSITY NEUROSURGERY SERVICE EXTENDED SYSTEM

(E)   **CUSTOMERS**

Private Insurance Patients
Managed Care Organization Patients
Medicaid/Medicare Patients
Self-pay Patients (Non-indigent)
Indigent Self-pay Patients
Referring University Clinical Services
Referring Outside Physicians
Referring Outside VA Hospitals
Emergency Room
Trauma Service
Neurosurgery GME House Officers
Rotating GME House Officers
University Medical School
University GME Lecture Series
Referral Hospital GME Departments

Figure 1.4   A list of internal and external customers for a university neurosurgical service's extended system (see *Fig.1.14,* and then *Figs. 1.5, 1.6, 1.8, and 1.15–1.17*). VA = Veteran's Administration; GME = Graduate Medical Education.

care contractors, and health and disability insurance companies.

In the total quality approach, customers should be the primary focus of a production or service organization because "quality" is defined in terms of customer needs and customer-defined quality characteristics. This is not to suggest that customer needs and quality characteristics are static, or that they always reflect more objective measurements of product or service excellence. The expression in politics that "perception is reality" holds true for the immediate customer perception of "quality." In an information vacuum, the two quality characteristics that always remain priorities for a service industry (including health care) are *timeliness* and *cost*. Any other quality attributes tend to be product or service dependent.

It should be the goal of organizational marketing to educate their customers about more substantive and objective quality characteristics for individual products and services, the appropriate objective measurements for these quality characteristics, and to compare and contrast these objective quality characteristics between service or product providers. It should be one of the goals of organizational research and innovation efforts to identify future customer needs and new quality characteristics that are reasonably likely to be important to the customer tomorrow. *Customers will insist on more than just timely and low-cost services if they know what characteristics to look for, and if the data for objective comparisons are readily available.*

In the past, physicians (including neurosurgeons) have feared and resisted any collection and publication of physician-specific objective outcome data. Much of this fear was legitimate, because only crude data (which could not be adjusted adequately for the medical risk of the patients or the complexity of the actual procedure) were available, and without proper risk and complexity adjustment, "apples could not be compared with apples." Differences noted between physicians might only be apparent differences, and quality judgments based on merely apparent differences might lead to unfair competitive advantage. Unfortunately, our lack of participation in improving this process and our resistance to any initiative that might lead to physician competition has perpetuated an information vacuum in which patients, hospitals, insurance companies, and managed care organizations have no choice but to judge us predominantly on the basis of cost and timeliness. As a profession, we need to realize that we are already in a competitive situation. Our best chance for fairness lies in getting involved to ensure that the playing field is indeed level, and that we are compared on matters that are most important to the actual objective quality of patient care (see Chapters 8 through 10).

Suppliers

In quality management terms, a *supplier* is the person or group who provides input to a process (*Fig. 1.5*). Suppliers can also be either internal or external suppliers. *Internal suppliers* are individuals or groups within an organization who

UNIVERSITY NEUROSURGERY SERVICE EXTENDED SYSTEM

 A

SUPPLIERS

Surgical Supply Companies	Clinical Laboratory
University Supply System	Hospital Administration
Affiliated Hospital Supply Systems	Medical School Library
Referring University Physicians	Medical Media Department
Referring Outside Physicians	Intraoperative Evoked Potential Services
Outside Referring VA Hospitals	Surgical Pathology
Am Assoc of Neurol Surgeons (AANS)	Radiology
Congress of Neurol Surgeons (CNS)	Anesthesia
Emergency Room	Pain Clinic
Main Operating Room	ENT
Short Stay Unit	Plastic Surgery
Post Anesthesia Care Unit	Critical Care Medicine
Inpatient ICU Nursing	Hematology/Oncology
Inpatient Ward Nursing	Radiation-Oncology
Outpatient Clinic Nursing	Neurology
Social Service Department	Pediatric Neurology
Pastoral Care Department	Physiatry
OT/PT/Speech Therapy services	Risk Management Office
Pharmacy	Patient Relations Office
Blood Bank	Information Resource Management Office

Figure 1.5   A list of internal and external suppliers for a university neurosurgical service's extended system (see *Fig. 1.14*, and then *Figs. 1.4, 1,6, 1.8, 1.15–1.17*). VA = Veteran's Administration; Am = American; Assoc = Association; Neurol = Neurological; ICU = intensive care unit; OT = occupational therapy; PT = physical therapy; ENT = ear, nose, throat.

provide input to another individual or group within an organization for use in a subsequent stage of a process that leads to the production of a final product or service. *External suppliers* are individuals or groups outside an organization who provide input to the receiving organization. In neurosurgery, examples of internal suppliers include support services such as radiology, pathology, the operating room, the emergency room, the clinical laboratory, the hospital inpatient wards, and the pharmacy. Examples of external suppliers include surgical supply companies, pharmaceutical companies, outside billing agencies, and national neurosurgical organizations.

Processes

A *process* is a set of causes and conditions that repeatedly come together to transform inputs into outputs (23) (*Fig. 1.6*). A process can be broken down on flow charts into definable individual decisions and steps (*Fig. 1.7;* see Chapter 5). Macrolevel flow charts are used to describe significant organizational processes as they relate to external suppliers and external customers. They usually include very few decision steps and often do not identify internal suppliers and customers. Microlevel flow charts define significant processes in more detail, describing

internal suppliers and customers across organizational functions, divisions, and departments. Minilevel flow charts describe every detailed step and/or decision within a process or, more commonly, within a stage of a process. In neurosurgery, examples of processes include performing different surgical operations (including preoperative and postoperative clinical management), performing inpatient and outpatient neurosurgical consultations, managing telephone consultations, scheduling patient appointments, executing patient billing, training medical students and house officers, and negotiating managed care contracts.

A *significant process* is a process that directly produces outputs that address customer quality needs and can be traced back through the organization to external suppliers. Improving these processes improves customer outcomes. A *critical process* is a stage within a significant process (a subprocess) that is deemed most important for improvement because of perception within the organization that incremental improvement during this stage will lead to the greatest incremental improvement in the overall significant process per unit investment.

A process is considered *stable* if it operates within statistical control limits according to objective measurement data expressed on a control

UNIVERSITY NEUROSURGERY SERVICE EXTENDED SYSTEM

(B)

ORGANIZATION PROCESSES

Performing Neurological Surgery
Performing Inpatient Neurosurgical
   Consultations/Evaluations
Performing Outpatient Neurosurgical
   Consultations/Evaluations
Performing Follow-up Outpatient
   Neurosurgical Evaluations
Performing Outpatient Disability Evaluations
Performing Patient Telephone Consultations
Performing Legal Brief Evaluations
Scheduling Outpatient Clinic Appointments
Processing Dictation Transcription and
   Correspondence
Patient Billing

Updating and Archiving Patient Office Files
Patient Database Data Entry
Training Neurosurgical House Officers
Training Rotating House Officers & Medical
   Students
Departmental Inventory Ordering
Departmental Budgeting and Budget
   Management
Research Grant Applications
Basic Science Research Protocols
Professional Lecture Preparation
Professional Poster Preparation
Professional Publication Preparation
Quality Assurance Monitoring

Figure 1.6 A list of organizational processes for a university neurosurgical service's extended system (see *Fig. 1.14,* and then *Figs. 1.4, 1.5, 1.8, 1.15–1.17*).

THE FLOW CHART

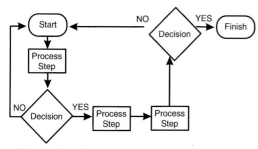

- Diagram that displays the steps and activities in a process or system and how they interact.

Figure 1.7 The flow chart visually reduces a process up into a starting point (*oval*), individual steps (*rectangles or boxes*), individual decisions (*triangles*), and a finishing point (*oval*) using geometric symbols.

chart (68, 77–80) (see Chapters 5 and 11). A *stable process* is one that has been standardized and one in which special cause variation has been eliminated (see the Knowledge of Variation section in this chapter). Standardization of a process involves reducing process complexity and ensuring that all participants carry out the process in a uniform and consistent manner. Redundant steps, nonvalue-added steps, and unnecessary process delay loops are examples of process complexity. The two most important attributes of a stable process are that it is consistently predictable in terms of future output and that it is ready for empirical attempts at improve-

ment through application of the PDCA cycle (explained in detail in the Process Knowledge section in this chapter). A *capable process* is one that is both stable *and* meets all customer needs.

Stakeholders

Stakeholders are groups and individuals inside or outside the organization who affect and are affected by the achievement of the organization's mission, goals, and strategy (23, 27, 28) (*Fig 1.8*). Stakeholders monitor performance, may themselves be evaluated based on organizational performance, adjudicate disputes, control access to resources, regulate the organization, and establish clinical options, standards, and guidelines.

Internal stakeholders are the key senior management figures within the organization as well as the directors of organizational departments and divisions that interface with external stakeholders. For neurosurgery, examples of internal stakeholders include more senior partners, neurosurgery division heads, neurosurgery or surgery department chairman, the director of surgical services in a hospital, hospital medical board members, the hospital medical director, key hospital administrators, and the dean of the medical school.

External stakeholders exist outside the boundaries of an organization and set environmental constraints on organizational practice. In neurosurgery, examples of external stakeholders include: state licensing boards, the American

UNIVERSITY NEUROSURGERY SERVICE EXTENDED SYSTEM

(F)   Environment & Other Stakeholders

University Policies	Malpractice Tort Law
University GME Committee	Managed Care Organizations
Credentials Office	Health Insurance Organizations
Laser Safety Office	Hospital Policies
State Disability Office	JCAHO
Social Security Office	ACGME
State Medicare Offices	CNS
Dean of the Medical School	AANS
IRB	HCFA
Animal Use Committee	AHA
Radiation Safety Office	ACS

Figure 1.8 A list of environmental constraints and internal and external stakeholders for a university neurosurgical service's extended system (see *Fig. 1.14,* and then *Figs. 1.4–1.6 and 1.15–1.17*). ACS = American College of Surgeons; ACGME = American College of Graduate Medical Education; JCAHO = Joint Commission Accreditation of Health Care Organizations; HCFA = Health Care Financing Administration.

Board of Neurological Surgery, national neurosurgical organizations, the American College of Surgeons, the American Medical Association, the American College of Graduate Medical Education, the Joint Commission on Accreditation of Health Care Organizations, the Food and Dug Administration, the sum total of malpractice tort law and precedent, the National Practitioner Data Bank, the Health Care Financing Administration, and individual contracting hospitals and/or managed care organizations. The need to comply with external stakeholder requirements or regulations is a frequent cause of complexity, leading to nonvalue-added steps in organizational processes.

Data-Driven Management Decisions

Surprisingly, most management and leadership decisions in the United States are still based on tradition, anecdotal experience, mimicking the course taken by others, or relying on personal intuition or instinct. New managers, often trained to pursue and to focus on short-term goals, frequently try to implement new ideas and institute changes with limited knowledge of the baseline performance of the process they are changing, or pursue administrative reorganization as a means of reflecting an illusion of positive change. In the first instance, without baseline performance data, changes might lead to worse performance, and management might be unaware of the performance degradation. Alternatively, performance might fluctuate randomly in a positive direction solely as a result of common-cause variation (unrelated to any benefit

from the change instituted), and management might erroneously conclude that their change was the responsible cause and maintain the change. In the second instance, valuable organizational resources and time are consumed to restructure an administration without any proved return from the investment.

In contrast, a fundamental principle of TQM is that management and leadership decisions should always be based on objective data measurements (23, 28). This principle has three corollaries. First, management must take the time, energy, and expense to determine current process performance and to ensure that the processes in question are defined, applied uniformly, and stabilized. This ensures that the results of any future changes can be compared objectively against this baseline to determine their effect. Second, changes should be tried initially and evaluated on a small scale (e.g., pilot project), to try and predict whether the proposed change on an organizational scale will justify the investment. Lastly, data should continue to be collected after committing to the change to serve as the new baseline for future improvements. Indeed, a popular total quality mantra has developed stating, "In God we trust, all others must bring data."

Quality Improvement Teams

Another fundamental tenant of TQM is reliance on quality improvement teams as the "engines" for total quality improvement within an organization (26, 53, 55, 66). These teams can be set up informally, as is the case with most *quality circles,* or they can be organized formally and chartered through managed participation, as is the case for *quality management boards* (QMBs) and *process action teams* (PATs). Both approaches have employee involvement at multiple organizational levels and cross-functional participation, data management decisions, the PDCA cycle, and decision through consensus as common features.

Quality circles tend to be voluntary participation teams open to all who are interested in participating. They develop within individual departments or services in an organization and have varying degrees of contact and guidance from higher organizational leadership. The advantage of a quality circle approach is that employee participation is maximized, no employee feels excluded, and the chances for innovation as well as employee support for any recommended changes are maximized. Disadvantages of this approach include lack of horizontal integration across departments with process interest, potential lack of authority from senior leadership outside the department to implement changes that would affect other departments, the potential for suboptimization within the organization as a whole, and a potential to waste valuable resources (especially time) on efforts not sanctioned by senior organizational leadership. Other

disadvantages include continually varying levels of employee participation and potentially unstable evolution of group dynamics (see Chapter 4). For these reasons most quality organizations adopt a more formal approach with managed participation.

In a managed participation total quality approach (23, 26, 27) (*Figs. 1.9 and 1.10*), permanent QMBs are chartered formally by the organization's Executive Steering Committee (ESC) around each organization's significant processes as identified by the ESC. The members of the QMB are the actual "process owners" across all relevant departments within the organization (usually middle-level management), are usually 7 to 10 in number, and are formally assigned to the QMB. Each QMB is provided with an "uplink" to the ESC to facilitate communication and to minimize suboptimization, adequate resources to perform their assignment, and a team facilitator or quality advisor for "just-in-time training" in quality tools (see Chapter 5). The QMBs meet on a frequent and regular basis, and are empowered to charter their own PATs. The leader for the QMB is also assigned by the ESC and works with the team's facilitator or quality advisor to organize the meeting agendas, run the meetings, and manage team dynamics (see Chapter 4). QMBs develop plans for pro-

Integrated Quality Improvement Team Structure

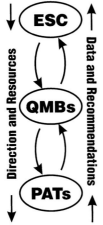

Strategic Quality Policy/Goals
What are our customers' needs?
What are our critical processes?
Do our processes meet customers' needs?
What changes are required for quality improvement?

Process Improvement
How does the process work?
Which process variables are most significant for quality?
How do we gather current performance data?
What resources are needed to analyze/improve the process?

Data Collection
What can we do to simplify the process?
What can we do to stabilize the process?
What did we learn from the data collected?
Are there special problems to be corrected?

Figure 1.9   With a planned and integrated quality improvement team structure, leadership direction and empowering resources flow downward from the ESC to the QMBs and PATs, whereas data and recommendations flow in the reverse direction. The ESC focuses primarily on strategic policy and goals for the organization. The QMBs focus on improvement of significant organizational processes. The PATs function primarily in a data collection and critical process evaluation role.

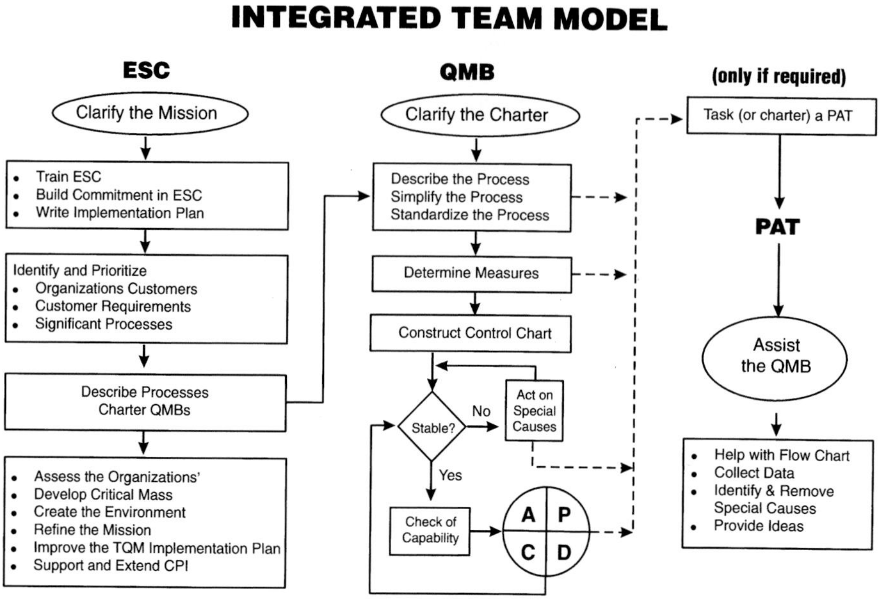

INTEGRATED TEAM MODEL

Figure 1.10   A process deployment flow chart depicting the various roles of each of the three types of quality improvement teams during implementation of TQM and ongoing process management.

cess improvement, initiate process analysis, evaluate the effects of process changes, and recommend major process changes to the ESC.

PATs can also be chartered by the ESC, but are usually chartered by a QMB. PATs are usually temporary teams that exist to gather data, or they are long-term teams with more expanded responsibilities chartered around a critical process. Their members are assigned and consist of workers within the process in question, are also organized horizontally across different departments (usually workers and first-level management), and are also usually 7 to 10 in number. Each PAT is provided with an uplink to the QMB to facilitate communication and to minimize suboptimization, adequate resources to perform their assignment, and a team facilitator or quality advisor for just-in-time training in quality tools (see Chapter 5). The PATs also meet on a frequent and regular basis. The leader for the PAT is also assigned by the QMB and works with the team's facilitator or quality advisor to organize the meeting agendas, run the meetings, and manage team dynamics (see Chapter 4). PATs develop measures, collect data, identify and remove problems when authorized, document process analysis and action, and make recommendations to the QMB for improving the process.

A managed participation approach to total quality has the advantages of minimizing the chance of suboptimization within an organization, maximizing cross-functional interdepartmental input to a quality program, minimizing the waste of resources in pursuit of total quality, and optimizing the chance of rapid and stable evolution of group dynamics. Disadvantages include the potential for some employees to feel left out of the process, the loss of potentially valuable input from excluded employees, and less grassroots support for recommended changes within the organization. Another potential disadvantage is that membership in quality improvement teams may eventually become a coveted end in itself, if it is perceived as a necessary step for accelerated advancement within the organization once the total quality movement becomes accepted and becomes self-sustaining within a particular organization. To avoid this problem, and to maintain morale, team membership may need to be rotated on a regular basis.

DEMING'S 14 POINTS

At the apex of Deming's philosophy of TQM (see *Fig. 1.3*) are his 14 points:

1. Create and publish to all employees a statement of the aims and purposes of the com-

pany or other organization. The management must demonstrate constantly their commitment to this statement.

2. Learn the new philosophy—top management and everybody.
3. Understand the purpose of inspection, for improvement of processes and reduction of cost.
4. End the practice of awarding business on the basis of price alone.
5. Improve constantly and forever the system of production and service.
6. Institute training (for skills).
7. Teach and institute leadership.
8. Drive out fear. Create trust. Create a climate for innovation.
9. Optimize toward the aims and purposes of the company the efforts of teams, groups, and staff areas.
10. Eliminate exhortations for the workforce.
11. (a) Eliminate numerical quotas for production. Instead, learn and institute methods for improvement. (b) Eliminate management by objective. Instead, learn the capabilities of the processes, and how to improve them.
12. Remove barriers that rob people of pride of workmanship.
13. Encourage education and self-improvement for everyone.
14. Take action to accomplish the transformation.

These 14 points are a set of management guidance principles for successfully achieving a quality transformation within an organization (21, 23, 52, 63, 64, 75, 76). To stress the primacy of management's responsibility in bringing about the quality transformation within an organization, Deming sometimes refers to his 14 points as the *14 obligations of management*.

Point 1: Create Constancy of Purpose

Within a quality organization, it is a leadership obligation to establish and to demonstrate to all employees unwavering commitment to the long-term purpose of the organization. The first step in this endeavor involves establishing a formal strategic framework for the organization that consists of a mission statement, a vision statement, and an organizational statement of guiding principles and/or core values that are usually developed by the organization's ESC (see Chapter 3). Ideally, these statements are published, distributed to all employees, and are

referenced consistently in any major organizational policy decision. Demonstration of constancy of purpose, despite changing environmental and economic conditions, is one of the best ways to drive out fear and to create trust among the employees within the organization. It important to realize that mission, vision, and core value statements are designed primarily for internal consumption, *not organizational public relations*. Free from flowery words, and unobtainable goals and superlatives, the mission statement should state exactly what the organization does and for whom. Organizations make a serious mistake if they use these items as front office advertisements or exhortations to the workforce (see Deming's point 10).

Point 2: Adopt the New Philosophy

Implementation of a total quality initiative within an organization requires that everyone in a senior leadership position must learn and adopt the new philosophy. Attempts to delegate this obligation to others, or simply to hire additional ''experts'' to perform the task, are doomed to failure. Although successful implementation requires leadership to adopt the new philosophy, sustaining the effort within the organization also requires that a critical mass of employees learns and adopts the philosophy. Ways of assessing whether the philosophy is indeed being adopted include evaluating whether total quality training is occurring at all organizational levels, and assessing whether supervisors are truly focusing on process performance data, or are still clinging to a focus on results.

Point 3: Cease Dependence on Mass Inspection

Mass inspections never ensure future performance or quality. They are expensive, disruptive, and time-consuming. Such inspection is an admission that duds are expected and, by extension, tolerated. Inspection only serves a useful purpose when it is performed on a limited sampling basis as part of efforts to measure and monitor process improvement (see Chapter 7). Inspection should only be performed as a means to finding out *what* you are doing, not *how* you are doing.

Point 4: End the Practice of Awarding Business on the Basis of Price Tag Alone

One of the most destructive policies for any total quality program is the practice of choosing

of public humiliation, fear of losing respect or prestige, fear of losing a leader's trust and loyalty, fear of appearing stupid, fear of punishment, fear of increased workload, fear of increased job stress, fear of a negative evaluation, and so on. Most managers underestimate both the amount and types of fear present in the workplace.

It is management's responsibility to create trust within the organization. This is best accomplished by clearly defining and publishing the organizational mission and guiding principles, by demonstrating constancy of purpose with respect to that mission and those principles despite changing environmental and economic conditions, and by promoting actions that demonstrate the value that management places in fairness, teamwork, new ideas, and innovation.

One of the most destructive impediments to eliminating fear in the workplace is the presence of employee evaluation systems that reward employees differentially for short-term measures of performance (65). On the one hand, clearly superior employees will *consistently* perform in the top quartile or top 10% among their peers, and it is a natural tendency in our capitalistic society to want to provide incentive for others to emulate this degree of productivity and for the individual involved to continue his/her efforts.

On the other hand, consider a group of employees with intrinsically equal aptitude and productivity. At any given time, there will always be a random spread of productivity such that 50% appear above average and 50% appear below average (when all are really equivalent). Because this variation is a result of common cause and is random, the relative performance position of each employee in relation to the rest of the group will fluctuate from evaluation interval to evaluation interval independent of their individual efforts to "try harder." Short-term performance rewards damage morale among the equivalent half that just happens to fall below the mean during that interval. In addition, over the course of several evaluation intervals, employees eventually come to realize that performance rewards are not causally linked to the level of their individual effort (because they fluctuate based on common cause). As a result, they become apathetic with regard to the effort they expend, and the performance reward becomes self-defeating. In behavioral psychology circles, this phenomena is known as the *rat-in-the-cage effect*.

A quality approach to performance evaluations requires gathering objective data on overall employee productivity over several performance intervals to establish a statistically interpretable control chart (65). All employees who performed in subsequent evaluation intervals within the performance control limits are treated equally (despite an equal distribution above and below the mean). By treating these employees equally despite statistically insignificant short-term fluctuations in performance, employees become more confident and secure in their position within the organization, and are more open to cooperating with each other as a team rather than competing with each other to the detriment of the organization. Employees no longer have a disincentive to collect accurate data for analysis of process performance (eliminating "cooked" books, inflated claims, and "gun decking"), and they are empowered to express new ideas for innovation. Employee morale improves and fear is greatly reduced.

Only those who performed above the upper control limit during one interval or who consistently performed above the mean but below the upper control limit in a nonrandom pattern over several evaluation intervals would be singled out for reward (see Chapter 5). Identifying these individuals should also lead to an investigation of how they are able to consistently excel. Superior aptitude will be readily apparent. However, if the performance is linked to superior training or knowledge, the specifics of these items can be identified and provided to the rest of the group to improve their performance as well.

At the same time, individuals who performed below the lower control limit during one interval or who consistently performed below the mean but above the upper control limit in a nonrandom pattern over several evaluation intervals should be singled out for special attention. If the problem is one of lack of training or knowledge, that can be provided. If the problem is personal and external to the organization, that can be identified and resources provided to help when appropriate. Unfortunately there will always be some occasions when the problem is one of lack of aptitude for the job despite the employee's best intentions and efforts. Demonstrating that discovering mismatches between job needs and job aptitude leads to employment in a different role with a better match, rather than loss of employment, is an important means of driving out fear within an organization and is a critical responsibility of organizational leadership (see point 7).

Point 9: Break Down Barriers Between Staff Areas

Most American organizations are organized around a vertical organizational concept in which individual departments have separate vertical chains of command, and information tends to flow up and down within a department rather than between personnel at equivalent "rungs" of the "ladder" in different departments (*Fig. 1.12*). Although the organizational bureaucracy is organized vertically, most processes within an organization function horizontally, requiring input from employees at similar levels across multiple departments.

This vertical bureaucratic organizational structure can potentially lead to two negative effects. The first, termed the *silo effect,* is when the absence of horizontal flow of important information and/or conflicts of jurisdiction and authority between separate departmental command structures leads to poor organizational process performance. The second effect, termed *suboptimization,* is when one department is able to excel as a result of adversarial competition for organizational resources at the expense of other departments, or when the individual department's goals are out of step with the overall goals and priorities of the organization as a whole.

It is the responsibility of organizational leadership to ensure that the organization's overall goals and priorities are well defined and publicized among department heads, that all departments are working together toward the same goals, and that resources within an organization are balanced according to needs in reference to these goals and priorities. The important ability to break down barriers between staff areas is sometimes referred to as *managing the whitespaces* (61), in reference to the whitespaces between the vertical arms of an organizational flow chart.

Point 10: Eliminate Exhortations for the Workforce

Lofty-sounding slogans or exhortations such as "If you don't have time to do it right the first time, how will you find the time to do it over," "Work smarter not harder," and the like, generate frustration and resentment within a workforce. Implicit in "sloganeering" is the assumption that a better product or service is simply a matter of the employee trying harder, rather than the reality, which is that improving the actual process is a function of management and is, for the most part, out of the employee's control. Motivation is rarely an issue, especially when managers are effective leaders. Rather than slogans, management needs to provide the means to their desired ends (tools, training, supplies, resources, system improvement). Resorting to slogans offends workers' intelligence and is a clear indica-

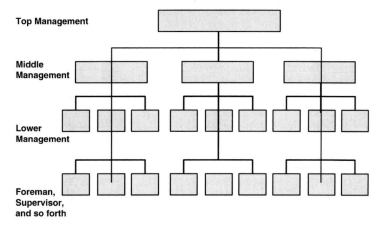

Figure 1.12 A diagram representing the traditional, vertically arranged structure and management organization within most businesses and institutions today.

tion that management either does not understand the reality of the situation or does not care.

Point 11: Eliminate Numerical Quotas and Management by Objective

Numerical quotas and management by objective involves setting short-term goals (often chosen arbitrarily) and then evaluating performance based on achieving those goals. If the process for producing a product or delivering a service that you have always used is not capable of achieving those goals, then no amount of effort and exhortation will be successful in achieving that goal. Only improvement in the process itself could potentially lead to success.

Let us assume that one achieves the desired performance goals over a given time period with the same process for producing a product or delivering a service that you have always used. The question then arises, Why didn't you produce or perform at that level before? If the current improvement was the result of a special cause and thus is not predictably reproducible, then you have not accomplished stable, sustainable improvement. The only assumption that appears to make any sense is that management believes that the processes for producing a product or delivering a service that you have always used are inherently capable, but are not currently performing to a desired level only as a result of lack of effort or motivation of the workers and supervisors involved. This is rarely the case, and is interpreted as misguided, arbitrary, patronizing, and insensitive by those tasked with meeting the quota or objective in question.

Rather than "whip the horses" that are already giving a good effort, management needs to learn and institute methods for process improvement. They first need to learn the empiric capabilities of their organization's processes, ensure that they are stable, and then initiate systematic, data-driven experiments to improve the processes. Improvement in productivity is a natural by-product of this endeavor, and will be predictably sustainable because the process itself will have improved.

Point 12: Remove Barriers to Pride in Workmanship

Pride in workmanship is a very strong performance reward with inherent value to the employee, inestimable value to the employer, and little cost to the organization. It is ultimately a more powerful and lasting incentive or inducement than monetary or time-off bonuses. Barriers to pride in workmanship include absence of the resources necessary to succeed at the position, defective or obsolete tools or equipment, lack of performance feedback except at periods of formal evaluation (when it's too late to change), lack of training in the methods and tools necessary to succeed, perceived lack of input toward improving the working environment and/or process improvement, and fear within the workplace (see point 8). Removing these barriers is the responsibility of management.

Point 13: Encourage Education and Self-Improvement for Everyone

It is not enough to have good people and to improve an organization's significant processes continually. The people themselves need to improve continually through the constant acquisition of new knowledge and skills. This requires a willingness by management to invest in employee education and training beyond the minimum training necessary to perform the job. In Japan, the balance of individual personal quality improvement as an integral component to quality improvement in the workplace is referred to as *Kaizen* (48). This approach not only pays off in better morale and higher quality employees, it also has the effect of minimizing an organization's employee turnover rate.

Point 14: Take Action to Put Everyone to Work to Accomplish the Transformation

Nothing will occur without motivational force applied consistently until inertia and friction are overcome, and the change becomes self-sustaining. This motivational force must come from management at all levels, beginning with the top leadership positions. Management must organize itself as a team to advance the other 13 points (75). Consultation with a statistician and/or a quality management consultant is usually both necessary and desirable. Management must not reduce its efforts and insistence until a "critical mass" is achieved within the organization, or the attempt at change will stall and ultimately fail.

THE SYSTEM OF PROFOUND KNOWLEDGE

Another point in the triangle forming Deming's approach to quality management (see *Fig.*

1.3) is the concept of *profound knowledge* (23) (*Fig. 1.13*). To Deming, profound knowledge could only be obtained by gaining knowledge of an organization's extended system, organizational process performance, the science of variation and statistics, and the art of human psychology. Although the latter two are common throughout all organizations and can be taught in school or a training program, the former two are unique to each organization and must be learned "on the job." The specifics of any system of profound knowledge differ from organization to organization.

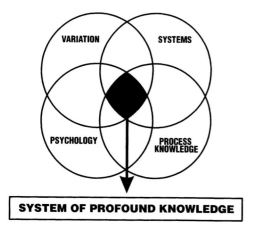

SYSTEM OF PROFOUND KNOWLEDGE

Figure 1.13 A Ven diagram depicting the emergence of profound knowledge from a balanced understanding of knowledge of variation, process knowledge, knowledge of systems, and knowledge of psychology.

Knowledge of an Organization as an Extended System

It is natural to consider an organization as a self-contained and enclosed structure separate from suppliers, stakeholders, and customers external to the organization. Although understandable, this view fails to appreciate the inseparable and intimate relationship that exists between all four of these elements. In understanding the organization as an extended system, the view of the organization is opened on either end to include external suppliers, stakeholders, environmental constraints, and customers in all organizational decisions and planning (28). This approach emphasizes the need to work and cooperate with all four external elements as part of process improvement and to maximize the chances of organizational success. Although some of the external elements are common among similar organizations, the individual specifics of the identity and relationship of each element to any given organization is usually relatively unique.

In addition, obtaining knowledge of external suppliers, stakeholders, and customers provides insight into inputs, outputs, and outcomes of the significant processes of the organization. These inputs, outputs, and outcomes can be measured objectively as part of the process improvement effort. A detailed example of an extended system for an academic neurosurgical department is outlined in *Figures 1.4 through 1.6,* and *1.14 through 1.17.*

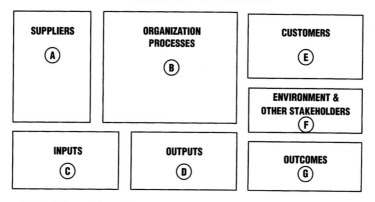

Figure 1.14 A graphic breakdown of the various components of a university neurosurgical service's extended system (see *Figs. 1.4–1.6, 1.8, and 1.15–1.17* for specifics regarding each of the lettered components).

UNIVERSITY NEUROSURGERY SERVICE
EXTENDED SYSTEM

Ⓒ **INPUTS**

Centralized Consult Requests
Direct Telephone Consult Requests
FAX Consult Requests
Emergency Pages
Patient Telephone Messages
Legal Brief Review Requests
Insurance/Disability Forms
Physician Dictation Tapes
Clinic Coding Face Sheets
Database Data Entry Sheets
Lecture Requests

Figure 1.15 A list of inputs for a university neurosurgical service's extended system (see *Fig. 1.14,* and then *Figs. 1.4–1.6, 1.8, 1.16, 1.17*).

UNIVERSITY NEUROSURGERY SERVICE
EXTENDED SYSTEM

Ⓓ **OUTPUTS**

Surgery
Neurosurgical Consultations
Non-operative Neurosurgical Care
Post-operative Neurosurgical Care
Legal Brief Reviews
Clinic Appointments
Transcription & Correspondence
Patient Bills
Patient Files & Updated Database
House Officer & Medical Student Training
Professional Lectures/Posters/Publications
Clinical & Basic Science Grants
Department Budget
Department Supplies
Completed Disability/Insurance Forms

Figure 1.16 A list of outputs for a university neurosurgical service's extended system (see *Fig. 1.14,* and then *Figs. 1.4–1.6, 1.8, 1.15, 1.17*).

UNIVERSITY NEUROSURGERY SERVICE
EXTENDED SYSTEM

Ⓖ **OUTCOMES**

Patient Health
Patient Satisfaction
Increasing Department Income
Society Work Force Productivity
Fair Patient Compensation
Well-trained Neurosurgeons
Medical Student/House Officer Education
Increasing Patient Referrals
Accurate & Current Records/Databases
Grant Funding for Research
Clinical & Basic Science Research
Reduced Legal Liability
Continuous Quality Improvement

Figure 1.17 A list of outcomes for a university neurosurgical service's extended system (see *Fig. 1.14,* and then *Figs. 1.4–1.6, 1.8, 1.15, 1.16*).

Knowledge of Psychology

You don't need to have a degree in psychology to be effective with TQM, but a baseline level of understanding and skill is essential for ensuring effective leadership, achieving consensus within a group, managing the dynamics of normal team evolution, and resolving interpersonal conflict (26). Of the four areas of knowledge that are components of profound knowledge, psychology is the most foreign to most neurosurgeons. It is the area farthest from the more comfortable arenas of medical science, scientific research, and the technical aspects of surgery. Furthermore, most neurosurgical training programs familiarize us only incidentally with these concepts. The rigorous training crucible through which we pass selects for rugged individualists who jealously guard individual autonomy, who are extremely successful individual competitors, and who often have not experienced the power and advantages of multidisciplinary "hybrid vigor" as well as group synergy (i.e., 1 + 1 = >2).

Knowledge of psychology requires one to become familiar with different individual human character types (*Fig. 1.18*) (49), how they relate to what an individual respects and cherishes, and how they relate to the approaches that persuade and motivate any given individual. It requires one to understand the four basic elements of communication (26), the skills required for active listening (7), and how to give effective feedback:

Four Basic Components

1. Sender
2. Receiver
3. Message
4. Feedback

Six Basic Factors

1. Words used
2. Nonverbal cues
3. Experience
4. Attitude
5. Abilities
6. Perception

In a group setting, knowledge of psychology includes the realization that any group of diverse individuals must go through stages of evolution or development before they can become an effective, optimally functioning team (26, 53, 55, 66, 74). These four stages of evolution, which are discussed in detail in Chapter 4, are often referred to as *forming, storming, norming,* and

---

The Four Temperament Axes

Extroversion (E) versus Introversion (I)	Equal Weighting (X)
Intuitive (N) versus Sensing (S)	Equal Weighting (X)
Thinking (T) versus Feeling (F)	Equal Weighting (X)
Judging (J) versus Perceiving (P)	Equal Weighting (X)

Sixteen Pure Character Types

INFP	ISFP	INTJ	ISTP
ENFP	ESFP	ENTP	ESTP
INFJ	ISFJ	INTJ	ISTJ
ENFJ	ESFJ	ENTJ	ESTJ

Thirty-two Mixed Character Types

XNTP	EXTP	ENXP	ENTX
XNTJ	EXTJ	INXP	INTX
XNFP	EXFP	ENXJ	ENFX
XNFJ	EXFJ	INXJ	INFX
XSTP	IXTP	EXSP	ESTX
XSTJ	IXTJ	ISXP	ISTX
XSFP	IXFP	ESXJ	ESFX
XSFJ	IXFJ	ISXJ	ISFX

Figure 1.18 Human temperament and character types (49).

TABLE 1.3
Stages of Team Development

Stage	Group Structure	Team Activity
Forming	Testing and dependence	Orientation
Storming	Intragroup hostility	Emotional response to task demands
Norming	Development of group cohesion	Expression of opinions
Performing	Functional role relatedness	Emergence of solutions

performing (*Table 1.3*). These stages cannot be avoided, but can be facilitated and managed by team leaders and quality advisors with knowledge of psychology. The effectiveness of any given quality tool (see Chapter 5) depends on the stage of maturation of the team, and some tools are difficult to use effectively during certain stages (e.g., the interrelationship diagraph is both disruptive and ineffective during the storming phase).

Two other areas in a group setting that require significant knowledge of psychology are working to achieve consensus and working to resolve conflict. Consensus can take hard work and considerable time to achieve (26). Strategies that may be effective depend on both the character types represented within the group and the current stage of team evolution. Although this is hard work and time-consuming to achieve, the importance of achieving consensus as a fundamental tenant of TQM cannot be overemphasized. Three important questions to ask when you are having trouble reaching consensus are as follows:

• What information do you need so you can support this decision?
• What results of this decision do you think we have neglected to consider?
• How can we build on this idea so we can reach a decision that you can support?

Conflict naturally arises whenever people get together to discuss important issues. It is not necessarily a bad occurrence because it can increase group energy and creativity as well as clarify ideas and increase understanding. However, if not checked and properly channeled and managed, conflict can decrease group productivity, lead to negative interpersonal relationships, and ultimately impair process improvement efforts. Conflict can arise within an individual or between individuals. It can be caused by different values, goals and methods, communication problems, issues of group control, established loyalties within groups, personality conflicts, individual status-seeking behavior, or frustration at lack of tangible progress. The five most common behaviors exhibited by people in conflict situations are:

1. Competing
2. Avoiding
3. Accommodating
4. Collaborating
5. Compromising

Knowing when and how to intervene and how to negotiate with a principled approach are all factors in the knowledge of psychology (26, 29, 70), which is discussed in detail in Chapter 4.

Knowledge of Variation

As neurosurgeons, most of us have some knowledge of statistics as it applies to scientific research. However, knowledge of variation extends beyond the statistics of clinical protocols, scientific experiments, and the question of statistical significance. It requires an understanding of variation inherent in all processes, whether they are production processes or service processes (23, 28, 58, 78–80). It requires an understanding of the difference between *common-cause variation* and *special-cause variation*. Common-cause variation is random variation, which is inherent in a process and cannot be reduced without changing the process itself. Special-cause variation occurs as a result of a cause outside the process. As a result, it can be eliminated without changing the process by simply removing the special cause. Knowledge of variation requires that one appreciate that trying to make changes in a process in response to common-cause variation is called *tampering,* and only leads to additional variability in common-cause variation.

The distinction between common-cause and special-cause variation can best be discerned through the use of control charts (28, 77) (see Chapters 5 and 11). A control chart is a run chart in which data measurements are plotted on the y-axis and time is plotted on the x-axis. For any set of data points taken from a process over time, a mean value can be established, and upper and lower control limits (three standard deviations

TABLE 1.4
Categories of Causes for Process Variation

Manufacturing Processes	Administrative or Service Processes
Environment	Environment
Manpower	Policies
Machines	Procedures
Methods	People
Materials	Plant

above and below the mean respectively) can be calculated and plotted on the y-axis. In the simplest case, data points falling between the upper and lower control limits are simply the result of common-cause variation, whereas those falling above or below the limits should be investigated for special causes. At a very minimum, knowledge of variation requires familiarity with the use and interpretation of process control charts (72) (see Chapters 5 and 11).

Potential causes of common-cause variation fall into the basic categories presented in *Table 1.4*. Sequentially identifying and modifying the most variable of these factors is the formula for CPI. Objective measures of the success or failure of CPI are readily reflected in changes in the data plot on the process control chart.

Process Knowledge

There is no substitute for knowing the actual objective performance attributes and variability of your own processes. This knowledge can only be discovered through empiric measurement and planned perturbations. This in turn requires an investment in time, introspection, CPI, and hard work. Many American managers try to avoid the amount of work and time inherent in this approach by trying to improve their processes through a distorted interpretation of the practice of *benchmarking*.

Benchmarking is the practice of comparing one's own process performance against that of a successful competitor in terms of objectively measurable outcomes to evaluate your own organization's progress with process improvement. Unfortunately, this concept has been perverted to suggest copying the process steps of another organization to begin quickly to approximate their results. This "bastardized" approach fails to consider that every organization has a unique extended system (with slightly different

environmental constraints, suppliers, customers, and stakeholders), and thus requires a customized process for optimal results. Even the specifics among the categories of potential factors leading to common-cause variation in a given process (see *Table 1.4*) are relatively unique to each organization. Deming refers to this practice a search for "instant pudding" (63, 75).

One also needs to make the distinction between process improvement and process refinement. *Process refinement* involves standardizing the process among all process workers and reducing process complexity by eliminating non-value-added steps and any unnecessary delay loops. *Process refinement* improves a process for an organization by stabilizing it (bringing it into predictable statistical control). However, process refinement only improves the performance of the existing process. It does not improve the process itself, and thus is not CPI as espoused in TQM.

THE PDCA CYCLE AND QUALITY TOOLS

The third point in the triangle forming Deming's approach to quality management (see *Fig. 1.3*) is the practice of using the PDCA cycle and the quality tools explained in detail in Chapter 5 to:

1. Provide the objective data necessary to make data-driven management decisions
2. Identify the most likely fruitful starting points for CPI efforts

As described in the Historical Background section, the PDCA cycle was invented by William A. Shewhart at Bell Laboratories (*Fig. 1.19*). It is a series of steps that brings scientific method to attempts to improve production

THE SHEWHART CYCLE

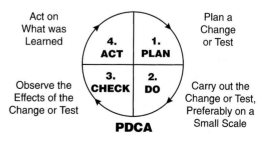

PDCA

Figure 1.19 The Shewhart PDCA cycle, which is the empiric engine of CPI.

and service processes. By repeatedly running through the PDCA cycle and making sequential adjustments between each cycle, one can continually improve a process, just like tuning in a radio signal. As process output common-cause variation is reduced, the upper and lower control limits on a control chart are brought closer and closer to the process output mean. If this mean is centered on a target value agreed to in an operational definition between the organization and its customers, then the process is not just stable (functioning predictably within control limits), it is also capable.

Quality management tools can be divided into quality graphic tools and quality management tools (3, 5, 23, 28, 33, 34, 54, 77), examples of which were listed earlier. These tools are presented and discussed in detail in Chapter 5. Not taught in most neurosurgical training programs, these tools are extremely useful for management purposes in general, and are indispensable for any TQM effort. They can be taught to quality improvement team members as the need for their use arises as part of just-in-time training provided by either team leaders or quality advisors.

DEMING'S SEVEN DEADLY DISEASES AND COMMONLY ENCOUNTERED OBSTACLES

Just as Deming's 14 points stand as the fundamental approach to TQM, he also describes seven conditions that will doom any TQM movement to failure. He calls these conditions *the seven deadly diseases* (75):

1. Lack of constancy of purpose to plan products and services that will have a market, keep the organization in business, and provide jobs (Deming's point # 1)
2. Emphasis on short-term goals and profits; short-term thinking that is fed by fear of an unfriendly takeover
3. Performance appraisal systems, merit ratings, or annual reviews that establish objectives or goals but lack a clear method for meeting the goal, instill fear, and discourage and/or eliminate needed teamwork
4. Mobility of management; personnel practices that encourage "job hopping" by management and labor
5. Managing with visible figures only
6. Excessive medical costs in the workforce
7. Excessive costs of warranty and liability,

fueled by lawyers that work on contingency fees

These are seven roadblocks to institutionalizing quality transformation, and they are inherent in most organizations in the western world. Their cure requires a complete change in management style.

Deming also describes multiple conditions that impede or impair a TQM movement without necessarily dooming it to ultimate failure. These he calls *obstacles* (75), and they are as follows:

1. Neglect of long-range planning and transformation
2. The supposition that problem solving, automation, gadgets, and new machinery will transform industry
3. The search for examples to copy
4. Offering the excuse, "Our problems are different!"
5. Reliance on quality control departments
6. Blaming the workforce for problems
7. Quality by inspection
8. False starts
9. The "unmanned computer"
10. Meeting specifications
11. Inadequate testing of prototypes
12. The assumption that anyone who comes to try to help us must understand all about our business

These commonly encountered obstacles are relatively self-explanatory and are not as "fatal" to an organization as the "seven deadly diseases." They represent management practice roadblocks to institutionalizing quality transformation that are harmful but still "curable" through the application of Deming's 14 obligations of management. A description of the seven deadly diseases follows.

Disease 1: Lack of Constancy of Purpose

The first disease is the opposite of the first of Deming's 14 points. How do you convince your employees that the changes you propose are not just the latest in a series of transient management "fads" except through consistent and repetitive demonstration of constancy of purpose? Two additional items that are almost as persuasive as unchanging, consistent repetition toward demonstrating constancy of purpose are demonstrated willingness to spend both money and time during working hours toward the acquisition of the necessary equipment and employee training in quality methods.

Disease 2: Emphasis on Short-Term Profits

Impatient and myopic focus on short-term paper profits does not allow room for real process improvement, which takes time and investment to achieve real and durable longer term profits. Pressures to produce short-term profits are not compatible with a TQM approach. Short-term paper profits give shareholders a "bigger piece of the pie," but do not "make the pie bigger" (75).

Disease 3: Evaluation of Performance, Merit Rating, or Annual Review

As discussed previously in point 8 (drive out fear), performance evaluations based on short-term productivity differences between employees (usually explainable by common-cause variation alone) are fatal to employee morale. They also eliminate any incentive for teamwork, and eliminate pride in workmanship.

Disease 4: Mobility of Top Management

Members of management who focus more on building their resume than the success of the organization, and who breed the concept that "you have to move out to move up," do not have the organization's long-term interests at heart. They are too ready to sacrifice real improvement over the long term on the altar of short-term profits that improve their short-term appearance. They will never truly be committed to a real quality improvement program.

Disease 5: Running an Organization on Visible Figures Alone

Visible figures tend to be monetary in nature. It is relatively easy to calculate visible costs, expenditures, and profits, and it is easiest to justify management decisions based on this type of objective data. The problem is that not all of our costs or profits are visible or easily measurable (except indirectly as increased or reduced business growth). For example, it is estimated that every satisfied customer yields repeat business for that individual, or perhaps the acquisition of new business from one to three people to whom the satisfied customer talks. On the other hand, it is estimated that every dissatisfied customer tells 8 to 12 people about his/her experience.

What is the cost to the organization of this negative publicity? How can we possibly know? Leaders in TQM need to include these invisible factors when they make decisions to succeed. Because they are not measured easily, the estimation and inclusion of these invisible factors in decision making involves some risk.

Disease 6: Excessive Medical Costs

This item is self-evident as a cause of ever-increasing costs to an organization. Is it any surprise who is driving the managed care movement in the United States, or why corporations turned to managed care companies when physicians alone demonstrated an inability to control these spiraling costs?

Disease 7: Excessive Costs of Warranty Fueled by Lawyers Who Work on Contingency Fees

This disease is so overwhelmingly self-evident to the medical community that it requires no further elaboration here.

IMPLEMENTATION OF TOTAL QUALITY WITHIN AN ORGANIZATION

Implementation of a fundamental philosophical management change throughout an organization is extremely difficult. The odds against success are very large. A detailed discussion of obstacles to implementation is presented in Chapter 14. Suffice it to say, TQM will not succeed without the unswerving commitment, courage, and perseverance of organizational leadership and a sustained commitment in terms of money and time. No approach has a higher, proven long-term return on an investment.

Implementation of TQM can be broken down into two stages:

The First Phase of Implementation of TQM

- Establish a critical mass.
- Ensure top leaders are trained and committed.
- Select and train an organizational TQM coordinator.
- Select and train the ESC.
- Design an organizationwide initial implementation plan (including a plan for training throughout the organization).
- Define the organization (mission statement, vision statement, and core values).
- Begin process management.

The Second Phase of Implementation of TQM

- Assess the mission of the organization.
- Identify and prioritize external customers.
- Identify customer needs.
- Identify and prioritize your significant processes.
- Establish output measures for the significant process.
- Identify and prioritize critical processes.
- Select in-process measurements.
- Standardize and refine the process and collect data.
- Analyze and improve the process through application of the PDCA cycle.
- Continue to monitor, improve, and search for innovation.

During the first stage, top leaders must train, commit to, and participate in the transformation. Leaders simply cannot lend their political support and delegate the planning and work of the transformation to others, or the transformation will fail. The second priority is to establish a critical mass of personnel within the organization that is trained in TQM principles and techniques and is committed to the transformation. From the group of trained leaders, an organizational ESC is chosen with the senior leader at its head (see *Figs. 1.9 and 1.10*). From the critical mass, an organizational TQM coordinator is chosen to serve as a quality advisor for the ESC. The ESC begins the formal portion of implementation by initiating strategic planning (see Chapter 3) and developing a formal organizational TQM implementation plan. The strategic plan includes an organizational mission statement, vision statement, and core values. The implementation plan includes a plan for completing and continuing TQM training throughout the organization as well as a phased, stepwise schedule for initiating process management by establishing QMBs for each of the organizations significant processes in order of priority. As part of the latter procedure, external customers are identified and prioritized by the ESC. By working with these customers, their needs and desired quality characteristics are identified and defined operationally.

During the second stage, total quality process management begins at the QMB level (see *Figs. 1.9 and 1.10*). Output measures for the significant process are identified. The critical process within the significant process (subprocess within the significant process) is defined and refined.

During process measurement, points and measurement instruments are chosen (see Chapter 8). The process is then refined and standardized, and baseline data are collected. If the data show that the process is not yet stable, then sequential pilot studies via the PDCA cycle are run until the process is stabilized. PATs may be established to assist with this phase. The stable process is then assessed for process capability relative to customer requirements. If the data show that it is not yet capable, then sequential pilot studies modifying additional causes via the PDCA cycle are run until the process is capable as well as stable. PATs may also be established to assist with this phase. Once the process is both stable and capable, process monitoring continues on a regular basis, and the search begins for new innovations, which are tested empirically. The overall systems approach to process improvement as well as a macrolevel flow chart for the steps of process management are presented and summarized in *Figures 1.10, 1.20, and 1.21*.

With smaller organizations, a more formal, nonintegrated team approach to CPI may be more desirable. This is often best achieved through establishing informal quality circles that may include everyone in the practice, if it is small enough (see the Quality Improvement Teams section in this chapter). In this less formal setting, a strategy developed by the Hospital Corporation of America may be more appropriate (*Fig. 1.22*).

The Hospital Corporation of America's Find–Organize–Clarify–Uncover–Start–PDCA (FOCUS–PDCA) cycle incorporates Shewhart's PDCA cycle (see *Fig. 1.19*) to allow for empiric, data-driven decision making, but is far less strategically directed or structured than an organizational integrated team model. As a form of spontaneous, ad hoc CPI, it can be very effective. However, to be most effective, it must include cross-functional participation integrated horizontally across departments, and it must maintain direct contact for bidirectional feedback with the external customers and suppliers of the extended system. If ad hoc FOCUS–PDCA is performed solely within the vertical columns of larger traditional organizational structures (see *Fig. 1.12*), it can lead to suboptimization. If ad hoc FOCUS–PDCA is performed disconnected from external supplier and/or customer input, it can lead to trivial changes that waste organizational resources, including time.

PROCESS MANAGEMENT FLOWCHART

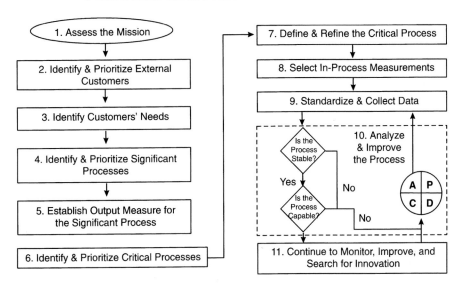

Figure 1.20 A flow chart depicting the basic steps involved in TQM implementation and ongoing process management.

SYSTEMS APPROACH TO PROCESS IMPROVEMENT

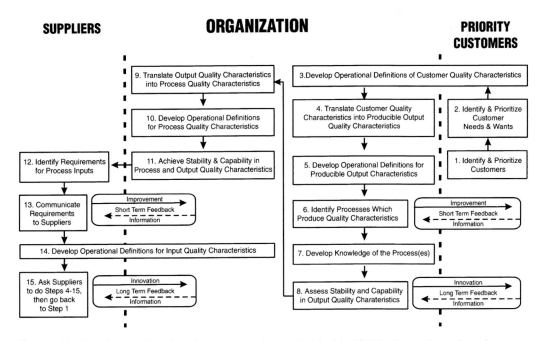

Figure 1.21 A deployment flow chart depicting the basic steps involved in TQM implementation and ongoing process management focusing on the interface steps with each member of an organization's extended system.

FOCUS-PDCA MODEL

Find a Process Improvement Opportunity
Organize a Team Who Understands the Process
Clarify the Current Knowledge of the Process
Uncover the Root Cause of Variation/Poor Quality
Start the "Plan-Do-Check-Act" Cycle

Plan the Process Improvement
Do the Improvement, Data Collection
Check the Results and Lessons Learned
Act by Adopting, Adjusting, or Abandoning the Change

Figure 1.22 The abbreviated CPI model developed by the Hospital Corporation of America for performing ad hoc (not centrally planned) process improvement.

REFERENCES

1. Aguayo R: Dr. Deming: The American who taught the Japanese about quality. New York, Lyle Stuart, 1990.
2. Akoa Y (ed): Quality function deployment: Integrating customer requirements into product design. Cambridge, MA, Productivity Press, 1990.
3. Asaka T, Ozeki K (eds): Handbook of quality tools: The Japanese approach (lesson 6). Cambridge, MA, Productivity Press, 1990.
4. Barker J: Discovering the future: The business of paradigms. Tape, 38 minutes, stock no. 0120-LF-020-8900. Joel Barker, Films Inc., 1-800-323-4222, extension 44.
5. Brassard M: The memory jogger plus +. Methuen, MA, GOAL/QPC, 1989.
6. Byham WC, Cox J: Zapp!: The lightening of empowerment. New York, Harmony Books, 1988.
7. Covey SR: The seven habits of highly effective people: Powerful lessons in personal change. New York, Simon and Schuster, 1989.
8. Crawford-Mason C, Dobyns L: The Deming library. Videotapes, vols. I–XX. Washington, DC, CC-M Productions, 1989, 1990, and 1991.
9. Crosby PB: The art of getting your own sweet way. New York, McGraw-Hill, 1972.
10. Crosby PB: Quality is free. New York, McGraw-Hill, 1979.
11. Crosby PB: Quality without tears: The art of hassle-free management. New York, McGraw-Hill, 1984.
12. Crosby PB: Running things: The art of making things happen. New York, McGraw-Hill, 1986.
13. Crosby PB. Quality Process Improvement Management College course materials. San Jose, CA, Philip Crosby Associates, 1987.
14. Crosby PB: The eternally successful organization. New York, McGraw-Hill, 1988.
15. Crosby PB: Let's talk quality. New York, McGraw-Hill, 1989.
16. Crosby PB: Leading. New York, McGraw-Hill, 1990.
17. Deming WE: Statistical adjustment of data. New York, John Wiley, 1943.
18. Deming WE: Theory of sampling. New York, John Wiley, 1950.
19. Deming WE: Sample design in business research. New York, John Wiley, 1961.
20. Deming WE: Quality, productivity and competitive position. Cambridge, MA, Massachusetts Institute of Technology, Center for Advanced Engineering Studies, 1982.
21. Deming WE: Out of the crisis. Cambridge, MA, Massachusetts Institute of Technology, Center for Advanced Engineering Studies, 1986.
22. Deming WE: The new economics for industry, government, education. Cambridge, MA, Massachusetts Institute of Technology Press, 1993.
23. Department of the Navy: Fundamentals of total quality leadership. Publication no. CIN P-500-0012. Washington, DC, Department of the Navy, Total Quality Leadership Office, November 1992.
24. Department of the Navy: Introduction to total quality leadership. Washington, DC, Department of the Navy, Total Quality Leadership Office, November 1992.
25. Department of the Navy: Department of the Navy total quality leadership glossary. Publication no. 94-01. Washington, DC, Department of the Navy, Total Quality Leadership Office, March 1994.
26. Department of the Navy: Team skills and concepts. Publication no. CIN P-500-0014. Washington, DC, Department of the Navy, Total Quality Leadership Office, October 1995.
27. Department of the Navy: Methods of managing quality. Washington, DC, Department of the Navy, Total Quality Leadership Office, December 1996.
28. Department of the Navy: Systems approach to process improvement. Publication no. CIN P-500-0004. Washington, DC, Department of the Navy, Total Quality Leadership Office, February 1997.
29. Deutsch M: The resolution of conflict. New Haven, CT, Yale University Press, 1973.
30. Gabor A: The man who discovered quality. New York, Times Books, 1990.
31. Garvin DA, March A: A note on quality: The views of Deming, Juran, and Crosby. Boston, MA, Harvard Business School, 1986.
32. Gitlow H, Gitlow S: The Deming guide to quality and competitive position. Englewood Cliffs, NJ, Prentice-Hall, 1987.
33. Gitlow HS, Gitlow S, Oppenheim A, Oppenheim R: Tools and methods for the improvement of quality. Homewood, IL, Richard D. Irwin, 1989.
34. GOAL/QPC. The memory jogger: A pocket guide of tools for continuous improvement. Methuen, MA, GOAL/QPC, 1988.
35. Gunter B: A perspective on the Taguchi methods. *Quality Progress* 20:44–52, 1987.
36. Ishikawa K: Guide to quality control. White Plains, NY, UNIPUB–Kraus International, 1982.
37. Ishikawa K, Lu D: What is total quality control? Englewood Cliffs, NJ, Prentice-Hall, 1985.
38. Joiner B: Total quality leadership versus management by result. Madison, WI, Joiner Associates, 1985.
39. Juran JM: Bureaucracy: A challenge to better management. New York, Harper Brothers, 1944.
40. Juran JM: Management of inspection and quality control. New York, Harper Brothers, 1945.
41. Juran JM: Case studies in industrial management. New York, McGraw-Hill, 1955.

42. Juran JM: Managerial breakthrough. New York, McGraw-Hill, 1964.
43. Juran JM: Management of quality. Course materials. Wilton, CT, Juran Institute, 1981.
44. Juran JM: The quality trilogy: A universal approach to managing for quality. *Quality Progress* 19:19–24, 1986.
45. Juran JM: Juran on planning for quality. New York, Free Press, 1988.
46. Juran JM: Juran on leadership for quality: An executive handbook. New York, Free Press, 1989.
47. Juran JM, Gryna FM (eds): Quality control handbook. New York, McGraw-Hill, 1988, ed 4.
48. Kaizen IM: The key to Japan's competitive success. New York, Random House, 1986.
49. Keirsey D, Bates M: Please understand me: Character and temperament types. Del Mar, CA, Prometheus Nemesis Book Company, 1984.
50. Lowe TA, Mazzeo JM: Three preachers, one religion. *Quality* 25:22–25, 1986.
51. Mann N: Keys to excellence: The story of the Deming philosophy. Santa Monica, CA, Prestwick Books, 1985.
52. McConnell J: Safer than a known way. Dee Why, Australia: Delaware Books, 1988.
53. Miller LM, Howard J: Managing quality through teams. Atlanta, GA, The Miller Consulting Group, 1991.
54. Mizuno S (ed): Management for quality improvement: The seven new OC tools. Cambridge, MA, Productivity Press, 1988.
55. Moosbruker J: Developing a productive team: Making groups at work. Team building: Blueprints for productivity and satisfaction. Alexandria, VA, NTL Institute for Applied Behavioral Science, 1988.
56. NBC producer. If Japan can . . . why can't we? Two videotapes, 80 minutes total. New York, NBC whitepaper, 1980.
57. Neave HR: The Deming dimension. Knoxville, TN, SPC Press, 1990.
58. Noln TW, Provost LP: Understanding variation. *Quality Progress* 23:70–78, 1990.
59. Reilly L: Deming WE: A lesson learned from the master? *Washington Technology* 6:23, 1991.
60. Ross PJ: The role of Taguchi methods and design of experiments in QFD. *Quality Progress* 21:41–47, 1988.
61. Rummler GA, Brache AP: Managing the white space. *Training* 28:55–70, 1991.
62. Ryan KD, Oestreich DK: Driving out fear in the workplace. San Francisco, CA, Jossey-Bass, 1991.
63. Scherkenbach WW: The Deming route to quality and productivity: Roadmaps and roadblocks. Rockville, MD, Mercury Press, 1987.
64. Scherkenbach WW: Deming's road to continual improvement. Knoxville, TN, SPC Press, 1991.
65. Scholtes PR: An elaboration on Deming's teachings on performance appraisal. Madison, WI, Joiner and Associates, 1987.
66. Scholtes PR, Joiner B, Braswell B, et al.: The team handbook. Madison, WI, Joiner and Associates, 1988.
67. Shewhart WA: Economic control of quality of manufactured product. New York, D. van Nostrand, 1932.
68. Suarez JG: Three experts on quality management: Philip B. Crosby, W. Edwards Deming, Joseph M. Duran. Publication no. 92-02. Washington, DC, Department of the Navy, Total Quality Leadership Office, July 1992.
69. Suarez JG: Managing fear in the workplace. Publication no. 93-01. Washington, DC, Department of the Navy, Total Quality Leadership Office, January 1993.
70. Tjosvold D, Johnson D: Productive conflict management. Coon Rapids, MN, Team Media, 1989.
71. Tribus M: Deming's redefinition of management. From selected papers on quality and productivity improvement. Washington, DC, American Quality and Productivity Institute, 1988.
72. Tribus M: Deming's way. From selected papers on quality and productivity improvement. Washington, DC, American Quality and Productivity Institute, 1988.
73. Tribus M: Reducing Deming's 14 points to practice. From selected papers on quality and productivity improvement. Washington, DC, American Quality and Productivity Institute, 1988.
74. Tuckman BW, Jensen MAC: Stages of small group development revisited. *Group and Organizational Studies* 2(4): 1977.
75. Walton M: The Deming management method. New York, Putnam Publishing Group, 1986.
76. Walton M: Deming management at work. New York, GP Putnam, 1990.
77. Wheeler DJ: Charts done right. Manuscript no. 56. Knoxville, TN, Statistical Process Controls, 1991.
78. Wheeler DJ: Understanding variation: The key to managing chaos. Knoxville, TN, SPC Press, 1993.
79. Wheeler DJ, Chambers DS: Understanding statistical process control. Knoxville, TN, SPC Press, 1992.
80. Wheeler DJ, Chambers DS: Advanced topics in statistical process control. Knoxville, TN, SPC Press, 1995.
81. Wilson L, Edmondson A: Deming's elusive eighth point: Why you can never drive fear out of the organization and what to do about it. Minneapolis, MN, Pecos River Learning Centers, 1991.

CHAPTER 2

What Is Quality In Neurosurgery?

ROBERT E. FLORIN, M.D.

EDITOR'S NOTE: As neurosurgeons, we all believe that we can readily recognize quality in neurosurgery. Yet when we are pressed for specifics, quality becomes a slippery term to define objectively. Quality is not the same as clinical excellence, because excellence only reflects surgical outcome and does not adequately address patient wellness, patient satisfaction, or cost of treatment. It is not the same as value, because value gives preeminence to cost over outcome. From a total quality perspective, quality is perceived and measured by the customer (e.g., patient, health care organization, contracting health management corporation) and not the physician. For an educated and enlightened customer with access to the necessary data for comparison, quality includes surgical outcomes, patient wellness, patient satisfaction, cost, and timeliness.

"I can't give you a definition of pornography [quality], but I sure know it when I see it!"

—Paraphrase of a prominent U.S. Supreme Court Justice on pornography

Quality involves the ability to achieve desirable objectives using legitimate means. In health care, this objective is usually an achievable state of health. Quality in neurosurgery is no different from quality as a concept in other medical specialties or in the general enterprise of health care.

The necessary means to achieving desirable health objectives vary according to the context of the definition of health as well as the chosen level of assessment. Health can be defined in many ways, but for our purposes, it is viewed in the context of its assessment. In a narrow sense, health is a measurable improvement in physical or physiological function, and in its broadest sense it also includes subjective assessment of the quality of life.

The level at which the assessment of quality is made is not in itself a measure of quality.

The importance of specifying the level of quality assessment is related to the need to match the measurable components of quality to their proper context. There is a progression of assessment levels that extends from the performance of health care practitioners, the performance of institutions, and the care received by patients in small groups, to entire populations enrolled in a health plan. At each level, health care concerns are different, and the attributes measured to assess quality are also different. The point is to select the proper level for analysis, be it the patient, physician, hospital, or health plan. These specifications of both context and the level of assessment are necessary because as the level broadens, our view of health care quality changes.

Despite the changing definitions of quality relating to the context and level of assessment, it *is* possible to measure quality in health care. The work of such pioneers in quality as Brook, Eddy, and Donabedian have helped define the problems in quality assessment as well as show the way toward practical application of these concepts (9, 17, 18).

In this chapter we first examine the philosophical basis for defining quality as a concept. Then we cover the relational aspects of quality assessment in terms of different health care contexts and assessment levels. We present a brief history of physician attitudes toward quality followed by the effects of different perceptions on its usefulness. The role of cost and value in appraising quality in health care and neurosurgery is examined. Finally, we explore steps to restore the primacy of quality in neurosurgery and health care policy. In summary, we offer a perspective on quality in health care and neurosurgery, and how its measurement and applications affect and are influenced by various factors in the health care continuum.

WHAT IS QUALITY?

In one sense, quality represents a degree of excellence, such as a grade or caliber, and implies conformance to a standard. It is distinct from the idea of quantity, although, as we will discuss, there are some crossovers in certain types of quality that blur this distinction. Quality is a concept that implies comparison with something else with attributes or characteristics that are represented as qualities of that object. Furthermore, quality implies a high ranking on a scale of comparative measures, which is obtained only after a certain level of excellence has been reached. Measures include traits or characteristics selected to reflect merit or superiority when compared with some standard. Such comparisons are made by applying subjective judgments to something that has special attributes or characteristics that can be identified as markers of quality. The level of quality of a given object can then be defined by the degree of adherence of such attributes or characteristics to a standard.

THE PHILOSOPHICAL BASIS OF QUALITY

Aristotle (3) suggested that the essential characteristic of quality is that it serves as the basis for saying that things are alike or unlike, analogous to quantity as the basis for saying things are equal or unequal. The idea of quality implies a comparative estimate of attributes or characteristics, rather than a quantitative measure of a physical property.

There seems to be little argument among the philosophers regarding the existence of qualities. This is in contrast with arguments about the existence of substances by those, like Hume (20), who question our ability to know whether substances actually exist. In this context, substances are the enduring things, material or otherwise, in which qualities are supposed to exist. They acknowledge such qualities as hot and cold, hard and soft, wet or dry, light or dark as attributes or characteristics of substances, but dispute other aspects of quality that leave a number of questions about quality incompletely answered.

Can Qualities Exist Alone?

The first question concerns whether qualities exist independently or whether they are only identifiable as attributes of substances. For example, are qualities attributes, and if so, do they exist only as qualifiers, only as belonging to something else? Or do they exist independently, in and of themselves? If qualities are attributes, do they belong to things apart from our experience of them, or do they belong to things only as experienced and have no separate reality?

There is general agreement among the many philosophers who have considered quality—such as Aristotle (4), Locke (24), and Spinoza (30)—that qualities do not exist (float freely) without any support in either reality or experience.

The Relationship Between Quality and Quantity

A second question deals with the distinction of quality from quantity. The assessment of a degree or amount of a quality assumes the notion of quantity. This leads to an examination of how quality and quantity are related to one another, including the order or precedence between these two attributes. Are quantities the more fundamental attributes of things and thus do they precede or underlie quality? Or do qualities precede quantities in certain respects and vice versa? Both Aristotle (6) and Aquinas (1) hold that ''quantity is in substance before sensible qualities are,'' which can be interpreted to mean that they believe that quantity universally precedes quality among the attributes of substance. Or this statement can be understood to mean that quantity precedes only *sensible* qualities, and then only among the physical attributes of bodies. Which interpretation is chosen depends, in part, on your view of whether *all* qualities are sensible.

Sensible Versus Insensible Qualities

A third question is whether all qualities are sensible; in other words, capable of affecting our senses directly. According to Aristotle (4) and Aquinas (2), certain types of quality are not sensible. Aquinas (2) enumerates a number of human qualities, such as knowledge and virtue,

TABLE 2.1
Philosophical Types of Quality

Type	Characteristics	Examples
Insensible		
Type 1, *natural*	Habit or disposition	Knowledge and virtue, beauty and health
Type 2, *properties*	Inborn capacity or incapacity	Good or poor athlete, healthy or sickly
Sensible		
Type 3, *dimensive*	Figure and shape	Square or triangle
Type 4, *principal affective*	Principal affective or sensible qualities	Hot or cold; sweet, bitter, sour; white or black

beauty and health, that are not sensible. These natural qualities, Aquinas writes, "may be in the intellectual part or in the body and its powers" (2). Clearly, the qualities inherent in the intellectual part of human nature are not sensible, and therefore do not precede every kind of quality among the attributes of substance. Aristotle (4) includes such human qualities as habits and disposition among these natural qualities that represent the first of four types of quality (*Table 2.1*).

A second type of insensible quality is the power or inborn capacities from which humans and other animals act to develop their natures. This includes rationality in humans and sensitivity in animals, which are considered qualities proper to these species and are, therefore, called *properties.* This second type of insensible quality is not restricted to living things, because inanimate bodies have among their properties certain fundamental powers of action and reaction. Aristotle (4) includes hardness and softness as an example of this type of insensible quality applied to inanimate objects because it reflects the inherent capacity or incapacity of the object to withstand disintegration.

Sensible Qualities

The third and fourth types of quality are sensible—in other words, capable of affecting the senses directly, and thus are sometimes called *affective qualities.* Of these, the third type deals with shapes and figures. This type of quality illustrates that not all qualities have opposites and not all admit to variations in degree. A shape such as a square represents a kind of quality that cannot become more or less square, and therefore cannot admit to "degrees of squareness." Shape or figure is a curious mixture of quality and quantity. It is an affective quality that can be viewed as a quantified quality or a qualified quantity. Aquinas (2) notes that shape appears to represent "a quality about quantity, since the

nature of shape consists in fixing the bounds of magnitude" (p. XX). This is evident in the fact that shapes, like quantities, do not admit variation in degree. In view of all of this, Aristotle (3) concluded that there is one characteristic alone that differentiates quality not only from substance, but also from everything else. Quality is the basis for saying that things are like or unlike, similar or dissimilar, whereas quantity is the basis for saying that things are equal or unequal.

The fourth type of quality includes the principal affective or sensible qualities, which include such attributes as color, sound, odor, taste, texture, and thermal qualities. These sensible qualities are the elements of human perceptual experience, and they represent the attributes of substance as actually perceived. These qualities are changeable as attributes of sensible substances (3, 5).

Given this classification of types of qualities, it is clear that quantity does not precede all attributes of substance. Because living things are a composite of body and soul, the qualities that are vital powers are usually regarded as properties that the thing has in virtue of having a soul. They are certainly not founded on the quantitative attributes of the organism's body. The moral and spiritual qualities of humans seem to afford another example of qualities that either precede or are at least independent of quantities. Even in the case of inanimate bodies, it may be that certain fundamental properties or powers are essentially qualitative rather than quantitative. The proposition that, in substances, quantities precede qualities—or that qualities are inherent in substances only by virtue of their quantities—may apply only to sensible qualities, as, for example, colors in relation to surfaces.

Does this philosophical exploration of the idea of quality answer the question of the relation of quality and quantity, and the priority of one or the other in the nature of things? According to one theory, difference in quality rather than quantity seems to be the defining characteristic of substances. Certain kinds of qualities are inherent in substances directly without being based on the quantitative aspects. However, it is rarely suggested that quality takes universal precedence over quantity. A key difference between quality and quantity is that qualities are subject to variation in degree within a given substance, and quantities are not.

THE IDEA OF QUALITY IN HEALTH

The idea of quality requires examination of the attributes or characteristics of some object rather than a quantitative estimate of a physical property of the same object. The question of how much an attribute is like or unlike an ideal standard for that attribute provides a measure of the quality.

This concept applies equally to quality in health care. According to Aquinas, health is one of the first type of qualities. It is not a sensible quality and it is not amenable to quantitative measurement regarding its attributes. Therefore, the practical application of efforts to measure or to assess quality in health care necessarily depend on comparisons between what currently exists and an ideal standard that represents the best estimate of what *could* exist under optimal circumstances. This is what Kathleen Lohr has called *the science of comparative quality measurement* (26).

USE OF QUALITY ASSESSMENT IN HEALTH CARE

Any health care quality assessment must be matched to the concerns pertinent and appropriate to each level of care. This requires defining the purpose of the assessment relative to the level of care to permit an appropriate and relevant judgment of performance as an attribute of care amenable to measurement.

Effect of the Level of Care on Measurable Components of Quality

At the practitioner level, the two most common components of care examined as measurable components of quality are the technical aspects of care and the interpersonal process. At the institutional level (e.g., a practice, clinic, or

TABLE 2.2
Level of Care and Quality Assessment

Level of Assessment	Components of Quality Measured
Provider/practitioner	Technical competence, performance measures; appropriateness of care; interpersonal process
Institutution	Amenities of care such as privacy, comfort, courtesy, staff behavior; adverse events
Health plan	Process end points such as mortality, morbidity, complications; cost, length of stay, patient satisfaction; efficiency of care management; effectiveness of intervention
Individual patient	Convenience, access, provider support; clinical outcomes, satisfaction, family support
Groups of patients, larger populations	Access to services; performance of providers, institutions, health plans; value of services for disease condition

hospital), the components of quality expand to include the amenities of care. These include privacy, comfort, access, and courtesy as the most commonly measured attributes. When the level of care expands to include the care actually received by a patient over an entire episode of care, the measured attributes include elements from clinical outcomes as a measure of what the health care encounters actually did to improve the health status of the patient. It also should include some measure of how much the patient and family helped and cooperated during the encounter, because this can have substantial effects on the clinical outcome. When the level of assessment expands to include the overall care received by large groups or a population, the scope of measured attributes expands to include patient health care access, provider performance, performance by the institutions and health care organizations (e.g., insurance plans, managed care organizations), and performance of the patient and family during the episode (*Table 2.2*).

Judgments of Care at Any Level

Two kinds of judgments are applicable at any level of health care quality assessment. The first is the expected contribution of care to the overall improvement of health of the population under examination. The second concerns the desirable properties of the care itself, as measured by social and patient preferences, appropriateness, and even efficiency.

Quality and Effectiveness

A central theme of quality in health care is that it is proportionate to the attainment of achievable improvements in health. The outcomes actually achieved in health care represent the effectiveness of the intervention provided for the patient. Actual outcomes of care seldom rise to the theoretical maximum achievable level. That goal is what is considered by the term *efficacy*. At a finer level of detail, efficacy reflects the best that can be achieved under theoretically ideal circumstances in which the appropriateness of the intervention and the technical skill of the care delivery meet the highest standard of accomplishment to which health care can be held. In practice, the ideal may not be achievable because of problems with patient or provider compliance, or should not be attempted because of an unacceptable cost–benefit analysis. In the assessment of quality, *effectiveness* is the term that reflects what is achieved by using the best or most appropriate intervention or test. The degree to which a care outcome approaches the theoretical maximum achievable (*efficacy*) is in itself a measure of the quality of that intervention and represents the *effectiveness* of that intervention.

Appropriateness

Appropriateness refers to care that is suitable or proper but not always necessary, required, or essential. In the context of quality assessment, appropriate care is defined as care for which the expected health benefit exceeds the expected negative consequences by a sufficient margin that it is worth providing.

The appropriate or best rate for use of procedures or tests depends on determining the appropriate clinical indications for performing that procedure or test. Determining appropriate rates for interventions requires the development of national standards for practice that can be used as a guideline by practitioners to help decide if and when to perform the procedures (10). Reviews of quality by examining appropriateness of procedures involves efforts to identify a mismatch in the care and services offered, and the care actually received. Measurement of underuse, overuse, and misuse of services all are included in this assessment. A fundamental reason that more

assessments of appropriateness of care have not been performed is in the absence of valid and accepted national practice standards for the majority of medical procedures. Such standards would ideally include indications regarding which options, among several diagnostic or therapeutic choices, would provide the greatest probability of a beneficial and satisfying outcome. Practice guidelines deal directly with these issues, but are equally difficult to develop by reason of insufficient reliable data on which to base such recommendations.

Practical Measures of Quality

The question of what to examine to provide some objective measure of the quality of the health care interventions was answered by Donabedian's formulation of an assessment triad (15). He proposed that health care quality can be assessed by using the following three categories to define the approach to the assessment: *structure, process, and outcomes (Table 2.3)*.

Structure defines the environment in which care occurs, including the physical setting, personnel, and organization of the delivery system. Process involves elements of the encounter between the patient and provider, which includes the technical components of the physician's skill and judgment plus the interpersonal skills applied to the relationship. Outcomes refer to the effects of the care on the health and welfare of the individual or population involved, and include not only the results of interventions but the functional and psychological consequences to the patient. Outcomes in quality assessment are not static measures of health, well-being, or some other state, but represent a change in status attributable to the intervention provided. As before-and-after comparisons, they offer clues that provide information in the assessment of process and structure that helps in understanding why outcomes depart from expectations, and suggest steps to improve the situation.

Components of Quality in Health Care

These three approaches toward quality assessment are seen as a judgment about quality and not as three different dimensions or attributes of quality. An approach that specifies structural characteristics increases the probability of providing specified kinds of care. An approach that emphasizes the particular properties of the process of care improves the probability of achiev-

TABLE 2.3
Measures of Quality

Structure	Process		Outcome
Characteristics of the setting and recipients of care	Elements of the encounter with the patient		Effects of care on the health and welfare of patients and populations
The environment in which care occurs	*Technical measures*	*Interpersonal process*	*The effects of care on the health status of patients*
Physical plant	Consult with provider	Access to provider information about therapy	Disease–specific health status
Credentials of facility			
Health care personnel			**Patient-reported status and satisfaction**
Organization of the system	Proficiency/skill	Communication	Functional status:
	Therapy factors	Concern/caring	1, physical function
			2, social function
			3, role function
			4, psychological function
Qualifications of providers	Complexity	Status of symptom	
	Ease of therapy		
Access to services	Discomfort	Patient preference	
	Convenience		
Comfort, convenience, and privacy			Health-related quality of life
Patient-related factors			General health status
Demographics, comorbidity, severity of illness	Disease-specific technical measures		***Procedural end points (intermediate outcomes)***
			Mortality, morbidity, complications, unplanned returns for services, costs, length of stay

ing specific changes in the health of individuals or populations so studied. The assumptions inherent in these two approaches are that there is existing knowledge that has been validated concerning the reliability of the relationship across structure, process, and outcomes. The current problem is that there is precious little data that support this critical assumption, and what data exist suggest an indirect rather than a direct relationship.

Of the three components, structure provides the weakest tool for quality assessment because the relationship between structure and either process or outcome is fundamentally weak. The relationship between process and outcome can provide useful information for nonclinical outcomes (e.g., cost, patient satisfaction). However, the relationship between process and clinical outcomes is poorly substantiated. This limits the usefulness of the attributes of both structure and process for assessing clinical health care quality.

Outcomes in the assessment of quality reflect a change in status that can be traced to an antecedent cause. Their use as the only measure of quality is limited because of the paucity of relia-

ble and valid outcome studies. A large amount of doubt remains about the causes of outcomes for patients not meeting the rigorous inclusion criteria of an outcomes study design. Outcomes are better used to provide clues to prompt the assessment of process and structure in search for causes that can be improved (11).

Patient satisfaction is currently not used much by physicians in quality assessment, largely because practitioners are strongly biased in favor of the technical aspects of care. However, from a market-based perspective, the attitudes of patients about their providers and the associated structures (and amenities) are becoming increasingly important. Service quality is becoming an important parameter to health plans because patients desire convenient access, timeliness, good service, politeness, consideration of their questions and fears, and reasonable cost (23).

Standards and Criteria

Standards and criteria are the actual measurement tools used in quality assessment. The more general concepts and definitions of quality need to be translated into specific criteria and standards that specify and calibrate the relevant attributes of structure, process, and outcomes.

There are two kinds of such criteria: implicit and explicit. Implicit criteria are what an expert uses when reviewing a medical record to rate the quality of care. Explicit criteria are previously specified without much latitude for the expert to adjust or change. Their main advantage is the standardization and ease of use, whereas their disadvantage is an inability to adapt to case variability (16).

DIFFERENT VIEWS OF QUALITY

Different views and definitions of quality by the principal stakeholders in health care must be considered because these will influence the expectations and value associated with different aspects of care. Each perspective calls for a different approach to measuring the aspects of quality most appropriate to that perspective, which tends to reflect those elements of care most important to that stakeholder (27) (*Table 2.4*).

Provider Perspective

For example, providers usually define quality in terms of the process of care, which deals with both technical competence and interpersonal skills. Provider competence is most often judged by performance measures, which include statistical rates of adverse as well as salutary outcomes of whatever intervention was provided. These are also beginning to appear on the report cards in use by various oversight groups that have positioned themselves to review individual and group performance for managed care organizations. The use of risk adjustment for such

TABLE 2.4
Perspectives on Components of Quality

Component	Provider	Patient	Purchaser/Payer
Structure	Med[a]	Med	Med
Process	High	Med	Med
Technical factors	High	Med	Med
Interpersonal factors	Low	High	Med
Outcomes	Med	Med	Low
Functional	High	Med	Low
Satisfaction	Low	High	Med
Cost	Med	High	High
Value	Med	Low	High

[a] Ranking of importance of the component of quality by each stakeholder.
Med = medium.

comparisons is essential and is slowly beginning to emerge as a part of such assessments.

The interpersonal skills of the physician are difficult to quantify, but have been subjected to estimation by psychometric survey techniques with some success. This turns out to be a very important factor from the perspective of the patient, who ultimately is the consumer of physician services. Satisfaction with the physician's skills in dealing with not just the medical or surgical problems but also the ease, comfort, and security of the encounter are of great importance to a majority of patients. It appears that a good "bedside manner" is still important and may even be marketable. Good communication skills and a caring manner contribute to the impression about "bedside manner," and have been found to be very important to the consumers of our services.

Patient Perspective

Patients tend to evaluate care in terms of its responsiveness to their individual needs. Unfortunately, their expectations have been shaped by the fee-for-service system in which most grew up, and access and economic restraints placed on their requests frequently and adversely impact their perception of quality.

The patient's perspective also includes some appraisal of their functional status at the end of the encounter, which is included as a subset of outcomes. A number of health status parameters to measure functional status have been examined, including biological and physiological factors, symptoms, physical functions, mental health, and general health perceptions. Patients usually focus on measures of satisfaction with the physician encounter, such as convenience, access, timeliness, and other amenities to a greater degree than the technical measures of competence described earlier.

Purchaser/Payer Perspective

The purchasers of health care began their efforts at monitoring quality by review of the usefulness of efforts at measuring the appropriateness of services provided. Currently, most managed care organizations and insurance companies rely on report cards to assess quality of care. The National Committee for Quality Assurance has developed a tool that focuses on a select group of performance and outcomes measures that are based loosely on clinical quality, access, satisfaction, use, and financial performance within the plan. With the increasing accountability imposed on the plans by regulatory agencies, the National Committee for Quality Assurance has promoted the development of the Health Plan Employer Data and Information Set, which examines a few outcomes measures as part of the package of evaluation tools it has employed (28). The goal has been to provide some standardized measure of quality that is useful when comparing health plans, although the measures employed to date do not yet fulfill that lofty goal.

Because of the growth and wide acceptance of the National Committee for Quality Assurance as a purveyor of a limited type of quality assessment, it has acquired substantial support among employers, purchasers, and even governmental agencies with oversight for publicly funded medical care. The hope is that such monitoring will reduce the tendency to cut costs at the expense of and risk to quality of service.

The Perspective of Value

A final perspective on the measurement of quality combines the various categories of outcomes into an estimate of the value of the service provided. This requires that a cost be attached to the encounter and that some judgment about the ratio of the outcomes (including patient satisfaction) to the actual costs be determined. This produces a measure of the value of the encounter and intervention in terms of actual dollars expended on behalf of the patient for a specified health problem. This has been used rather loosely by a number of insurance companies by coupling the report card performance measures to the average costs per patient episode of care, resulting in a cost per patient with a specified condition or procedure for each physician examined. The validity of this type of measure is very low, yet the insurance companies continue to produce such data and presumably make provider selection decisions aided by such shaky information. With more valid outcomes and accurate cost data, a more useful determination of value is possible.

A SHORT HISTORY OF QUALITY IN HEALTH CARE

The Health Care Market

In the modern arena of health care, the concept of quality and its assessment and management have consumed an ever-increasing amount of attention and budget, largely as a result of the increasing awareness that quality is the key to both improved services as well as value in the enterprise. When value is defined as the ratio of quality to the cost of a health intervention, it becomes clear that an increase in value requires either better quality or lower cost, or both. Because many markets have already been squeezed down to the bone regarding cost reductions, the focus has gradually shifted to strategies to improve the quality and thereby the value of services. After two decades of cost reductions, the cost cutters have now begun to focus on the quality of health care. Employer groups as well as managed care companies and insurers have begun to discuss ways to measure and to improve quality.

History of Physician Attitudes Toward Quality

Most physicians still remain on the sidelines in this game. Perhaps it is a consequence of the failed efforts dating from the 1960s to improve quality of care, which began by increasing access to care for specific populations by subsidizing health insurance for the poor and the elderly. In the 1970s, peer review organizations were instituted to improve quality of care, whereas in the 1980s, the mantra turned to quality assurance. All of these programs, which typically consisted of checking hospital documentation and statistics, with punitive potential, were viewed as regulatory agency harassment that rarely dealt with issues physicians felt were important for patient care.

Another negative influence on physician attitudes toward quality assessment was the lack of evidence that quality assurance programs actually did anything to improve patient outcomes. Physicians by nature and training expect to see compelling evidence to justify any requirement that alters how they care for patients.

Finally, many physicians became disillusioned with efforts to improve quality that were simply disguised schemes to cut costs, expand market share, or reduce staffing and length of stays. Some plans promoting ''excellence'' were simply missing any efforts to document outcomes and improvements consequent to the package of care advertised.

A major impediment to quality assessment as a useful means of judging and improving health care services has been the absence of standards against which to compare attributes and elements of such services. This was a consequence of the tradition that monitoring and improvements in quality were generally left to individual clinicians. Hospitals simply monitored poor outcomes such as deaths or infections as a means of quality control. Most providers assumed they were providing the best care (i.e., "quality"), and saw no need to bother with a concept of quality too difficult to warrant their time and efforts.

The Era of Accountability

In an editorial in the *New England Journal of Medicine* in 1988, Arnold Relman (29) described several changes in the health care system that he termed *the third revolution in medical care*. He called it the *Era of Assessment and Accountability* (29). This was based on a growing awareness that decisions about funding and the organization of health care required a better understanding of the relative costs, safety, and effectiveness of what physicians do, while trying to explain the wide variations in performance between equivalent providers and hospitals.

Studies by the RAND Corporation on carotid endarterectomy, and reported by Chassin et al. (12, 13, 14), showed apparent inappropriate surgery in the range of 30%, which got the attention of many, including the Health Care Financing Administration and their policy planners. Wennberg and Gittelsohn (31) found unexplained differences in the use of surgical management of reasonably matched populations in different communities for the same condition. These studies raised questions about whether the medical profession actually knew what was right to do for many conditions.

Concurrent with the availability of such information, several basic changes occurred. Patient expectations for good results increased rapidly, and payers began to realize that all medical care was not beneficial or appropriate. Another change was that the purchasers of health care services shifted from patients to health plans, employer groups, and government. Medicine's authority for judgments about quality was eclipsed by information that revealed there was no real evidence to use in making decisions about the comparative quality of similar services. Medicine had been spared from external

accountability for so long that, when challenged, it was unable to defend itself based on facts.

The move to managed care as the instrument chosen by payers to change the culture of medical care and to control costs had some unintended consequences. One of these was the negative impact it has had on quality. Managed care plans contain an inherent conflict of interest between their agreement to provide care for the enrollees and their dependence on providing as little care as possible for financial success. Because most physicians are currently trying to deal with the conflicting demands of the system and the risks to their patients as well as their own financial interests, it is important to consider methods to counter the incentives of the health plans to ration care. This is where monitoring of quality can be applied with a tangible benefit for patients.

The way that the delivery of medical services is changing obliges physicians to understand how the systems of health care delivery affect quality (19). These changes in turn have a direct influence on understanding how the interaction of providers, the system, and the patients view and affect the outcomes of any intervention.

THE SOCIAL BASIS OF QUALITY IN HEALTH CARE

Health care quality should be defined in terms of benefits to consumers: High-quality health care is care that best maintains and improves beneficiaries' health and satisfaction. Because health care is the primary product of the health care system, how can that system be designed and operated rationally unless the quality of that product is measured, understood, and controlled? Does knowledge of cost matter if the quantity or quality of the product is unknown?

The Institute of Medicine defined quality as "the degree to which health services for individuals and populations increase the likelihood of desired health outcomes and are consistent with current professional knowledge" (25, p. 21). In general terms, quality consists of the ability to achieve desirable objectives using legitimate means, for which the goal specified is an *achievable* state of health. The concept of quality in this context is a social construct that includes the idea and valuation of health, expectations of the provider–patient relationship, and views of the roles of different players in the health care enterprise. Quality assurance reflects our attempt to oversee individual and public responsibility, and includes the degree of commitment to equal access to and the enjoyment of health. A simple but persuasive definition of quality in health care is care that meets or exceeds expectations (21).

These definitions of quality illustrate the complexity of the concept and the need to consider it from a variety of perspectives when viewed by different stakeholders.

Perceptions of Quality Regarding Expectations

The perception of quality by various stakeholders in the system needs to be considered in relation to the expectations and values held by different groups, because the concept of quality differs from the perspective of different parties.

Physicians' views are already tainted by apprehension as a result of the development of measures of quality outside organized medicine. These measurements often challenge the belief of many physicians that professional judgment should be authoritative in matters of quality of care. This belief is further threatened by the reduced importance of physician judgment and autonomy resulting from the intrusion of third parties in decision making. When patients' values are included in the selection of a treatment plan, the physicians feel a loss of their professional status and control.

Patients evaluate quality in terms of responsiveness to their own needs. Medical and other technological advances have led to expectations of the ability to solve almost any health problem. The traditional fee-for-service system that paid physicians for doing everything possible for the patient has influenced the patient's perception of quality and sometimes inflated their expectations to unachievable levels. Recent studies have shown that a critical desire among patients is to retain some control over their choice of physicians, which has largely been ignored by managed care.

For purchasers, quality represents a way of evaluating how well premium dollars are being spent for the clients of the purchaser. In considering the value of services for their employees or members, they are gradually shifting from quantity measures to measures of efficiency and appropriateness of the care delivered. Although this approach includes unneeded services, it should also examine and guard against underuse or lack of access to needed and appropriate services.

Cost-Effectiveness

The effectiveness of an intervention can also be measured in terms of its cost, when the alternative therapies and their respective costs are compared, to determine which therapy achieved the best result at the least cost. However, the judgment about the appropriate cost–benefit ratio is really a question of economic and ethical policy, because it depends on the thresholds of cost and effectiveness established.

Perceptions of Value in Outcomes

Value, as perceived by the consumers of health care services, is gradually becoming a prime mover in the new health care economy. The influence of cost is beginning to diminish relative to considerations of quality. The role of value lies in its definition: *Value* = quality + patient satisfaction/cost. Quality can be defined as the degree of conformance to a standard, and requires that a standard exist for a comparison to be made. Outcomes measurement is the basis for identifying components of quality amenable to measurement and capable of serving as a standard or benchmark. Patient satisfaction is measured by a variety of survey techniques that target various aspects of the patient's perception of the intervention employed and the service encounter. The cost is the divisor in this formula and roughly represents the cost–benefit ratio of the encounter. As such, it tends to drive the consumer's perception of the value of the service.

Value plays a significant role in the business of neurosurgery by influencing the perceptions of the parties that are involved in a medical encounter. This can range from the health maintenance organization that may feel that a provider is too costly and therefore an undesirable entity to hold a contract to care for their patients, to the patient that may feel he was not treated courteously by the staff in the physicians office. Both of these perceptions track back to a judgment that the involved physician is not providing quality care. The impact of these perceptions of value frequently results in adverse effects on the physician's practice, and hence require attention.

There are a variety of problems that influence the business of neurosurgical practice that will not go away. They affect all of our members in

CHAPTER 3

Strategic Planning: Establishing the Framework for Total Quality Management

JOHN F. ALKSNE, M.D., AND JULIANNE R. HOWELL, Ph.D.

EDITOR'S NOTE: Strategic planning is a fundamental early step in the implementation of total quality management within an organization. It serves the purpose of focusing and ranking organizational goals and priorities to minimize "suboptimization" within the organization. It serves as a first step toward obtaining "buy-in" of key personnel within the organization for initiating and adopting the total quality philosophy as well as the changes that will accompany its implementation. It establishes organizational "first principles" that provide the basis for future growth and development, and that can be referred to in efforts to resolve potential future conflicts within the organization.

"Do you know that doing your best is not good enough? You have to know what to do. Then do your best."

—W. Edwards Deming

The concept of strategy traces its origins to political and military history, from Sun Tzu to Euripides. The Greek verb *stratego* means "to plan the destruction of one's enemies." Many of the basic terms associated with strategic planning—*mission, objectives, strengths, weaknesses*—derive from military applications. In the civilian sector, strategic planning has been used in business since the 1960s, when companies such as General Electric developed systematic approaches for tying annual financial budgeting processes to managing business units (10).

In health care, strategic planning dates to the 1970s, applied initially by hospitals as part of their response to regional and state comprehensive health planning regulation that required demonstration of community need to justify new facility construction and major equipment purchases (1). The use of strategic planning in health care waned in the 1980s as attention shifted inward to identifying and improving internal processes through reengineering and total quality management (TQM) (10).

Strategic planning experienced a resurgence in the 1990s as organizations sought an approach to position themselves for long-term success in the midst of the complexity and turbulence that now characterize the health care industry. The 1990s also brought an integration of external and internal perspectives because many organizations and consultants recognized the interdependency of strategic planning and TQM, and developed organizational processes that link these key approaches (5, 8). As *Figure 3.1* demonstrates, 3M's "total strategy" captures the essence of this linkage: doing "right things right" as the organization's "way of life."

In this chapter we consider the fundamental elements of strategic planning, both in concept and in practical examples derived from our experience within the Health Sciences at the University of California at San Diego (UCSD). "UCSD Health Sciences" includes both the UCSD School of Medicine, founded in the mid 1960s on an innovative model that integrated basic scientists and clinicians in a small number of clinical departments to encourage interdisciplinary research, and UCSD Health Care, the integrated delivery system created in 1995 to bring together

Total Strategy

Strategic Planning
- Do Right Things

Quality Strategy
- Do Things Right

Total Strategy
- Do Right Things Right

A Way Of Life

Figure 3.1   Total strategy.

UCSD Medical Center, the UCSD Medical Group, and UCSD Managed Care. In the early 1990s, UCSD Medical Center began to link its strategic planning and quality management processes, and is providing the foundation for bringing this linkage to all of UCSD Health Care. Our intent is to offer an overview of strategic planning and its role in creating the organizational context for TQM. We do not attempt to provide a step-by-step guide on how to conduct a strategic planning process and how to develop a strategic plan because several excellent and relatively brief recent texts fulfill this purpose (6, 8, 10).

WHAT IS STRATEGIC PLANNING? AN OVERVIEW

In its essence, strategic planning is the process by which an organization creates the framework for guiding all decisions made by senior leadership regarding priorities, resource allocation, and organizational development. Strategic planning entails periodically establishing overall goals and direction for the organization in light of the fundamental purposes for which it exists, the opportunities and challenges posed by the external environment in which it operates, and the resources that it can marshall.

To be truly *strategic,* this process must be oriented externally and future directed. As Hamel and Prahalad (7), two noted business strategists, have emphasized, an organization's ability to create its future depends on a clear and shared understanding of how the industry will be different in 10 years. What skills and capabilities will make the organization unique in the future?

Which customers will be served? What will be the basis of competitive advantage (7)? The answers to fundamental questions such as these define the "right things" for the organization to be doing, and hence indicate where the focus of quality management efforts should lie.

The strategic planning process itself creates the context for gaining a shared understanding of the organization and its environment, and therefore provides maximum benefit if it is broadly inclusive of key internal and external stakeholders at various levels throughout the organization. Many years of organizational experience have demonstrated that the most effective way to generate "buy-in" to the new directions and approaches that often result from a strategic plan is to include the key internal stakeholders in the plan's development. Nonetheless, because the strategic plan sets the organization's overall agenda, the planning process must be led by executive management.

With this overview, let us now consider each component of strategic planning, and organization of the planning process in more detail. It is important to recognize that, regardless of whether you are planning for a corporation, a medical school, a department or division of neurosurgery, a private multispecialty group practice, or a solo or group private neurosurgical practice, the process is the same.

BASIC COMPONENTS OF STRATEGIC PLANNING

Although various authors advocate different planning models, all models include seven basic components:

1. Clarification of mission, vision, and values
2. External assessment
3. Internal assessment
4. Strategic assessment: strengths, weakness, opportunities, and threats (SWOT)
5. Formulation of core strategies
6. Development of action plans to implement core strategies
7. Creation of monitors to evaluate plan outcomes

Figures 3.2 and 3.3 illustrate models developed by two different consulting groups with broad experience in strategic planning for health care organizations. *Figure 3.4* provides an ex-

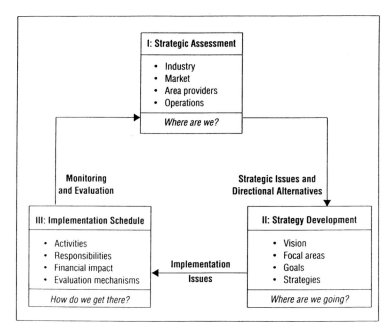

Figure 3.2   Model utilizing basic components of strategic planning.

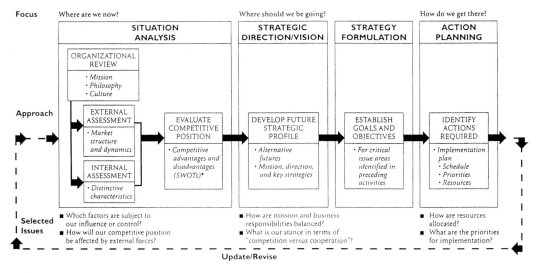

Figure 3.3   Another model utilizing basic components of strategic planning.

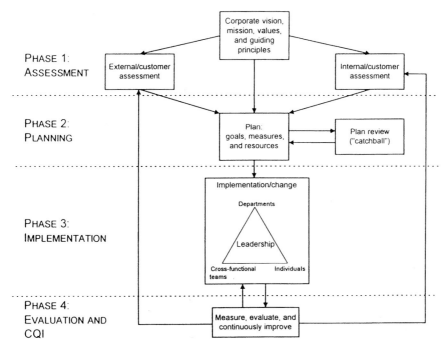

PHASE 1:
ASSESSMENT

PHASE 2:
PLANNING

PHASE 3:
IMPLEMENTATION

PHASE 4:
EVALUATION AND
CQI

Figure 3.4   Example of a process that integrates strategic planning and TQM.

ample of a process that specifically integrates strategic planning and TQM.

Vision: The Synthesis of Mission, Core Values, and Goals

Prevailing wisdom and practice acknowledge the importance of grounding strategic planning in an organization's *mission* and *vision.* The challenge comes in identifying and articulating these fundamental precepts because vision and mission are often confused, thus creating confusion rather than clarity around organizational purpose and future direction.

We have found that the model of vision developed by Collins and Porras through their research of such corporations as Hewlett–Packard, 3M, Johnson & Johnson, and Merck provides a useful construct for resolving any confusion between the concepts of mission and vision. As presented by Collins and Porras (3, 4) in their widely acclaimed book *Built to Last: Successful Habits of Visionary Companies* (3) and a subsequent *Harvard Business Review* article (4), vision has two key components: core ideology and envisioned future. *Figure 3.5* depicts the elements within each component.

Core ideology defines the enduring and un-

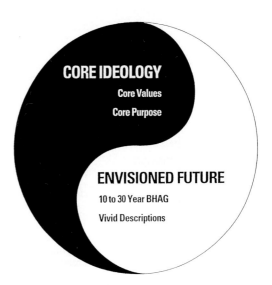

Figure 3.5   Articulating vision.

changing character of an organization—''the glue that holds an organization together through time'' (4). Core ideology, in turn, consists of two parts: *core values,* the guiding principles and tenets of an organization, and *core purpose* (or *mission,* as it is more commonly called in health care), the fundamental reason for existence that is unchanging and timeless, and provides the foundation for the organization.

Envisioned future is the second primary component of the vision framework and it also includes two parts: *10- to 30-year audacious goals* and *vivid descriptions* of what the future will be like if these goals are achieved. *Big Hairy Audacious Goals* or BHAGs, as Collins and Porras refer to them, apply to the entire organization and are intended to stretch it beyond current capabilities and the current environment to provide a compelling focal point for effort. The National Aeronautics and Space Administration's goal to put a man on the moon by the end of the 1960s, articulated by President Kennedy in 1961, is a classic example of such a goal. Vivid descriptions of achieving this end point help to characterize the future state. *Vision* changes over time as the organization achieves major goals and pursues new opportunities created by changes in the external environment and its own resources and capacity.

As Collins and Porras (4) summarize these concepts, "think of core purpose as the star on the horizon to be chased forever; the BHAG is the mountain to be climbed. Once you have reached its summit, you move on to other mountains''.

To provide an example from our own experience, *Figure 3.6* presents the vision for UCSD Health Care that has evolved since 1990 through several rounds of strategic planning first for UCSD Medical Center, then for UCSD Health Care, and finally for UCSD Health Sciences. The vision incorporates our mission and core values, which date to the founding of the School of Medicine and Medical Center in the mid 1960s, and the goal established in 1995 to become an integrated health care system, an organizational transformation necessitated by the challenges of managed care in the San Diego market. We are currently in the process of making this goal more specific as we evaluate options for providing necessary hospital capacity in "stand-alone" versus partnership arrangements with other San Diego health care systems.

Approaches to discovering core values and mission, and generating vision are considered in the section on the strategic planning process.

External Assessment

The external assessment provides the opportunity to examine all key environmental factors

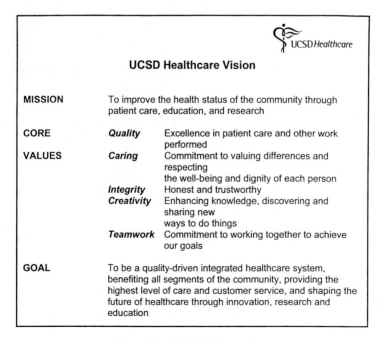

Figure 3.6   UCSD healthcare vision.

that influence the organization's present and future reality. At a minimum for a health care organization, these factors include

• Health care technology and information system technology trends
• Organizational structure and service delivery trends, both industrywide and in the local market
• Reimbursement and regulatory trends in the public and private sectors
• Human resource trends for physicians, nurses, and other personnel, both industrywide and in the local market
• Demographic, economic, and health status trends and forecasts for the population and region served
• Competitor analysis for other hospitals and health systems, organized physician groups, and other providers in the market

The external assessment is conducted using a variety of market information available through public sources; interviewing key payers, government officials, employers, and others familiar with the specifics of the market; and conducting consumer research to gain insight into the organization's current position relative to its competitors and into consumer preferences for future services. From the perspective of establishing priorities for TQM, careful attention to customer expectations regarding access, service, cost, and other aspects of the care delivery process is particularly important.

Internal Assessment

The internal assessment addresses the spectrum of organizational characteristics and performance that defines its current position and determines its capacity for future development. Essential elements include

• Use trends, quality and cost performance, and market position of the organization overall, its major components (hospital, medical groups, etc.), and its principal programs and services
• Service scope, including education and research as well as clinical services provided
• Organizational structure, processes, and the ''culture'' that results
• The number, specialty distribution, and distinctive capabilities of the medical staff and other essential ''human'' resources
• The location, condition, and competitiveness

of physical facilities and equipment, information systems, and other key physical resources
• Financial status, including operating performance, reserves, debt capacity, and ability to attract philanthropy
• Relationship to the community, including current patients served, potential patients who might be attracted to the organization's services, and the population in the service area overall who help to shape the organization's role

The internal assessment is conducted using information maintained in the organization's management systems, market share and benchmarking data available from a variety of external sources, and market research to gain qualitative and quantitative insight into the organization's performance as viewed both by those working within it and from key external stakeholders. Periodic reviews conducted by the Joint Commission on the Accreditation of Health Care Organizations and annual surveys of patient satisfaction and other performance studies increasingly being conducted by managed care organizations provide important input from the perspectives of accrediting groups intimately familiar with other health care providers and from current ''customers.''

An objective internal assessment is vital to defining the organization's *core competencies* and to identifying areas of focus for TQM.

STRATEGIC ASSESSMENT: STRENGTHS, WEAKNESSES, OPPORTUNITIES, AND THREATS

The external and internal assessments provide the basis for developing a key input to strategy formulation—a succinct and honest evaluation of the organization's competitive strengths and weaknesses, and of the opportunities and threats it confronts currently and into the foreseeable future. This *SWOT analysis,* as it is frequently called, gives organizational leadership a clear assessment of where the organization stands in its competitive marketplace and assists in determining what planning issues it must address in its future development (10).

As noted by Zuckerman (10), competitive analysis in health care has traditionally focused on historical data regarding market share. It is becoming more future oriented through the use of market size modeling and companion evaluation of organizational performance using information on industry best practices and benchmarks. Market size modeling involves estimating the health care service demands and capacity requirements for a given population and/or geographic service area under a variety of different scenarios regarding managed care penetration, population changes, economic conditions, and so forth. It provides the opportunity to explore the implications of various possible external environments on the organization's development. Best practice analysis and benchmarking identify performance levels the organization must achieve to be competitive; for example, case-mix adjusted cost per case or time to first available new appointment. Comparing current organizational performance to future expected levels yields important findings about future competitive needs and the competitive fitness of the organization (10).

Four critical outputs result from this strategic assessment:

1. The potential future impact of major market trends on the organization
2. The organization's strategic resources and core competencies
3. The needs and perceptions of key constituency groups
4. The critical planning issues facing the organization as a result of changing market dynamics and current organizational core competencies

This understanding provides the foundation for strategy development (6).

Core Strategies

Strategy is the vehicle through which an organization pursues its vision. It is developed in the context of the future environmental conditions and required organizational competencies identified by the strategic assessment. *Core strategies* become the specific approaches through which the organization plans to address the environmental opportunities and to overcome competitive disadvantages.

Moving from vision to the specific strategies to attain it is one of the most challenging and difficult parts of strategic planning. As Zuckerman (10) has noted, "strategic planning at its essence is the process of making difficult choices among competing priorities and focusing the organization's limited resources in those

areas with the greatest payoff". In our experience, these choices do not have to be fully confronted during the process of developing the strategic plan because the plan should provide an agenda that covers a range of core strategies to be addressed over a number of years. The difficult choices become most apparent and potentially contentious during implementation, as annual action plans are prepared and resources are committed.

The strategic choices confronting most health care organizations as they look to the 21st century frequently fall into the following areas:

• What type of affiliation and/or strategic alliance, if any, should be developed to maintain and to develop further market position?
• What delivery system integration models are appropriate, given organizational capabilities and market dynamics?
• What scope of services should be offered? To which market segments (6)?

When TQM is linked to strategic planning, then essential issues of customer focus, access to service, and organizational performance are incorporated into the strategic agenda and are recognized appropriately as vital to achieving organizational vision (8).

Figure 3.7 presents the core strategies developed as part of the UCSD Health Care Strategic Plan in 1995. Core strategy 2, Deliver High-Quality Care and Service at Low Cost, has provided the framework for setting the agenda of our continuous quality improvement program, UCSD's approach to TQM.

Action Plans

As Goldman and Nolan (6) have noted, "the output of planning is not a plan; the output of planning is action". The final step in the strategic planning process is, therefore, to create explicit implementation/action plans that identify the tasks to be accomplished, the roles and responsibilities of key players, and the timetable for completion. Action plans translate core strategies into what the organization will do to accomplish them, providing "the task-level direction necessary for the organization to grow into its envisioned 'future state' " (6). Typically, action plans are developed on a yearly basis, and ideally they are linked to the annual operating and capital budget processes of the organization so that resources required for implementation can be identified and committed.

UCSD Healthcare Core Strategies

1. Create Effective Governance, Leadership, and Organizational Structure for UCSD Healthcare and Its Components

2. Deliver High Quality Care and Service at Low Cost

3. Establish the Market Position for UCSD Healthcare and Healthcare Network Required to Fulfill Our Missions

4. Develop UCSD's Distinctive Clinical Capabilities as Centers of Emphasis and Excellence

5. Achieve Enhanced Recognition and Support for UCSD Healthcare as an Essential Resource to the San Diego Community

---

Figure 3.7 UCSD healthcare core strategies.

Action plans are also a key link between strategic planning and TQM. UCSD Health Care's core strategy on quality care and service, for example, generated an action plan that created Project Access, a comprehensive effort to "reengineer" the many aspects of our telephone, appointment, and registration systems that make obtaining ambulatory care a major source of patient and physician dissatisfaction.

The creation and implementation of action plans is the point during the planning process at which priorities and tradeoffs most often become apparent. The commitment of funds to an institutionwide initiative, such as UCSD Health Care's Project Access, may compete with an initiative important to a single department. Within an academic medical center, giving priority to providing funds to support faculty time for clinical teaching may compete with providing the resources to recruit new faculty outstanding in basic research. The vision and strategies articulated in the strategic plan, and the inclusive process by which the plan is developed, provide the foundation on which to make these difficult choices. Strong leadership is essential, nonetheless, to guide these choices and to generate the organizational support required to sustain them.

Monitoring and Evaluation

Establishing the "dashboard" or "scorecard" of key measures to monitor the organization's progress toward achieving its strategic goals is an essential component of implementation and action planning. Periodic review of these measures is a critical responsibility of management, and it provides the feedback that supports necessary modification to plans over time (8). TQM's emphasis on continuous improvement and the importance of measurement to achieving goals has brought heightened attention to this aspect of planning—an important contribution to strategic planning methodology and application.

THE STRATEGIC PLANNING PROCESS

The prevailing opinion among many planning professionals and participants in strategic planning efforts is that the strategic planning process itself is often more important than the resulting strategic plan. Given the increasing complexity of the health care environment, the growing vulnerability of health care organizations to environmental and competitive threats, and the resulting challenges to both managing these organizations and developing strategies for them, Zuckerman (10) comments:

The planning process can be an important bridge to the many constituencies involved in the organization. . . . The planning process presents important opportunities for improving communications across the organization and forges new and stronger bonds among stakeholder individuals and groups to help ensure the organization's future viability.

The principles of TQM have been important

in generating this perception. Traditionally, strategic planning was viewed as the province of an organization's board and executive management with limited involvement of other elements of the organization. The focus of strategy was on the market. As health care organizations have begun to link TQM and strategic planning, important cultural changes have occurred in the traditional strategic planning process. Including an understanding of the needs of internal and external customers as critical components of strategic assessment, developing strategies to address these needs, and opening the process to wider involvement by physicians, managers, and staff are key changes that have occurred. TQM has also brought systems thinking to strategic planning, resulting in the recognition that the organization must be viewed as a system and that plans must be developed and implemented to get all parts working together to meet and exceed customer expectations (2).

In light of the importance of the process itself, several critical issues must be addressed in its design and conduct:

- Organization of the process
- Roles, responsibilities, and involvement in the planning process
- Open forums, retreats, and other methods of communication
- Crafting mission and vision

Organization of the Strategic Planning Process

As Zuckerman (10) comments, "One of the common mistakes in an organization's strategic planning process is the failure to organize before the 'work' of strategic planning begins".

Critical issues to address in preparation for planning revolve around who will participate, how the process will be structured and phased, whether outside consulting assistance will be involved and for what tasks, and what mechanisms will be used for communicating with key stakeholders, both internal and external. Resolving these questions before the actual launch of the strategic planning process and communicating this information to the organization helps to ensure active, engaged participation.

Roles, Responsibilities, and Involvement in the Planning Process

Current planning practice emphasizes the importance of including as many elements of orga-

nizational leadership and as many perspectives as possible. To guide the planning process and ultimately to develop the strategic plan, a Strategic Planning Committee is usually created with members drawn from the board (or other governing structure), executive management, and physician leadership selected for their ability to represent the perspectives of their colleagues/constituency as well as to take an institutional view. Management is the coordinator of the strategic planning process—structuring it, staffing it, keeping it moving, and overseeing implementation. Regardless of how responsibilities to conduct the process are assigned within the organization, those who occupy positions of ultimate approval and decision-making authority must be closely involved (6).

To broaden participation in addressing the key strategic issues that emerge during the assessment phase, creation of task forces that report to the Strategic Planning Committee is a valuable approach. Participation on a task force constructively engages important stakeholders in defining organization strategy in areas of significance and relevance to them. In selecting task force members, it is important to gain broad representation from potentially affected constituencies, have enough diversity that the group is not biased toward any single perspective, choose members interested enough to participate, and choose a leader who will lead but not dominate. It is also essential that members understand that their charge is time limited and that they are examining alternatives and making recommendations to the Strategic Planning Committee, not making decisions (10).

To gain input from key constituency groups, both internal and external, and to provide a vital sense of inclusion in setting organizational direction, a variety of primary research techniques can be useful. *Figure 3.8,* from Goldman and Nolan (6), illustrates some of the major techniques used to obtain the insights, perceptions, and suggestions from an organization's constituency groups. Interviews and focus groups, in particular, provide mechanisms for obtaining important qualitative information and perceptions from a large number of key individuals and groups.

Regarding the use of consultants, in our experience some outside assistance, selectively employed, is essential. UCSD Health Sciences has an in-house planning function that organizes and

Constituency Group	Research Technique				
	Personal Interview	Telephone Interview	Telephone Survey	Mail Survey	Focus Group
Board	X	X			
Management	X				
Medical staff	X		X	X	X
Department directors				X	X
Employees				X	X
Community leaders	X				
Consumers			X		X
Employers	X	X		X	
Insurers	X	X			

Figure 3.8   Techniques used to obtain the insights, perceptions, and suggestions from an organization's constituency groups.

staffs all planning efforts, conducts much of the internal and external assessment, organizes and orchestrates all retreats and similar events, and drafts strategic plans and action plans. We use consultants for five specific purposes:

1. To provide the "organizational development" perspective in structuring and guiding strategic planning
2. To facilitate all retreats and critical meetings of the Strategic Planning Committee
3. To provide perspective and expertise on major health care policy issues
4. To interview key stakeholders as part of both the internal and external assessments, and to conduct other primary research, including surveys and focus groups
5. To address critical and sensitive issues that require outside objectivity; for example, whether to seek a partner for inpatient facilities

Regarding the "organizational development" role, an outside organizational development professional has proved invaluable in establishing a constructive environment that encourages open dialogue, in assisting executive management to address controversy, and in providing guidance and insight on group process and dynamics. In our experience, those faculty members and managers who have participated in TQM efforts through UCSD Health Care have acquired critical group process skills. The School of Medicine does not yet have a TQM program; therefore, many members of the faculty and management of the School of Medicine lack the group process experience that TQM participation can provide.

Open Forums, Retreats, and Communication

Communication before, during, and at the completion of the strategic planning process is vital to the success of the effort. We have found that open forums for all faculty, managers, and staff are effective in announcing the start of a planning process, informing all stakeholders about the details of the process, and soliciting involvement. Throughout the process, this mechanism is also valuable for communicating key insights gained and obtaining feedback as the strategic assessment is completed, the vision drafted, and initial strategies developed. Open forums are designed to be informal opportunities for presentation and dialogue of 1 to 2 hours' duration. Members of executive management and participants of the Strategic Planning Committee and its task forces lead the sessions—an important vehicle for demonstrating and ensuring that ownership of the process and its products extends to all of those involved, not just to executive management.

Retreats provide the opportunity for concentrated effort at key junctures in the planning process for the Strategic Planning Committee, its task forces, and senior management. Lasting a half day to a weekend, retreats have proved to be an invaluable mechanism for launching and structuring the work of task forces, for developing core strategies and outlining the strategic plan, for reviewing and gaining buy-in to a draft strategic plan, and for developing an annual action plan. We always use an outside facilitator to ensure effective design and management of the process and to free UCSD staff to be active participants.

During the course of developing the UCSD Health Sciences Strategic Plan during 1997/1998, we discovered a very effective tool for exploring the perspectives of a large group and obtaining immediate quantitative feedback to guide discussion. OptionFinder is an interactive polling technology that uses a wireless radio fre-

UCSD Health Sciences Strategic Planning
General Faculty Retreats: June11 & June 16, 1998
Examples of Option Finder Polling Statements & Distribution of Responses

Achieving Clinical Excellence

1. UCSD must develop, recognize, and reward a critical mass of clinically active faculty to foster a culture of clinical excellence.

Strongly agree				Strongly disagree
1	2	3	4	5
86%	8%	4%	2%	0%

Number of Voters = 84

2. Encouraging the ongoing development of the UCSD Medical Group to promote effectiveness and excellence across clinical disciplines is an essential strategy for achieving clinical excellence.

1	2	3	4	5
62%	13%	14%	6%	3%

Number of Voters = 86

Providing Exemplary Education

1. A commitment to develop, recognize, and reward faculty who teach is a necessary strategy for creating a culture of educational excellence.

1	2	3	4	5
80%	16%	4%	0%	0%

Number of Voters = 85

2. The size of and support for current graduate biomedical research programs and the Medical Scientist Training Program should be increased.

1	2	3	4	5
44%	20%	24%	11%	1%

Number of Voters = 86

Fostering Outstanding Research

1. Selected research areas should be identified for emphasis and development.

1	2	3	4	5
34%	30%	13%	10%	10%

Number of Voters = 88

3. New interdisciplinary programs and centers should be encouraged to promote synergy and collaboration.

1	2	3	4	5
56%	31%	8%	1%	4%

Number of Voters = 88

Figure 3.9　Sample statements used during faculty retreats.

quency response system and standard personal computer-based software (9). Statements and questions to be presented to the group are programmed in advance of the meeting and are displayed one at a time on a screen. Each participant is given a hand-held keypad with which to indicate his/her responses, which are captured electronically and displayed in a histogram or other graphic format. *Figure 3.9* presents a sample of statements that we used during our faculty retreats conducted in June 1998 to get input to the draft UCSD Health Sciences Strategic Plan, and the distribution of responses to these statements. By immediately displaying audience response to a statement, it was easy to determine the degree of support for a proposed strategy, ensuring that the tendency to interpret the most vocal participants as representative of the group did not occur. In addition, the response histogram provided the opportunity to ask for volunteers who had voted at various points on the spectrum to share their perspectives with the group, providing an opportunity for further discussion of different points of view. This technology was received enthusiastically and added a novel, futuristic element that was very appropriate to the creation of a strategic plan.

Crafting Mission, Core Values, and Vision

In our experience at UCSD, when a strategic planning process is launched, approximately half the participants are adamant that mission, core values, and vision should be addressed immediately, and half feel that these concepts are ''psychobabble'' and of no value whatsoever

anywhere in the process. Because industrywide experience (as well as our own) emphasizes the importance of mission, core values, and vision to strategic planning, we have found it most productive to defer addressing these concepts until the internal and external assessments are well underway and the Strategic Planning Committee has begun to appreciate the range of strategic issues confronting the organization. By this time, the need to clarify core values and mission, and to craft a compelling vision begins to become apparent to all participants.

Collins and Porras (4) note that identifying core values and core purpose (mission) is essentially a discovery process, but setting the envisioned future is a creative process. They imply that the discovery of core values and core purpose precedes the articulation of vision, and recommend that it is often best to begin with vivid descriptions of a desired future, perhaps 20 years hence, before trying to specify goals. In our experience, trying to characterize the desired future helps to bring forth values, mission, and ultimately strategic goals. It is an ongoing task of the Strategic Planning Committee that continues throughout the process, with periodic drafts developed to clarify the Committee's own thinking, which is then shared in open forums for input from the whole UCSD Health Sciences community. Our first use of OptionFinder was during an open forum approximately midway through the planning process to share components of the vision statement—Achieving Clinical Excellence, Providing Exemplary Education, and Fostering Outstanding Research—that was developed during two evening retreats for the Committee and its three task forces. *Figure 3.10*

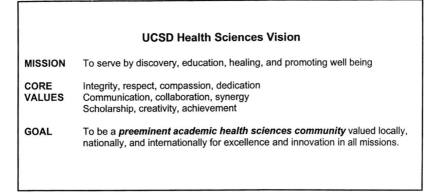

UCSD Health Sciences Vision

MISSION   To serve by discovery, education, healing, and promoting well being

CORE   Integrity, respect, compassion, dedication
VALUES   Communication, collaboration, synergy
               Scholarship, creativity, achievement

GOAL   To be a ***preeminent academic health sciences community*** valued locally,
               nationally, and internationally for excellence and innovation in all missions.

Figure 3.10   UCSD Health Sciences vision.

presents the vision for UCSD Health Sciences that emerged from this process. The endorsement by even our basic bench scientists that UCSD must achieve excellence in *all* missions, not just research, if we are to achieve preeminence was one of the most important outcomes to emerge from strategic planning for UCSD Health Sciences. It is already influencing our ability to make important strategic choices in the commitment of resources to our education and clinical missions.

CONCLUSION

In this chapter we provided an overview of current thinking on the components of strategic planning, its link to TQM, and the strategic planning process itself. We shared references that we have found useful in our planning, as well as some of our own experiences in planning for both UCSD's "clinical enterprise" and UCSD Health Sciences overall.

Strategic planning has been an essential process in establishing organizational direction in UCSD Health Sciences, and the plans developed have been important in providing a framework for key initiatives and for enhancing the daily work of the organization. The strategic planning process has been of value because we have customized industry practice to meet our own unique circumstances, and have been flexible in applying various techniques and concepts. We have not rigorously followed any one model presented in the literature, but instead have used elements from many to develop approaches that work for us. We also apply the concept of "continuous improvement" to strategic planning itself, modifying our process with each iteration as we learn from the mistakes and successes of previous efforts.

EPILOGUE

Between our first submission of this chapter and its return to us for minor revisions, an event occurred that demonstrates the power of strategic planning and potential consequences of implementation when the plan involves significant change. Both the strategic plan for UCSD Health Care completed in 1995 and the strategic plan for UCSD Health Sciences completed in 1998 represented major departures from the status quo. A key component of the UCSD Health Care

Strategic Plan involved restructuring the UCSD Medical Group by creating a board of governors elected by the clinically active faculty. This change challenged the traditional prerogatives of the department chair to manage the clinical practice in his department independent of any institutional requirements. The vision articulated in the UCSD Health Sciences Strategic Plan that all missions are essential to achieving future preeminence—education, clinical service, as well as research—is a widely acknowledged accomplishment of the planning process. Nonetheless, efforts initiated as part of the 1999 action plan to develop a basis for providing additional resources to faculty committed to the educational and clinical missions were viewed as a major threat to powerful senior basic science faculty.

UCSD has a periodic review process for senior academic leaders, including deans and department chairs, and Dr. Alkne's review as dean of the School of Medicine occurred this year. The review provided the opportunity for chairs and faculty displeased with the new directions established by the strategic plans to voice their opposition. The Review Committee recommended that Dr. Alksne not be reappointed as vice chancellor and dean, a recommendation accepted by the chancellor. Dr. Alksne returned to his position as professor of neurosurgery and his commitments to clinical medicine and education on August 1, 1999. A national search for his successor is underway.

A strong clinical enterprise and Medical Group, and a strategic plan for achieving UCSD's Health Sciences vision of preeminence are important legacies of Dr. Alkne's leadership. The chancellor has committed to finding a successor who will continue to pursue these directions.

REFERENCES

1. Altman D, Greene R, Sapolsky HM: Health planning and regulation. Washington, DC, AUPHA Press, 1981:20–3l.
2. Arvantes JC: Using TQM to forge customer-driven strategic planning. *Quality Letter for Health Care Leaders* 5:2–12, 1993.
3. Collins JC, Porras JI: Built to last: Successful habits of visionary companies. New York, Harper Business, 1994.
4. Collins JC, Porras JI: Building your company's vision. *Harvard Business Review* 74:65–77, 1996.
5. Durbin S, Haglund C, Dowling W: Integrating strategic

planning and quality management in a multi-institutional system. *Quality Management in Health Care* 1:24–34, 1993.

6. Goldman EF, Nolan KC: Strategic planning in health care: A guide for board members. Chicago, American Hospital Publishing, 1994.

7. Hamel G, Prahalad CK: Competing for the future. *Harvard Business Review* 72:122–128, 1994.

8. Horak BJ: Strategic planning in healthcare: Building a quality-based plan step by step. New York, Quality Resources, 1997.

9. Option Technologies, Inc. 389 W. 2nd Street, Suite B, Ogden, UT 84404.

10. Zuckerman A: Health Care strategic planning: Approaches for the 21st century. Chicago, Health Administration Press, 1998:2.

CHAPTER 4

Team Procedures for Neurosurgeons

ERIC J. HUMMEL, Ph.D., AND BARBARA J. STREIBEL, Ph.D.

EDITOR'S NOTE: Of the four areas contributing to profound knowledge (knowledge of variation, systems knowledge, process knowledge, and knowledge of psychology), knowledge of psychology is the area that is usually most deficient in the training of neurosurgeons. As driven, decisive, and analytical surgeons, we are often less comfortable with the "softer" science of human character and interpersonal dynamics than we are in performing surgery, making patient care decisions, or performing and/or analyzing clinical or basic science research. Yet good leadership is founded firmly on a broad and thorough understanding of human psychology. This chapter focuses on knowledge of psychology as it applies critically to working effectively in quality improvement teams, and as it applies to leading and facilitating quality improvement implementation.

"There are principles of leadership just as there are principles of war, and these have to be studied."

—*Field Marshal Viscount Montgomery*

Like every other type of business, health care is evolving. The environment in which neurosurgeons work is affected and reshaped by forces such as managed care, mergers and acquisitions, government regulations, medical malpractice, and a market-share mentality. And like all other medical professionals, neurosurgeons are expected to keep their footing in the shifting terrain and continue to provide quality health care.

Probably one of the most fundamental and far-reaching changes is the fact that health care has been more clearly defined as a service-oriented business. Neurosurgeons must continue to do more than perform surgical procedures. They have to perform their work in a way that satisfies a variety of customers.

Meanwhile, more people and entities than ever are managing health care by scrutinizing and compiling data on outcomes. The purpose:

To make the outcomes more consistently positive and to achieve them more efficiently. As a result, medical providers at every level must attend to the medical and surgical procedures they perform as well as to the process that surrounds those procedures—the whole set of causes and conditions that contribute to the final outcom—and the part they play in it. They need to work together seamlessly and to communicate tirelessly at the bedside, in the operating suite, and in meeting rooms to set, maintain, and improve standards and practices.

THE NEED FOR TEAMS

To do this successfully, health care organizations—from private practice groups and clinics to hospitals and medical schools—are creating growing numbers of cross-functional teams and ongoing work groups. Like nonmedical businesses, health care organizations rely increasingly on teams because they need to make improvements and achieve results more quickly and efficiently, often with fewer resources. These teams bring together the knowledge, skills, experience, and perspectives of the wide range of people who provide patient care, as well as those who support it.

The team approach is not new in health care. From the emergency room to the operating suite, groups of doctors, nurses, and other professionals work together to treat patients. What is less common is the practice of bringing these same people together on teams that assess and improve the process of medical care. So, for example, members of the team who provide postoperative patient care must work together to decide how to provide that care at a lower cost and/or with a lower rate of complications.

Also new for some health care workers is the distinction between working as part of a group and working on a team. Groups share information and coordinate their work. However, the actual work that is done and its outcomes are mainly individual. Teams, on the other hand, collaborate and share fully in the overall outcome.

This chapter examines what it takes to build a group that works like a team. Common principles apply to most work groups, including project and ongoing work teams such as caregiving and surgical teams, practice committees, and standing administrative committees. The characteristics of genuine teamwork are the same in most every arena, from manufacturing to government to education to health care: a diverse group of people with clear purposes and goals that is mutually accountable for achieving those goals and that works collaboratively to do so. The terminology and titles may be different, but the processes are essentially the same. So is the mind-set: Every one contributes to the success of the mission.

THE SURGEON'S ROLE IN TEAM BUILDING

Surgeons are not exempt from health care's focus on process as well as procedure, and on service beyond procedure. Nor can they leave teamwork to others. In fact, surgeons should be at the forefront of these efforts. Although some outside the profession may think that teams and surgeons are mutually exclusive, we know that the neurosurgeon's role in the continuum of patient care is that of a team leader and sometimes team member.

The new realities of medical practice and administration have affected surgeons' autonomy and authority. However, they continue to be regarded as leaders, in and out of the operating suite. Thus, in addition to their work at the apex of the caregiving team, surgeons are often called on to serve on peer review and residency review committees, to work on quality and improvement projects, and to take part in administrative and policy-making groups in their practices, medical schools, and hospitals.

By joining these team efforts, surgeons make them more credible. By supporting them, they can help them succeed. And surgeons can do more. They can demonstrate the value of highly functioning teamwork and promote the team mind-set in the operating suite and in all their other professional activities. By doing so, they'll use their time more efficiently, improve the quality of work among the people on whom they depend, and provide improved quality of care to their patients.

As a neurosurgeon, you probably already serve as the leader, or at least ex-officio leader, of many "teams" related to your practice and other roles. You have led teams for some time and think you do an adequate, perhaps even a fine, job. Nevertheless, we invite and challenge you to read this chapter to see what you can add to your leadership skills to increase the efficiency and focus of your current team experiences. The material here may also prove helpful to you for those occasions when you are a team member. Finally, we recommend that you share this material with your administrative assistant or secretary, because he or she is probably integrally involved in coordinating the logistics that support you and your teams.

THE MODEL TEAM

As a neurosurgeon, you regularly lead and take part in a model team: the operating team. When it works well, the operating team is an efficient, technically skilled, cost-effective work group that collectively supports, assists, and manages delivery of the highest quality patient care.

Because of the complexity and intricacy of neurosurgical cases, your operating team usually consists of a network of teams, including smaller teams of anesthesiologists, surgeons, circulating nurses, scrub technicians, radiologists, and other technical support people. And that operating room network is linked to the pre- and postoperative care teams, probably more closely than some other surgical groups. This is a very complex system that works only by the full cooperation of each of its components.

As we develop the themes of team building in this chapter, keep this model in mind. And as you work on other teams, try to replicate the dynamics and the mind-set of a high-performance operating room team. These will serve you and your team members well, whatever your role.

KEYS TO A SUCCESSFUL TEAM

No team exists or functions flawlessly. Human nature, along with the normal and unexpected course of events, interferes with smooth progress. However, if the following 10 conditions exist, your team can avoid many of the problems that hinder groups and manage the ones it can't avoid.

Ten Conditions for a Successful Team

1. The team must have clearly defined purposes and goals that serve the organization.
2. Teams need clearly defined parameters within which to work.
3. The roles of the team members must be clearly defined.
4. Teams need to have clear and consistent communication.
5. Teams need to adopt and practice beneficial team skills.
6. A team needs a well-defined decision-making process.
7. Every team member should participate in the team's work.
8. A team needs ground rules that all team members support.
9. All team members share the responsibility for the group process.
10. A team must draw its conclusions from and base its decisions on data.

Condition 1: The Team Must Have Clearly Defined Purposes and Goals that Serve the Organization

A team works best when everyone understands what they are trying to accomplish and why. On the ideal team, all team members work together to integrate their diverse perspectives so they can agree to the group's purpose. They must see the goal as being one they can attain; otherwise, they need to redefine the goal. Team members also need to agree to the process they will use to reach the goal, including phases or steps, meeting schedules, decision making, and so forth

The team's purpose must be clearly linked to larger organizational missions, goals, and strategies that ultimately deliver added value to patients. When the team is working on something that is clearly important to the organization, people are more likely to feel that their time is being well spent.

Think back to the neurosurgical operating team. Its purpose is clear. And if a question regarding process arises—for example, which anesthesia technique to use—the team has ground rules in place for resolving the issue promptly. Other teams and committees need similarly well-defined goals and ground rules. When you are a member or a leader of one of those other teams, the time you spend up front getting clarity and unity of purpose makes the team more efficient in the long run.

Condition 2: Teams Need Clearly Defined Parameters Within Which to Work

A team works most effectively and efficiently if it has a work plan. The plan defines the expertise, consultation, training, materials and equipment, and other resources it may need. It identifies the steps of the team's work, as well as the schedules, deadlines, and mileposts of the project or procedure. The team also needs to know the limits of its authority, including budget and decision making. These parameters are usually defined by the sponsoring organization such as the practice group, department, hospital, or medical school.

Condition 3: The Roles of the Team Members Must Be Clearly Defined

A team operates best when everyone knows who is responsible for each issue or task. In addition, a team must have people with the necessary knowledge and skills to accomplish its purpose, and must tap the talents of all its members.

On the surgical team, members' duties and responsibilities seem evident; they almost "go without saying." On other types of teams, members must define and agree explicitly to their roles and duties regarding the work of the team and "housekeeping" tasks such as note taking and timekeeping at meetings.

Condition 4: Teams Need to Have Clear and Consistent Communication

Meaningful discussion and rational decision making depend on how well information is passed among team members. Team members should pay extra attention to the level of their communication skills and work to improve them. Everyone needs to be able to speak and write clearly and succinctly, listen actively, and be mindful of their own nonverbal communication and that of others. The team needs to have ground rules to manage the content and tenor of meeting discussions so that they are cogent and civil, and needs to encourage the exchange of differing ideas. In addition, guidelines should determine how members will be kept informed of team work status between meetings. For example, e-mail should make it possible for even the most far-flung teams to stay in touch between meetings.

It is also vital for a team to be able to communicate with the larger organization to get the data, equipment, and other resources it needs, and to inform others of its progress.

Condition 5: Teams Need to Adopt and Practice Beneficial Team Skills

All team members should be encouraged to use the skills and practices that make discussions and meetings more effective. These include initiating discussions, seeking diverse opinions and information, clarifying ideas, summarizing, testing for agreement, checking opinions with data, and accepting praise and complaints.

Condition 6: A Team Needs a Well-Defined Decision-Making Process

You can tell a lot about how well a team works by watching its decision-making process. A team should know about the different ways it can reach a decision and when they are appropriate. There is no single "right" way to decide an issue; a lot depends on the context of the decision.

- Consensus, a decision that all group members can support, takes time and, often, repeated exchange of ideas. A team might want to have consensus on major decisions that affect a lot of people or that have widespread ramifications.
- Voting, in which the majority rules, is appropriate for smaller decisions that involve less complex issues or matters that don't generate strong feelings or opinions. The team may also choose to vote on larger issues if it doesn't have the time to devote to reaching consensus. Voting regularly on large issues involves risks, however, especially if the team has not made a sincere effort to reach consensus. Majority support can become majority tyranny, in

which the concerns of the minority are disregarded and member buy-in is limited. The team needs to understand these possible drawbacks at the outset, and the team leader must be prepared to deal with them if they arise.

- A subgroup or subcommittee might make a decision for the team when it has all the information and expertise to do so.
- One person may make a decision for the team. This often happens in an emergency, when that person has full responsibility for the decision and accepts all the consequences, or the team may put the decision in that person's hands because he or she is an expert in the area.

In addition, the team should know how to explore issues, use data as the basis of its decisions, and test for agreement. If a team has difficulty reaching decisions, it should consider having a facilitator or outsider observe its process and offer feedback for improvement.

Condition 7: Every Team Member Should Participate in the Team's Work

Because every team member has a stake in the team's achievements, each one should take part in its discussions and decisions, share commitment to the project's success, and contribute his or her talents. If participation is unbalanced, the team can end up being dominated by the ideas and opinions of a few members. The meeting leader should use brainstorming and other techniques to structure discussions and to encourage full participation.

Condition 8: A Team Needs Ground Rules that All Team Members Support

Successful teams invariably have ground rules that define the behavior that will and will not be tolerated on the team. Some of the issues typically covered by team ground rules are attendance, promptness, participation, conversational courtesies, confidentiality, assignments, and rotation of responsibility. Attendance can be a particular problem for neurosurgeons, who have tremendous demands on their time. Nevertheless, poor attendance by a neurosurgical team member or team leader will surely doom his or her team to failure. Some examples of ground rules for participation and discussion are as follows:

- Meetings will start on time and end on time.
- Team members will make attendance at team meetings a top priority.

- All team members will participate in discussions and decision making.
- Team members will treat each other with respect.
- There will be no side conversations during meetings. Anything you have to say should be shared with the entire team.
- All team members will act on facts, not on opinions or assumptions.
- All ideas will be considered.
- There are no stupid questions.
- Team members are responsible for completing their assignments on time.
- All discussions between team members are confidential.

From the start, the entire team should discuss the ground rules and agree to them. Once they are established, the team leader should have them written up and distributed to all team members for continued reference. Then, throughout the life of the team—especially when new members join—the team should review the ground rules and revise them as they see fit.

When drifting develops around one of the ground rules, the team can address the problem promptly. The ground rule itself is usually not the problem. Instead, the problem may stem from a weakness in the team's process or the organization's commitment to the team. For example, if attendance at meetings is consistently low, it may be because the meeting leader doesn't manage discussions effectively or because some members aren't given the time by their supervisors to attend.

Condition 9: All Team Members Share the Responsibility for the Group Process

Ideally, all team members should be aware of how the team works together, should strive to maintain a positive dynamic, and should work to resolve problems with the process. To accomplish this, members need to be aware of nonverbal communication as well as processes like decision making and participation. The team can assess its process periodically as part of its self-evaluation.

Condition 10: A Team Must Draw Its Conclusions From and Base Its Decisions on Data

Team decisions are best when they are grounded on data. A team that abides by this

statement can avoid many team problems and disagreements. In keeping with this key to success, many teams in the health care arena include a representative from the medical records department (4).

VIRTUAL TEAMS

A team often consists of members who work in different parts of a large campus, a city, the country, and even the world. If you are the leader of such a team, you need to think about how some of these keys to success apply to your team.

Communication and building team spirit can be particularly challenging when geography makes frequent face-to-face meetings impractical or impossible. Clearly, meetings are crucial when the team is forming and setting ground rules, making major decisions, or being slowed by internal differences. Also, if you sense that personality, rank, or territorial issues are creating distrust among members, you may want to hold more rather than fewer meetings.

Virtual teams rely heavily on e-mail, voice mail, and telephone communication to get their work done. As a result, they may need special ground rules, such as not doing other work while ''attending'' a team meeting by teleconference. These teams may also need to be especially mindful of confidentiality.

JUST-IN-TIME TRAINING

To contribute to their team's success, team members need a number of skills in addition to their particular professional knowledge. Everyone on the team should have good communication skills and knowledge of common problem-solving tools and processes like decision making. Members who lead meetings need to have planning and facilitation skills, and should be comfortable speaking to a group. The organization that sponsors the team should provide members with the tools they need to gain and/or hone those skills.

Traditional training takes place when employees take one or several days away from their work to attend class to learn a skill they may need in their job. This ''just-in-case'' training is often ineffective. People rarely retain what they learn during training unless they use it promptly and regularly on the job. In the case of teams, traditional training may be impractical as well. Even if the training was immediately available, team members may not be able to devote several days to a training course.

The solution is *just-in-time training,* in which people are taught new techniques or skills only when they need to use them. So, for example, people assigned to a team for the first time might need a ''refresher course'' in meeting skills or an overview of data collection and analysis. They get what they need when they need to use it.

BUILDING THE TEAM

Building a team involves more than pulling some names out of a hat or taking anyone who volunteers—at least it should. In this section we look at the roles and relationships on teams, as well as criteria and considerations to take into account when choosing team members.

Most organizations have a system for identifying work priorities and special projects, and assigning them to individuals and teams or committees. This direction is usually linked to the organization's strategic plan and comes from a management group made up of department heads or other key leaders of the organization. This group often chooses the team leader and works with him or her to choose team members.

Team Roles, Responsibilities, and Relationships

For all team members to work together effectively, they need to understand the various roles and relationships within the team structure.

Team Leader

This is probably the role in which you most often find yourself. As the team leader, you manage the team: calling and sometimes facilitating meetings, handling or assigning administrative tasks, orchestrating team activities, and overseeing preparation of reports and presentations. The team leader is also responsible for maintaining the official team records, including copies of correspondence, records of meetings, and data related to the project.

You also need to be reasonably good at working with individuals and groups. Once again, your clinical work provides an excellent model. If you take the time when the team is forming to understand your team members the way you

do your patients, you can form the basis of a smooth working relationship. You will need a thorough knowledge of decision-making methods and approaches to problem solving.

Because you are often senior in rank to other team members, you must consciously leave your rank outside the meeting room and take extra precautions to avoid dominating the group during meetings. Because of your status and experience, you could easily sway the team to your thinking or cause members to self-censor their opinions or questions. Take care to encourage diversity of thought and show your respect for the range of perspectives on the team.

The team leader serves as the contact point between the team and the rest of the organization. This involves more than keeping others informed of the team's progress and status. You may also have to speak to a team member's supervisor if the team member is having problems finding time to work on the project.

The team leader is also a team member, and must fulfill the responsibilities of a team member. This involves attending meetings, carrying out assignments between meetings, and generally sharing in the team's work. An exception is that you may want to restrain your participation in some discussions so that others will be more active.

Coach

Although health care workers often work as part of a caregiving ''team,'' many of them focus on their own area of care without working collaboratively with the other members of the team. Thus, team members probably are not highly skilled in project management, group processes, data collection and analysis, problem solving, and process improvement. The absence of these skills can seriously impede the smooth working of a team.

Some organizations have employees who are specially trained in these techniques and who can coach or teach others to use these skills in their work. If your organization does not have such a person or the training resources, then the team leader may also have to fulfill these responsibilities.

If your team has a coach, he will attend some team meetings. The coach is an outsider to the team in many ways, so he can remain neutral as far as the content of the meeting is concerned. One of the coach's most important jobs is to observe the team's progress and to help the team work more effectively. The coach looks at the team's *process* rather than its *product*. In other words, the coach looks at *how* the team discusses a topic or makes a decision, not *what* the topic or decision is. A coach needs to have excellent people skills, including techniques for encouraging and guiding participation, resolving conflict, and giving feedback.

The coach's second major focus is to help the team become more comfortable using statistics and other nonmedical tools needed to accomplish its purpose. If necessary, he can teach the team data collection and analysis techniques, showing the conclusions that may or may not be drawn from the data and suggesting alternative ways of looking at the data.

The coach is not a subject matter expert. If the team needs subject matter expertise, the coach can help identify and locate a resource person for the team.

Team Members

Team members do the work of the team. Team members represent some or all of the major groups that are likely to be affected by the project or that contribute to the team's work. Team members are likely to be of various ranks, professions, classifications, and shifts. So, for example, a team looking at ways to reduce costs in the neurosurgical intensive care unit might include a neurosurgeon, a registered nurse, a clinical social worker, a physical therapist, as well as representatives from medical records, purchasing, and finance.

Team members must view the team's work as a priority, not as an intrusion on their "real jobs." This means being willing to contribute fully to the team's work and carrying out their assignments between meetings. A team's success often depends on how well members reach a common understanding of the issues, so members must be willing to listen to others and be open to their ideas.

Choosing Team Members

The sponsor of the project or improvement initiative should collaborate with the team leader and coach (if any) to determine the disciplines, work units, and job classifications that should be represented on the team.

As a neurosurgeon, you know the value of a multidisciplinary team. The neurosurgical pro-

cedure, however complex and lengthy, is only one part of a continuum of care that stretches from diagnosis and assessment of the patient, through preoperative testing and preparations, into the operating room, and beyond to the recovery room, the intensive care unit, and disposition planning. Most improvement initiatives don't require as much specialized knowledge and experience as the neurosurgical patient. However, any project or work activity that spans departments or disciplines needs a team that does the same.

Ideally, team members should represent each area affected by the project. However, the need to manage the size of the team may preclude full representation. Typically, teams should have between five and eight members in addition to the team leader and coach. A team of more than eight people definitely challenges the team leader's ability to manage "air time" during meetings. The team does not have to include everyone who might possibly contribute something worthwhile. Team members can always consult with stakeholders and others as the project unfolds.

The team membership does not have to represent different levels of the organization. Even when the nature of the project requires a slice of the hierarchy, be cautious. High-level managers on a team can intimidate lower level personnel. On the other hand, organizations that endorse open communication believe that mixing levels is an excellent way to practice what they preach and to improve leadership methods. Ultimately, team members should be picked based on the knowledge and expertise they can bring to the project, not their titles.

Do not limit consideration to people who have time for the project. You may deprive yourself of some of the most valuable people in the organization. In the case of improvement efforts and priority projects, the organization should support all team members to adjust and delegate some of their regular workload to make time for the team project. One of the team leader's responsibilities is to help bring that about.

The range of skills and knowledge required of team members includes medical expertise as well as team skills. So, for example, teams need people with skills in planning, applying logic and data in problem solving, decision making, running effective meetings, and communicating. It probably also means bringing together people from a number of disciplines such as anesthesiology, radiology, surgery, and social work, and departments such as medical records, public relations, and finance.

Personality Types and Personal Styles

Undoubtedly, one of the greatest sources of friction and conflict on a team is the mix of personality types and personal styles of its members. The temperaments of the team members, as well as their styles of processing and using information, can have a dramatic impact on team interactions and results. We'll look at these factors from several angles throughout this chapter and give an overview of two models used to categorize personal styles. Here, we address personal styles in the context of choosing team members.

A multidisciplinary medical team is rich in expertise. Similarly, a team with many personality types and personal styles is rich in viewpoints and opportunities. It is up to the team leader to make sure that those viewpoints don't become sore points and that the opportunities aren't all troublesome.

You don't accomplish this by picking team members who all have the same style. Assuming this were possible, the result would be a group of people who think the same way—all inside the same box. So, for example, let's say you put together six people who are exacting, steady workers; who like to gather and organize facts and details; and who honor rules and traditions. You may get a lot of information about current conditions and have no impetus to implement changes.

An effective team needs diversity of styles as well as skills. So if, along with a couple of steady fact gatherers, you also have a big-picture thinker who looks for new possibilities, and a pragmatic risk taker who can negotiate agreements, you have a team that will generate energy, ideas, and results.

As the leader of such a diverse team, your task is to learn about some of the different personality models so that you understand your team members. This should help you manage your impatience with styles that are different from your own and should help you to find ways to help the people with uncomplementary styles work together. For example, you may get impatient with a member who thinks out loud, rambling around before getting to the point. You need to make

the mental shift to understand that this is how that member needs to organize his or her thoughts; it is not a sign of inattention. If you prompt the member by asking for a summary, you can reach the desired result while accommodating his style.

THE TEAM AT WORK

The team at work is a complicated creature. Members must work out personal differences, find strengths on which to build, and balance commitments to the project against the demands of their everyday jobs. And, of course, they also have to do their work for the team.

Dealing with internal group needs that arise from these pressures is as important as the group's task of solving problems, improving processes, or completing daily work. Teams often underestimate the need for team development. When a team works well together, members can concentrate on their primary goal. In contrast, a team that fails to build relationships among its members will waste time on struggles for control and endless discussions that lead nowhere.

Stages of Team Growth

The more you know about what to expect as your team grows, the better equipped you will be to handle challenges as they emerge. With a strong foundation in place, you can recognize and avoid many disruptions, and work as a group through the ones that cannot be avoided.

The team goes through four fairly predictable stages as it grows. Obviously, as team leader, you need to be familiar with the team's developmental stages. The team's meeting leader or facilitator also needs to understand them so she can deal with their dynamics during meetings.

Stage 1: Forming

When a team is forming, members explore the boundaries of acceptable group behavior. They shift from individual status to member status and test the leader's guidance directly and indirectly. During this stage, a lot is going on to distract members from their tasks, so progress toward team goals may be slow.

During the forming stage, members' reactions include

- Anticipation, optimism, and stimulation
- Initial tentative attachment to the team

• Uncertainty about the job ahead and how the team will accomplish its purpose

During the forming stage, members often exhibit the following behaviors:

• Working to define the task and deciding how it will be accomplished
• Setting ground rules for acceptable team behavior and dealing with team issues
• Discussing the information needed by the team
• Talking in abstract terms about concepts and issues or, for some members, being impatient with these discussions
• Talking about symptoms or problems that aren't relevant to the task; having difficulty identifying the relevant problems
• Displaying frustration about the organization and its barriers to completing the task

If you are the team leader, you need to concentrate on building trust and confidence during this stage. You can do this by helping members get to know each other. You should also provide clear direction and a sense of purpose by quickly involving members in making plans and clarifying roles and ground rules. You should also make sure the team has the information it needs to get started.

For the meeting leader, there are specific exercises and tools that can be used during the forming stage to help team members get engaged. Warm-up exercises, during which members introduce themselves and talk about their interests in and concerns about the team, are very helpful. They satisfy members' need for information and bring some doubts and concerns to the surface, where they can be addressed. The process of setting explicit team ground rules, which is led by the meeting leader, also informs and guides the team's structure.

Stage 2: Storming

Storming can be the most challenging stage for the team. Think of the team at this stage as a patient who believes his condition will never improve. As team members begin to realize the amount of work ahead of them, it's normal for them to become demanding, testy, or overzealous.

Impatient about the lack of progress and having limited experience in team decision making and the data-driven approach, members argue about what the team should be doing. Still wary of the team dynamic, they resist the need to collaborate and try to rely on their personal and professional experience. As a result, team members still have limited energy to devote to the team's goals, so progress in that direction remains slow. With good team dynamics, however, people can begin to understand one another even in the midst of this chaotic stage.

Storming brings out the following reactions:

• Reluctance to perform tasks and use methods that are unfamiliar
• Uncertainty about the team's chances for success, leading to sharp fluctuations in attitude

Behaviors typical of the storming stage include

• Disputes among members even when they agree on the main issue
• Acting defensive and competitive, forming factions, and taking sides
• Questioning the makeup of the team or the wisdom of the people who chose the project
• Setting unrealistic goals

Many leaders will become impatient with what appears to be the sloppiness of the storming process. However, trying to push the team through it is a waste of energy. Instead, as team leader, you can help the team work through it as efficiently as possible. Allow for some controlled chaos, maybe even making some time for members to "blow off steam." At the same time, help the team see its uncertainty for what it is—a natural stage of growth. In that way, you can keep the team moving toward being productive while it attends to its internal process.

The meeting leader can firmly enforce structure and direction at this stage. However, she should be careful not to push for more cooperation than the group can handle at this time. For example, a team that is deeply divided philosophically may find it impossible to agree on groupings in an affinity diagram. Instead, each "camp" can complete its own affinity diagram. Then the entire team can compare both sets of results.

Stage 3: Norming

During this stage, members accept the team, team ground rules, their roles on the team, and the individuality of fellow members. Emotional conflict is reduced as previously competitive relationships become more cooperative. In other words, as team members realize they aren't going to drown, they stop thrashing about and start helping each other to stay afloat. Team members have time and energy to spend on their work, and they start to make meaningful progress. Team members start to enjoy and take pride in being part of the team, and come to appreciate their fellow team members.

Reactions that are part of the norming stage include

- A sense of cohesion, a common spirit and goals
- Acceptance of membership in the team
- Relief that things appear to be working out

Behaviors during the norming stage include

- Working to achieve harmony and avoid conflict
- Confiding in each other, sharing personal problems
- Discussing the team's dynamics
- Expressing criticism constructively
- Agreeing to and maintaining team ground rules and boundaries

As team leader, you can take advantage of the team's calmer state to build cooperation and mutual respect. Make full use of team members' skills, knowledge, and experience, and encourage members to do the same with each other.

During this period of new-found calm and appreciation, the team may find itself in the pitfall of *groupthink.* This "habit of consent" can also develop during the performing stage. As team members settle into their roles, they may conform too readily to team values and ethics in making decisions. Or they may be too willing to accept and support the opinions of one person because of his expertise. To guard against this tendency, the meeting leader or facilitator can encourage team members to stretch beyond their comfort levels and even question their consent. For example, the team leader can challenge the team by using a tool such as failure modes and effects analysis, in which the team has to find the weaknesses in their proposed solutions.

Stage 4: Performing

By now, the team has settled its relationships and expectations. They can begin performing—diagnosing and assessing the problems, and choosing and implementing changes. Team members have discovered and accepted each other's strengths and weaknesses, and under-

stand their role. The team is now an effective unit. You can tell when your team has reached this stage because you start getting a lot of work done.

Reactions that are evident during the performing stage include

- Appreciation and understanding of the group process as well as the strengths and weaknesses of individual members
- Satisfaction with the team's progress
- Desire to succeed
- Attachment and loyalty to the team

Behaviors seen during this stage include

- Communicating openly and effectively
- Being positive about the team's ability to produce useful results
- Being able to prevent or work through group problems

At this stage, the team is ready to take responsibility for the direction, work, and processes of the team. As team leader, you monitor the team's progress and stand ready to facilitate when necessary.

The duration and intensity of these stages vary from team to team. Sometimes a team can reach the performing stage in a meeting or two; other times it may take months. The team may go through the stages repeatedly as it works through each major decision or starts a new phase of the project. Use the descriptions here to compare your team with the normal pattern for maturing groups. Understanding these stages will keep you from overreacting to normal problems and setting unrealistic expectations that only add to frustration (4).

Highs and Lows—Ebbs and Flows

Knowing about the team's typical growth stages should relieve much of the fear members have about the project's success. It is also helpful to be aware of the roller coaster of highs and lows every team experiences.

A team's mood usually reflects its fortune. With every step forward, the future looks bright and team members grow optimistic. But no matter how well team members work together, progress is never smooth or steady. As progress swings from moving forward to stalling, and then from stalling to going backward, the team mood swings as well. These swings are only partly linked to the stages of growth, so they are not as predictable. The degree to which a team's spirit ebbs and flows depend on factors such as

Purpose of the team—The more the team's purpose affects team members or causes significant change, the greater the stress among team members.

History of the people involved—As elsewhere, past personal relationships of team members can be a powerful source of positive and negative emotion.

External factors over which you have no control—The team may have some problems with trust or acceptance if their work is affected by a situation that is out of their control, such as staff layoffs in their department.

The team begins with enthusiasm and optimism. These positive reactions often change to boredom and impatience as the project gets underway. Members begin to feel overwhelmed when they realize how much work lies ahead. This is the time that storming begins.

When they finally begin collecting data, team members again feel encouraged—at last they are getting somewhere! This elation rarely lasts. Because few people are experts in scientific methods the first time out, team members almost always uncover mistakes in data collection procedures, and realize they have to do it again. The mood swings down. Recovery comes as the team learns from the experience, tries again, and gathers reliable data.

Ongoing teams also experience highs and lows regarding the progress of their work. Initial excitement about defining how work will be done can shift to frustration or defensiveness when work methods are examined and changed. The team recovers as it adjusts to the new methods and processes. Then new deadlines, the loss or addition of members, or other setbacks can cause the team to get discouraged again. Any time you sense a change in mood, take time to review what's going on and give the team time to readjust.

The best way to deal with this cycle is to understand and accept it with a "this-too-shall-pass" attitude. Changes in attitude, like growth stages, are normal. The team must cultivate patience. Eventually, everyone will see how the work unfolds and will be able to set more realistic expectations for themselves (4).

As team leader, you need to monitor the team's patterns so you know what is "normal."

You can do this by taking several "photographs" of the team at each meeting. Note specific interactions among team members; rate attributes such as cooperation, energy, and humor; and record your own reaction to these events and situations. You may even want to sketch rough diagrams. By writing down the details, you have a record to which to refer and won't have to rely on your memory of isolated incidents. You will begin to see a pattern emerge, from which you can determine what is a "normal" range for your team. Keep in mind, too, that a lack of fluctuation can mean the team has a problem. It could be a sign that team members are working too hard at being harmonious, or it could mean the team lacks the diversity of thought and approach it needs (3).

Guidelines for Good Meetings

Although individual team members carry out assignments between team meetings, some of the team's work must be done when all team members are together—during meetings. Most people groan at the thought of attending another meeting, and in reality many meetings result in little more than wasted time and energy. This is because few people know and practice the techniques for running productive meetings. This section briefly discusses three key guidelines for good meetings:

1. Have a clear purpose.
2. Fill key meeting roles.
3. Improve the meeting process.

One of the team's ground rules should state that people are expected to be on time for team meetings. A meeting should start within a few minutes of the scheduled time, regardless of whether all of the players are present. When most of the team members are present, it's time to start. If latecomers miss something important, they can be brought up to speed *after* the meeting.

Guideline 1: Clear Purpose

Each meeting should have a clear purpose that team members understand before the meeting starts. The tool for defining and achieving the purpose is the meeting agenda.

The team leader should develop and distribute an agenda for each team meeting, preferably before the meeting. The agenda tells team members what to expect and how to prepare. Regard-

Figure 1: Sample Agenda

Meeting Date: Wednesday, July 7, 1999

Place: Conference Room B

Time: 11:00 AM

Purpose: To identify two standard scopes that will be available to surgical teams in the performance of carpal tunnel procedures.

Time	Topic	Person	Method	Outcome
5 min.	Agenda review	Mark	Discussion	Changes?
10 min.	The reasons for standardizing to two scopes	Mark	Presentation	Understanding
10 min.	Review of scopes currently used	Janet	Presentation	Awareness
30 min.	Pros and cons of scopes currently used	Mark	Discussion	Shared knowledge
15 min.	Identify two scopes	Mark	Discussion	Decision
5 min.	Next steps for implementation	Janet	Discussion	Understanding
5 min.	Evaluate meeting	Mark	Discussion	Improvement

Figure 4.1 Sample agenda.

less of whether the agenda was sent out in advance, it should be displayed for all to see at the start of the meeting. The group should spend the first few minutes of the meeting reviewing it, and refer to it during the meeting as a way of checking progress.

An agenda is more than a list of topics. It defines the purpose and methods of the meeting. It is a tool for managing discussions and decision making. *Figure 4.1* presents a sample meeting agenda. The following is a list of items that should be included in a meeting agenda:

- Purpose of the meeting
- Topics, including a phrase or sentence that defines each item and why it is being discussed (Topics should support the purpose of the meeting.)
- The lead person for each topic, usually the person who will introduce it and manage any discussion

- Method or process for each topic, to indicate whether there will be discussion, a report, and so forth
- Desired outcome for each topic, such as a decision, a plan, a list of options, information only, and so on
- Time estimates for each topic

Even if the items on your agenda stay the same from one meeting to the next, the content will certainly vary and new topics will be added. Also, the purpose of the meeting will greatly affect its design and structure. For example, a meeting intended to reach a decision will involve more discussion than a meeting meant to present and identify options.

Guideline 2: Key Meeting Roles

Team members should fulfill the roles of meeting leader, timekeeper, note taker, and scribe. These people are jointly responsible for making sure the meeting runs smoothly.

The *meeting leader* or *facilitator* keeps the meeting focused and moving forward. The team leader often fills this role; however, your team may choose to rotate the responsibility among its members. Specific tasks of the meeting leader are as follows:

- Begin and end the meeting on time.
- Review the agenda.
- Move through the agenda one item at a time.
- Keep the team focused on the agenda.
- Facilitate discussion and mange participation.
- Help the team use appropriate decision methods.
- Help the team evaluate the meeting.
- Gather ideas for the next meeting.

The meeting leader generally does not get involved in the content of team discussions. She needs to concentrate on the process to make sure all members are participating, following ground rules, and so forth. The meeting leader may help the process by asking questions, summarizing, suggesting different methods, and so on. For this reason, the same person probably will not lead all the team's meetings. Several team members may fulfill the role of meeting leader during the life of the team, and even during a single meeting. It's not uncommon—and is actually advisable—for a designated meeting leader to hand the role over to another person for one meeting or part of a meeting when he wants to be part of the discussion. If the team is working through a particularly thorny issue, in which all team members want to have a say, the team leader should find someone from outside the team to act as meeting leader.

The *timekeeper* helps the group keep track of time during the meeting. He alerts the group when the allotted time for a topic is almost up. Then the group can decide whether to continue the discussion or cut it short. This keeps the team from spending all its meeting time on the first few agenda items and not completing its agenda. Depending on the complexity of the discussion and size of the team, the meeting leader may also keep time.

The *note taker* records key topics, main points raised for each agenda item, decisions made, action items (who will do what by when), and items to be discussed at future meetings. The team may want to develop a standard form for note taking. These notes comprise the meeting minutes, so they must reflect the content and outcomes of the meeting completely and accurately. The note taker is also responsible for having these minutes distributed to team members and other interested parties promptly after the meeting.

The *scribe* writes ideas on a flip chart or whiteboard as discussions unfold so that everyone can see them. Posting ideas helps the team stay focused and keeps the team memory from changing as the dialog continues. This approach also shows members that their ideas have been captured for consideration, which encourages participation and discourages "broken records." The scribe must write legibly and large enough for all to see, but doesn't need to be overly concerned about spelling or grammar. He should also check with team members to be sure that what is written accurately reflects what was said (4).

Guideline 3: Improve the Meeting Process

Meetings are processes that can be studied and improved like any other process. The meeting process includes planning the meeting (including preparing the agenda and setting up the room), conducting the meeting (starting, running, and ending the meeting), and following up (including distributing minutes, filing the agenda, and completing assignments). Evaluating the meeting should be part of every meeting agenda. It gives members a chance to identify and address problems before they become serious.

The evaluation should include what worked well and what will be done to improve the next meeting. You can use a number of methods to evaluate your meetings, from round-robin comments or open discussion to written evaluation (4). Some questions the team can use to evaluate its meetings are as follows:

- How did the meeting go?
- How were the pace, tone, and flow of the meeting?
- Did we handle the agenda items in a logical sequence? Did we get stuck?
- How well did we stay on topic?
- How clearly and accurately did we discuss the topics?
- Did we observe the team's ground rules?
- How well did we respond to each other's questions?

TABLE 4.1
Dos and Don'ts for Active Listening

Do	Don't
• Attend and be silent. Let the silence be an invitation to the speaker to continue, rather than an opportunity for you to interject. You can signal your attention with verbal and nonverbal cues: eye contact, ''uh-huh,'' a nod, and so forth.	• Give advice. The listener's role is to help the speaker come up with his own answers.
• Summarize. A skilled listener will occasionally summarize what the speaker has said and reflect it back to him for comment, reaction, or clarification.	• Judge. Avoid words like good or bad, right or wrong, should, and so forth.
• Sort out. Help the speaker separate the solutions and problems, the important from the trivial.	• Discount. Don't downplay the speaker's concerns or sense of urgency.
• Find patterns. An active listener can identify patterns that occur in discussion, as when the same problem occurs in certain situations.	• Sympathize. Be supportive instead of sympathetic.
• Attend to gaps. The attentive listener can identify gaps in the speaker's logic or narrative and ask for clarification.	• Invade or take over. Don't shift the focus of the discussion to your experience or thinking. Let the speaker explore his own ideas.
• Test responsibility and commitment. The listener can check out how much responsibility the speaker takes for his comments or assumptions.	
• Express feelings. Check out any feelings you hear in the speaker's tone of voice.	

• What was just right and should continue as is?
• What do we need to improve for the next meeting? How can we do that?

The "Meat" of the Meetings

Most of the meeting time is taken up with discussion and decision making. To facilitate these activities, the meeting leader must have well-honed skills that include listening, summarizing, testing for agreement, and managing participation. The team will be more successful, however, if every team member learns and practices these skills. This is an area in which just-in-time training is invaluable. The team's coach can also give team members pointers to improve their communication techniques.

The art of listening is particularly valuable, for the meeting leader and team members alike. A skilled listener listens *actively*; she does not sit silently and passively. The active listener is genuinely interested, and truly curious and eager to understand what the speaker means to say. A skilled listener helps the speaker gain insight and explore his ideas more fully by asking questions and summarizing. Some dos and don'ts for practicing active listening are summarized in *Table 4.1*.

WORKING TOWARD CONSENSUS

As explained earlier, a group reaches consensus when it makes a decision that all team members can support. This doesn't mean that everyone is totally pleased with the result. It means that each person sees enough value in the choice to support it. The result is a solution that is easier to implement because it has the team's full support.

Reaching consensus is time-consuming. So, the first requirement for consensus is to make sure you have enough time to devote to the process. You have to consider the ideas, feelings, and situations of all team members, not just the few who object or the majority in support. Those in the minority have to clarify the key elements of their points of view and describe their concerns or reservations. Those in the majority need to explain the reasons for their support. Everyone has to listen actively, be open to new perspectives, and be mindful of potential problems.

The process for reaching and testing consensus works best when a facilitator and scribe are used. Each team member should have a chance to relate her position and opinion. The facilitator should allow questions aimed only at clarifying what someone has said. After everyone has spoken, the facilitator should summarize to point out where the team is in agreement and where it disagrees. He can then lead a discussion to look for solutions or greater unity on the points of difference. Once again, each person can give his opinion on the issue. Remember, if even one person is unwilling to support a decision, you do not have consensus. This process continues until the whole team understands and agrees to the terms of the decision.

UNDERSTANDING PERSONALITY TYPES

People on your team will have varying personal styles. These styles become apparent in the way the people interact with others, look at the world, and process information. People with seemingly incompatible styles can actually work well together and produce excellent results. To do so, they need to understand and appreciate their own styles and those of others.

It is invaluable for the team leader to know the strengths and weaknesses of the different types on the team and, when possible, make assignments accordingly. For example, a detail-oriented person who processes information visually is ideal for working on data collection and analysis. The creative, intuitive type will be a source of ideas and options during decision making and problem solving, but may need to be reminded about completing his or her action items.

There are countless models for categorizing personality types. These models define the characteristics that typify certain personality types, including their communication styles, typical behaviors and attitudes, preferred activities and professions, and approaches to relationships. Teams and other groups often use these models to assess their members and improve the way they work together. In this section, we look briefly at one of the more widely used models—the Myers–Briggs Type Indicator—as well as the concept of sensory dominance (1).

Myers–Briggs Type Indicator

Myers–Briggs explores personality type in four dimensions, each one of which is a continuum (*Table 4.2*).

From Extroversion (E) To Introversion (I)

This set of qualities influences where people direct their energy, their attitude and orientation, and their preferred work environment. For example, extroverts direct their energy outward on people, are generally relaxed and confident, and like work that involves lots of activities with people. Introverts are more thoughtful; they try to understand the world rather than change it. They are often reserved and work best in situations in which they can be quiet and on their own.

From Sensing (S) To Intuition (N)

This dimension relates to how people perceive their experiences, what they care about, and how they work. Strong sensing people experiences life through their senses, focus on details and practical matters, take life as it is, and are good with detail-oriented work. People with high intuition score pick up on possibilities, see patterns and potential, tend to like change and learning new skills, and are good at dealing with the big picture and complex issues.

TABLE 4.2
Four Dimensions of the Myers–Briggs Personality Types

Extroversion ↔ Introversion Where people direct their energy; their attitude and orientation		Sensing ↔ Intuition How people perceive their experiences; what they care about		Thinking ↔ Feeling How people relate to others		Judgment ↔ Perception People's attitudes and styles	
Extroversion	Introversion	Sensing	Intuition	Thinking	Feeling	Judgment	Perception
Energy directed outward to people	Inward focus on concepts and ideas	Experience life through senses	Use "sixth sense" to pick up on things	Focus on logic and higher truth	Focus on human values and needs	Decisive, self-disciplined, exacting	Curious, tolerant, flexible
Relaxed, easy-going	Reserved	Live in the moment, practical	See patterns and potential	Businesslike, fair	Tactful, enthusiastic, naturally friendly	Want to complete tasks, make decisions	Good at starting tasks, put off decisions
Prefer a lot of activity and people	Like quiet, to work independently	Use current skills, detail-oriented	Learn new skills, work on complex problems	Problem solver	Loyal supporter, caretaker	Just the relevant facts	Everything there is to know

From Thinking (T) To Feeling (F)

This dimension indicates what people care about and how they relate to others. Thinking people, not surprisingly, focus on the logic of a situation and look for the truth. They are fair in their dealings with others, but are usually terse and impersonal, and seek to find solutions and right wrongs. Feeling people care about people and their needs and values. They are naturally friendly, enthusiastic, and empathetic, and seek to care for others.

From Judgment (J) To Perception (P)

This dimension influences people's attitudes and the way they work. A judgment-type person is decisive, self-controlled, purposeful, and exacting, and focuses on reaching a decision and completing a task. The perception-type person, on the other hand, is spontaneous and continually curious, flexible, and adaptable; likes to start tasks; and tends to postpone decisions.

Each person is assessed on each of these dimensions to see where they sit on the continuum. Based on the scores for each dimension, a person has a four-letter type indicator, such as INFP—introvert, intuition, feeling, perception (1).

Sensory Dominance

We use all five of our senses. However, sight, hearing, and touch are the ones we use most often. Each person instinctively prefers to use one of these three senses to *take in* information, another to *organize* the information, and a third to *use* the information. In other words, our dominant sensory modes—visual, auditory, and kinesthetic—influence how we perceive, relate to, and act in our environment.

Visual people relate to pictures and think in pictures. In meetings, these people need graphics and charts, not just the spoken word. They talk a mile a minute, tripping over their words, to keep up with the images that are in their "mind" as they talk. They often look up or squint as they talk, trying to get a better look at that image. They are animated and don't like to be interrupted. Words and phrases that identify a visual person include, "I *see* what you mean," "That *looks* good to me," "*Show* me . . ."

Auditory people are oriented to sound. They love spoken words, theirs and other people's. They think in dialog and often talk to themselves or move their lips as they read. People who use

hearing to organize their thoughts literally "think out loud." They talk through and around ideas until they make sense of them. The auditory person's byword is "*Tell* me."

Kinesthetic people can be focused either inward, on their emotions, or outward on their touch. Inward kinesthetic people are in tune with how they feel about something and may act on "gut instinct." Outward kinesthetic people are literally in touch, always fiddling with something, needing to be "hands on." Kinesthetic people may need to move around to think, so don't force them to stay seated during discussions. Their conversation contains phrases like, "Keep in *touch*," "This just doesn't *feel* right," "I've got a good *feeling* about this" (2).

GIVING AND GETTING CONSTRUCTIVE FEEDBACK

Members of any group committed to quality improvement needs to be able to give constructive feedback and receive it so that both parties have their needs met. The team's ground rules should acknowledge the need for feedback.

Effective feedback recognizes strengths and achievements. It also offers help for processes and behaviors that need improvement. It is not an opportunity for you or someone else to demonstrate superior insight or authority.

When giving feedback, first pay attention to the timing and the context. Be sure both you and the person to whom you are talking are prepared to be attentive and thoughtful. Establish an understanding that a difference exists and then define that difference. Be descriptive without using judgmental words, and cite specific examples that reflect your experience. Don't use second-hand reports. Invite discussion so that you can explore the other person's feelings about the difference and possible solutions. When putting forth suggestions for change, focus on behavior or situations that the other person can control and on which you can follow up.

If you are receiving feedback, your greatest challenge is probably to avoid getting defensive so that you can hear and respond to the feedback. Be an active listener. Pay close attention to what is being said and make sure you understand *why* the other person is offering this feedback to you. Summarize what you have heard and ask questions so you get specific examples and facts. Take time to think about what you have heard and to assess it; don't reject or accept it out of hand. If you are willing to change as a result of the feedback, say so. Ask for the other person's suggestions or make one of your own. If you disagree with the feedback, explain your viewpoint and be open to other ways of resolving the difference.

WORKING THROUGH GROUP PROBLEMS

No matter how well you practice positive team behaviors and observe the team process, problems and conflict arise on the team. Members polarize, legitimate differences of opinion become win–lose struggles, and progress stops. Sometimes one person's behavior disrupts the team; other times the entire team behaves in ways that prevent work from getting done. Whatever the source of the problem, team members need to deal with it so they can get back to work.

When a problem develops, think of it as a *group* problem. It is a natural tendency to blame someone for causing the problem. The truth is that many problems arise because the group lets them happen or even encourages them in some way. For example, if the same team member repeatedly derails team decisions at the last minute, it is because the team is allowing that to happen. The team needs to examine each problem in light of how it encourages or allows the behavior and what it can do to encourage more constructive behavior.

When you are team leader, you should not overreact or underreact. This means you have to take time to assess what's going on so your response will match the seriousness of the problem. Some behaviors are only fleeting disruptions in the team's progress. Other behaviors are very disruptive and can impede, halt, or reverse the team's progress. Some behaviors are chronic, occurring again and again. Experienced leaders develop a range of responses to typical problems. This way they can "crank up" the response as the problem gets more disruptive, just as physicians may use more aggressive treatments as a patient's condition worsens.

The range of responses to team problems usually includes

Do nothing (nonintervention)—Ignore the offensive behavior, particularly if it is not chronic or doesn't inhibit the group. Some-

times you don't need to intervene because other group members deal with the offending behavior. In such cases, you should be available to facilitate when one member confronts another.

Off-line conversation (minimal intervention)—Talk to the disruptive members outside the group meeting. Find out what would increase their satisfaction with the group and offer constructive feedback. For example, you may have one member who consistently interrupts another member who does a lot of thinking out loud. You can help the interrupter understand the other person's need to talk through things, and encourage the other person to be more concise.

Impersonal group time (low intervention)—Take some time at the start of the meeting to talk about general concerns with group process and team ground rules. Don't name names. Do list some potential problem areas on the flip chart, including the disruptive behavior you want to address. This puts the problem in the context of the group, not an individual. Then at the end of the meeting, during the evaluation, the team can evaluate its conduct for each item on the list. It is usually difficult to deal with problems without referring to the offenders. One way to get around this is to describe the context of the problem, as in, "Each time we talk about preoperative issues, we get sidetracked."

Off-line confrontation (medium intervention)—This is an off-line conversation with the problem members during which the team leader is more assertive. Use it when other attempts have failed, especially when the disruptive behavior continues even after the group has tried to change. This confrontation may lead to an informal contract, in which you and the member agree to certain changes. For example, "I know you don't get along with Joe, and I will do everything I can to avoid pairing you up on assignments. Meanwhile, I want you to stop discounting all his comments during meetings."

In-group confrontation (high intervention)—As a last resort, you may have to deal with the offending behavior in the presence of the group. This disrupts the team's business and exposes the person's behavior to open critique. You must prepare carefully for this type of intervention: how to word the confrontation, what reactions to anticipate, and how to avoid defensiveness or hostility from the offending member. Using ''I'' statements and constructive feedback techniques can help accomplish the goal of changing the behavior without punishing the member.

Expulsion from the team (very high intervention)—Kicking someone off the team should be a rare occurrence. The stigma will attach to the team and to the expelled member for a long time. It makes an enemy of the expelled member and creates an unfavorable impression throughout the organization of the team and its leadership. A possible alternative is to exclude the member from team meetings and find other ways for him or her to contribute to the team's work.

As the preceding examples illustrate, there will be times as team leader when you need to intervene with members of your team. You may also be asked by groups or individuals outside your team to mediate for them. The following are some questions to help you think through your decision to intervene:

- Do you have enough credibility with the parties involved?
- Can you remain neutral?
- How much time, energy, and skill are needed for success? Do you have these resources?
- Can you focus on one issue or element of the conflict?
- Is the timing right?
- Which is more risky—intervening or staying out of it?

If you decide to intervene, choose a meeting place that is on neutral territory. Make sure the setting is informal and that all the people involved in the conflict can attend. Set an agenda and ground rules and stick to them. Use active listening and constructive feedback skills to keep people from getting defensive, playing games, or blaming.

When the meeting is underway, referee the process conscientiously. Allow each participant to make a short, timed opening statement, like in a debate. When everyone has made their statements, try to restate the views and issues in neutral terms. This helps all parties to hear and understand the key elements of the conflict. Try to help them uncover the core issue in the conflict and move them toward a resolution that meets each person's needs (4).

TEN COMMON TEAM PROBLEMS AND WHAT TO DO ABOUT THEM

When people work together on a project, it's unreasonable to expect everything to go smoothly. For that reason, it is best to be prepared for what might go wrong. Encourage team members to get to know one another early on the project. Discuss and establish ground rules for behavior before work starts. It is also important to discuss and develop strategies for dealing with the ten most common problems:

1. **Floundering**—The team doesn't know where to start or what to do next.
2. **Overbearing participants**—Certain team members wield a disproportionate amount of influence over the team.
3. **Dominating participants**—Certain team members monopolize the air time at meetings.
4. **Reluctant participants**—Some team members don't contribute to team discussions and decisions.
5. **Unquestioned acceptance of opinion as facts**—Team members fail to support personal beliefs or assertions with data.
6. **Rush to accomplishment**—One team member's impatience for decision undermines the team's decision process.
7. **Attribution**—Team members suspect the motives of others on the team and within the organization.
8. **Discounts and "plops"**—One or more team members ignore or ridicule comments or contributions of another team member.
9. **Wanderlust: digressions and tangents**—Meeting discussions go astray.
10. **Feuding team members**—Feuding team members make team meetings and activities their battleground.

The following examples provide some suggestions for working through common team problems.

Problem 1: Floundering

Teams commonly have trouble starting and ending a project, or even moving between different project stages. They flounder, wondering what to do next.

Problems at the beginning suggest that the team is either unclear about or overwhelmed by its task. Startup problems may also arise because members are not yet comfortable enough with each other to engage in meaningful discussion and decision making.

Floundering when trying to make decisions may indicate that the team's work doesn't have full team support and that, in fact, some members are reluctant to say they disagree with the team's conclusions.

Floundering at the end of a phase of the project could mean that the team doesn't have a clear plan and doesn't know where to go next. Floundering at the end of the project may reflect reluctance to disband the team or concern about exposing their work to outside review and possible criticism.

The following are some feedback questions and comments that can help the team deal with floundering:

- Let's review how this project is being run. Let's review the team's work plan or create one if one isn't already in place.
- Let's review our purpose and make sure it's clear to everyone.
- Let's review our work plan and see what we have to do next.
- What do we need so we can move on? What is holding us up? Data? Knowledge? Assurances? Support?
- Are we being held up by unfinished business? Does anyone feel we've missed something?
- Let's set some time aside at the next meeting to talk about how we will proceed. In the meantime, each of us should write down what we think is needed to get us moving.

Problem 2: Overbearing Participants

The health care profession can be a hierarchical domain. And on a team made up of doctors, nurses, technicians, medical professionals, and administrators, that hierarchy can make its biases felt. However much you extol the team spirit, some members may wield a disproportionate amount of influence on the team. These people usually have a position of authority or base their authority an area of expertise—or both.

Teams need the resources of authorities and experts, but their presence can be harmful if they

- Discourage or forbid discussion of topics that encroach on their area of authority or expertise. "I don't think you need to involve yourself in the technicalities of our choice of equipment for that procedure. We're taking care of

that in our department. Let's move on to something else."
- Make their area "untouchable" by using jargon or holding up current procedures, regulations, or policies as the only and ultimate authority. "Hospital policy is clear . . . ," "You obviously don't grasp the relationship of the nonincidental seizing response to hypermiasma."
- Regularly discount any proposed activity as being unworkable, based on their previous experience. "We tried that at NIH. The best people in the field couldn't make it work! Don't even think about it!" Other members soon get the message that they are too naive and shortsighted to come up with a workable solution.

The team leader has a number of options for dealing with an overbearing member:

- Reinforce the ground rule that says no area is sacred. All team members have a right to explore any topic that pertains to the team's purpose.
- Because you can probably identify the problem participants before they start running roughshod over the team, take steps ahead of time to rein them in. Talk to them about how important it is for everyone to understand the entire process. Ask them if they'd be willing, at specified and appropriate times, to act as subject matter experts and share their knowledge with the team.
- Talk to the offending "expert" off-line to ask for cooperation and patience.
- Enforce the primacy of data. If the data contradict the "expert's" opinion, the data prevails.

Problem 3: Dominating Participants

Some members, with or without authority or expertise, consume a disproportionate amount of airtime. They talk too much. Instead of concise statements, they tell long anecdotes. They assume that the normal moments of silence that occasionally occur are invitations for them to speak. Their talk keeps the team from building a sense of joint accomplishment or momentum. Other team members are discouraged from trying to participate, whereas others find excuses to skip meetings.

To deal with dominators, the team leader or meeting leader can

- Structure discussion on key issues in a way that encourages equal participation. For example, have members write down their thoughts and then share them with all other members at the table.

- Practice gatekeeping: "We've already heard from you on this, Joe. I'd like to hear what the others have to say."
- List "balance of participation" as a general group concern to critique during the meeting evaluation.
- Get the team to agree on a ground rule stating the value of balanced participation and the need limit and focus in discussions.

Problem 4: Reluctant Participants

At the other end of the spectrum are participants who rarely speak. Each of us has a different threshold of need to be part of a team (tribal versus loner instincts) and a different level of comfort with speaking in a group (extrovert versus introvert). Like other personal styles, there is no right or wrong with these preferences. However, problems can develop in a team that has no built-in activities that encourage introverts to talk while the extroverts listen.

The meeting leader can deal with reluctant participants by

- Structuring discussion to encourage full participation
- Dividing tasks into individual assignments and reports so that introverts are forced to take part
- Acting as gatekeeper. Try to draw the introverts into the discussion: "Does anyone else have some ideas about this?" (while looking straight at the reluctant member). Or more, directly, "Sam, what's your experience in this area?"

Problem 5: Unquestioned Acceptance of Opinions as Facts

Some team members express personal beliefs and assumptions with such confidence that listeners assume they are hearing a presentation of facts. This can be dangerous, and leads to an unshakable acceptance of various "earth-is-flat" assertions. This tendency in particular is evident with clinical opinions or philosophies that may not be supported by evidence-based medicine.

Most team members are reluctant to question self-assured statements, such as "patients prefer it that way" from other members. Besides wanting to be polite, they think they need to have data before they can challenge someone else's assertions. However, an axiom of debate states that if a speaker presents something as fact without legitimate supporting evidence, the listener doesn't need to have evidence to respond with skepticism.

To deal with this problem, the meeting leader can ask or state

- Is what you said an opinion or a fact? Do you have data?
- How do you know that is true?
- Let's accept that what you say is possible, but let's also get some data to test it.
- Let's have the team agree on the primacy of the scientific approach.

Problem 6: Rush to Accomplishment

Most teams will have at least one "do something" member who is either impatient to act (a dominant personality type perhaps, or someone with a high judgment score) or sensitive to pressure from managers or other influential people or groups. This type of person typically reaches an independent decision about a problem and its solution before the group has had time to consider different options. He urges the team to make hasty decisions and discourages any further efforts to analyze or discuss the matter. His nonverbal behavior and direct statements constantly express impatience.

Too much of this pressure can lead a team to a series of random, hasty decisions. Like hunters shooting at dim targets in a heavy fog, they hope that at least one shot will find a target.

Teams must realize that results do not come easily, and rarely can the team make significant progress overnight. Quality takes patience. After making sure that she is not exerting undue pressure on the team to produce, the meeting leader can reinforce this mind-set by

- Reminding team members of their ground rule not to compromise or circumvent data-based decision making
- Confronting the rusher using the techniques of constructive feedback. Give examples of rushing and explain the effects of this impatience on the team's work.

Problem 7: Attribution

As individuals and teams, we tend to attribute motives to other people when we disagree with them or don't understand their opinion or behavior. This is a substitute for the difficult and sometimes uncomfortable task of seeking real explanations. It is faster and easier to "make something up" than to ask questions and explore possibilities. Attribution can create resentment. It is perfectly normal to bristle when someone else tells you why you did something.

Within a team, attribution can lead to hostility when it is aimed at other team members: "He's just trying to get out of doing the work." When it is aimed at people or groups outside the team, attribution can lead to misguided efforts: "They don't want to help. They're busy protecting their own budget."

The following are some steps the team leader can take to deal with attribution:

- Reaffirm the team's commitment to data-based decisions. Do not act on anything unless and until it is supported by fact.
- Identify and respond to a statement of attribution: "That's a possible explanation for what they did. But how do we know? What have we seen or heard that supports that idea? Can we confirm that with data?"
- If the attribution is from one team member to another, don't let it pass without checking it out: "Jim, I heard Sally describe your approach as 'catering to the administration.' How would you describe it?"

Problem 8: Discounts and "Plops"

We all have values and viewpoints that are important to us at conscious and unconscious levels. When someone else ignores or ridicules these values, we feel discounted. Being discounted can cause hostility on a team, especially if it happens a lot.

For instance, there will be time when someone makes a statement that "plops." No one acknowledges it, and the discussion resumes on a totally new tact, leaving the speaker to wonder why no one responded.

Discounting happens for many reasons. Maybe the discounted member said something that was truly irrelevant to the discussion, or maybe he didn't express the idea clearly. Maybe the rest of the team missed the meaning. Whatever the reason, every member deserves respect and attention from the team. So team members must help each other identify and articulate what is important to them.

The team leader or meeting leader can help this effort by

- Including training in active listening and other constructive communication skills early in the team's life
- Supporting the discounted person: "Nancy, it sounds like that thought is important to you and we weren't giving it enough consideration." "I think Jerry was getting at something worthwhile and that we should spend some time on it before we move on." "Bill, before we move on, is there some part of what you said that you'd like the group to discuss?"
- Talking off-line with anyone who frequently discounts, puts down, or ignores previous speakers' statements

Problem 9: Wanderlust: Digressions and Tangents

If you spend any time in meetings, this scenario will sound familiar to you: A team working on improving recovery room procedures is told of how one hospital addressed a particularly thorny problem. This reminds someone of how that same hospital solved a problem in another area, which reminds someone else of an incident in the operating suite at that hospital, which leads to a discussion of whatever happened to that anesthetist, which leads to a discussion of the job market, and so on. When the meeting ends, everyone wonders where the time went.

Such unfocused conversations are an example of wanderlust, our natural tendency to stray from the subject. Sometimes these digressions are innocent journeys from the conversation. But if they happen often, digressions may be the team's way of avoiding a subject it needs to address or a problem it can't solve. In either case, the meeting leader has to bring the conversation back to the agenda. She can do that by

- Using a written agenda with time estimates for each item and referring to the topic and time when discussion begins to stray
- Writing topics or items on a flip chart page so that team members can refer to them during the discussion
- Directing the conversation back on track: "We're getting away from the topic of ✂✂✂✂. We've only got five more minutes to wrap this up."
- Focusing the team on what it is trying to avoid: "We've had trouble sticking to this point. Is there something about this particular topic that makes it hard to talk about?"

Problem 10: Feuding Team Members

Sometimes a team becomes a field of combat for members who are vying with each other. Usually, the contest itself is more important than the subjects about which they choose to argue. Other members feel like spectators at a sporting event. They avoid interceding for fear of getting swept into the battle on one side or the other.

Usually, these feuds predate the team and will outlast it. The best way to deal with this situation is to prevent it by choosing members who are not known adversaries. If that's impossible, then bring the combatants together before the first meeting to work out some agreement about their behavior. This agreement should probably be in the form of an up-front contract (''If you agree to do X, I'll agree not to do Y'') for managing their differences without disrupting the team. If confrontations do occur during a meeting, remind them of the contract and instruct them to finish their discussion off-line (4).

CLOSING DOWN THE TEAM

When your team's work is complete, it is time to close down the team. This, of course, means that your team must be able to recognize when it has achieved its purpose.

Problems arise if the team's charter is too broad and general, or if the team takes it upon itself to expand its charter to include issues or problems it thinks are related to the original charter. A team may also be reluctant to ''close up shop'' if they feel their gains will be lost when others take over.

If your team's charter was clear and specific, closing down won't present a problem. Before starting its work, the team should have identified clear data-based criteria for measuring its success, as well as a timeline. Along the way, the management group should review the team's progress regularly. The group should also work with the team leader to make sure the team documents its results and has a process for handing over ongoing responsibility for monitoring and maintaining the solution. Team members can help develop new documentation such as procedural manuals or work instructions, or make a presentation to the work group that will implement the change. They can also suggest a plan for implementing the new procedure, including training and communication materials. These activities give team members a clear signal that their work is done. They also give team members the satisfaction of knowing that their gains will be preserved.

CONCLUSION

Teamwork—the collaborative effort by a diverse group toward a common goal—is fast becoming a required skill for neurosurgeons in and out of the operating suite. Health care organizations need to adapt quickly and effectively to their changing markets and missions, and they are creating teams to help them do this. Because of their place at the apex of the caregiving team, neurosurgeons often serve on these teams as leaders or valued members. Their ability to build and work effectively on teams can enhance improvement initiatives as well as the standard of care and teaching in their organizations.

SUGGESTED READINGS

Burchill G, Brodie CB: Voices into choices: Acting on the voice of the customer. Madison, Oriel Incorporated, 1997.

GOAL/QPC-Oriel Incorporated: The Team Memory Jogger®. Methuen, GOAL/QPC-Oriel Incorporated, 1995.

Joiner BL: Fourth generation management: The new business consciousness. New York, McGraw–Hill, 1994.

Katzenbach JR, Smith DK: The wisdom of teams: Creating the high-performance organization. Boston, Harvard Business School Press, 1993.

Lipnack J, Stamps J: Virtual teams. New York, John Wiley & Sons, 1997.

Oriel Incorporated: Plain & Simple® learning and application guides. Madison, Oriel Incorporated, 1995.

Oriel Incorporated: The Team® trail guide. CD-ROM. Madison, Oriel Incorporated, 1998.

Reddy B: Intervention skills: Process consultation for small groups and teams. San Diego, Pfeiffer & Company, 1994.

Sampson E, Marthas M: Group process for the health professions. Albany, NY, Delmar Publishers, 1990.

Scholtes PR, Joiner BL, Streibel BJ: The Team® handbook. Madison, Oriel Incorporated, 1996, ed 2.

Stone D, Patton B, Heen S: Difficult conversations: How to discuss what matters most. New York, Viking Press

REFERENCES

1. Kroeger O, Thuesen J: Type talk at work. New York, Dell Publishing, 1992, pp 15–25.
2. Markova D: The art of the possible. Conari Press, 1991, pp 124–158.
3. Oriel Incorporated: The Team® trail guide. CD-ROM. Madison, Oriel Incorporated, 1998.
4. Scholtes P, Joiner B, Streibel B: The Team® handbook. Madison, Oriel Incorporated, 1996, ed 2, pp 7-7–7-10.

CHAPTER 5

Practical Methods and Tools for Improving Quality in Neurosurgery

STEPHEN L. DAVID, M.B.A., TERRY HOWELL, Ph.D., AND
AARON FAUSZ, Ph.D.

EDITOR'S NOTE: Bringing empirical science to management, business, and leadership requires different tools than we are used to using from clinical neurosurgery or neurosurgery clinical and basic science research. Because we are usually not exposed to or taught these tools or techniques in neurosurgery residency, we are somewhat on our own when it comes to acquiring these competencies. This chapter focuses on commonly used quality graphic and management tools from a very practical "how-to" standpoint. The purpose is to introduce and demystify these techniques and to demonstrate their potential practical use.

"Statistical thinking will one day be as necessary for effective citizenship as the ability to read and write."

—H. G. Wells

WHY DO WE NEED QUALITY IMPROVEMENT?

Poor quality in health care affects patients, families, payers, physicians, administrators, and staff adversely. It is not only unhealthy and potentially dangerous, it is also expensive. This should be of primary concern to all physicians who care for the well-being of their patients and their profession. Furthermore, as data become increasingly accessible to the public, there will be a concomitant increase in demands for improvement by forces outside of health care. It has been estimated that 180,000 preventable deaths occur per year in hospitals (6). If this is true, it makes a hospital visit the number one cause of preventable death in America. Additional estimates state that 25% to 30% of health care revenues are wasted because of the inefficiencies

found throughout the health care system (6). These inefficiencies are "treatable" through the tools and ideas found in the rather substantial body of literature that describes continuous quality improvement. Whether we are looking to reduce mortality rates, readmission rates, late starts in surgery, medication errors, postoperative infections, missed diagnoses, or slow lab results, the tools discussed in this chapter can help. The tools help us focus on processes and systems that need improvement, instead of on which physicians or staff to blame. Because physicians are often held solely accountable for the results of a system of processes over which they have little control, they perhaps should be the ones most interested in tools and methods to improve processes across the continuum of care.

QUALITY IMPROVEMENT AND THE SCIENTIFIC METHOD

The scientific method starts with a problem or a question. The scientist generally reviews the literature, creates a hypothesis, performs careful experimentation, evaluates the findings, and makes a decision based on the findings. Often, depending on the complexity of the question, the process cycles repeatedly because the initial findings create new questions and deeper probing into the issue. Over time, new facts emerge, leading to new and better theories that benefit humankind in a variety of ways, materially, emotionally, and culturally.

The discipline of quality improvement is

based on the scientific method. Basically, one uses the Plan–Do–Check–Act cycle repeatedly throughout efforts to improve.

It should be made plain at the outset that there is no particular mystique about quality management. Every field invariably develops a jargon—medicine included. Individuals who promote the improvement of quality are no different. In writing this, we explain as clearly as possible how one can use straightforward tools to improve the practice of medicine, or anything else for that matter.

WHY TOOLS?

To perform neurosurgery, one needs the right tools to clip aneurysms and cut off the blood supply from tumors. The most skilled surgeon is handicapped without the tools needed to perform certain tasks. Similarly, there exists a well-defined set of quality improvement tools that help one explore, experiment, analyze, decide, and improve. There are more than 50 different, commonly used tools. Fortunately, some are more helpful and more frequently employed than others. These tools are the focus of this chapter.

In addition to picking the most useful tools from the full armamentarium, it is helpful to classify them, to make it easier to decide which tools should be deployed in a given situation. We suggest classifying the tools as follows:

• Project management tools
• Meeting support tools
• Just-in-time learning tools
• Creative-thinking tools
• Logical-thinking tools
• Decision-making tools
• Data analysis tools

PROJECT MANAGEMENT TOOLS

Some improvements are easy to make. Some can be made immediately by one person. Whenever this is possible, it should be done. At other times, a team may be required. In this instance, an organized project, a designated team, and a series of meetings may be required. This is particularly true when trying to improve a complex process or system of processes. In these instances, using an established project support system will save time, money, and unnecessary

frustration. There exists a well-established science of project management, and the Project Management Institute offers one of the best reference sites on the subject (http://www.pmi.org). Project management tools range from simple, basic organizational ones to some very arcane but powerful software.

The nature of improvement teams in health care is that they are generally organized on an ad hoc basis for the purpose of solving specific problems or reviewing a particular process. Improvement teams generally do not require high-end project management tools. Rather, simple Gantt or Performance Evaluation and Review Technique (PERT) charts are usually adequate for controlling, scheduling, and monitoring the progress of a team.

Our experience in health care process improvement suggests that it is essential to track the sequence of steps that the team will follow. Data for the project should be stored in a single place where it is accessible to team members and other interested parties. Health care teams are often interested in sharing results, so there is a need for easy publication or display of the team's improvement journey. There are three project management tools that teams have found most useful: project pathway, Gantt chart, and storyboarding.

Project Pathway

There are many variants of the basic Plan–Do–Check–Act cycle. Most consulting firms in the industry have proprietary variations that they teach, but in our view the common elements of these far outweigh their differences.

First, most pathways begin with defining the goal of the project. For example, we want to reduce postoperative infection rates to those achieved by some benchmark hospital. Second, the current process is put under the microscope. What data exist now to show the current performance of the process? Where does the process begin and where does it end? How does the process flow? Who is involved in the process? What materials, equipment, supplies, facilities, and information affect the output? Third, the team looks for problems and inefficiencies in the existing process. What are the most likely causes for postoperative infections? Are there patterns in the data that reveal clues? Fourth, the team looks for improvements in the literature, in other organizations, or within their own team for identified trouble spots. The best ideas are chosen, and detailed plans for change are formulated. Lastly, the planned changes are carried out, and all necessary data are collected and analyzed. Did the changes work as expected? Do infection rates decline? Do they meet the target value? Will the improvement be sustained over time?

Sometimes the first round of improvements will work as planned, the target will be met, the team will make final notes on its findings, and then it will publish them internally or externally. Sometimes the team will generate other improvement ideas that are worth pursuing. Sometimes the changes will not work as hoped, and the team must go back to the drawing board.

The steps that the team takes are best captured in a project pathway. It can be a paper document—many hospitals use a paper checklist for quality teams. It is more flexible to use software, with the pathway stored on a network server where team members can have access to it. A typical project pathway software package is shown in *Figure 5.1*.

Gantt Chart

The Gantt chart is the most popular tool for tracking the progress of a project along its planned schedule. It provides a quick picture of progress made on tasks and allows for adjustments as the project goes along.

Although ''Gantt charting'' can be done by hand, it is much easier to use one of at least six major Gantt chart software packages, or one of the several simpler ones that are combined with management software toolkits (*Fig 5.2*).

Often in a project, one task depends on others. If task 2 cannot start until task 1 is complete, this dependency is noted on the Gantt chart, and the bar that represents the length of task 2 will start just below and to the right of task 1.

When all the dependencies between tasks have been established, it is easy to see how long the whole project will take. In modern Gantt charts, the critical path (the set of tasks that takes the longest to complete) may be highlighted in color so that project managers can identify it easily and can actively seek ways to shorten overall project duration.

Gantt charts can tell their users which tasks have the most impact on project length, which ones are late in starting or finishing, and which

ones must be finished before others can begin. More sophisticated Gantt charts include ways to assign manpower to various tasks, reallocate man-hours to critical tasks, and adjust loads so that no one is overloaded.

Gantt charts compete with PERT charts and the Critical Path Model for acceptance, but the best features of these other charts have been largely absorbed into the Gantt chart. The tool of choice for people who need either a quick-and-easy project scheduling tool or a very sophisticated one, is still—87 years after its invention—the Gantt chart.

Storyboarding

Walt Disney first used storyboards to animate cartoons. He was perceptive enough to see that the visual sequencing that worked so well to bring out creative ideas could apply to business planning too. Mike Vance, Dean of Disney University in the 1960s, refined the process, which had been used primarily for brainstorming. He added an action planning step so that teams could translate creative ideas readily into concrete plans.

The highlights of the team's project pathway are usually displayed: the mission, a picture of the original process, the trouble spots that were identified, the experiments tried, and the results achieved. The storyboard in this use has two roles: to emphasize what is really important and to communicate quality gains so that others need not reinvent the wheel.

People use a variety of paper-based and computer-based tools for storyboarding. Most word processors and presentation packages work well for this purpose, and some, more dedicated to quality improvement work, make it very easy to arrange the results of various tools in a storyboard format.

MEETING SUPPORT TOOLS

A 1994 study of meetings in private-sector companies showed that 30% of managers spend at least 16 hours per work week in meetings. Most of the meetings did not have a written agenda, less than half recorded the discussion that took place, and 54% included people who weren't essential to the meeting. Approximately 33% of the meetings had no defined purpose and 41% had follow-up actions assigned (1).

Because meetings will always be necessary,

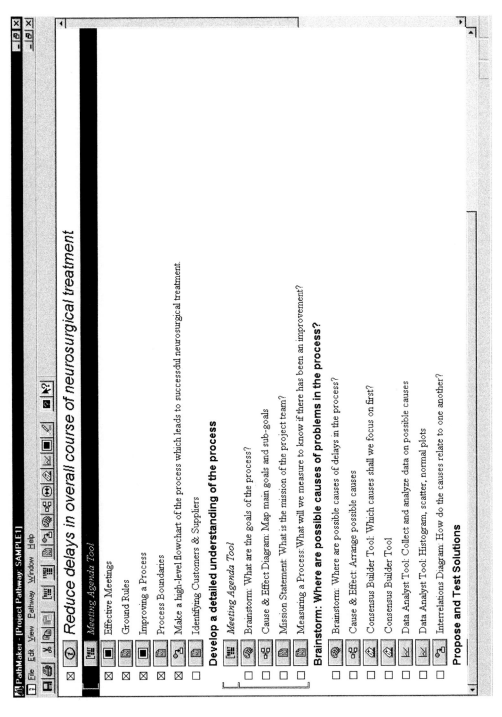

Figure 5.1 This screen capture from SkyMark Corporation's PathMaker® software depicts a project pathway, with the steps that a quality team has planned or completed.

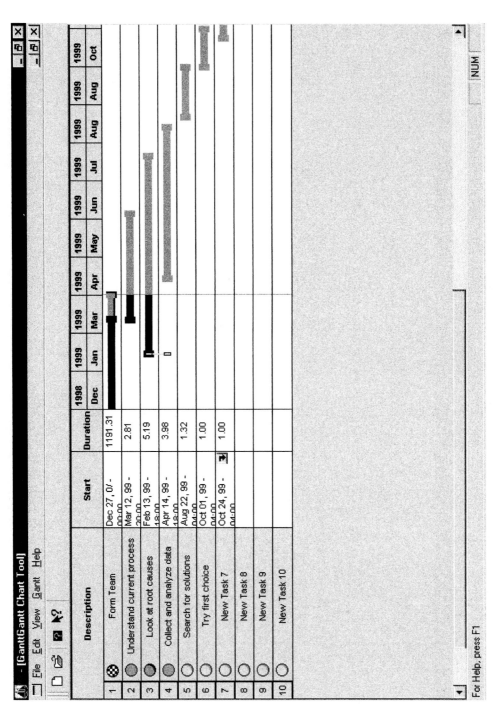

Figure 5.2 In a Gantt chart, all the anticipated tasks in a project are listed, one per row, down the left column. Each task is accompanied by a timeframe (i.e., how long it will take to accomplish the task). Moving left to right, across the chart, is a time axis, with the past toward the left, the present marked by a vertical line, and the future extending toward the right.

well-run meetings should be the goal. Most meetings suffer from a poorly designed meeting process. Meeting and teamwork tools and skills are considered in depth in another chapter of this monograph, so we will just touch on a few issues here.

First, good meeting facilitation and leadership skills are as important to the success of a quality improvement effort as any of the other tools. Meetings should be considered a quality improvement tool in and of themselves.

Second, good meeting processes exist and are widely known. These skills can be learned; health care leaders who have gone through formal training report good results—shorter meetings, better decisions, and faster action. Shortcuts in following a sound meeting process will almost invariably result in waste.

Third, there are good tools available for meeting support. The leading word processors include templates for meeting agendas. Microsoft's NetMeeting and Lotus's Sametime software are two leaders in the emerging virtual meeting market, but there are many competing entries in the market. Finally, and we must declare a bias here, SkyMark's PathMaker software is unique in tying together meeting agendas with project pathways and the major quality improvement tools for local or virtual meetings.

JUST-IN-TIME LEARNING TOOLS

Neurosurgeons and operating room nurses and anesthesiologists typically do not have time to become expert in all aspects of quality improvement. Neither do specialists in most other fields. It is, therefore, incumbent on the experts in the field to make the necessary knowledge granular, self-explanatory, and easy to get. This is happening. Indeed it is the purpose of this chapter.

CREATIVE-THINKING TOOLS

One of the biggest obstacles to improvement is previous experience—both successes and failures. Because of our experience, we assume, often unconsciously, that what worked or failed in the past will continue to do so in the future. We therefore perpetuate patterns of thinking that don't always make the most of our brainpower. Continuous improvement usually requires that new ideas and approaches be explored, and there are specific tools that can be used to stimulate creativity.

Two of the tools discussed in this section—brainstorming and nominal group technique—will help you generate numerous creative ideas about a given question or issue, including possible causes of problems, approaches to use, and/or actions to take. The third tool, the affinity diagram, provides an excellent way to organize those ideas into meaningful clusters for further elaboration. Used together, these tools provide a powerful way to harness the creative energies of your team for improvement.

Brainstorming

Brainstorming consists of listing all ideas put forth by a group in response to a given problem or question. In 1939, a team led by advertising executive Alex Osborn coined the term *brainstorm*. According to Osborn (7), brainstorm means using the brain to storm a creative problem, and to do so in an appropriate fashion requires each ''stormer'' to attack the same objective audaciously.

Brainstorming can help a group break free from old, ineffective ideas. By not allowing ideas to be evaluated or discussed until everyone has exhausted their suggestions, this freewheeling technique for generating ideas can lead to new and original solutions to problems. During brainstorming, any and all ideas are considered legitimate, and often the most far-fetched prove to be the most fertile.

As stated, brainstorming is a useful way to produce numerous creative ideas about a given question or issue, including possible causes of problems, approaches to use, and/or actions to take. When performed properly, brainstorming taps the mind's capacity for lateral thinking and free association. The major benefits of brainstorming are that it:

- **Encourages creativity**—It expands thinking to include all aspects of a problem or a solution and enables participants to identify a wide range of options.
- **Rapidly produces a large number of ideas**—It helps groups develop many ideas quickly by encouraging people to offer whatever ideas come to mind.
- **Equalizes involvement by all team members**—It provides a nonjudgmental environ-

ment that encourages everyone to offer ideas, and all ideas are recorded.

- **Fosters a sense of ownership**—When all members actively participate in the brainstorming process, a sense of ownership in the topic being discussed and in the resulting activities is fostered.

For all participants to enjoy a creative and productive brainstorming experience, the following ground rules should be observed:

- **Participate actively**—Everyone should be encouraged to express his ideas, even if they seem silly or far out.
- **Do not enter into discussion**—No criticisms, compliments, or other comments should be made during the brainstorm session.
- **Build on ideas**—Participants should build on and elaborate ideas generated by other group members.
- **Record ideas as stated**—All ideas generated during the brainstorming session should be written exactly as presented and displayed where everyone can see them.
- **Set a time limit**—A limit on the amount of time to be spent generating ideas should be agreed to by the group before beginning the brainstorm.

The recommended steps for conducting an effective brainstorm session are as follows:

1. Review the ground rules. Describe how this session will be conducted by going over the points described earlier.
2. Set a time limit. Assign a timekeeper and data recorder, and start the clock. Brainstorming should be a rapid generation of ideas, so do it quickly. Five to 15 minutes works well. If the time limit has expired and ideas are still being generated, you can extend the time limit at 5-minute intervals.
3. Clarify the central question of the brainstorm. Every brainstorm answers a question. For example, What are the main quality problems in our neurosurgery practice? What ideas do we have for reducing complications in a given procedure? What would the ideal operating room be like? Make sure everyone understands and is satisfied with the central question before you generate ideas. Write down the question and post it where everyone can refer to it.

4. Collect ideas. After giving participants a few minutes to think about the question, ask them to give their ideas. Establish either a structured or unstructured format for calling out ideas:
   - **Structured**—The facilitator establishes a rotation that enables each person in the group to contribute an idea in turn. Any individual who is not ready with an idea when his or her turn comes can pass until the next round, when he or she may offer an idea or pass again.
   - **Unstructured**—Team members call out ideas as they come to mind. This method calls for close monitoring by the facilitator to enforce the ground rules and ensure that all team members have a chance to participate.
5. Record ideas. Write ideas on a flip chart as they are called out, collect ideas written by team members on Post-its, or enter ideas into a brainstorming software package. Display the ideas where everyone can see them. Having the exact words visible to everyone at the same time avoids misinterpretation and duplication, and helps stimulate creative thinking by other team members. When recording ideas, ensure that they are written down exactly as spoken by the team member; don't interpret or paraphrase. Try to generate as long a list as possible and keep brainstorming until all participants have run out of ideas or the allotted time has expired. Encourage creative thinking, including radical ideas and piggybacking.
6. Clarify each idea. After all ideas have been presented, review the list to make sure that all team members understand the ideas. If there are questions or uncertainties, have the contributor explain the idea in a different way. Remember that you are only clarifying the ideas, not making judgments about them.
7. Eliminate duplicates. If two or more ideas appear to mean the same thing, try to combine them, and eliminate duplicate ideas. Before combining similar ideas into a single item or eliminating items, those who contributed the ideas in question must agree that they mean the same thing. Otherwise, the ideas should remain as separate items.

Brainstorming is an excellent way to elicit a large number of ideas regarding potential problems, possible causes, possible solutions, and implementation alternatives. However, brainstorming cannot help you identify positively causes of problems, rank ideas in a meaningful order, select important ideas, or check solutions. Brainstorming starts with a clear question and ends with a raw list of ideas. Some of these ideas will be good and others will not. Additional analysis of the ideas should be performed with other quality improvement tools. In particular, affinity diagramming, which is designed to sort a raw list into categories, is very often the next step after brainstorming.

Nominal Group Technique (NGT)

The NGT, developed by Delbecq et al. (2), uses an individualized brainstorming method to generate ideas, and then some simple discussion and voting methods to choose the most important ideas.

The name itself describes how the process works: The participants are only nominally a group. They generate ideas individually and then look at them as a group.

The purpose of the NGT is to eliminate social and psychological dynamics of group behavior that might inhibit individual creativity and participation during group decisions. Some people can be more creative if some of the factors that inhibit free thinking are eliminated. Such factors include shyness, unwillingness to float an idea that isn't perfect, fear of reprisal, and groupthink.

The disadvantage of the NGT relative to simple brainstorming is that people don't get the immediate benefit of each other's thinking, and thus some creative chemistry can be lost.

In practice, either a simple group brainstorm or the NGT can be followed by the discussion and selection methods described in steps 3 through 7 listed in the following pages.

A successful NGT experience depends on careful planning and preparation. During the NGT process, people will respond to an initial question by the NGT leader. The nature and quality of the response is determined as much by the nature of the question as it is by the NGT process itself. Therefore, the type of information desired should be determined well before the NGT process begins. The quality of the NGT output also depends on the composition of the group. Heterogeneous groups provide different perspectives on a given situation whereas homogeneous groups reduce communication barriers.

The NGT requires 2 to 3 hours to complete the entire step-by-step process, and works best with 6 to 12 people. Larger groups should work in subgroups and share results later. There are many variations in the NGT; however, the following steps outline a general approach to using the process:

1. Generate ideas in silence. Group members, working silently and independently, should be given 5 to 10 minutes to write their ideas in response to the nominal question.
2. Record ideas. Group members should read one of their ideas in turn, with each idea recorded on a flip chart or in an appropriate software package as it is read. Continue this procedure until all members have exhausted their list.
3. Enter into a brief discussion and clarification. Discuss each idea in order. The leader should point to each idea beginning with the first, read it out loud, and ask the group if there are any questions, statements of clarification, or statements of agreement or disagreement that members would like to make.
4. Take a preliminary vote. Have group members select a specific number (five to seven is best) of ''priority'' items from the entire list of ideas. Ask members to place each priority item on a separate 3×5 index card. After members have their set of priority cards completed, have them place their cards in rank order. Collect the cards and record the votes on a flip chart or projected screen in front of the group.
5. Discuss the preliminary vote. The purpose of this discussion is to examine inconsistent voting patterns and to provide the opportunity to address items that are perceived as receiving too many or too few votes.
6. Take a final vote. Silently and independently, repeat step 4 to determine a final list of group priorities. If desired, a more refined voting technique such as rating may be used here.
7. Agree on prioritized items. List the results from the final vote on the flip chart to provide a permanent record of the group's agreement.

The NGT provides a useful alternative or extension to the more familiar technique of brainstorming. In selecting which problems to deal with and in what order, it is often the person who shouts the loudest who has the most authority. The NGT is useful in situations in which individuals feel vulnerable because of a dominant personality or social pressure, when there are others in the group who inhibit them for whatever reason, or when people are particularly new to group problem solving and therefore are less confident. Because the NGT reduces the pressure on individuals, it can be more effective in generating ideas than if the group members were allowed to interact, as in a typical brainstorming session.

But like brainstorming, the NGT cannot help you to identify positively causes of problems and to check solutions. Additional analysis of the ideas is generally required and should be performed with other quality improvement tools. As with brainstorming, affinity diagramming is very often the next logical step.

Affinity Diagrams

In quality improvement efforts, affinity diagrams are used to sort and refine the results of idea generation (via brainstorming or the NGT), moving from a single long list of ideas to more manageable groups or sets of related ideas that have an affinity for one another. It's a very simple and obvious tool, and like many simple tools, it is very effective.

Affinity diagrams have become one of the most widely used of the Japanese management and planning tools, but its origins are in anthropology (9). A Japanese anthropologist, Kawakita Jiro developed them in the 1960s to help identify meaningful patterns in the mountainous amount of notes he had made on the societies he was studying. He found that the simple prerational sorting of large amounts of language data (ideas, opinions, issues) into groupings enabled new patterns of information to rise to the surface.

The affinity process is a good way to get people to work on a creative level to address difficult issues. It may be used in situations that are unknown or unexplored by a team, or in circumstances that seem confusing or disorganized, such as when people with diverse experiences form a new team or when members have incomplete knowledge of the area of analysis (*Fig 5.3*).

The affinity process is formalized in an affinity diagram and is useful when you want to:

- **Sift through large volumes of data**—For example, a process owner who is identifying customers and their needs might compile a very large list of unsorted data. In such a case, creating an affinity diagram might be helpful in organizing the data into groups.
- **Encourage new patterns of thinking**—Creating an affinity diagram is an excellent way to get a group of people to react on a "gut" level rather than mulling things over intellectually. Because idea generation (e.g., brainstorming, NGT) is the first step in creating an affinity diagram, the team considers all ideas from all members without criticism. This stimulus is often enough to break through traditional or entrenched thinking, enabling the team to develop a creative list of ideas.

NOTE: As a rule of thumb, if less than 15 items have been identified, you should skip the affinity process. Instead, clarify and combine the ideas, and then use one of the decision-making tools to identify the highest priority items.

A group or team usually performs the affinity diagramming process. The idea is to meld the perspectives, opinions, and insights of a group of people who are knowledgeable about the issues. The process of developing an affinity diagram seems to work best when there are no more than five or six participants.

Before we address the steps used to create an affinity diagram, we should consider several unique features of the affinity process that are important to its success:

- **Sort silently**—The most effective way to work is to have everyone organize the displayed ideas at will, without talking. This will be a new experience for many people, and it has two positive results. First, it encourages unconventional thinking (which is good) while discouraging semantic battles (which are bad). Second, it helps prevent one person from dominating the affinity process.
- **Go for initial reactions**—Encourage team members to react quickly to what they see and not to agonize over the details of the sort. Speed rather than deliberation is the order of the day, so keep the process moving.
- **Handle disagreements simply**—The process provides a simple way to handle disagreements over the placement of ideas: If a team member doesn't like where an idea is grouped, he should move it. This is intended to create an environment in which it is okay to disagree with people who have a different viewpoint. If consensus cannot be reached, make a duplicate of the idea and place it in each group.

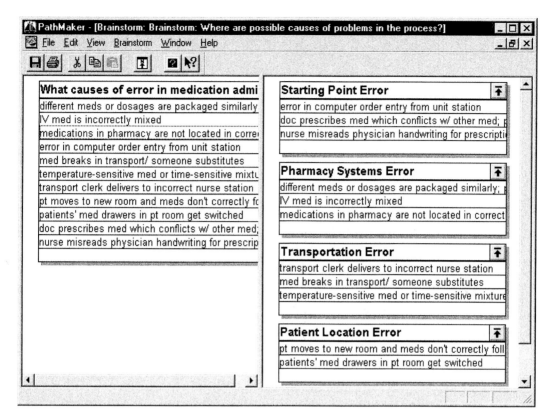

Figure 5.3 The brainstormed list of ideas on the left is being sorted into groups called *affinity sets*. The titles of the affinity sets are only added late in the sorting process. The lines on which the sorting is done are supposed to be ill defined.

Now let's walk through the step-by-step process of creating an affinity diagram:

1. Display the ideas. Take the ideas generated from a brainstorming or NGT session and post them on a flip chart, a wall, or a table in a *random* manner. The remaining steps in the affinity process will be easier if these ideas are written on Post-its. Better yet, use one of the available quality improvement software packages, project the brainstormed list on a screen, and sort the ideas into affinity groups within the software.

2. Sort the ideas. Sort each idea into groups of ideas that belong together. At this point it isn't important to define why certain ideas belong together. Begin by looking for two ideas that seem related in some way and place them together in a column off to one side. Look for additional ideas that are related to those you've already set aside and add them to that group. Next, look for other ideas that are related to each other and establish new groups. Repeat this process until the team has placed all of the ideas into a group. *NOTE:* Ideally, all the ideas can be sorted into related groups. However, ideas that don't fit into the existing groups should not be forced where they don't logically belong. These ideas should stand alone under their own headers.

3. Create group headers. Headers describe the essential link among the ideas contained within a group. Each header should be written on a single Post-it note and should consist of a word, phrase, or sentence that clearly conveys the meaning of the group of ideas. The team should develop headers for each group by identifying a key idea within each group that will serve well as a header, and should place these headers at the top of each group. Team members can discuss and agree on specific wording for the headers.

4. Draw the finished affinity diagram. Write a problem statement at the top of the affinity

diagram. Place the headers above the groups of ideas, and review and clarify the ideas and groupings. Document the finished affinity diagram.

Although affinity diagrams are most powerful when used in conjunction with other tools and techniques, they have proved to be tremendously useful as a stand-alone tool. Their ability to help sift through large volumes of information and identify new patterns is an asset in any improvement effort. The affinity process may appear to be very structured and inflexible, but this is not the case. When performed properly, the creation of an affinity diagram encourages participants' creative energies to flow freely, distilling ideas and information into rough chunks that can be subsequently refined using other tools or through discussion.

LOGICAL-THINKING TOOLS

Some things we can do in our heads. More complex things can be better understood if they are diagrammed, sketched, or analyzed systematically. There are lots of tools to help the human brain with this sort of thinking. Some of the most useful ones are described in the following subsections.

Flowcharts

Flowcharts are maps or graphical representations of a process. Steps in a process are shown with symbolic shapes, and the flow of the process is indicated with arrows that connect the symbols. Computer programmers popularized flowcharts in the 1960s, using them to map the logic of programs. In quality improvement work, flowcharts are particularly useful for displaying how a process currently functions or could function better. Flowcharts can (1) help determine whether the steps of a process are logical, (2) uncover problems or miscommunications, (3) define the boundaries of a process, and (4) develop a common base of knowledge about a process. However, flowcharts will not work if they are inaccurate, if team members are afraid to describe what actually happens, or if the team is too far removed from the actual workings of the process to document it.

Although there are scores of symbols that can be used in flowcharts to represent different kinds of steps, accurate flowcharts can be created using very few (*Table 5.1*).

TABLE 5.1
Common Flowchart Symbols and Their Meanings

Symbol	Definition
Ovals	Starting and ending points in a process
Rectangles	Steps in a process
Diamonds	Decisions, or gates, where a choice is made or where there is a branch in the process
Delays	Where there is a waiting period
Clouds	Not an ANSI standard symbol, but are used to indicate areas of uncertainty, where the process is not well understood by the people constructing the chart

Flowchart Types

There are many varieties of flowcharts, and scores of symbols that one can use. Experience has shown that there are three main types that work for almost all situations:

1. High-level flowcharts (*Fig. 5.4*) map only the major steps in a process for a good overview.
2. Detailed flowcharts show a step-by-step mapping of all events and decisions in a process.
3. Deployment flowcharts organize the flowchart by columns, with each column representing a person or department involved in a process.

To construct an effective flowchart, adhere to the following steps:

1. Define the process boundaries with starting and ending points.
2. Complete the big picture before filling in the details.
3. Clearly define each step in the process. Be accurate and honest.
4. Identify time lags and nonvalue-added steps.
5. Circulate the flowchart to other people involved in the process to get their comments.

Using Flowcharts Effectively

The point of making a flowchart is to create an accurate picture of the process, which will then suggest areas in which the process could be improved. The trouble spots in a process usually begin to appear as a team constructs a detailed flowchart.

As stated earlier, flowcharts do not work if

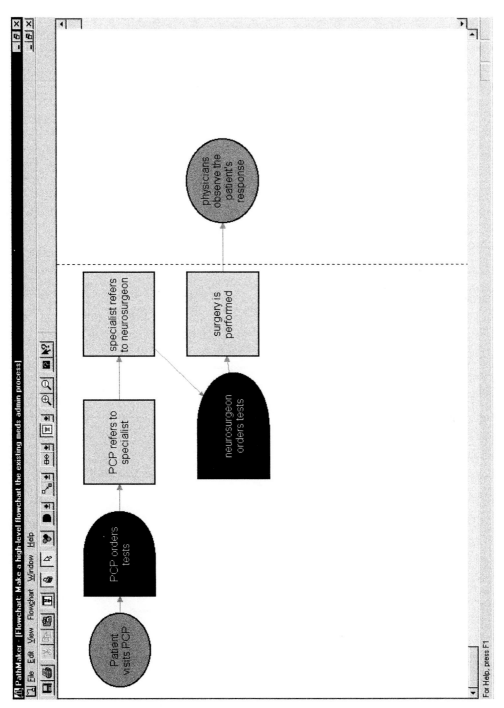

Figure 5.4   This screen capture shows a high-level flowchart of the process by which a patient is referred for neurosurgical treatment.

they are not accurate or if the team is too far removed from the process itself. Team members should be true participants in the process and should feel free to describe what really happens. A thorough flowchart should provide a clear view of how a process works. With a completed flowchart, you can accomplish the following:

- Identify time lags and nonvalue-added steps.
- Identify responsibility for each step.
- Brainstorm for problems in the process.
- Determine major and minor inputs to the process with a cause-and-effect diagram.
- Choose the most likely trouble spots with the consensus builder.

Cause-and-Effect Diagrams

The cause-and-effect diagram is the brainchild of Kaoru Ishikawa (3), who pioneered quality management processes in the Kawasaki shipyards of Japan, and in the process became one of the founding fathers of modern management. Ishikawa called the cause-and-effect diagram a *fault tree.* It is also called an *Ishikawa diagram* and a *fishbone diagram.* This last name has obvious origins, because main causal categories are drawn as "bones" attached to the spine of the fish, as shown in *Figure 5.5.*

Cause-and-effect diagrams can also be drawn using right angles (*Fig. 5.6*). From a single outcome or trunk, branches extend that represent major categories of inputs or causes that create that single outcome. These large branches then

lead to smaller and smaller branches of causes all the way down to twigs at the ends. The tree structure has an advantage over the fishbone-style diagram. As a fishbone diagram becomes more and more complex, it becomes difficult to find and compare items that are the same distance from the effect because they are dispersed throughout the diagram. With the tree structure, all items on the same causal level are aligned vertically.

The cause-and-effect diagram is used to explore all the potential or real causes of some effect—usually a problem. Causes are arranged according to their level of "rootness," or detail, resulting in a depiction of relationships and a hierarchy of events. This can help you search for root causes, identify areas where there may be problems, and compare the relative importance of different causes.

We often recommend creating the basic structure of the cause-and-effect tree from the titles of the affinity sets determined in a completed affinity diagram. There's no "one-size-fits-all" way to categorize causes, but you will often see

- Manpower, methods, materials, and machinery
- Equipment, policies, procedures, and people

These guidelines can be helpful but should not be used if they limit the diagram or are inappropriate. The categories you use should suit your needs.

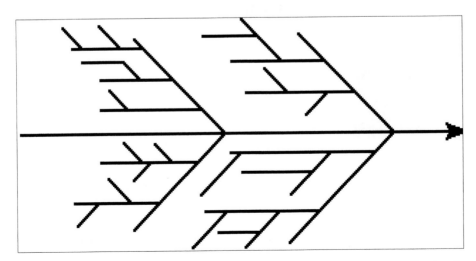

Figure 5.5 Depicted is the classic Ishikawa fishbone diagram, or fault tree. The problem, or main effect, is written to the right of the arrow, and each bone, or root, is a cause or subcause of the problem.

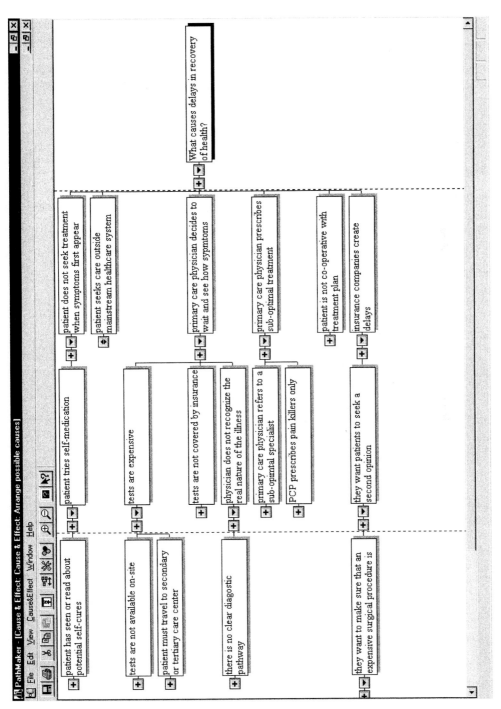

Figure 5.6 A right-angle cause-and-effect diagram is used to understand the reasons that delays occur in treating disorders that require neurosurgical treatments.

To build a cause-and-effect diagram successfully, be sure to adhere to the following:

- Be sure everyone agrees on the effect or problem statement before beginning.
- Be succinct.
- For each node, brainstorm its causes and add them to the tree.
- Pursue each line of causality back to its root cause.
- Consider grafting relatively empty branches onto others.
- Consider splitting up overcrowded branches.
- Consider which root causes are most likely to merit further investigation.

Tree Diagrams

The tree diagram uses the same treelike structure as the cause-and-effect diagram, but for a different purpose. Instead of starting with an observed problem, or main effect, and working backward to root causes, one begins with a goal and then traces all the strands of effort that will make that goal a reality.

For example, if your goal is to reduce the turnaround time for ordering magnetic resonance imaging tests and receiving test results, you could construct a tree diagram that traces all the elements of the process that need to change (*Fig. 5.7*).

It is very important to have a clear goal statement at the outset. You will also want to have people on the team who are knowledgeable of the various disciplines involved in progressing toward the goal.

You will find that the tree diagram will help you discover and therefore plan for complexities and roadblocks that would otherwise have taken you by surprise. You will also find that it may spark new ideas because it pushes the group to expand its thinking. It's much better to see a roadblock at the tree-diagramming stage, and go back to look for an alternative solution, than it is to invest time and money in a project, only to hit this insurmountable problem later.

The tree should provide as much detail as is practical. Others who have the needed expertise should fill in areas that aren't well understood by the team. The tree can be posted on a bulletin board or, if it is diagrammed in a software tool, on a company intranet so that team members and others can follow progress. Color coding can be added to track progress, and branches can be filled in as different steps are completed.

DECISION-MAKING AND CONSENSUS-BUILDING TOOLS

We have considered tools for generating lots of ideas, and tools for exploring root causes and flow bottlenecks. Usually, though, there comes a time when, from a list of good ideas or potential root causes, the group must choose one or two on which to act. This is usually when people start to disagree, and when meetings can degenerate in their effectiveness.

There are, of course, tools for winnowing lists, rating different ideas, and reaching consensus. Some are simple; others are fairly elaborate. Often, the size of the list with which you are working, the size of the group, and the impact of the decision determine the tool you need.

Before we get into the specifics of the various tools, we want to discuss consensus briefly. The word consensus comes from Latin roots meaning *shared thought*. Consensus does not imply complete agreement. Rather, it implies a sense that:

- Everyone involved in the decision has had a fair chance to be heard
- Everyone can live with and support the decision
- The group has truly gone through the process required to make a responsible decision
- Latent issues have been explored

Where consensus exists, actions can be swift and results solid. If minorities remain unheard or unhappy, actions may be undermined and success may be short-lived.

Consensus-building tools are designed to help groups reduce a list to a handful of options or to make thoughtful decisions. To be effective, such tools should:

- Protect against reprisals for open disagreement
- Reduce the urge to conform to group opinion
- Discourage ''gaming the system,'' when one faction tries to outweigh another
- Structure the discussion and keep it moving forward
- Encourage respect for strong opinions
- Downplay the link between an idea and its author
- Support decision making in a manageable framework
- Follow valid mathematical rules when applicable

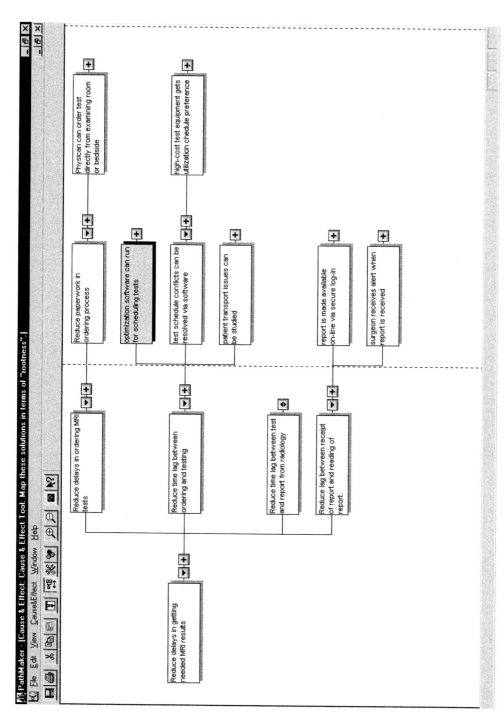

Figure 5.7 The tree diagram is used to think through all the elements of a solution, from broad concepts to fine details.

There are two key elements to building consensus. One is the effective use of rating systems to reduce lists and to quantify opinions. The second is the recognition that such quantitative methods are limited and that structured discussion is just as important.

Multivoting

For long lists of ideas, say 10 or more, a multivote is a quick way to narrow the list (*Fig. 5.8*). Each team member gets some votes—usually one third or one half the number of ideas in the whole list. All team members then cast a vote for the ideas in the list that they think are the most important. No one can cast more than one vote for any idea.

When all members have voted, the votes are counted, and the candidates with the most votes go forward to the next round. The group can determine the cutoff point. If someone feels strongly that an item should be included, even though it didn't get many votes, keep it on the list and have this person explain his or her thinking.

Multivoting is accomplished easily with flip charts and markers. Group members armed with markers simply put dots beside the ideas for which they vote. This process is also easy to do with some of the software tools that are on the market.

Rating Systems

For shorter lists (10 items or less), binary multivoting is too crude. Rating each item on a wider scale—possibly 1 to 3 points, 1 to 5 points, or as many as 1 to 10 points—tends to be the best way to evaluate short lists. Rating scales allow items to be rated as equal, and they permit intervals between items to vary. In comparison, rank ordering, another common voting mechanism, is markedly inferior because it forces regular intervals where they usually don't apply, and therefore severely limits the mathematical analysis that can follow.

Rating Using Several Criteria

When striving for consensus, it is often helpful for team members to rate options with respect to different criteria chosen by the group. For example, you could rate several cars, each with respect to price, safety, cargo capacity, performance, and styling.

Weighting the Criteria

You can also weight the ratings for each item by rating the criteria themselves. For example, each voter would rate the importance of price, safety, cargo capacity, and so on, as factors that influence a purchase decision. This division of decision making into bite-size pieces often elicits latent ideas or opinions (*Fig. 5.9*).

The bottom line in consensus building is to:

- Vote to reduce a list to a manageable size and to illustrate the distribution of opinion.
- Reach consensus on the most important or relevant issues.
- Discuss to gain insight into the opinions of team members.

A vote should not be the final step in making a decision. To gain real consensus, use voting to guide and structure discussions, and to seek a course of action that everyone can support.

Structured Discussion

Before, during, and after voting, you will be discussing different candidates. Take notes as you proceed to capture the points people make and to avoid discussions that go in circles. It helps to have a three-column list, with candidates in the left column, "pros" or strengths in the middle column, and "cons" or weaknesses in the right column. This not only makes it easier to capture key points during discussion, but it makes it easier for voters to keep all the issues in mind as they cast ballots. It also makes it possible to effect contingency planning for the winner. For example, say you choose a new medical equipment supplier, and you pick one with a good track record of quality and low prices, but you have some lingering concerns about innovativeness. You might set up semiannual meetings with the supplier to talk about the latest innovations in the industry, and to have input into new product development.

Force Field Analysis

Force field analysis was first articulated by social psychologist Kurt Lewin (5). According to Lewin, human behavior is caused by forces—beliefs, values, cultural norms, expectations, and the like—within the "life space" of an individual or society. These forces can be positive, urging us toward a behavior, or negative, propelling us away from a behavior.

We need to understand the forces that make

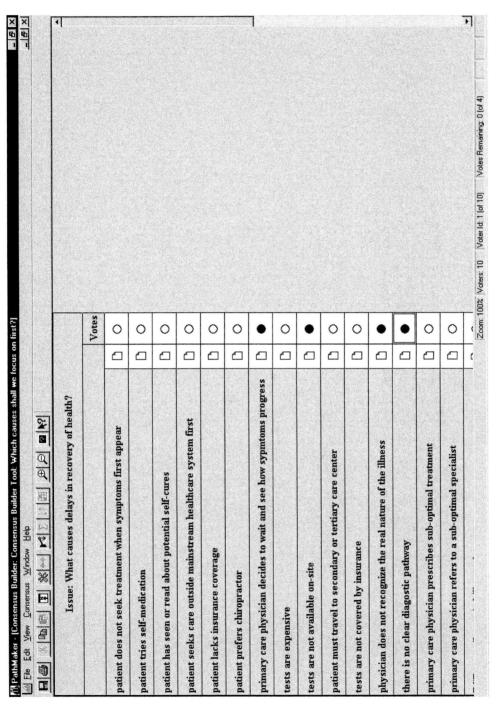

Figure 5.8 A multivote ballot is being used to narrow down a long list of causes of delay in treatment. The goal is to select the few causes that are most likely to give a lot of leverage in solving the problem.

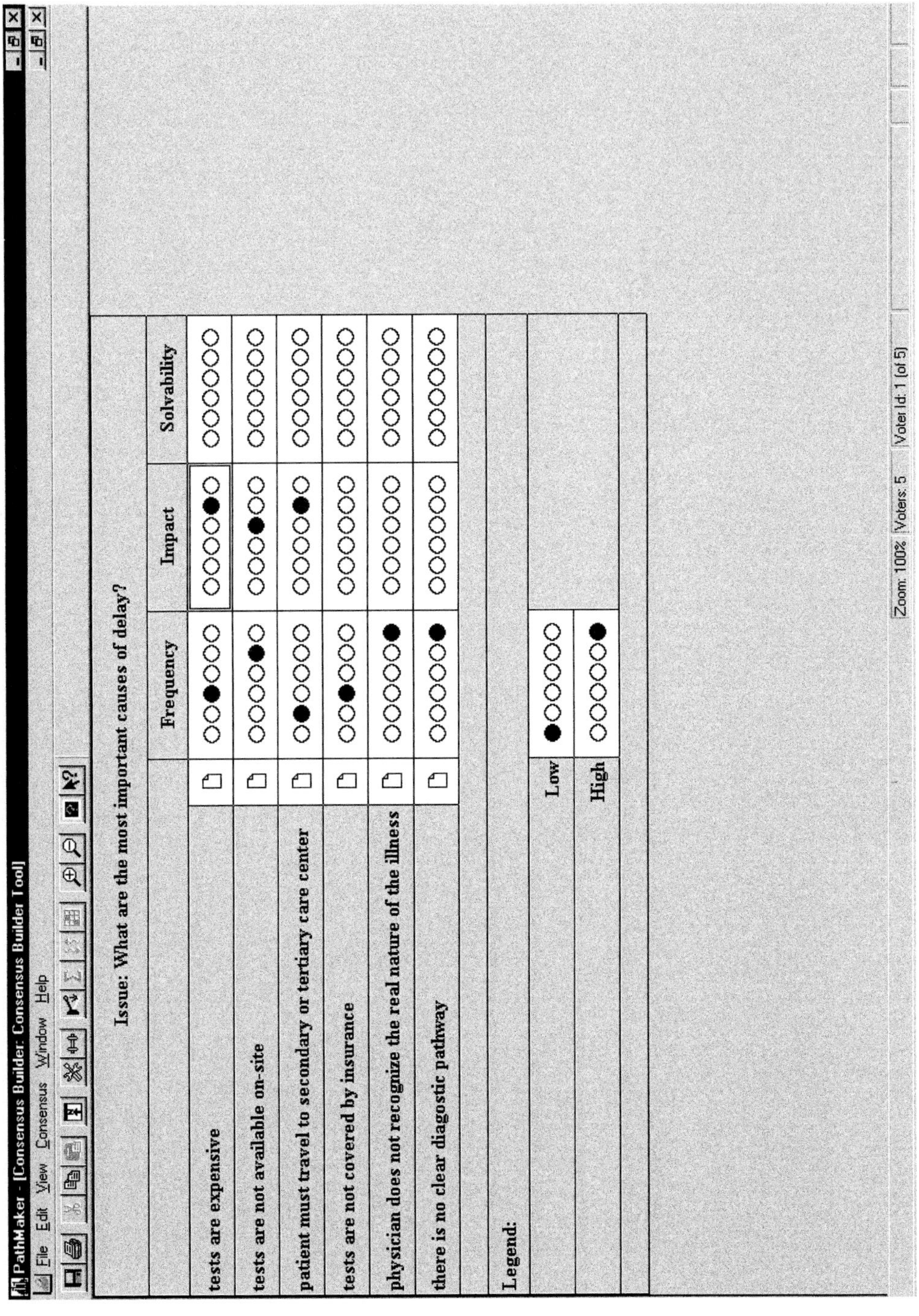

Figure 5.9 A multicriteria rating vote is represented using, in this case, a 6-point scale to rate different issues regarding their frequency, impact, and solvability.

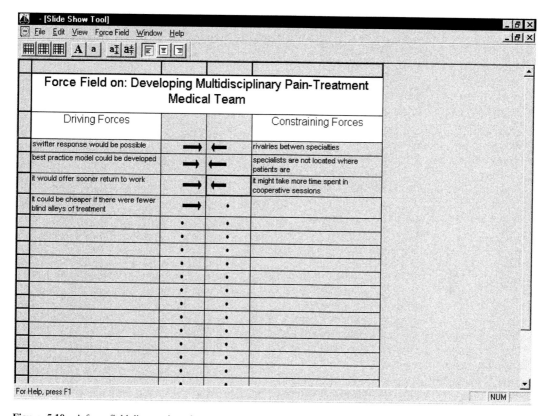

Figure 5.10 A force field diagram is under construction, with driving forces on the left and restraining forces on the right.

change possible. The force field diagram maps these forces and is constructed, as shown in *Figure 5.10,* with driving forces on the left and restraining forces on the right.

Change will not occur when the restraining forces are equal to or stronger than the driving forces. Usually, the most effective way to implement change is to diminish or remove restraining forces. It can be tempting to try to strengthen the driving forces instead, but this often tends to intensify opposition as well.

When using force field analysis, keep in mind the following:

• Encourage creative but realistic thinking.
• Encourage change by creating asymmetry between forces.
• Look for the most important restraining forces. Of these, which can be removed or weakened?

Lewin (5) also focused on forces affecting behavior within a group, and several of his experiments investigated the effects of changes in the workplace on groups of workers. The results showed that psychological forces, such as fear of authority, a sense of belonging, self-fulfillment, and the power of group decision making, play a very real role in the workplace. These psychological forces should be considered along with structural forces when managing change.

The balance structure of the force field diagram makes it useful for comparing more than opposing forces. You can also do the following:

• List pros and cons.
• List actions and reactions.
• List strengths and weaknesses.
• Compare ideal situations and reality.
• During negotiation, list the desires of each party.

The goal of force field analysis is to understand the reality of making a change and to highlight the hindering factors. When you have completed a force field diagram, you can do the following:

• Use the consensus builder to identify forces to be strengthened or removed.

- Brainstorm ways of dealing with the forces identified.
- Use the tree diagram to plan implementation and make contingency plans to deal with likely problems.

DATA ANALYSIS TOOLS

Countless times a day we make decisions. We rarely have all the information we would like, so we make judgment calls. The human brain has an amazing capacity to weigh factors and probabilities and to make informed choices, but it *is* limited.

There are some data analysis tools to help collect real, "hard" numbers from a process and display them in graphs to make it easier for us to see what is really happening. Some of them will be familiar; others are important but not as well known. The most important ones for use in health care are described in the following subsections.

Health care is inundated with numbers: length of stay, cost per case, clinical outcomes, staffing, patient satisfaction, procedure times, turnaround times, testing volumes, net income, monthly expenses, and many others. Every time you make a chart from data, you are trying to find clues about the process. In every case, you gain a picture of your data that was not clear from the underlying table, but you also give up some detail. There's no one perfect chart for every use, and some processes can only be understood properly by using two or more charts for analysis. Choosing the right charts is obviously important, as is proper chart construction.

There are two main types of charts for looking at these data. In what we call *snapshot charts*—pie, radar, Pareto, histogram, normal plot, scatterplot, and some bar charts—time is not considered. If you make a pie chart of the types of neurosurgery cases treated in your hospital during the past year, you get a snapshot of the data. You can tell, say, that you had a higher infection rate with metastatic tumors than with aneurysms, but you can't tell whether the rates changed over time.

The second type is the time series chart. In time series charts—primarily run and control charts—the x-axis usually represents the passage of time, with earlier data points to the left, and the most recent ones to the right. You can plot the readings from a process over time, and see how they vary. Some variation is, of course, to be expected. How, then, can we tell when the variation we are seeing is a trend that we should note? The traditional ways of examining these numbers are badly flawed and, as a result, the customary responses to both "good" and "bad" numbers are usually misguided. Happily, the simple run and control charts developed by quality engineers can help us react the right way at the right time, saving enormous costs and wasted effort.

Both types of charts are important for quality improvement. The snapshot charts are probably more familiar, and simpler, so we'll discuss them first. Before we do, however, let's briefly visit the subject of data collection, which is the foundation for all data-based decisions.

Data Collection

Data analysis begins with data collection. All data are flawed to some extent by sampling problems, measurement errors, changes in the process resulting from observation, and so on. And yet, you want the data you collect and analyze to be as "clean" as possible. Otherwise, you will see yet another illustration of the "garbage in–garbage out" principle.

What are "clean" data? They must be relevant (i.e., they must measure something important). They must be recorded without mistakes. They must be representative of reality in that they are typical of the process. The act of measuring must not have a material impact on the process itself.

Planning for data collection can be structured around the following questions:

- What do we want to know about the process?
- What information will help us know this?
- What can we measure that would give this information?
- What information do we need for future analysis, reference, and traceability?
- How can we take the measurements without disrupting the process?
- How can we collect the data with a minimum of error?
- Who will do the collection? Who will do the input?
- Who is responsible for the data after they have been collected? Who will do the analysis?
- How long should we collect data? What time periods do we need to include?

A software spreadsheet or database is the preferred location for your collected data. A database usually provides the central storage you normally require, and multiuser access. From the database, the data can be imported to other programs for analysis, or the database report generator can be used instead. For some of the charts that we recommend, a statistics program is almost a must. There are many good ones available.

It also helps, when you are planning to collect data, to anticipate what charts you will want to see as outputs. This can help you make sure that you collect all the details you need from the outset. This, of course, requires some familiarity with the various common charts, which are described in the following subsections. Let's begin with the snapshot charts.

Pie Charts

Pie charts show classes of data as percentages of the whole dataset. For example, a company could record customer complaints. To make a pie chart of these data, complaints would be divided into classes, and a count would be taken for each class. When the pie is drawn, each slice represents a different class, with its percentage of the whole indicated by its size (*Fig. 5.11*).

When working with pie charts, there are a number of things for which to look:

1. Look for the largest piece to find the most common class.
2. Notice relative sizes of pieces. Some classes might be unexpectedly similar or different.
3. Try looking at a two-dimensional view of the pie. Three-dimensional charts are attractive, but they can make pieces at the front of the picture look bigger than they really are.

For the pie chart, the statistics of most interest are shown in *Table 5.2*.

TABLE 5.2
Statistics Relevant to Pie Charts

Statistic	Definition
Mean	The average of all the data points in the series
Maximum	The maximum value (biggest slice) in the series
Minimum	The minimum value (smallest slice) in the series
Sample size	The number of values (slices) in the series
Range	The maximum value minus the minimum value

Bar Charts

Like pie charts, bar charts are useful for comparing classes or groups of data. With simple bar charts, each class or group is represented by a single bar. For example, you could draw a bar chart showing how much money you spend each week (*Fig. 5.12*).

Bar charts can also be broken down further into multiple categories for greater depth of analysis. To graph more than one category within each class or group, you can use a:

- **Grouped bar chart**—In a grouped bar chart, the week's spending can be broken down into categories of food, car expenses, and miscellaneous, each represented by its own bar within the class. This arrangement emphasizes changes between categories.
- **Stacked bar chart**—Here the bars for the different categories are placed on top of one another. This lets you see changes easily in both the categories and the total. Like pie charts, bar charts are useful for comparing classes or groups of data. In bar charts, a class or group can have a single category of data, or they can be broken down further into multiple categories for greater depth of analysis.

Interpreting bar charts depends largely on the information for which you are looking. You might look for:

- The tallest bar
- The shortest bar
- Growth or shrinking of the bars over time
- One bar relative to another
- Change in bars representing the same category in different classes

Other tips include the following:

- Watch for inconsistent scales. If you're comparing two or more charts, be sure they use the same scale. If they don't use the same scale, be aware of the differences and how they may trick your eye.
- Be sure that all your classes are equal. For example, don't mix weeks and months, years and half-years, or newly invented categories with ones that have trails of data behind them.
- Be sure that the interval between classes is consistent. For example, if you want to compare current data that are collected monthly with older data that are only available every 6 months, either use current data for every 6

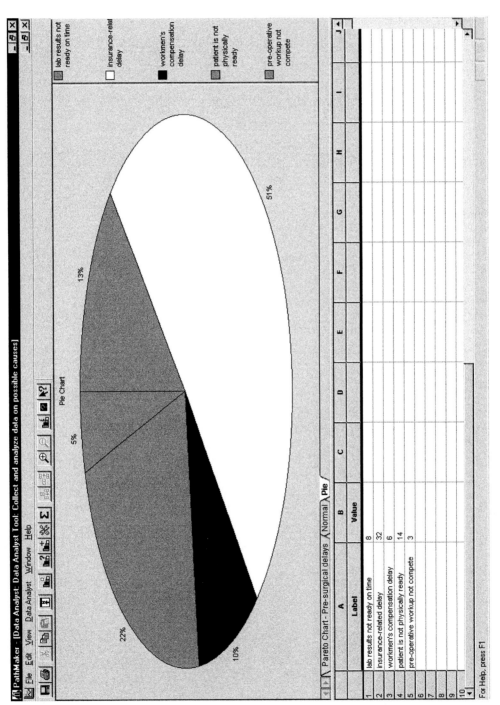

Figure 5.11 A pie chart is shown. The data are fictitious.

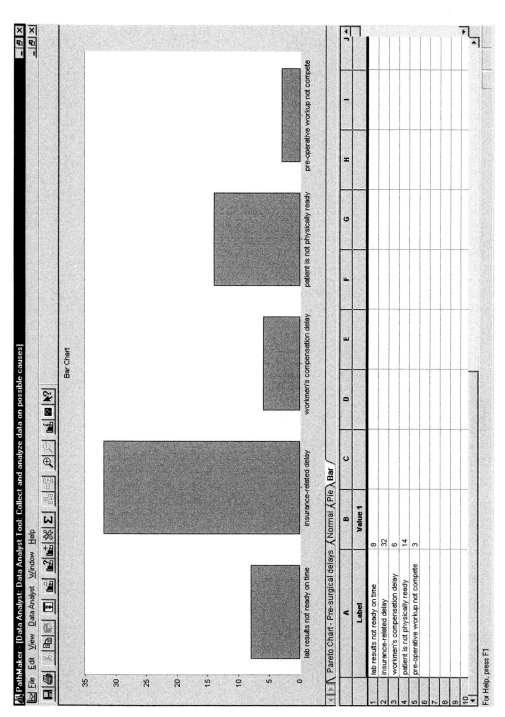

Figure 5.12   A simple bar chart is shown. The data are fictitious; the figure serves merely to illustrate the construction of a bar chart.

TABLE 5.3
Statistics Relevant to Bar Charts

Statistic	Definition
Mean	The average of all the data points in the series
Maximum	The maximum value (tallest bar) in the series
Minimum	The minimum value (shortest bar) in the series
Sample size	The number of values (bars) in the series
Range	The maximum value minus the minimum value
Standard deviation	How widely data are spread around the mean value

months or show the older data with blanks for the missing months. For each series in the bar chart, the most useful statistics are shown in *Table 5.3.*

Pareto Charts

Vilfredo Pareto, a turn-of-the-century Italian economist, studied the distributions of wealth in different countries, concluding that a fairly consistent minority (approximately 20%) of people controlled the large majority (approximately 80%) of a society's wealth (8). This same distribution has been observed in many other arenas, and has been termed *the Pareto effect.*

The Pareto effect even operates in quality improvement: Eighty percent of problems usually stem from 20% of the causes. Pareto charts are used to display the Pareto principle in action, arranging data so that the few vital factors that are causing most of the problems reveal themselves. Concentrating improvement efforts on these few areas will have a greater impact and be more cost-effective than undirected efforts.

For example, in an automobile manufacturing plant, defects in finished cars are tracked. These defects are classified by type (e.g., paint defects, body panel fit defects). When the categories of data are displayed in a Pareto chart, the most frequent types appear as the tallest bars on the left. Focusing efforts on these few areas is far more effective in improving overall quality than untargeted efforts.

Pareto charts also use a cumulative percentage line to show what portion of the overall situation the categories represent (*Fig. 5.13*). When working with Pareto charts, there are a number of things for which to look. In most cases, two or three categories will tower above the others. These few categories that account for the bulk of the problem will be the high-impact points on which to focus. If in doubt, follow these three guidelines:

1. Look for a breakpoint in the cumulative percentage line. This point occurs where the slope of the line begins to flatten out. The factors under the steepest part of the curve are the most important.
2. If there is not a fairly clear change in the slope of the line, look for the factors that make up at least 60% of the problem. You can always improve these few, redo the Pareto analysis, and discover the factors that have risen to the top now that the biggest ones have been improved.
3. If the bars are all similar size or more than half of the categories are needed to make up the needed 60%, try a different breakdown of categories that may be more appropriate.

Often, one Pareto chart will lead to another: before-and-after charts, charts that break down the most important factors discovered in an earlier chart, and charts that use different scales, such as number of complaints and the cost to respond, with the same categories. For the Pareto chart, the most useful statistics are shown in *Table 5.4.*

Scatterplots

Scatterplots are used to search for a possible relationship between two variables that both relate to the same "event." For example, we could study reading scores for people of all ages. With either variable on either axis, we would plot a point at the intersection of age and reading score for each person. As more points are plotted, a pattern may or may not begin to emerge (*Fig. 5.14*).

TABLE 5.4
Statistics Relevant to Pareto Charts

Statistic	Definition
Mean	The average of all the values in the series (i.e., the average bar height)
Sum	The sum of all the values in the series
Total	The number of items in that class (bar)
Percentage	The percentage of the whole dataset for which that bar accounts.

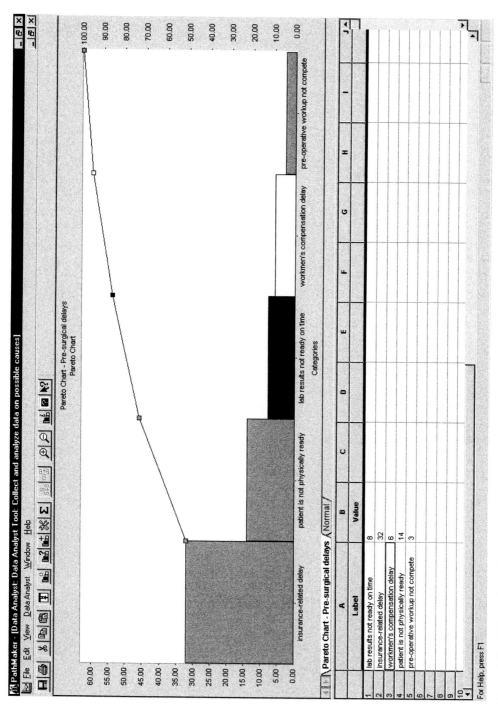

Figure 5.13 A Pareto chart of reasons for presurgical delays. The data are for illustrative purposes only; they are not based on any actual results. Clearly, in this example, an improvement effort aimed at the leftmost bar will have more impact than one aimed at one of the shorter bars.

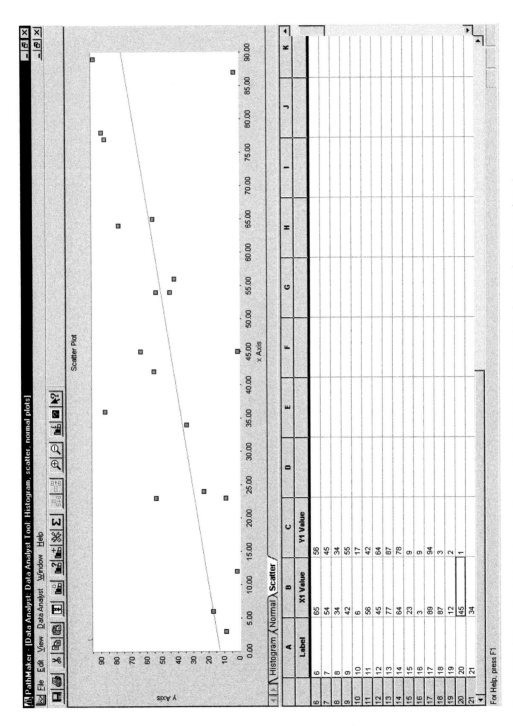

Figure 5.14 This scatterplot indicates a positive correlation between the x and y values (i.e., as x increases, so does y). Bear in mind that it cannot be deduced from this plot that increases in x cause increases in y, or vice versa. All we can tell is that the data seem to move together.

Often, in scatterplots, the plotted points cluster along a straight line. If the line slants up to the right, the two factors are said to have a positive correlation. If the line slants down, they are said to be negatively correlated. Some seem to be scattered randomly, indicating that there is little or no correlation between the two factors being charted.

Scatterplots (also called *scatter diagrams*) are used to investigate the possible relationship between two variables that both relate to the same "event." When using scatterplots, the things for which to look include the following:

- If the points cluster in a band running from lower left to upper right, there is a positive correlation (if x increases, y increases).
- If the points cluster in a band from upper left to lower right, there is a negative correlation (if x increases, y decreases).
- Imagine drawing a straight line or curve through the data so that it "fits" as best as possible. The more the points cluster closely around the imaginary line of best fit, the stronger the relationship that exists between the two variables.
- If it is hard to see where you would draw a line, and if the points show no significant clustering, there is probably no correlation.

For the x data and the y data, the statistics calculated most often are shown in *Table 5.5.*

Caution! There is a maxim in statistics that states, *Correlation does not imply causality*. In other words, your scatterplot may show that a relationship exists, but it does not and cannot prove that one variable is causing the other. Either one could be causing the other, there could be a third factor involved that is causing both, or there could be some other systemic cause. Nevertheless, the scatterplot can give you a clue that two things may be related and, if so, how they move together.

Radar Charts

Radar charts (sometimes called *spider web charts*) are used to plot data along many axes in a single view. They have become widely used for showing the status of progress toward strategic goals.

For example, you could use a radar chart to compile data about the wide receivers on a professional football team. On one axis, you could plot the percentage of passes caught. Another axis would show yards per completion; another, completions per 100 plays; another, speed; and a final axis may show interceptions. If a team did this for all their wide receivers, they could easily spot each player's strengths and weaknesses, and set up a coaching plan that capitalizes on strengths, and strengthens weaknesses (*Fig. 5.15*).

In a radar chart, a point close to the center on any axis indicates a low value. A point near the edge is a high value. In the football example, we would want high marks (near the outside) because of the nature of what is being measured. In other scenarios, you may want points near the center, or low values. When you're interpreting a radar chart, check each axis as well as the overall shape to see how well it fits your goals. For the radar chart, the statistics generally used are shown in *Table 5.6.*

Histograms

Variation can be difficult to detect when it is just a bunch of measurements in a table. You can use a histogram (a specialized bar chart) to

TABLE 5.5
Statistics Relevant to Scatterplots

Statistic	Definition
Mean	The average of all the data points in the series
Maximum	The maximum value in the series
Minimum	The minimum value in the series
Sample size	The number of values in the series
Range	The maximum value minus the minimum value
Standard deviation	How widely data are spread around the mean

TABLE 5.6
Statistics Relevant to Radar Charts

Statistic	Definition
Mean	The average of all the values in the series
Maximum	The maximum value in the series
Minimum	The minimum value in the series
Sample size	The number of values in the series
Range	The maximum value minus the minimum value
Standard deviation	How widely data are spread around the mean

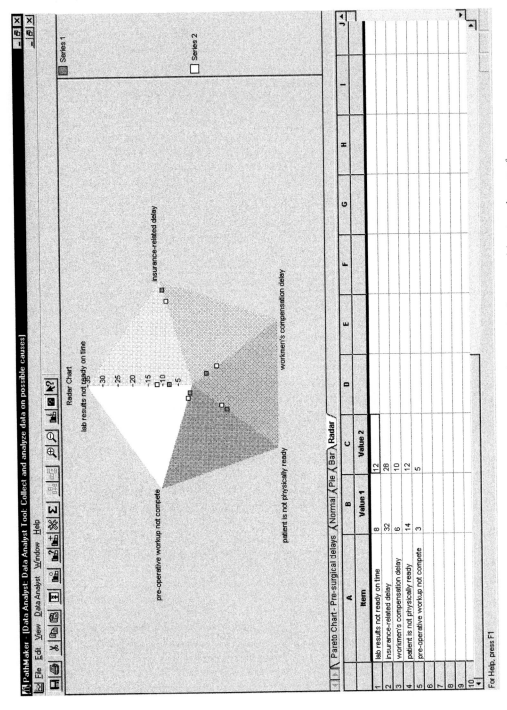

Figure 5.15 In this radar chart, two series are shown. The radar chart format makes it easy to pick out weak areas of performance, and relative differences.

graph the data and make sense of the variations. Each bar in a histogram represents a range of measurement. The bar height indicates how often values in that range occur. The strength of a histogram is that it provides an easy-to-read picture of the location and variation in a dataset (*Fig. 5.16*).

Four aspects of a histogram are important: its spread, its center, its skewness, and its kurtosis. Imagine measuring furnace temperature variations in a steel mill. In a histogram of these data we would see the following:

- The spread will show the entire range of temperatures.
- The center is the peak of the pattern and should fall near the target temperature.
- The skewness measures whether the pattern is symmetrical around the mean.
- The kurtosis measures the pointiness/flatness of the pattern.

There are two weaknesses, however, that you should bear in mind. The first is that histograms can be manipulated to show different pictures. If too few or too many bars are used, the histogram can be misleading. This is an area that requires some judgment, and perhaps some experimentation, based on the analyst's experience. Histograms can also obscure the time differences among datasets. For example, if you looked at data for number of births per day in the United States in 1998, you would miss any seasonal variations, such as peaks during full moons. Likewise, in quality control, a histogram of a process run tells only one part of a long story. You must keep reviewing the histograms and control charts for consecutive process runs over an extended time to gain useful knowledge about a process. For the histogram, the most useful statistics are shown in *Table 5.7*.

Process Performance

Histograms can be used to measure the performance of a process during a given timeframe. You can compare what a process is producing—process performance—with what it should be producing. This is done by overlaying process specification limits on the histogram, with the target value and upper and lower specification limits drawn as vertical lines. If the histogram fits comfortably within specification limits, the process is producing mostly ''in-spec'' product. If one or both tails of the histo-

TABLE 5.7
Statistics Relevant to Histograms

Statistic	Definition
Mean	The average of all the values
Minimum	The smallest value
Maximum	The biggest value
Standard deviation	How widely spread the values are around the mean
Class width	The x-axis distance between the left and right edges of each bar in the histogram
Number of classes	The number of bars (including zero height bars) in the histograms
Skewness	Is the histogram symmetrical? If so, skewness is zero. If the left tail is longer, skewness is negative. If the right tail is longer, skewness is positive. Where skewness exists, process capability indices are suspect. For process improvement, a good rule of thumb is to look at the long tail of your distribution; this is usually where quality problems lie.
Kurtosis	A measure of the peak of a distribution. The standard normal curve has a kurtosis of zero. The Matterhorn, has a negative kurtosis, whereas a flatter curve has a positive kurtosis. A positive kurtosis is usually more of a problem for quality control, because with big tails, the process may well be wider than the specified limits.

gram are near spec limits, some out-of-spec parts may be being produced.

If the histogram shows that your process is wider than the specification limits, then it is not currently capable of meeting your specifications. Perhaps you are willing to tolerate some out-of-spec results. Perhaps your specifications can be relaxed. Usually, though, the best choice is to reduce the variation of the process.

Also, if the process is not centered on the target value, it may need to be adjusted so that it can, on average, hit the target value. Sometimes the distribution of a process can fit between the specification limits if it is centered, but it spreads across one of the limits because it is not centered. Again, the process needs to be adjusted so that it can hit the target value most often.

Normal Test Plots

A well-constructed histogram will, when you have enough points, give you a rough idea of

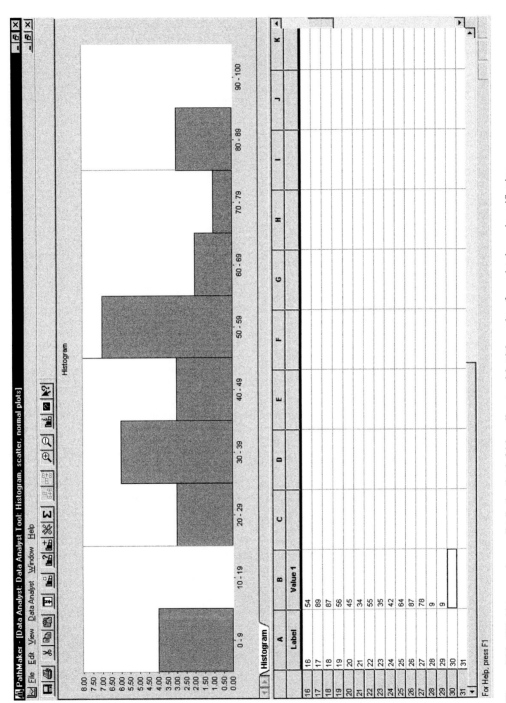

Figure 5.16   This histogram shows a distribution that is fairly well centered, but it has quite a few points beyond specification limits. It also appears to be skewed to the left.

the shape of the curve, or density function, that your process is producing. Sometimes, particularly when there are specifications that the process has to meet, you need to try to project how many out-of-spec events there will be in a large sample (e.g., the number of nonconforming parts per million). This isn't always easy to know. Most processes display some sort of curved distribution, with a peak, and with tails sloping downward. Unless the process is badly centered, the out-of-spec units lie mostly in one or both tails. Until you have hundreds of points, or more, you may not have enough data in the tails to be able to guess at the number of out-of-spec units in the population. So . . . the tails are very important, but we often know little about them. One thing we can do easily is test whether our data are distributed normally; that is, whether they fit the standard normal frequency distribution, or *bell curve,* as it is commonly known (*Fig. 5.17*).

In the normal test plot, the x-axis is changed so that if your data points are distributed normally, they will plot in a straight line. If your points bend away from the straight line, your process is characterized by some abnormal function. Until you understand the nature of that function (which requires expert help), you won't be able to project with any confidence how much of your output is outside specification limits. For the normal test plot, the statistics in *Table 5.8* are of most general interest.

TABLE 5.8
Statistics Relevant to the Normal Test Plot

Statistic	Definition
Sample size	The number of points in the data
Mean	The arithmetic average of the points in the data
Median	The number that has as many points above it as it does below it
Maximum	The highest value in the dataset
Minimum	The lowest value in the dataset
Range	The maximum value minus the minimum value
Standard deviation	How the data are spread around the mean
Anderson–Darling Statistic	An estimator for the closeness of fit to the normal distribution

Understanding Variation

At this point, we've completed our review of what we call the *snapshot charts,* and we now turn our attention to the two important types of time series charts. First, we'll set the stage with examples that illustrate the problems that good time series charts can solve.

Imagine the following scenario. You get a monthly report that shows the postoperative infection rate for several common procedures. The rate isn't always going to be the same; some months will be better than others. If an administrator was to scream every time the infection rate went up, would that help? If, in this report, you get a table that shows you three numbers—the rate this month, the rate last month, and the rate a year ago—would that be very helpful? Not really. You can't tell from that few data what is really going on with the infection rate.

Consider this second scenario. Because the director of patient services was concerned about the high cost of intravenous (IV) waste, he began monitoring the amount of IV waste from all units. The volume of IVs administered per week remained relatively constant across the units, so it was fairly easy to track and compare the overall percentage of IV waste from week to week. Looking at the numbers for the first week, the average amount of IV waste for all units was approximately 11.7%. Wanting to take immediate action, the director decided to send a memorandum to the head nurses of all units admonishing them for having so much IV waste and demanding that they improve immediately. During the following week, the overall percentage of IV waste dropped to 7.0%. The director of patient services concluded that his memo was effective and that he would have to send it out again if the percentage of IV waste rose too high. He is, unfortunately, wrong.

The study of variation has been of critical importance in the runaway success of the quality movement. If you understand the way that your process varies, you will know when the data are telling you that something is happening that demands attention, and when the variation you are seeing is within an expected range.

Variation refers to the way the performance of a process changes over time. There are fluctuations in all processes over time (e.g., day to day, week to week, month to month). This variation is usually the result of a myriad of sources such as equipment, materials, procedures, and people that are present in a process and that af-

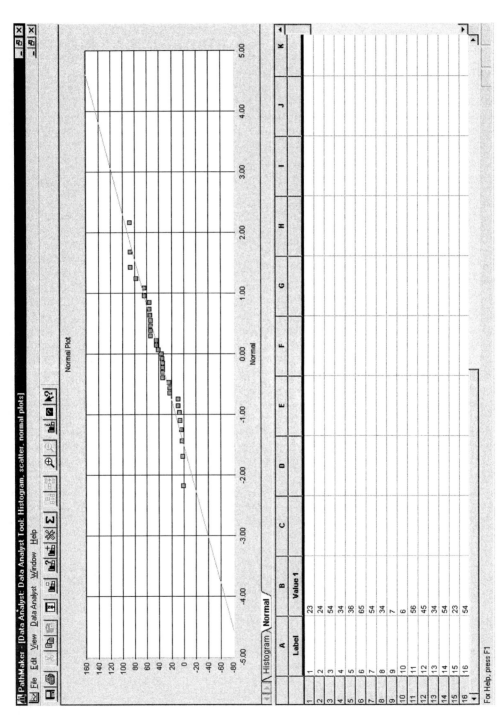

Figure 5.17 This normal plot appears to be somewhat abnormal. The low values begin to move away from the normal line to the left, and the higher values appear to curve to the right of the line. We would expect to see tails that are shorter than they would be in a normal distribution.

fect all elements of a process. This inherent variation in a process is referred to as *common-cause* (or *random*) *variation*. Consider your home telephone bill. It is probably different every month because the cost of long-distance calls varies from month to month. But you probably have a range of cost that's normal for your family. Within this range, we see common-cause (random) variation because such fluctuations are normally present in your family's telephone calling "process."

In addition to the common-cause variation inherent in all processes, special circumstances sometimes throw a process out of its normal range. These circumstances are unusual, abnormal, or intermittent influences that lead to erratic or unpredictable process behavior, which is known as *special-cause variation*. Because such unusual fluctuations can often be attributed or assigned to a specific factor or factors, they are also referred to as *assignable-cause variation*.

Suppose one month your telephone bill is unusually high and outside the normal range. When you examine the bill more closely, you notice that your teenager made a 4-hour long-distance call, or you got moved to a new long-distance carrier. This is very different from the normal, random fluctuation in your monthly bill. The increase in this month's bill is attributable to a specific circumstance—a special cause.

Consider the two situations presented at the beginning of this section. One basic comparison was being made in both situations: the current value versus some previous value. Although the comparisons made in each situation are technically correct (i.e., the infection rate has changed from last month, and from a year ago), none is conclusive. Simple comparisons between two values, no matter how easy they are to make or how intuitive they appear to be, cannot fully convey the behavior of any data collected over time. Both numbers are subject to the common-cause variation that is inevitably present in all data. Because both the current value and the comparison value (e.g., previous month, year to date) are subject to this variation, it is impossible to determine how much of the difference is the result of common-cause (random) variation and how much is the result of true differences in the underlying process. Furthermore, the way data are usually presented—in tables of numbers—does not help us to see how the numbers change (i.e., the variation in the data).

The best way to see variation and get a picture of what's happening in your organization is to graph data over time. Two basic graphs have proved their usefulness in displaying variation and in detecting the presence or absence of special causes—run charts and control charts. Run charts and control charts offer a more fundamental and more comprehensive approach to analyzing and interpreting numbers by helping people concentrate on the behavior of the underlying process rather than on individual data points. These charts help filter out the common-cause (random) variation in a process that clouds comparisons between single values and obscures special causes.

Run Charts

Run charts (often known as *line graphs* outside the quality management field) display process performance over time. Upward and downward trends, cycles, and large aberrations may be spotted and investigated further. In a simple run chart, one variable (such as IV waste or an infection rate) is measured and graphed over time. Connecting these measurements creates a simple run chart (*Fig. 5.18*).

There are several alternatives with run charts:

- An average line, representing the average of all the y values recorded, can be added easily to a run chart to clarify movement of the data away from the average. An average line runs parallel to the x-axis.
- Several variables may be tracked on a single chart, with each variable having its own line. The chart is then called a *multiple run chart*.
- Run charts can also be used to track improvements that have been put into place, checking their success.

Questions to ask about a run chart include the following:

- Is the average line where it should be to meet customer requirements?
- Is there a significant trend or pattern that should be investigated?
- Look at data for a long enough period of time, so that a "usual" range of variation is evident.
- Are the recent data within the usual range of variation? Is there a daily pattern? Weekly? Monthly? Yearly?

There are two ways to misinterpret run charts:

1. You conclude that some trend or cycle exists, when in fact you are just seeing normal pro-

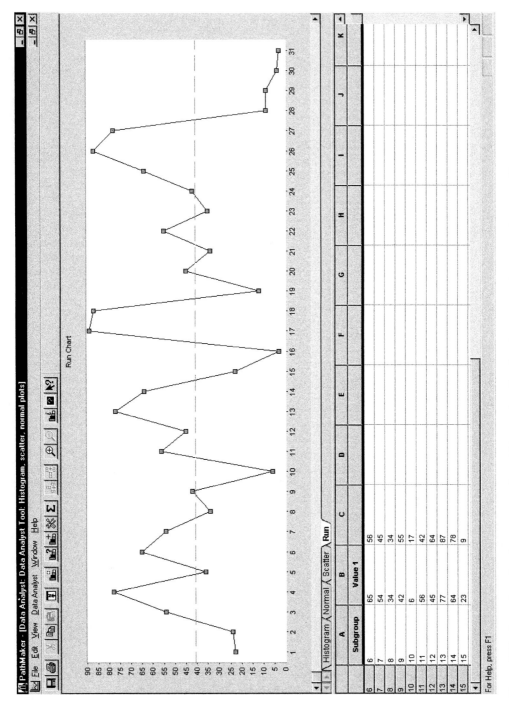

Figure 5.18 A run chart plots the movement of a variable over time. Trends and patterns can be seen much more readily with a run chart than in a table of data.

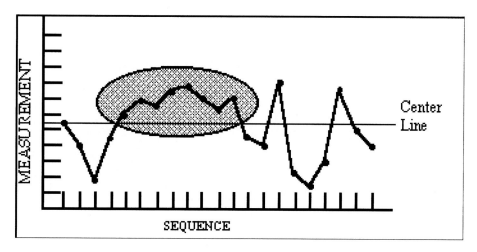

Figure 5.19   If seven or more consecutive values are either above or below the average line, this is known as a *shift* or *run,* and it indicates that a special cause is effecting the process.

cess variation (and every process will show some variation).

2. You do not recognize a trend or cycle when it does exist.

Both of these mistakes are common, but people are generally less aware that they are making the first type, and they tamper with a process that is really behaving normally. To avoid mistakes,

use the rules of thumb presented in *Figures 5.19 through 5.21* for run chart interpretation.

Notice that all of these conditions require many numerical values (i.e., the previous values) to discern an unusual current value. Thus, when taken together, the previous values create the context for examining the current value. Notice that the run chart in *Figure 5.18* does not contain any conditions that indicate the presence

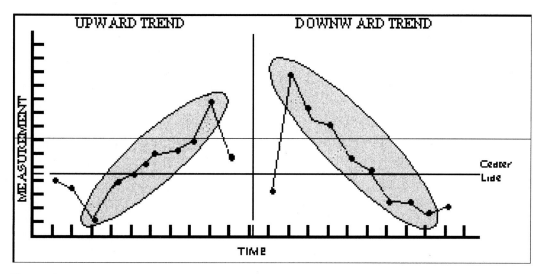

Figure 5.20   If seven or more consecutive values are all going up or all going down, this is called a *trend,* and it also indicates that a special cause is effecting the process.

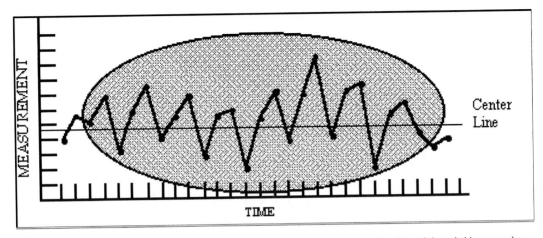

Figure 5.21   If any pattern, in this case a regular zigzag, recurs seven or more consecutive times, it is probably not random, but rather is the result of a special cause.

of special-cause variation. If this run chart had been used to track infection rates or IV waste, it would have been clear whether the variation was expected common-cause variation or not.

The manual construction of run charts is fairly straightforward. The steps include the following:

1. Draw vertical and horizontal axes on a piece of graph paper. Be sure to leave room on all sides of the axes to label and title the graph.
2. Label the vertical axis with the name of the value being plotted.
3. Label the horizontal axis with the unit of time or sequence in which numbers were collected.
4. Determine the scale of the axis. Pick a number 20% larger than the largest value and 20% smaller than the smallest value. Label the axis in intervals between these two numbers.
5. Plot the data values in the sequence in which they occurred.
6. Draw lines to connect the points on the graph. A graph completed to this point is known as a *line graph*. A line graph is often used to begin to observe data over time. However, if the graph is to be used to analyze variation, a mean should be added.
7. Calculate the mathematical mean of the plotted numbers and draw a mean line on the graph. In cases when it is suspected that the data are asymmetrical, a median line may be a more appropriate measure of central tendency

because median values are less sensitive to extreme values and skewed distributions.
8. Title the chart and note the source of data, date, and data collector.

For more robust monitoring of a process, and better information about when your process is showing variation beyond what is expected, try using a control chart.

Control Charts

Like run charts, control charts are used to measure and track variation in processes. The distinguishing characteristic of control charts is the presence of a statistically determined upper control limit (UCL) and a lower control limit (LCL). These limits, drawn above and below the average line, are computed from the data—not set arbitrarily. The control limits represent the range of the variation expected in the measurement of a process. They are set at a point where it is rare for a point in a stable process to be outside the limits. Therefore, if a point does get plotted outside the control limits, it indicates that a special cause of variation is present in the process that demands immediate investigation.

Variation is essentially the phenomenon of nothing occurring the same way twice. No two snowflakes, no two ball bearings or cars or patients are exactly alike. Each new result of every process will be different from the last result. In work settings, we tend to ignore special-cause variation or overreact to common-cause variation. To avoid these two wasteful practices and to create a very practical middle ground, we use *statistical process control* (SPC). SPC is a broad term used to include the various data analyses and charts used in quality-related activities, but it depends particularly on control charts.

SPC distinguishes between two types of variation: those caused by "special causes" and those caused by "common causes." Special causes of variation are factors that disrupt the usual flow, or are out-of-the-ordinary events. Special causes are not inherent in the process. In the process of commuting to work, the time it takes may be varied by special causes such as car trouble, a blizzard, an accident, or a detour. Special causes require immediate, stopgap measures (such as calling the tow truck).

Common causes of variation are factors that are inherent in the process but that have an impact that varies from day to day or month to month. This is also known as *normal variation.*

When you are trying to improve a process, you first need to remove special causes of variation as much as possible, so that you can get a good idea of the underlying, common-cause variation. Once the special causes are out of the way, common-cause variation can be reduced by changing the underlying process. For example, the improvement of traffic flow would require changes in modes of transportation, reprogramming traffic lights, or building new roads.

A control chart has three essential components, which are visible in the chart in *Figure 5.22.* These components are:

- Process data plotted over time
- Upper and lower statistical control limits that define the expected boundaries of common-cause variation. These limits are determined statistically, not determined arbitrarily or taken from design specifications.
- A centerline, usually the average of all the sample averages plotted

If a process contains only normal or random variation (i.e., no runs, no shifts, no patterns, no points beyond the control limits), the process is operating as consistently as possible and is said to be "in control" or "stable." On the other hand, if a process contains special-cause variation (i.e., a run, shift, pattern, or point beyond the control limits), the process is not operating

consistently and is said to be "out of control" or "unstable."

There are several types of control charts, which vary depending on the type of data they contain. Certain data are based on measurements, such as time, temperature, pressure, and cost, for which each observation yields a number that may represent any value along a continuum. These are known as *continuous* or *variables data.* Other data are known as *discrete, count,* or *attributes data.* You can count errors, number of arrivals, and infections. There are seven major types of control charts based on these two categories of data; however, two of these charts suffice for the vast majority of the data generated in the health care environment. These charts are the individual and Moving Range chart (iMR or xMR) and the *p* chart.

iMR and xMR Charts

iMR charts are a pair of control charts used to track individual values or measures taken on a process or its output. xMR charts are used for variables data (data that are both quantitative and continuous in measurement, such as a measured dimension or time). The x chart monitors the process location over time, based on the current subgroup, containing a single observation. The MR chart monitors the variation between consecutive subgroups over time.

xMR charts are generally used when you can't group measurements into rational subgroups, or when the process distribution is very skewed or bounded. Each subgroup, consisting of a single observation, represents a "snapshot" of the process at a given point in time. You should have data that are time ordered; that is, they are entered in the sequence from which they were generated. Axes are time based so that the charts show a history of the process. The steps to construct xMR charts are as follows:

1. Collect the data. List the data sequentially in the x value column. Include the date, time, or sequence at which each data point was obtained.
2. Calculate the ranges (MR values) by taking the absolute value of the difference between sequential x values.
3. Calculate the average range by summing the range values and dividing by the number of range values. When calculating, remember

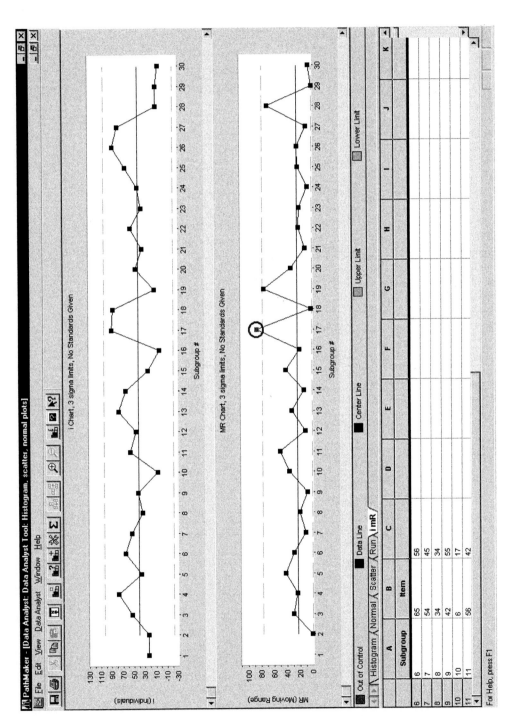

Figure 5.22 The iMR chart is used to track a variable over time. This chart is actually a pair of charts. The upper chart tracks the variable itself. The lower chart tracks the moving range, or the difference between each successive pair of readings. In this example, the lower chart shows an out-of-control point, which is circled. This indicates that a special cause effected the process at the time that the reading was taken.

that there are fewer range values than there are x values.

4. Calculate the UCL for the MR chart. There is no LCL for this chart.
5. Scale the range chart to allow room for the UCL and data. Plot the ranges, draw the average range as a solid line, and draw the UCL as a dashed line. The average and UCL should be labeled and their values noted on the chart.
6. Calculate the average of the x values by summing the x values and dividing by the number of x values.
7. Calculate the UCL and the LCL for the x values.
8. Scale the x chart to allow room for the control limits and data. Plot the x values, draw the average x as a solid line, and draw the control limits as dashed lines. The average and UCL should be labeled and their values noted on the chart.

p Chart

The p control chart is used to track nonconforming items arising from a process in which each item can either have the nonconforming condition, or not. These charts are effective for either fixed or varying sample sizes, but are generally used when a constant sample size cannot be maintained. For example, we might choose to examine job openings filled by internal applicants. Because the number of job vacancies varies from period to period, it would be misleading to simply chart the number of job openings filled internally. The percentage of jobs filled internally would be more accurate because it would account for the varying number of position openings from period to period. Consider medication errors as another example. Because the total number of medications administered from period to period varies, simply counting the number of medication errors would not provide an accurate picture of the medication error problem. Again, it would be much more useful to chart the percentage of medication errors from period to period.

The p chart differs from other control charts in that a set of control limits must be calculated for each data point obtained from the process to account for fluctuations in sample sizes. In most other respects, the p chart is similar to other control charts (*Fig. 5.23*).

The steps to construct p charts are as follows:

1. Collect the data. Record both the number of nonconforming items and the sample size.
2. Calculate and record the fraction of nonconforming items for each sample by dividing the number of nonconforming items by the sample size.; If desired, the values can be expressed as percent nonconforming by multiplying the fraction by 100.
3. Calculate the average fraction nonconforming by summing the individual fraction nonconforming and dividing by the sum of the sample sizes.
4. Calculate and record the UCL and LCL for each sample.Calculate and record the upper and lower control limits for each sample.
5. Scale the vertical axis of the chart to fit the control chart with which you are working, using the control limits as a guide. Be sure to leave some space above the UCL and below the LCL in case out-of-control conditions exist. Plot each fraction nonconforming on the chart and draw the centerline as a solid line on the chart. Then draw the control limit values as lines above and below the point for each fraction nonconforming. If the LCL is calculated to be less than zero, then there is no LCL. If an out-of-control condition does change the process' fraction nonconforming, the more data collected, the easier it will be to see the effect of the change (i.e., as a point outside of the control limits).
6. Interpret the control chart using the rules for detecting out-of-control conditions. Take action as appropriate.

When interpreting the "variation" in the control limits, look at the equation for the UCL and the LCL. Note that because the sample size is in the denominator, the larger the sample size, the tighter the control limits. Note that since the sample size is in the denominator, the larger the sample size, the tighter the control limits. The larger the sample size, the less uncertainty there is about the "true" value of the fraction nonconforming coming from the process. If an out-of-control condition does change the process' fraction nonconforming, the more data collected, the easier it will be to see the effect of the change (i.e., as a point outside of the control limits). Interpret the control chart using the rules for detecting out-of-control conditions. Take action as appropriate.

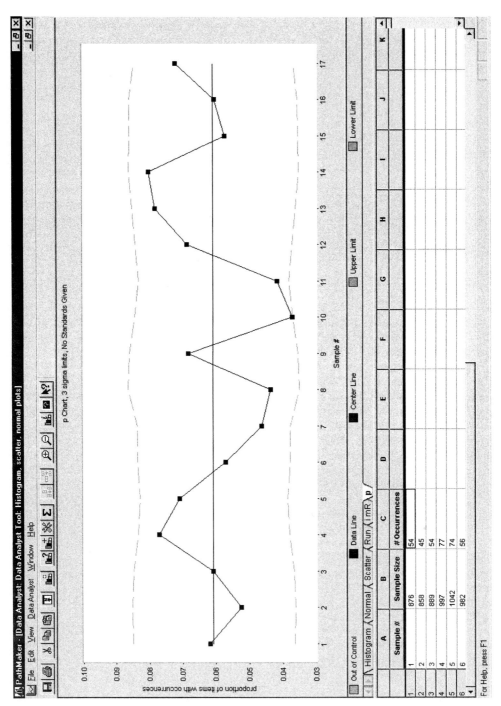

Figure 5.23   In this *p* chart the varying control limits are the result of varying sample sizes. In this case, all points are between the control limits, indicating that the process is in a state of statistical control.

Responding to Variation

Once you have identified the type of variation present in the process, you need to decide what to do about it. With run charts and control charts, the state of control (i.e., the type of variation present) determines the appropriate actions to take. If special-cause variation is present (i.e., if the process is out of control), immediate action should be taken to identify the cause of the unusual variation. You can do this by finding out what unusual event or series of events occurred that caused the out-of-control conditions. Next, you should take action to reduce or eliminate special causes that impact the process negatively, or build special causes into the process if they impact the results positively.

If the process is in control (i.e., only common-cause variation is present), reacting to changes from one data point to the next—regardless of how much they change—is inappropriate. You should not react to the inherent variation present in a stable process as if it was special and required adjustment. Processes that are in control are behaving consistently, and will require fundamental changes in the underlying system to change the output of the process. Setting goals, exhorting employees, or looking for alternative ways to examine the data will not change a stable process permanently. *Table 5.9* summarizes the appropriate actions to take in response to common- and special-cause variation.

The stability of a process indicates its predictability. That is, a stable process is predictable within a given range of values. However, just because a process is stable does not necessarily mean that the performance is acceptable. If the process itself needs to be improved—because it is not meeting customer expectations—we must change the capability of the entire process. To do this requires more in-depth study of the process itself and significant changes in how the work is actually performed.

As we work to improve continually, it is necessary to learn new strategies that will give us better ability to predict future performance and to minimize mistakes and related costs. The value of run and control charts has been proved over and over in numerous industries, and the reasons are straightforward. First, run and control charts offer an effective way of synthesizing important information so it can be readily understood. Because these charts are pictorial displays of information, everyone concerned can have the same level of understanding of the situation, be

TABLE 5.9
Types of Variation and Appropriate Actions

Type of Variation	Appropriate Action to Take
Special-cause variation	1. React to the special cause if it is causing defective product to be made. Consider stopping the process. 2. Identify the assignable cause. 3. If the assignable cause has a negative impact, identify ways to prevent it from recurring or develop a plan to minimize its impact. 4. If the assignable cause has a positive impact, build it into the process.
Common-cause variation	1. Recognize that the process has an inherent capability that will not change unless the process is changed. 2. Work to reduce variation resulting from common causes. 3. Do not react to individual occurrences or try to explain the difference between high and low numbers. 4. To improve, find out what to change.

it good or bad. Second, run and control charts will reveal opportunities for improvement by directing scrutiny to events that involve special causes of variation. In this sense, they make it clear when corrective action is necessary and, even more importantly, indicate when no action is appropriate. Finally, once a key process is tuned to eliminate special-cause variation, it is as well suited as it can be for alterations aimed at reducing common-cause variation or for producing more desirable mean values of a process variable.

CONCLUSIONS

The methods and tools of quality improvement have been shown to be useful in many areas of clinical medicine. The chapters in this monograph describe and explore the power of this methodology for neurosurgery. What is needed is a more widespread application of this improvement science, with extramural teams of surgeons collaborating on ways to break through the barriers to clinical progress.

Some of the work will be the stuff of headlines; these tools can be deployed to speed the development of new products and techniques. Most of the work will most likely be less glamorous, but it will pay off in better outcomes for patients, and less hassles for neurosurgeons.

Dr. Brian Joiner (4), one of the leading thinkers of the quality movement, says that in his experience, most organizations waste anywhere from 25% to 50% of their time and money in poor quality, rework, reacting to variation when they shouldn't, and ignoring data that really do indicate that something new is happening. From our work in the health care systems of the United States, Dr. Joiner's estimate holds true here as well.

ADDITIONAL READING

Delbecq AL, Van de Ven AH: A group process model for identification and program planning. *J Appl Behav Sci* 7: 466–492, 1971.

Delbecq AL, Van de Ven AH, Gustafson DH: Group techniques for program planning. A guide to nominal group technique and delphi processes. New York, Scott Foresman, 1975.

Deming WE: Out of the crisis. Cambridge, MIT Center for Advanced Engineering Study, 1986.

Deming WE: The new economics: For industry, government, education. Cambridge, MIT Center for Advanced Engineering Study, 1993.

Kilian CS: The world of W. Edwards Deming. Knoxville, SPC Press, 1990.

Walton M: Deming management at work. New York, G.P. Putnam's Sons, 1990.

Walton M: The Deming management method. New York, Perigee Books, 1996.

Wheeler D: Understanding variation: The key to managing chaos. Knoxville, SPC Press, 1993.

REFERENCES

1. Cronin MP: Benchmark: Meaningful meetings. *Inc. Magazine* September:122, 1994.
2. Delbecq AL, Van de Ven AH, Gustafson DH: Group techniques for program planning: A guide to nominal group technique and delphi processes. New York, Scott Foresman, 1975.
3. Ishikawa K: Guide to quality control. Tokyo, Asian Productivity Organization, 1989, pp 18–29.
4. Joiner BL: Fourth generation management: The new business consciousness. New York, McGraw-Hill, 1993.
5. Lewin K: Resolving social conflicts and field theory in social science. Washington, American Psychology Association, 1997.
6. Millenson ML: Demanding medical excellence: Doctors and accountability in the information age. Chicago, University of Chicago Press, 1977.
7. Osborn A: Applied Imagination. New York, Scribner's, 1953.
8. Pareto V: Manual of political economy. New York, Augustus M. Kelley Publishers, 1969, reprinted ed.
9. Scupin R: The KJ method: A technique for analyzing data derived from Japanese ethnology. *Hum Org* 56: 233–237, 1997.

CHAPTER 6

Defining, Standardizing, Refining, and Stabilizing Processes

MARK E. LINSKEY, M.D.

EDITOR'S NOTE: Applying empiric science to management, business, and leadership first requires an understanding of where you are now, how you actually produce what you do, and how good and consistent that product is today. Discovering how processes currently work in your organization requires a certain degree of healthy reflection and introspection among process owners and workers in an open and receptive atmosphere. Stabilizing these processes once they are defined, refined, and standardized can be a very positive experience for everyone involved, because visible improvement in the consistency of the results of current practices is usually apparent to all. It is important at this point not to be misled into complacency by confusing improvement of current process performance with actual process improvement. Defining, standardizing, refining, and stabilizing processes are only the first steps in continuous process improvement, which proceeds through repeated iterations of the plan–do–check–act cycle to create actual beneficial changes in the process.

"Anyone who stops learning is old, whether at twenty or eighty. Anyone who keeps learning stays young. The greatest thing in life is to keep your mind young."

—Henry Ford

A *process* is a set of causes and conditions that repeatedly come together to transform inputs into outputs (5, 6, 14, 22, 23, 27, 18). Individual neurosurgeons, neurosurgical group practices, multispecialty group practices, academic neurosurgical divisions and departments, hospitals and clinics, and national and international organizations all rely on processes for their function. Examples of processes one might find in an academic neurosurgical division or department include the following:

- Performing neurological surgery
- Performing inpatient neurosurgical consultations and evaluations
- Performing outpatient neurosurgical consultations and evaluations
- Performing follow-up outpatient neurosurgical evaluations
- Performing outpatient disability evaluations
- Performing patient telephone consultations
- Performing legal brief evaluations
- Scheduling outpatient clinic appointments
- Processing dictation transcription and correspondence
- Billing patients
- Updating and archiving patient office files
- Entering data into the patient database
- Training neurosurgical house officers
- Training rotating non-neurosurgical house officers and medical students
- Performing inventory and ordering for each department
- Budgeting and managing budgets for each department
- Preparing research grant applications
- Preparing basic science research protocols
- Preparing professional lectures
- Preparing professional posters
- Preparing professional publications
- Monitoring quality assurance

Each process extends in a continuous system from a supplier to a customer. The output of these processes defines what we do as private practice or academic neurosurgeons. Most processes in neurosurgery, and in health care in general, depend on the coordinated efforts of people with different training, roles, and skills who often come from different divisions or departments within an organization.

Surprisingly, most management and leadership decisions in neurological surgery are still based on tradition, anecdotal experience, mimicking the course taken by others, or relying on personal intuition or instinct. Neurosurgical residency is a rigorous training crucible through which we pass. It selects rugged individualists who jealously guard individual autonomy and who are extremely successful individual competitors. We tend to be most comfortable in the arenas of direct patient care, medical science, scientific research, and the technical aspects of surgery. In addition, neurosurgical residency is often more a mentorship than an educational curriculum, and as a result we often tend to emerge as faithful disciples, rather than open-minded, free-thinking, and independent future leaders.

Successful management is the science of leadership (namely, the ability to work effectively with others and, more importantly, to motivate and empower others effectively to achieve important and/or common goals), coupled with the application of scientific methods to decision making. Success as a neurosurgeon often thrusts us into positions such as senior partner, division or department head, program director, or officer in a neurosurgical organization, where we are expected to succeed as business persons, managers, and leaders. Unfortunately, the qualities that led us to become successful individual neurosurgeons do not ensure success in these new roles, and most neurosurgical training programs familiarize us only incidentally with the concepts and tools necessary to achieve this success.

New managers (either neurosurgeons or hired neurosurgery office or business managers) are often trained to pursue and focus on short-term goals, and frequently try to:

1. Implement new ideas and institute changes with limited knowledge of the baseline performance of the process they are changing.
2. Pursue administrative reorganization as a means of reflecting an illusion of positive change.

In the first instance, without baseline performance data, changes might lead to worse performance, and management might be unaware of the performance degradation. Alternatively, performance might fluctuate randomly in a positive direction solely as a result of common cause variation (unrelated to any benefit from the change instituted), and management may erroneously conclude that the changes executed were responsible, and may maintain the change. In the second instance, valuable organizational resources and time are consumed to restructure an administration without any proved return from the investment.

In contrast, a fundamental principle of total quality management (TQM) is that management and leadership decisions should always be based on objective data measurements (5, 6, 9, 14, 22, 23, 27, 28). This principle has three corollaries. First, management must take the time, energy, and expense to determine current process performance and to ensure that the processes in question are defined, applied uniformly, refined, and stabilized. This ensures that the results of any future changes can be compared objectively against this baseline to determine their effect. Second, initially changes should be tried and evaluated on a small scale (e.g., pilot project) to try to predict whether the proposed change on an organizational scale justifies the investment. Finally, data should continue to be collected after committing to the change to serve as the new baseline for future improvements. The purpose of this chapter is to outline the means to fulfill the first of these corollaries successfully.

THE WORLD OF PROCESSES

A process can be broken down on flow charts into definable, individual decisions and steps (*Fig. 6.1*) (1, 2, 6, 9, 12, 13, 16, 29, 31). Start and end points are marked with an oval, process steps are indicated by rectangles or boxes, and decisions are identified by diamonds (see Chapter 5). Macrolevel flow charts are used to describe significant organizational processes as they relate to external suppliers and external customers. They usually include very few decision steps and often do not identify internal suppliers and customers. Microlevel flow charts define significant processes in more detail, describing internal suppliers and customers across organizational functions, divisions, and departments. Minilevel flow charts describe every detailed step and/or decision within a process or, more commonly, within a stage of a process (processes can contain *subprocesses;* see the section entitled Critical Processes).

THE FLOW CHART

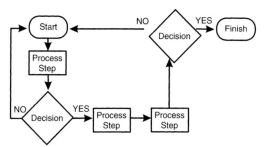

- Diagram that displays the steps and activities in a processor system and how they interact.

Figure 6.1 The flow chart visually reducing a process up into a starting point (oval), individual steps (rectangles or boxes), individual decisions (triangles), and a finishing point (oval) using geometric symbols.

THE SHEWHART CYCLE

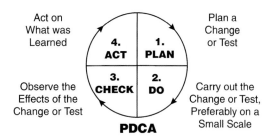

Figure 6.2 The Shewhart Plan–Do–Check–Act (PDCA) cycle, which is the empiric engine of CPI.

Significant Processes

A *significant process* is a process that produces outputs directly that address customer-defined quality needs, and can be traced back through the organization to external suppliers. Improving these processes improves customer outcomes. They are usually few in number because many more organizational processes only involve internal suppliers and customers. Because significant processes reach from one end of the extended system to the other (external suppliers and customers), they are the most important for the organization's success and survival, and should be given priority for any improvement effort.

Critical Processes

A *critical process* is a stage within a significant process (a *subprocess*) that is deemed most important for improvement because of perception within the organization that incremental improvement at this stage will lead to the greatest incremental improvement in the overall significant process per unit investment. Critical processes represent the most fertile starting point for continuous process improvement (CPI).

During the initial stages of CPI (in the absence of data), critical processes are identified through gauging quality improvement team member perceptions. However, this initial perception should be revisited and examined critically when process data are available. If a subprocess is critical to a significant process, then changes in it will lead to changes in measured process outcomes. If subsequent iterations of the Plan–Do–Check–Act (PDCA) cycle (*Fig. 6.2*) show that this is not the case, then the identified subprocess was not critical, and attention and efforts should be shifted to the next likely candidate.

Capable Processes

A process is considered *stable* if it operates within statistical control limits according to objective measurement data expressed on a control chart (5, 7–9, 11–29) (refer to Chapters 5 and 12). A stable process is one that has been standardized and one in which *special-cause variation* has been eliminated (see Stabilizing Processes later in this chapter). The two most important attributes of a stable process are that it is consistently predictable in terms of future output, and that it is ready for empiric attempts at improvement through application of the PDCA in successive cycles of CPI. A *capable process* is one that is both stable and meets all customer needs.

DEFINING PROCESSES

As stated previously, most processes in neurosurgery, and in health care in general, depend on the coordinated efforts of people with different training, roles, and skills who often come from different divisions or departments within the organization. *Process owners* are individuals who make money from the process in question, are themselves evaluated based (at least partially) on the performance of that process, and/or control the personnel or other resources that go into the process. *Process workers* are individuals who participate physically in the steps of the process in question. In many neurosurgical processes, the surgeon is both a process owner and a process worker at the same time.

Assembling the Team

The first step in properly defining a process is assembling a cross-functional team of individuals that represents both process owners and process workers, as well as all departments and divisions within the organization that participate substantively in the process in question. In general, for reasons of logistics and team dynamics, team membership should be limited to six to eight people. Additional representation can always be achieved through ad hoc consultation on an as-needed basis or through periodic rotation of team members at a later date. Assembling the representative cross-functional team is critically important to:

- Tap all potential sources of current process knowledge
- Keep improvement efforts moving and on target
- Empower the organizational movement toward change
- Obtain owner and worker buy-in proactively for both future process change and process measurement efforts

Once formed, the team must be provided with sufficient time, resources, leadership, facilitation, tools, and training to be able to accomplish their task successfully. The unwavering and unambiguous support of organizational leadership is absolutely critical (see Chapter 14). The team needs a convenient location for their meetings and must keep regular meeting hours, with dutiful attendance by all members (especially the neurosurgeons). Leadership must have the patience to allow the team sufficient time to progress through the expected stages of team evolution (*Table 6.1*) inherent in the dynamics of all human group relations (see Chapter 4) (7, 15, 17, 24, 25).

TABLE 6.1
Stages of Team Development

Stage	Group Structure	Team Activity
Forming	Testing and dependence	Orientation
Storming	Intragroup hostility	Emotional response to task demands
Norming	Development of group cohesion	Expression of opinions
Performing	Functional role relatedness	Emergence of solutions

"As-Is" Mapping

At this stage in process definition, no attempt should be made to change the process. The process should simply be defined in an extremely detailed manner as it currently exists, with all its potential idiosyncrasies and foibles left in place for analysis. This type of mapping is known as *as-is "flow charting,"* as opposed to *ideal-world flow charting*. As-is flow charting starts at a "macro level" and then proceeds all the way through the "micro" level to the most detailed "mini" level. Minilevel process flow charts for involved processes can become very large and detailed. In this situation, it is often best to break things down into more digestible subprocesses.

If, as is commonly the case, it turns out that different process workers are actually doing things differently to achieve the same process outcome, each method should be mapped for comparative purposes. Process owners need to sit back at this stage and refrain from commenting on how things are currently being done in their organization for fear of intimidating, disrupting, and potentially stifling the process. This exercise represents a tremendous opportunity for all team members to obtain process knowledge and insight if it is performed openly, honestly, and with unconditional support from leadership.

In addition to defining the steps and decision points in a process, flow charting can also be used to examine personnel use efficiency and space use efficiency. Personnel use is best defined and examined using *as-is functional deployment flow charting (Fig. 6.3)*. In this type of exercise, personnel involved in a process are arranged in vertical columns, and then process steps are mapped from side to side and verti-

Personnel Involved

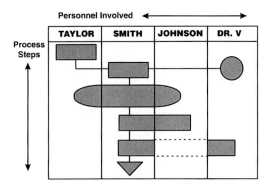

Figure 6.3 A functional deployment flow chart of an organizational process. Process steps are represented by boxes or ovals. However, ovals now indicate meetings or collaboration, whereas a circle represents an inform loop. A triangle indicates a return to the main flow chart.

Space Involved

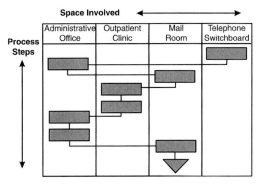

Figure 6.4 A space deployment flow chart for an organizational process. Process steps are represented by boxes or rectangles, whereas ovals represent wait loops, diamonds represent inspections, and circles represent rework.

cally. Steps remain boxes or ovals. However, ovals now indicate meetings or collaboration, and a circle represents an inform loop. A triangle indicates a return to the main flow chart.

Organizational space use is best defined and examined using *as-is space deployment flow charting* (*Fig. 6.4*). In this type of exercise, different locations or work spaces are arranged in vertical columns, and process steps are mapped from side to side and vertically. Once again process steps are represented by boxes or rectangles, but this time ovals represent wait loops, diamonds represent inspections, and circles represent rework.

ACHIEVING PROCESS INSIGHT

The very exercise of defining and refining a process yields tremendously valuable insight for both process owners and process workers. Team members may find that one reason for the previous unpredictability of their process performance, and the failure of the process to improve despite their best intuitive efforts, was that there was no uniformity of the process among process workers. Instead of one process, they had multiple similar processes going on simultaneously. Process workers will grow in process knowledge as well as morale and motivation by understanding and appreciating their own role in the larger overall process. Different process worker backgrounds and perspectives may lead to early identification of potential areas for improvement by having them review the process as a whole, rather than just their relevant portion.

Standardizing the Process

Many organizations have published *standard operating procedures* (SOPs), or "policies" produced, published, and promulgated by management. Most of these SOPs or policies sit unread, gathering dust, in notebooks or file drawers waiting to be brought out at times of inspection or new employee orientation. Management often labors under the erroneous conclusion that processes in the workspace are actually functioning according to those published guidelines, and they are often shocked to find out that this is not the case.

Process workers are intelligent and motivated to succeed. When an idealized SOP is presented that fails to function effectively to achieve the desired end, the process workers usually modify it to "fix" it in various creative ways to make it work. Different staff members may even use different means of fixing the "problems," and thus one process may in fact become a series of similar, but not identical, processes. Multiple processes will never achieve a statistically predictable outcome because increased variability is inherent in their very existence. The first step in stabilizing a process thus becomes having the process workers and owners standardize the processes jointly into a single process that all agree to support and follow (consensus) in a uniform and consistent manner.

For processes in which neurosurgeons are predominantly process owners (e.g., patient scheduling, patient billing), simplification through standardization to a single process makes obvious sense. However, processes in which neurosurgeons are also process workers (e.g., performing a certain neurosurgical procedure, developing a multidisciplinary inpatient clinical pathway for a specific patient diagnosis) usually involve clinical choices for patient care. Here one must be very careful to only insist on uniformity for steps for which adequate scientific evidence exists to confirm the superiority of that approach.

This is an area in which the powerful tool of evidence-based medicine can be immensely useful (*Tables 6.2 and 6.3*) (10, 11, 19–21, 26,

TABLE 6.2
Classes of Medical Evidence for Therapeutic Interventions

Evidence	Definition
Class I	Prospective, randomized clinical trials
Class II	Clinical studies in which the data are collected prospectively, and undergo retrospective analysis based on clearly reliable data; examples include observational studies, cohort studies, prevalence studies, and case–control studies
Class III	Most studies based on retrospectively collected and analyzed data; examples include clinical series, databases or registries, case reviews, case reports, and expert opinion

TABLE 6.3
Degrees of Certainty for Recommendations for Clinical Care

Type of Care	Definition
Standards	Accepted principles of patient management that reflect a *high degree of clinical certainty*; generally based on class I evidence and rarely on very strong class II evidence
Guidelines	A particular strategy or range of management strategies that reflect a *moderate degree of clinical certainty*, generally based on class II evidence or a preponderance of class III evidence
Options	The remaining strategies for patient management for which there is *unclear clinical certainty*, based on class III evidence

33). Only steps that have sufficiently strong class I and/or class II evidence to be considered "standards" or "guidelines" (and some would say only standards) should be standardized for uniformity among neurosurgeons. For steps for which only clinical "options" exist, the process must be engineered to allow neurosurgeons the freedom to choose among the available options (see Chapter 7). To do otherwise could potentially and negatively affect patient outcome despite good intentions, and will certainly undermine neurosurgical acceptance, buy-in, and support of the standardized process. One must always remember that clinical neurosurgery is both an art and a science, and that very strong feelings exist in areas in which data are most lacking.

Refining the Process

Once the process is defined as it is currently and actually performed in the workplace, and reasonable levels of uniformity and standardization have been achieved, the process is ready for refinement. Process refinement involves *identifying process complexity* and simplifying the process by removing or reducing this complexity whenever possible. Process complexity includes redundant steps, nonvalue-added steps, and unnecessary process delay loops. Redundant and/or unnecessary steps are usually readily apparent to process workers once all the steps of the process are mapped out in detail through as-is flow charting. Process owners are often amazed that they never noticed these wasted steps until the process was presented graphically as a whole. These steps can also include redundant and/or unnecessary transfer of process product between personnel or the need to transfer process product across excessive distances within the organization.

Value-added steps are those that contribute substantively to the outputs and/or outcomes of the process. Steps that do not contribute to the outputs and/or outcomes of the process are termed *nonvalue-added steps,* and they are ripe for streamlining if they do not serve environmental requirements imposed on the process by external stakeholders (usually regulatory agencies and/or liability concerns). Process delay loops are usually decision loops in which the process must halt pending a decision by a process owner or process worker. They can also be delays imposed by transfer of the process prod-

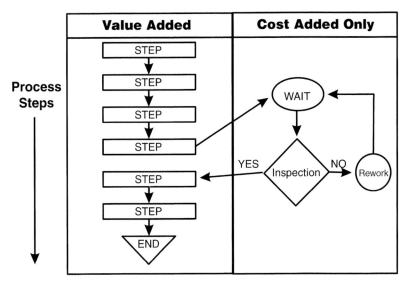

Figure 6.5 An opportunity flowchart for an organizational process. Process steps are represented by boxes or rectangles, ovals represent wait loops, diamonds represent inspections, and circles represent rework. Nonvalue-added process complexity becomes glaringly apparent using this quality tool.

uct from one process worker to another or from one organizational space to another.

Process complexity can often be best displayed and identified through opportunity deployment flow charting (*Fig. 6.5*). In this type of exercise, the chart is divided into two vertical columns for "value-added" and "cost-added-only" steps. Process steps are mapped from side to side and vertically, with individual steps represented by boxes or rectangles, wait loops represented by ovals, inspections represented by diamonds, and rework represented by circles.

Process complexity is sometimes the result of environmental factors outside the actual process. These environmental factors include public laws, tort liability concerns, and stakeholder regulations. Stakeholders are groups and individuals inside or outside the organization who affect and are affected by the achievement of the organization's mission, goals, and strategy (6, 8, 9). Stakeholders monitor performance, may themselves be evaluated based on organizational performance, adjudicate disputes, control access to resources, regulate the organization, and establish clinical options, standards, and guidelines. A more extensive list of academic neurosurgical environmental constraints and stakeholders includes:

- University policies
- University graduate medical education committee
- Laser safety office
- State disability office
- Social Security office
- State Medicaid offices
- Dean of the medical school
- Human research internal review board
- Animal Use Committee
- Radiation safety office
- Malpractice tort law
- Managed care organizations
- Health insurance organizations
- Hospital policies
- Health Care Financing Administration (HCFA)
- Joint Commission on Accreditation of Health Care Organization (JCAHO)
- American College of Graduate Medical Education (ACGME)
- CNS
- AANS
- AHA
- American College of Surgeons (ACS)

Although it is desirable to eliminate as much process complexity as possible, depending on environmental circumstances, a certain irreducible

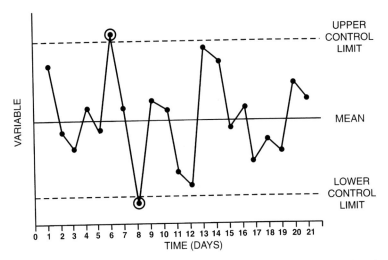

Figure 6.7 An example of part of a process control chart showing the mean (solid line) as well as the upper and lower control limits (dashed lines), which lie three standard deviations on either side of the mean value. The two circled data points represent special-cause variation because they fall outside the specified control limits. There are no other instances of special cause indicated, even using the six rules listed later in this chapter.

is plotted on the x-axis. For any set of data points taken from a process over time, a mean value can be established, and upper and lower control limits (three standard deviations above and below the mean respectively) can be calculated and plotted on the y-axis (*Fig. 6.7*). In the simplest case, data points that fall between the upper and lower control limits are simply the result of common-cause variation, those who was those that fall above or below the limits should be investigated for special causes (13, 29) (Chapters 5 and 12).

Even if all the data points fall within the upper and lower control limits on a control chart, there is still a chance of forming a pattern that is statistically unlikely to be random (implying the possibility of special-cause variation). The six rules for identifying these patterns and uncovering additional, potential special-cause variation are as follows:

1. Two points, out of three successive points, are on the same side of the center line at least two standard deviations from the mean.
2. Four points, out of five successive points, are on the same side of the center line at least one standard deviation from the mean.
3. Nine successive points are on the same side of the center line.
4. There are six consecutive points, either increasing or decreasing.
5. There are 14 points in a row that alternate up and down.
6. There are 15 points in a row one standard deviation from the mean (above and below the center line).

When one identifies one or more of these non-random patterns, they should be treated just like a data point that falls outside the control limits. At the very minimum, knowledge of variation requires familiarity with the use and interpretation of process control charts.

Each data point (or points) identified as representing a special cause requires consideration and investigation by the quality improvement team. The specific special cause leading to each aberrant data point may differ in each instance. However, it is only through identification and elimination of each special cause that a process can eventually be stabilized and brought under statistical control. Particularly egregious special causes are often termed *fires,* and eliminating them is often referred to as "putting out fires" or "fighting fires" in business and management jargon.

CONCLUSION

Once the measured output of a process falls consistently between the upper and lower control limits, with the data distributed randomly between these limits, the process (as it is currently performed) is in statistical control (i.e., stabilized). You now have an objective measure of "where you are" currently, and you can go on to evaluate objectively the impact of any future changes you may care to make. This processing of information forms the basis for data-based decision making, which brings science to the fields of management and business, which is part of the very essence of TQM. Your process is now reliably predictable and can be evaluated for it's inherent variability and its capability for meeting customer needs.

Defining, standardizing, refining, and stabilizing a process can be an exciting, enlightening, and gratifying exercise that leads to valuable process insight, identification of potential fertile targets for future process improvement, improved morale, and improved consistency of performance of the current process. However, process refinement and stabilization only improves the performance of the existing process. It does not improve the process itself and thus should not be confused with CPI as espoused in TQM. CPI is very different from problem solving, crisis management, or "putting out fires." As Deming stated, "Putting out fires is not improvement. Finding a point out of control, finding the special cause and removing it, is only putting the process back to where it was in the first place. It is not improvement of the process."(27)

Once your process is defined, standardized, refined, and stabilized, you are ready for CPI. CPI has two statistical goals. The first is to reduce the common-cause variation of your process continuously through improving the process itself. This will be visible on your process control chart as decrease in the distance between your upper and lower control limits on either side of your mean performance value. The second goal is to make your process more capable by making process changes that shift the performance mean toward the customer-defined optimal value. Both of these goals are achieved by addressing sequentially each of the potential causes of process variation identified during the process, definition, standardization, and refinement steps, and empirically "fine-tuning" each of these causes through sequential application of the Shewhart PDCA cycle. Both of these goals are part and parcel of "world-class quality" (*Fig. 6.8*).

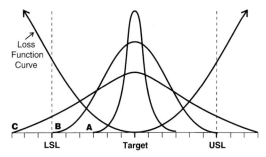

Continual Improvement

Measurement of Quality Characterisitic

Figure 6.8 Graphical representation of process improvement. As the quality improvement team progressed through successive PDCA cycles, they moved the process from point C, to point B, to point A, reducing output variability with each iteration, and thereby improving quality and lowering both measurable and unmeasurable costs. LSL = lower specification limit; USL = upper specification limit.

REFERENCES

1. Asaka T, Ozeki K., eds: Handbook of quality tools: The Japanese approach (lesson 6). Cambridge, Productivity Press, 1990.
2. Brassard M: The Memory Jogger Plus+. Methuen, GOAL/QPC, 1989.
3. Deming WE: Theory of sampling. New York, John Wiley, 1950.
4. Deming WE: Sample design in business research. New York, John Wiley, 1961.
5. Deming WE: Out of the crisis. Cambridge, Massachusetts Institute of Technology, Center for Advanced Engineering Studies, 1986.
6. Department of the Navy: Fundamentals of total quality leadership. Publication no. CIN P-500-0012. Washington, DC, Total Quality Leadership Office, November 1992.
7. Department of the Navy. Teams skills and concepts. Publication no. CIN P-500-0014. Washington, DC, Total Quality Leadership Office, October 1995.
8. Department of the Navy: Methods of managing quality. Washington, DC, Total Quality Leadership Office, December 1996.
9. Department of the Navy. Systems approach to process improvement. Publication no. CIN P-500-0004. Washington, DC, Total Quality Leadership Office, February 1997.
10. Eddy DM: Designing a practice policy: Standards, guidelines, and options. *JAMA* 26:3077–3084, 1990.
11. Field MJ, Lohr KN: Guidelines for clinical practice, from development to use. Washington, National Academy Press, 1992.
12. Gitlow HS, Gitlow S, Oppenheim A, Oppenheim R: Tools and methods for the improvement of quality. Homewood, Richard D. Irwin, 1989.
13. GOAL/QPC: The Memory Jogger: A pocket guide of tools for continuous improvement. Methuen, GOAL/QPC, 1988.

14. McConnell J: Safer than a known way. Dee Why, Australia, Delaware Books, 1988.

15. Miller LM, Howard J: Managing quality through teams. Atlanta, The Miller Consulting Group, 1991.

16. Mizuno S (ed): Management for quality improvement: The seven new OC tools. Cambridge, Productivity Press, 1988.

17. Moosbruker J: Developing a productive team: Making groups at work. Team building: Blueprints for productivity and satisfaction. Alexandria, NTL Institute for Applied Behavioral Science, 1988.

18. Nolan TW, Provost LP: Understanding variation. *Qual Prog* 23:70–78, 1990.

19. Rosenberg J, Greenberg MK: Practice parameters: Strategies for survival into the nineties. *Neurology* 42:1110–1115, 1992.

20. Sackett DL, Haynes RB, Tugwell PX: Clinical epidemiology: A basic science for clinical medicine. Toronto, Little, Brown, 1985.

21. Sackett DL, Richardson WS, Rosenberg W, Haynes RB: Evidence-based medicine. How to practice and teach EBM. New York, Churchill Livingstone, 1997.

22. Scherkenbach WW: The Deming route to quality and productivity: Roadmaps and roadblocks. Rockville, Mercury Press, 1987.

23. Scherkenbach WW: Deming's road to continual improvement. Knoxville, SPC Press, 1991.

24. Scholtes PR, Joiner B, Braswell B, et al.: The team handbook. Madison, Joiner and Associates, 1988.

25. Tuckman BW, Jensen MAC: Stages of small group development revisited. *Group Org Studies* 2(4), 1977.

26. Walters BC: Clinical practice parameter development in neurosurgery, in Bean JR (ed): *Neurosurgery in Transition: The Socioeconomic Transformation of Neurological Surgery.* Baltimore, William & Wilkins, 1998, vol 9, 99–111.

27. Walton M: The Deming management method. New York, Putnam Publishing Group, 1986.

28. Walton M: Deming management at work. New York, G. P. Putnam's, 1990.

29. Wheeler DJ: Charts done right. Manuscript no. 56. Knoxville, Statistical Process Controls, 1991.

30. Wheeler DJ: Understanding variation: The key to managing chaos. Knoxville, SPC Press, 1993.

31. Wheeler DJ, Chambers DS: Understanding statistical process control. Knoxville, SPC Press, 1992.

32. Wheeler DJ, Chambers DS: Advanced topics in statistical process control. Knoxville, SPC Press, 1995.

33. Woolf SH: Practice guidelines: A new reality in medicine. II: Methods of developing guidelines. *Arch Intern Med* 152:946–952, 1992.

CHAPTER 7

Establishing Clinical Pathways

JOHN B. WALDMAN, M.D., F.A.C.S., AND MARY B. MCLAUGHLIN, R.N., M.B.A.

EDITOR'S NOTE: Clinical pathways are standardized and refined "tracks" for inpatient care that specify steps and decision points in an inpatient process. Clinical pathway processes can be built around clinical procedures or patient diagnoses. Clinical pathways are cross-functional and multidisciplinary and involve physicians, nurses, social services, allied health therapists, pharmacists, and many others. It is important to keep in mind that the establishment of a clinical pathway is only the first step in continuous process improvement. Data from the established pathway should serve as the empiric baseline against which subsequent process improvement efforts are measured and compared. The pathway must be a dynamic and living entity that evolves and improves over time with repeated iterations of the plan–do–check–act cycle, rather than an arbitrary, stagnant, and rigid obstruction to innovation and progress. Creating a clinical pathway requires a great deal of planning and effort, as well as a cross-functional team composed of a representative from each of the major disciplines involved. It is critical for neurosurgeons to actively participate in this team planning and, ideally, take a leadership role.

"The key is not to prioritize your schedule, but to schedule your priorities. Do the important things first—because where you are headed is more important than how fast you are going."

—*Stephen R. Covey*

THE NEED FOR AND BENEFITS OF CLINICAL PATHWAYS

Why develop clinical pathways? It is clear that the impetus to develop clinical pathways has come from the sweeping changes occurring in health care delivery systems. The cost of medical payment programs to industry and the federal government has led to attempts to control and actively manage medical expenditures (24). At the same time, workforce excess in many specialties has led to increased competition for patients among providers in many geographical re-

gions (14). Increased competition has helped physicians realize that patient and referring-physician satisfaction are critical to success. These two factors, cost and satisfaction, have stimulated more efficient processes for medical decision making. A third factor, quality, frequently touted in the past as the foremost concern in patient care, has often been given only lip service. In fact, horror stories of patients being denied care have received national media attention (6, 25). In the midst of continuing pressures to increase patient and physician satisfaction in an environment of cost containment, it is critical that heath care providers maintain their focus on the quality of care. After all, providing the best possible patient outcomes should be the priority of every physician. Clinical pathways attempt to codify best practices, with the goal of increasing the likelihood of best outcomes.

Traditionally, from a physician's perspective, the only factor that mattered in providing the best care for individual patients was the physician's own concept of how to provide that care; cost and satisfaction were discussed rarely. More recently, the discrepancy between how a physician practiced and how insurers perceived that physician's practice in terms of the potential for cost savings led to confrontation. The result of this conflict stigmatized efforts at clinical pathway development. Comments such as "It's just cookbook medicine," "I don't want to be told how to practice," "All the insurers care about is the bottom line," and "I've always practiced this way and it works for me" were heard from physicians throughout the United States.

Why do physicians need to embrace the concepts of clinical pathway development? The reason is compelling: When developed properly, clinical pathways can lead to better patient outcomes. Although the practice of medicine is still very much an art, it is also a science. Surprisingly, what is in essence the scientific aspect of medicine often takes a backseat to what is perceived to be the "art" or individual physician's own way of practice (11). The process of pathway development uses the scientific literature or an evidence-based medicine approach to determine the best practice, uses consensus of the team when science does not provide a conclusive answer, and omits issues for which the scientific evidence is not available nor consensus achievable. If the team develops a pathway that reflects the best practice, and participants follow that pathway, variation in care will be reduced and results will improve. The prospect of better outcomes for their patients should encourage willing participation by all physicians. Often, as a byproduct of this process, reduction of cost, improvement in efficiency, and higher levels of patient and referring-physician satisfaction occur. When the primary objective of clinical pathway development is better patient outcomes, it is mandatory that physicians, not hospital administrators or insurers, take the lead. Conversely, if physicians abrogate their responsibility to assure that their patients receive the best care during pathway development, then others, with agendas that might be in conflict with best practice, can determine the course of patient care.

The priority of a clinical pathway must be understood by all the participants, physicians, nurses, other health care workers, and administrators. The goal of a pathway is to:

1. Maximize patient health and satisfaction; and
2. Minimize resource consumption.

The overriding objective, however, is to improve quality of care. Reduction in cost, although not a given, is a secondary goal. Pathways may additionally provide opportunities for enhancement of education and research. In the quest for reducing the cost of delivering care, services cannot be reduced below what it takes to deliver the best care. Thus, the best care becomes the cheapest care allowable to produce the best outcomes. The quest for quality determines the cost; cost must not determine the quality.

In summary, when approached from the proper perspective, clinical pathways accom-

plish something for everyone: improved patient outcomes, more efficient use of resources, lower costs, time savings for physicians and staff in terms of documentation, and higher levels of satisfaction for patients and physicians.

ESTABLISHING THE TEAM AND CHOOSING THE PATHWAY

It is important and crucial to the meaningful establishment of a pathway the selection of the team members and their acceptance of the pathway process. Few health care providers who believe that they are experts in a given area will eagerly participate in a process that is imposed on them. Therefore, thoughtful inclusion of those experts is the first step. Although physician involvement and participation are mandatory, so is the inclusion of other "front-line" health care personnel who are experts in their areas of care. To keep the size of the team at a manageable number, certain experts, whose roles may involve only a segment of the care, can be added to the team as temporary consultants when their portion of the plan is under development. Such an arrangement makes for better use of all providers' valuable time.

Team members are expected to represent their area of expertise, to communicate with their peers, and to bring back to the team representative opinions from their constituents. Team members should also have certain characteristics if they are to be productive in their role (see Chapter 4). Open mindedness and the ability to respect others' ideas and to actively listen to those ideas are essential. Members must be willing to work at consensus building, to adhere to a timeline, and to be prepared for the meetings (10). The only mandate by the organizational leader who sanctions the pathway team is that nonparticipation by an individual or service is not an option.

From an institutional perspective, pathways should be developed by a group on the basis of the patient population served and not the clinical service or hospital unit. Many pathways in which neurosurgeons participate involve multiple specialties. For example, an institution should have one pathway for patients undergoing carotid endarterectomy regardless of whether a neurosurgeon, vascular surgeon, or general surgeon performs the procedure. Likewise, a single pathway should be in use on all hospital units for that population of patients. There can only be one level of care for each patient population. Therefore, representation on the team should come from all services and units that will be involved in the care of that patient population.

Because the pathway process may challenge the way in which physicians practice, success can hinge on the presence of an institutional culture that supports continuous quality improvement techniques and that provides the resources to see these endeavors flourish. To this end, identifying a quality specialist with experience in consensus building, and preferably pathway development, is desirable. Most physicians are experts in the field of medicine that they practice; they feel in control when dealing with problems within their medical domain. However, when in unfamiliar territory, the loss of control can be intimidating. This feeling may manifest itself in unproductive behavior. A skilled quality specialist can preempt these issues and ease the physician who is a pathway development novice through the process. Most physicians enjoy learning; this is an opportunity for those participants to acquire useful knowledge, see positive results, and feel good about the team's accomplishments. From this achievement another convert is born.

In our institution, one of the surgical specialty groups was asked to participate in the development of a clinical pathway. Diverse complaints and excuses were offered for physician nonparticipation. Despite their delinquency at the meetings, the other members of the team persevered. Once the physicians realized that the pathway was soon to be finished without their input, they suddenly had an interest. After implementation (with their ultimate participation), they discovered that their patients sailed through their hospitalization much faster, with fewer complications, and with marked savings of physicians' time. The result was that they could now admit more patients and do more surgery—efficiency was greatly enhanced. Having recognized the benefits, this group is now unstoppable in their quest to create pathways for all of their procedures.

Choosing the right clinical procedure or episode of illness to develop into a pathway is essential, particularly when first embarking on this process. Consider where the greatest opportunities for improvement exist and where the greatest likelihood of success might be found. Data frequently can assist you in choosing the correct starting place; analyzing and comparing lengths of stay (LOS) for specific admitting diagnoses, outcomes, or costs between your institution and others (benchmarking) can help to make the choice readily apparent. Patient satisfaction survey results may also direct ones' efforts toward a particular procedure or diagnosis. In general, the most useful procedures or treatment episodes to create pathways for are those where the greatest opportunities for improvement exist. These commonly are the entities that involve high volume, high complexity, high resource use, or high cost. For example, in neurological surgery, lumbar discectomy is a high-volume procedure; therefore, even a small improvement could result in a large gain. Similarly, for spinal instrumentation procedures, where the cost of the instrumentation to the institution is high, consensus during pathway development on limiting the inventory of instrumentation equipment (with discounts from the manufacturer) might produce major cost savings. Of course, the process chosen must be within the control of the assembled group. One cannot change the way others (e.g., departments or specialties) do what they do without their inclusion in the pathway development process. The choice for development should receive a sanction from the department or institutional leader. Although anyone can suggest an area for improvement, the most common method in our institution (Albany Medical College, Albany, NY) for identifying a pathway development opportunity is through one of our service-based quality improvement teams (QITs) (*Fig. 7.1*).

After the choice of the pathway is made and team members are chosen, ground rules of participation must be accepted by the team (see Chapter 4). It is essential that the members understand the goals of the entire team and what is expected of each individual. Members must participate. They must attend meetings, and they must be engaged in the process. This may mean scheduling the meetings at odd hours to accommodate individual members or making special coverage arrangements to allow for attendance. Keep to a timeline; set a work schedule and maintain it. Time is a valuable commodity, and, therefore, no one should tolerate wasting it. To facilitate staying on schedule, members must be prepared for meetings. Minutes and handouts

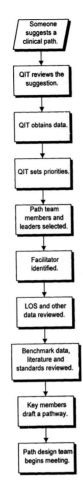

```
┌──────────────┐
│  Someone     │
│  suggests a  │
│  clinical path. │
└──────────────┘
        │
        ▼
┌──────────────┐
│ QIT reviews the │
│  suggestion.  │
└──────────────┘
        │
        ▼
┌──────────────┐
│ QIT obtains data. │
└──────────────┘
        │
        ▼
┌──────────────┐
│ QIT sets priorities. │
└──────────────┘
        │
        ▼
┌──────────────┐
│ Path team    │
│ members and  │
│ leaders selected. │
└──────────────┘
        │
        ▼
┌──────────────┐
│ Facilitator  │
│ identified.  │
└──────────────┘
        │
        ▼
┌──────────────┐
│ LOS and other │
│ data reviewed. │
└──────────────┘
        │
        ▼
┌──────────────┐
│ Benchmark data, │
│ literature and │
│ standards reviewed. │
└──────────────┘
        │
        ▼
┌──────────────┐
│ Key members  │
│ draft a pathway. │
└──────────────┘
        │
        ▼
┌──────────────┐
│ Path design team │
│ begins meeting. │
└──────────────┘
```

Figure 7.1 Albany Medical Center (Albany, NY) clinical pathway development flowchart, which shows an example of a process for determining which patient population to path.

should be read in advance and team members should complete any homework assignments.

Members must respect others' ideas and actively listen. Open mindedness is critical. Because participants are generally experts and experienced in the management of the process under development, each brings to the meeting a history, including preferences, agendas, and anecdotes that differ from the others who may have equally valid notions of how things should be done. Conflict resolution is the biggest challenge facing the team (see Chapter 4). Having an experienced quality specialist facilitating discussion and mediating differences is important, but equally important is the commitment of each

member to the principle of respecting and listening to other opinions. Decisions are made by consensus. This does not mean by majority rule. All members must ultimately agree and accept the pathway segment under development. Agreement is most likely to be reached when the element under discussion can be scientifically proven. For example, is the use of prophylactic antibiotics in a particular procedure associated with a lower infection rate? If data or the literature do not offer irrefutable scientific proof, consensus development is necessary. If, through this process, consensus cannot be reached, that particular element must be left off the pathway and up to individual decision and preference. Remember that after consensus is reached, members may not leave the meeting and expound another viewpoint. Consensus means that they accept the group opinion and will support that viewpoint. Each team member is a representative of his or her peers and must communicate with them and bring back to the group the opinions and ideas of their peers. Eventually the pathway will affect other health care providers whose representative will be held accountable to them for the result. When physicians lack input into the pathway process, poor compliance can be anticipated.

STAGES OF PATHWAY DEVELOPMENT

After the pathway choice is made, the appropriate pathway team members are assembled, and their acceptance of the ground rules obtained, the real work begins. The first task is an analysis of prior performance data. How long are patients currently in the hospital? What is the range of LOS? How many computerized tomography scans are ordered? How much does it cost to deliver the care? How many days do the patients spend in the intensive care unit (ICU)? Understanding the current practice, the current variations in care, the numbers of tests, procedures, days, and so forth, gives the group a sense of where the improvements may be made. Benchmark data are reviewed as well as other established national standards. For example, the team may examine Milliman and Robertson's (12) LOS information, University Health Care Consortium (UHC) data, and national standards from such sources as the Agency of Health Care Policy and Research Guidelines and National Institutes of Health (2, 13, 20–22). After the review of various data sources is complete, estimates can be made and agreed on regarding the general design and length of the pathway and its segments.

A useful method for understanding the process of pathway development is to chart patient flow. Flow diagrams (see Chapter 5) assist participants' understanding of the sequence of events involved in the care of patients and allow the group to see the process through the patient's eyes (*Fig. 7.2*) (4). Flow charts help organize the approach to the fundamentals of the pathway while maintaining a patient focus. These diagrams frequently help the team recognize a natu-

ral structure or organization to the path that translates into the pathway itself. For example, there may be a prehospitalization phase, an operating room segment, an ICU stay, a regular floor unit segment, and a rehabilitative phase before discharge to the home. At each segment, decision trees may come into play that might confuse the process unless recognized. An accurate patient flow chart obviates these confusions and keeps the group in focus (23, 26).

After the group is prepared and focused on the patient, the actual mapping of the orders and outcomes of the pathway begins. The following list illustrates the steps in mapping a clinical pathway:

1. Orders and interventions;
2. Discharge outcomes;
3. Daily outcomes;
4. Insert days; and
5. Order sheets.

Although there are many ways of proceeding, we have found that beginning with the orders and interventions is easiest (*Fig. 7.3*). It is this portion of the pathway that is more readily understood by physicians and nurses who are most familiar with health care delivery in terms of daily written orders and various interventions. The initial process begins with a draft that is created by a subgroup outside of the meeting. Starting from a blank page can be daunting; therefore, converting an existing nursing care plan or standing order set into the clinical pathway format is useful. Orders and interventions are developed for each day of the pathway. Each day is reviewed, and the decision process described above is used to reach consensus for each item and each day. Every item added to the pathway should undergo scrutiny. Is the test necessary? Does it alter care if the result is abnormal and, if so, how often is it abnormal? Including a particular test or intervention for a rare event is generally not useful. Do not accept orders or interventions without evidence that they are necessary for better outcomes. For example, daily hemoglobins and hematocrits (H & H) in routine lumbar discectomy patients are not warranted if your experience suggests that 99% of the time patients do not require transfusion after this procedure. However, excluding postoperative H & H determinations from the pathway does not preclude ordering one on a particular

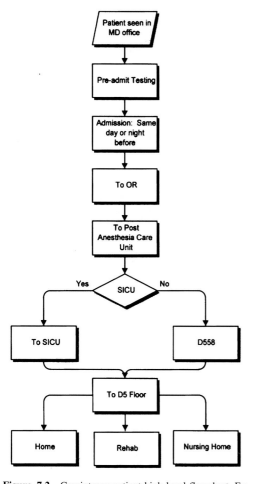

Figure 7.2 Craniotomy patient high-level flowchart. Example of patient movement through an episode of care demonstrating critical decision points. PT = patient; MD office = doctor's office; SICU = surgical intensive care unit; D558 = neurosurgery stepdown unit (or intermediate care unit); D5 Floor = neurosurgery floor; Rehab = rehabilitation.

ADDRESSOGRAPH

ORDERS/INTERVENTIONS				
ONGOING CARE				
Comfort/ Communication	Ongoing			Communicate plan of care to patient/significant other and encourage participation. Encourage patient to ventilate feelings.
Teaching	Ongoing			Encourage patient to report to nurse changes in neurovascular status. Explain all procedures and rationale for all medications prescribed.
POD	Date/ Time/Init			
Specimens/ Tests	D	E	N	
Treatments				Incentive spirometry q 1 h while awake. 40% O2 via humidified face mask. Scott Cannula at bedside for posterior fossa. Monitor dressings for drainage and reinforce. Notify MD if dressing has evidence of bleeding or drainage. If JP, empty JP q shift or when ½ full, be sure to clamp JP prior to emptying. Notify MD if it requires emptying q 2 h. Use orbital moisture chamber or artificial tears if unable to protect eyes. Sequential teds remove q shift for skin care for 30 mins. Foley to straight drainage.
IVs				D5 and .9 NS at 75/h.
Medications				See Medex
Activity/ Safety				Bedrest. Reposition q 2 h. HOB 30 unless patient is hypotensive. Maintain head in neutral position.
Nutrition				Clear liquids as tolerated with positive bowel sounds.
Protocols				O2 Therapy ☐ Ventriculostomy Peripheral IV ☐ CVL ☐ Seizure Protocol Fall Prevention ☐ Hemodynamic Monitoring Post-op ☐ Foley Management Pain Management ☐ Confusion/Agitation
Consults				PT consult for motor weakness, gait disturbance. OT consult if upper extremity weakness, cognitive deficit, need for splinting/positioning, ADL deficit. Speech consult if aphasia, swallowing disturbance, slurred speech or cognitive/linguistic deficit.
Teaching				Review plan of care with pt/SO.
Assessment				VS and neuro checks q 1 h. Assess dressing, Temp, O2 Sat and I & O q 2 h. Check for CSF leak q 2 h (salty taste in mouth, rhinorrhea, otorrhea, halo sign). Systems assessment q 8 h.
Report to MD				Notify MD if JP requires emptying > q 2 h or if JP inflates with air (indicates leak). Notify MD if decline in neuro status, CSF leak, seizure.
Additional Orders/ Interventions				

PLACE IN NURSING KARDEX/BINDER DURING USE

Figure 7.3 Example of a page from the Adult Craniotomy Pathway demonstrating typical organization of orders and interventions into similar subgroups. JP = Jackson Pratt drain; MD = doctor; D5 = neurosurgery floor; NS = normal saline; HOB = head of bed; CVL = central venous line; ADL = activities of daily living; PT = physical therapy; OT = occupational therapy; VS = vital signs; CSF = cerebrospinal fluid.

patient in whom excessive blood loss occurred at the time of surgery.

Practitioners caring for the same disorders or performing the same surgeries have different ways of doing nearly every detail of the care, from the medications in the "bowel routine," to the use of drains, to the time patients are allowed out of bed after surgery. These differences may become contentious issues because individ-

uals wish to stubbornly adhere to their own routine. The skillful facilitator is adept at dealing with the interpersonal dynamics that play out during these discussions (see Chapter 4) (17). One can learn a great deal about oneself and others by participating in such activities.

Discharge outcomes need to be determined: What criteria do the patients have to meet to be discharged? This seemingly simple question is sometimes controversial. Team members may have very different and conflicting viewpoints on these criteria. For example, while developing a congestive heart failure pathway at our institution some pathway team members felt that a complete safety evaluation was necessary prior to discharge. The member from home health care agency, however, pointed out that this could easily be accomplished as an outpatient and that it was not necessary to keep the patient in hospital for this purpose. In another group, surgeons insisted that patients could not be discharged until after their surgical drains were removed. Again, this was managed in the outpatient setting, including antibiotic coverage. Bringing professionals from different disciplines together in a collegial environment allows for nonthreatening challenges to long-held beliefs that may reflect nothing more than old habits and be unrelated to improved patient outcomes. It may be useful to divide discharge criteria into functional groups that are based on discharge disposition. This strategy encourages early referrals to appropriate facilities or services (*Fig. 7.4*).

After discharge outcomes have been created, expected daily outcomes are developed (*Fig. 7.5*). These outcomes are the intermediate expectations for the typical patient: Do we expect the patient to be out of bed on the night of surgery? How far should they be able to ambulate? When are the patients first fed? What should their neurological condition be? These expecta-

CLINICAL PATH: Adults Craniotomy
Page 14 of 16

Discharge Disposition Criteria (Case Manager Initial and Date Planned Disposition)						
	EXTENDED CARE NRSG. FACILITY		**REHABILITATION**	**HOME WITH SERVICES**		**HOME**
I. Clinical Status	1. Failed rehab screen. 2. Not appropriate for home with services. 3. Not appropriate for home. 4. Referral made to: ___ ___ ___ ___ ___ ___		1. Requires assistance for transfer/ambulation. 2. Requires assistance with ADL that exceeds family support available at home. 3. Afebrile x 24 hours. 4. Medically stable. 5. Referral made to: ___ ___ ___ ___ ___ ___ ___	1. Intervention(s) required that can be provided at home. 2. Vital signs stable. 3. Referral made to: ___ ___ ___ ___ ___ for: ☐ Nsg. ☐ PT ☐ OT ☐ HHA ☐ SW ☐ Lab ☐ Nutrition ☐ Speech		1. Wounds require no intervention beyond available support. 2. Independent ADLs or independent with available support. 3. Independent transfer/ambulation for 50 feet or independent with available support. 4. Independent on stairs if required or independent with available support. 5. Medically stable. 6. Patient understands diet, medical regimen.
II. Psycho-social Status	Support in place for extended care/nursing facility.		Support in place for rehab placement.	Support in place for home with services.		Support in place for home without services.

TO BE KEPT IN PROGRESS NOTE SECTION OF CHART AT ALL TIMES.

Figure 7.4 Example of a page from the Adult Craniotomy Pathway demonstrating criteria for level-of-care requirements at discharge. NRSG = nursing; rehab = rehabilitation; ADL = activities of daily living; Nsg = nursing; PT= physical therapy; OT = occupational therapy; HHA = home health aide; SW = social worker.

CLINICAL PATH: Adults Craniotomy
Page 16 of 16

DAILY ANTICIPATED OUTCOMES					
POD 2	DATE /INIT /WHEN MET	POD 3	DATE /INIT /WHEN MET	POD 4	DATE /INIT /WHEN MET
Wound dressing dry and intact		No signs of infection		Wound is clean and dry	
Afebrile					
Neuro status at baseline or improving.		Neuro status at baseline or improving.		Neuro status at baseline or improving.	
Tolerates nutrition		Wound edges approximately well without drainage		No signs of CSF leakage	
Pt is able to communicate effectively		Pt states knowledge of d/c instruction wound care, medications follow-up		Pt states knowledge of d/c instruction wound care, medications follow-up	
Pt/family asking pertinent questions regarding d/c		Pt/family asking pertinent questions regarding d/c		No signs of infection	
Voiding qs		Home care needs addressed and met (including transportation home)		Home care needs addressed	
Ambulates with assist		Ambulates independently			
No signs of CSF leakage		No signs of CSF leakage			
Pain score 3 or less in scale 1 to 10 after analgesics					

TO BE KEPT IN PROGRESS NOTE SECTION OF CHART AT ALL TIMES.

Figure 7.5 Daily anticipated outcomes. POD = postoperative day; INIT = initially; CSF = cerebrospinal fluid; Pt = patient; d/c = discharge; qs = quantity sufficient;

tions are based on desired patient outcomes, not staff tasks.

Because not every patient is the same, variations in LOS will invariably occur. Within limits, patients can continue on the pathway despite some patients' requiring extra days in the ICU or at the end of their stay. These variations can be managed technically by the use of "insert-day" and "end-of-stay insert-day" forms (*Fig. 7.6*). These forms are similar to the last regular ICU day in the normal pathway or a repetition of the last day of the regular pathway in the case of an extra end-of-stay day, with the addition of a menu listing the reasons why the extra day(s) occurred. These insert-day reasons are collected and the variances examined on a regular basis. The forms allow the improvement team, which is responsible for the long-term management of the pathway, to identify further opportunities for improvement. Pareto chart analysis (see Chapter 5) of these reasons helps prioritize the problems and direct one's focus on specific interventions (*Fig. 7.7*) (5). At our institution, the cardiac surgery pathway team recognized that 15% of pa-

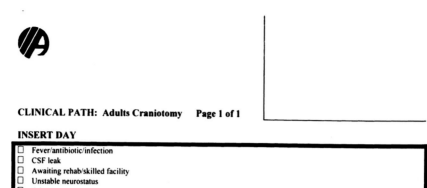

CLINICAL PATH: Adults Craniotomy   Page 1 of 1

INSERT DAY

☐	Fever/antibiotic/infection
☐	CSF leak
☐	Awaiting rehab/skilled facility
☐	Unstable neurostatus
☐	Other:_____

ORDERS/INTERVENTIONS

POD Date_____	Date/Time/ Init			
Specimen/ Tests	**D**	**E**	**N**	
Treatment				Straight cath q 6-8 hrs prn if no void Incentive spirometry q 1 h x 10 while awake Assess wound Dressing by MD until progress to OR cap, then change prn Thigh high TEDS remove q shift for 30 mins
IVs				D/C saline well when IV meds complete, collaborate with MD to change meds to PO
Medications				See Medex
Activity/Safety				OOB, ambulating
Nutrition				Usual diet as tolerated
Protocols				☐ Pain Management Fall Prevention ☐ Seizure Protocol ☐

Consults				PT consult for motor weakness, gait disturbance
				OT consult if upper extremity weakness, cognitive deficit, need for
				   splinting/positioning, ADL deficit
				Speech consult if aphasia, swallowing disturbance, slurred speech or cognitive
				   liquinstic deficit.

Teaching				☐ Post-op Craniotomy Care Instruction Sheet ☐ Seizure Instruction Sheet ☐
Assessment				VS, neurochecks and CSF leakage q 4 h and prn I & O q shift until IV discontinued
Additional orders/ Interventions				Discharge pt if outcomes are met

H#95557   (2/99)

PLACE IN NURSING KARDEX/BINDER DURING USE

Figure 7.6   Insert day. Note that the reason for an extended LOS is required at top of form. POD = postoperative day; D = days; E = evenings; N = nights; prn = as needed; MD = doctor; OOB = out of bed; PT = physical therapy; OT = occupational therapy; ADL = activities of daily living; VS = vital signs; CSF = cerebrospinal fluid; pt = patient.

tient discharges were delayed because of inadequate anticoagulation at the time the patients were otherwise meeting the discharge criteria. A protocol was developed to address this issue by earlier institution of oral anticoagulation therapy and more active management by a home health care worker to monitor therapeutic levels;

this protocol resulted in a reduction in LOS. Lumbar laminectomy patients (and other neurosurgical patients) were frequently discharged late in the day or even the day following their meeting of the expected discharge outcomes. Pareto charts revealed that the most frequent cause for the delay was there was no one avail-

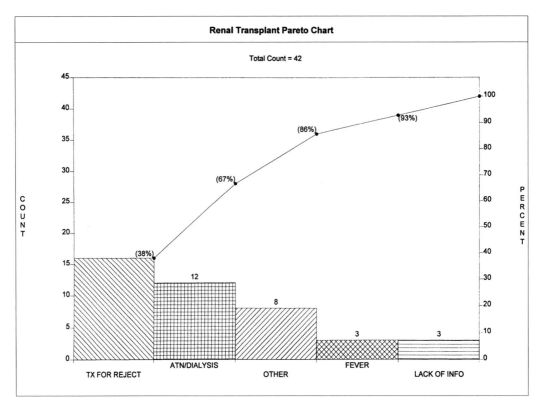

Figure 7.7   A Pareto chart example from renal transplant data, which were obtained from an insert-day-variance report. The chart suggests the focus for improvement on treatment for rejection and acute tubular necrosis (ATN). TX = treatment.

able to pick them up from the hospital. Patients were not told far enough in advance of their impending discharge to make necessary arrangement for a ride home! The team developed a strategy to actively deal with this issue, which greatly reduced this cause for delay and positively impacted the LOS and patient throughput.

Initially, in mapping orders and interventions, standard order sets are included; however, not all orders are standard or can be written in advance (e.g., medications requiring mg/kg dosing). Most pharmacy orders are put on a separate order form because of the complex nature of the pharmacy ordering process (and, in our institution, a lack of automated, computer order entry) and the patient-specific nature of many medication orders (*Fig. 7.8*). Some orders are determined at decision points along the pathway and others require direct physician input because consensus was not achieved. However, these order forms can allow for a prompting for specific orders that is particularly helpful in a teaching environment.

Once the pathway has been mapped and before it is fully implemented, it should be tested in a limited setting. Invariably, flaws are discovered that need to be corrected. Revisions, additions, deletions, and other changes are inevitable. Producing a smoothly running pathway in practice is difficult to accomplish solely on paper and in theory. Real-life experience is the real test of the document, and the choice of where the trial should be conducted is important. Initiation of the trial on a unit where some pathway team members work is helpful. Unit education is more easily accomplished when members of the pathway development team are part of the trial. You can increase the chances of success by polishing the pathway in a limited real-world trial. Full implementation prior to a limited trial can lead to frustration, cynicism, and rejection of the pathway process itself.

After completing the trial, after the revisions are incorporated, and prior to full implementation, staff education is necessary to further increase the chances of a smooth introduction of

**PHYSICIAN'S ORDER
SHEET/DEPENDENT PROTOCOL**

Instructions:
1. Imprint patient's plate before placing in chart.
2. The order must be dated, timed, and signed by the ordering credentialed practitioner.
3. Check all boxes that apply.
4. Cross out all orders that are not applicable.
5. Fax to pharmacy.

ALLERGIES:	WEIGHT:	LB.	KG.

CRANIOTOMY CLINICAL PATH ORDERS
(Page 1 of 1)

Post-Op Craniotomy:

1. Implement Craniotomy clinical path (excludes: intra cerebral or subarachnoid hemorrage, skull based procedures, and intubated patients).   Diagnosis:_____
2. Transfer to _____
3. Medications:
   a. Cefazolin 1g IV, if not allergic, q 8 h x 2. If drain in place, continue for 1 dose after drain removed. Notify pharmacy when drain removed.
      In a patient with penicillin allergy history, risk of cross-allergy with cephalosporin is negligible if reaction was either:
      1. Limited to rash and/or itching <u>only</u>   2. Not consistent with hives
      3. Not consistent with allergy   4. Vague, with no reaction in past 10 years
      5. Present, but subsequent cephalosporin use without reaction
      In such patients, use of cefazolin is recommended as drug of choice.
      ☐ **Do not** give cefazolin: ☐ penicillins allergic and does not meet above criteria or ☐ cephalosporin allergic)
      Order alternate antibiotic on Antibiotic Order Sheet.
   b. Acetaminophen 650 mg PO q 6 h prn for pain, temp >101.5F.
   c. Pain med:_____
   d. Droperidol 0.625 mg IV q 6 h prn, may repeat x1 in 30 mins.
   e. Ortho Bowel Regime
   f. Steroid_____
   g. Antacid and/or H2 blocker_____
   h. Post-op anti-convulsant_____
   i. Post-op anti-hypertensive and blood pressure parameters_____
   j. Calcium channel blocker_____
   k. Other Meds_____
4. PT/OT/Speech Therapy evaluate and treat if patient meets criteria in path.
5. Eye Care: ☐ lubricant ophthalmic ointment _____ eye q hs and prn   ☐ artificial tears 1-2 qtts_____ eye q 2 h
6. Additional Assessment: ☐ continuous BP monitoring via arterial line
                              ☐ continuous CVP
                              ☐ continuous Cardiac Monitoring
                              ☐ continuous ICP Monitoring
7. Other:_____

Credentialed Practitioner Signature		/ /
Print	Pager#	Date Time

PT evaluate and treat	RN Signature:	/	/
OT evaluate and treat	RN Signature:	/	/
Speech Therapy evaluate and treat	RN Signature:	/	/
For Swallow ☐ Speech ☐		Date	Time

(To activate consultations, please fax form to Rehab Department, ext. 4492)

Approval:

REVIEW:
DISTRIBUTION:
H#95557 (2/99)

Protocol Committee:
Medical Record Forms & Guidelines:
REVISION:

TO BE FILED IN PHYSICIAN ORDER SECTION OF CHART

Figure 7.8 A physician's order form, which can be faxed to the appropriate ancillary service to initiate treatment. PT = physical therapy; OT = occupational therapy; prn = as needed; BP = blood pressure; CVP = central venous pressure; ICP = intracranial pressure.

the pathway. Time spent introducing the goals, objectives, and rationale of the pathway process, as well as the anatomy of the pathway itself, to the health care workers will avoid many pitfalls. It is best to have the team members assist in this education phase: a nurse pathway team member for the nurses and a physician team member for other physicians who will be admitting patients included on the pathway. This encourages ownership by the users and sends a clear message that the pathway is a product developed by the very people who care for the patients. The feeling of an imposed set of rules generated by outsiders is avoided. In addition, a knowledgeable resource person should be available to answer questions both before and during the initial stage of full implementation.

The implementation phase requires attention, as it undoubtedly produces many changes for the personnel. A clear understanding of when and where the pathway begins, who is excluded, and what the exceptions are prevents confusion and incomplete inclusion of appropriate patients. The pathway team must continue to meet and review the performance of the pathway and discuss and solve ongoing problems. After the pathway is fully integrated into day-to-day operations, the pathway team's job is complete; however, the process is not finished.

Continuous quality improvement techniques must be applied to the pathway effort. Long-term responsibility for the pathway, maintaining the gains achieved, and making future improvements should be transferred to a responsible standing committee, such as a departmental quality improvement team or other interdisciplinary team that cares for that patient population. The role of this group is to monitor and manage the continuing performance of the pathway. This monitoring process should be part of the normal operations of the QIT. Monitoring entails analyzing variations in performance and measuring outcomes and satisfaction. Emphasis should focus on group rather than individual performance. Monitoring can identify future opportunities for improvement. The use of standard quality tools such as control charts and Pareto charts (see Chapter 5) can assist the team in identifying special causes for investigation or common problems in the process and assist in determining priorities for the focus of future improvement efforts (3, 5).

One method for analysis of performance uses a balanced scorecard approach that measures categories in a consistent manner with the institution's mission, vision, and strategic priorities (7, 8). At our institution, we evaluate a pathway's performance in terms of quality out-

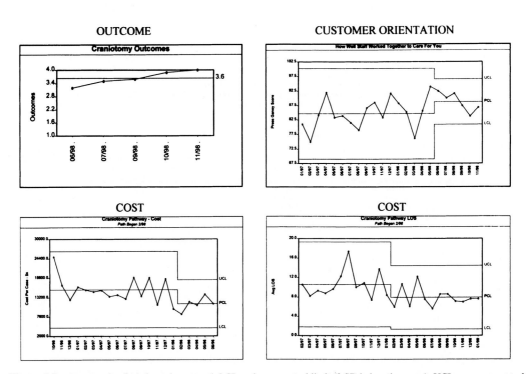

Figure 7.9　An example of a balanced scorecard. LCL = lower control limit (3 SD below the mean); UCL = upper control limit (3 SD above the mean); PCL = process center line mean. Note that the control lines were recalculated at the time of implementation of a critical process change and that the LOS control limits narrow, indicating that the process is coming under greater control.

comes, customer satisfaction, and cost or efficiency (*Fig. 7.9*). By looking at a balanced spectrum, we hope to avoid a situation in which a pathway inadvertently has a negative impact on one or another of these categories. For example, a pathway might result in reduced cost but cause a higher morbidity and lower patient satisfaction. Every pathway must assure the team members that, first and foremost, patient outcomes do not suffer as a result of the changes instituted in the management of patients. Whenever possible, benchmark data should be used to compare progress with national standards and trends.

The scorecards are tracked on individual x-bar control charts over time (see Chapter 5). Monthly data are analyzed in relation to the arithmetic mean and the control limits. Several run tests are performed on the data to establish whether the process is in control or changing as a result of improvement implementations (3, 5). These test include the following:

- Six consecutive points going up, or six consecutive points going down;
- Six consecutive points above or below the mean; and
- One point outside either the upper or lower control limit.

Pareto charts-of-variance explanations allow prioritization of the effort in correcting LOS extensions, as previously mentioned.

EXAMPLES OF SUCCESSFUL PATHWAY DEVELOPMENT

Several pathway efforts at our institution are presented to illustrate the principles outlined in this chapter. Craniotomy procedures were chosen as a high-complexity, high-resource–utilizing operation with a large potential for improvements. The team consisted of two neurosurgeons, two staff nurses from the neuroscience unit, the nurse manager and a clinical nurse specialist, occupational therapist, case manager, and quality facilitator. Others (e.g., speech therapist) were consulted for their specific expertise during segments of the process. The team met, agreed to a convenient future monthly meeting time and place, set ground rules, and began the development process. Previous year's data were analyzed, including minimum, average, and maximum LOSs. A high-level flow chart was

developed (*Fig. 2*). Several complexities were quickly identified. The diversity of the diagnoses for which craniotomy was performed often significantly altered the type of care the patient received. Review of this information allowed for a lumping of several diagnoses together and the exclusion of others from the pathway. For example, skull base procedures and patients with severe head injuries had very different courses and treatment requirements from patients with brain tumors. The team elected to path all craniotomy patients, except those who required ventilatory support postoperatively, underwent skull base operations, and suffered from subarachnoid hemorrhages. From the physicians' perspective, the patients lumped into the pathway still seemed very nonhomogeneous, but from the nurses' perspective the care was similar. On the basis of institutional data and Milliman and Robertson's (12 data, a LOS was set at five days (with discharge on postoperative day 4).

During the mapping of the orders and interventions, many issues arose that required resolution. Research and discussion on the topic of monitoring requirements and level of care generated a consensus that these patients did not require an intensive care setting in the postoperative period (16, 18). When it was determined that different units assessed patients differently, a subgroup devised a universal neurological assessment form and educated those units in its use. During the development of the discharge outcomes, it was determined that many patients met the discharge criteria except that they still had their sutures in place. Arrangements with home health care agencies to provide this service satisfied this issue and allowed for earlier discharge in some cases.

After a limited trial, pathway revisions, education, and implementation, the team remained together for two additional months to assure a smooth transition. Several operational issues, further education, and other minor problems were resolved or accomplished. The continued monitoring then passed to the permanent QIT of the Neuroscience Institute. This team added craniotomy LOS, cost, and patient satisfaction data to its scorecard. A simple outcome tool that was based on ideal operative goals was developed to follow patient outcomes (*Fig. 7.10*).

The craniotomy pathway decreased the LOS by 1.06 days per patient and the cost of providing

NEUROSCIENCE INSTITUTE QUALITY IMPROVEMENT TEAM

CRANIOTOMY PATIENT OUTCOME SCORE

Patient Name: _____ DOB: _____

MR#: _____ DOS: _____

Met Surgery Goal	Expected Patient Outcome	Neurologic Complication	Other Complication
No - 0	No - 0	Yes - 0	Yes - 0
Yes- 1	Yes- 1	No - 1	No - 1

Total overall score: _____

Figure 7.10   An example of a craniotomy outcome tool, which the surgeon completes. DOB = date of birth.

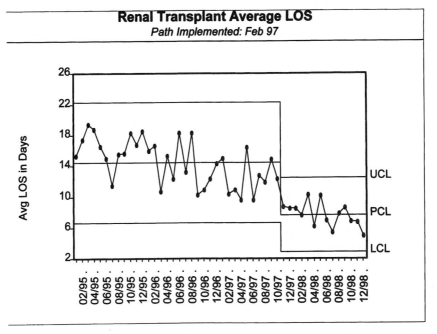

Figure 7.11   A renal transplant average LOS control chart. UCL = upper control limit; PCL = process center line; LCL = lower control limit.

care by $1,458. This will lead to a projected savings of $200,000 to $500,000 per year. Patient satisfaction remains at high levels compared with national standards (15). The neurological outcomes, mortality rate, and other morbidities have not changed. The life of the pathway development team was six months.

The renal transplant team was convened when national benchmark data revealed that the LOS for these patients was excessively long (22). Because our graft survival rates were among the best in the nation, the transplant surgeons were reluctant to alter their procedures. With encouragement and assurance that outcomes would be closely monitored, the surgeons agreed to participate in development and implementation of a renal transplant pathway. After full implementation, the care team was able to reduce the average LOS by seven days, reduce cost by $10,000 per patient, maintain a high level of patient satisfaction, and maintain a graft survival rate of 98.5% compared with the national average of 84% (20). Critical scrutiny of the use of laboratory testing resulted in significant reductions in costs of ancillary services. The pathway resulted in an initial reduction in LOS of two days. After six months of experience and an analysis of end-of-stay variance data, the team determined that, by moving portions of the intravenous therapies required to treat for rejection into the outpatient setting, further reductions could be realized. This achieved a lowering of LOS an additional five days. This effort required institutional support for outpatient lodging for out-of-town patients and the use of the hospital outpatient observation and infusion center (OOIC) for intravenous infusions (*Fig. 7.11*).

The vascular surgery team developed a lower-extremity revascularization pathway and was able to decrease LOS by 3.81 days and decrease cost by $1,840 per patient. This team was able to accomplish these outcomes by removing the unwanted variation in the timing of the initiation of rehabilitative services. If the patient cannot ambulate on postoperative day 1, a physical therapist is automatically consulted and begins moving the patient toward independence or begins planning home therapy. Similarly, patients with joint replacements have early rehabilitative services and preoperative home assessments for their postoperative needs, thereby avoiding delays at the time of discharge.

PEARLS AND PITFALLS: LESSONS LEARNED

Quality Before Cost

Interestingly, although physicians and other health care workers complain about cost cutting rather than quality outcomes as the focus of pathway development, it is often the physicians who become fixated on cost. Quality outcomes and best practice must remain the focus of pathway development. This is where the expertise of the group lies. Health care workers are not experts in cost savings.

Perfect Data

During the analysis and development phases of the project, data on current practice are used to assist in decision making. Physicians often find inaccuracies in the data provided that then may consume an inordinate amount of time in discussions and attempts to "improve" the data, thereby delaying if not paralyzing the process. Information may never be perfect; the team must accept this and move on. Of course decisions made on erroneous information might lead to erroneous conclusions; however, some degree of error is acceptable and can allow proper decision making without jeopardizing the result. Data that can display trends and assist in consensus building are what is required. The quest for perfect data can be a never-ending search.

Improvement versus Judgment

The process of pathway development inevitably reveals significant variations in performance among practitioners. The purpose of pathway development is to move the group toward the best practice. Focusing on individual performance, especially in a punitive way, undermines a major principle of quality improvement (5, 9). Data should be used for learning and improvement, not for judgment. Usually individual behavior, when obviously deviating from that of the peer group, will be altered simply by reporting the pathway variations to the physicians. The effects of tacit peer pressure are powerful. Years ago, well before pathways, our neurosurgical group presented data on LOS for lumbar discectomy by physician (coded). Each physician knew the code but not that of the other neurosurgeons. One physician's LOSs were several days longer than the other physicians' LOSs. After that meeting, the outlying physician's LOSs became the same as the groups' as a whole. Not a word had been said and that individual soon realized that, not only were his outcomes not adversely affected, but that by reducing LOS, he was able to make much more efficient use of his time, which had been previously spent following up with patients who were hospitalized for extra days.

Be the Patient's Best Advocate

By keeping the patient's best interest in mind, a pathway will produce results that are good for the doctor as well. Healthy and satisfied patients use fewer hospital resources and less physician time and energy. Focus on the process through the patient's eyes rather than the providers. Use patient satisfaction surveys to confirm the patient's response to the implementations.

Manage Change

Change is difficult for most humans, particularly physicians who consider themselves to be experts in what they do. This is paradoxical because physician education is built on the principle that medical science is ever changing and requires continuous education for a lifetime of practice. Consideration of the difficulties physicians experience when their ''tried and true'' practices are challenged and the management of those issues require a skillful facilitator. Because physician participation is the critical ingredient to the success of the process, attention to allaying physician concerns regarding the process at the initial stage will help assure physicians' productive involvement.

Manage Time

Physician and other patient care workers' most precious commodity is their time. No one will remain engaged in the process of pathway development to its conclusion if time is wasted. The inefficient use of time increases the likelihood that focus will be lost and that an inferior pathway will result. Choose acceptable meeting times and stick to agendas and timelines.

Educate the Staff

After the completion of the pathway process, the team must still remain active in the implementation phase. Insufficient education of those unit members with whom the pathway is to be initiated may lead to frustration, noncompliance, and outright rejection of the pathway. Time spent educating staff will smooth out this transition period.

Decide and Move On

Once consensus is reached on a given element in the pathway, it is nonproductive to revisit it continually. The tendency, for the members who differed in their opinion during the discussion of that element but who were ultimately persuaded to accept a differing viewpoint and a consensus position, is to revisit that element at the next meeting. The group must insist that this behavior is inappropriate. It is important to remember that a pathway is not written in stone. Future experience may allow for alteration and even reversal of initial positions. However, during the development phase, once sufficient data, analysis, and discussion have occurred and consensus is reached, the team must move on.

Substituting the Pathway for Thinking

An additional pitfall with pathway development is the tendency to allow the pathway to dictate all aspects of care for an individual patient. The pathway represents the care for a hypothetical patient. Real patients may or may not follow the flow that the pathway outlines. Thoughtful daily evaluation of patients, whether they are on a pathway, determines what orders and interventions are appropriate. For patients on a pathway, additions and deletions to the orders, interventions, and other decisions should be amended when warranted. However, habitual alterations of the pathway by individual physicians reneging on their previous commitment to a consensus agreement should be discouraged.

Administrative Support

Important to the success of any quality management program, of which pathway development is a part, is the atmosphere in which the effort is fostered. The top-down commitment of the administration and physician leaders of the organization is critical, and their support must be tangible. Every employee should believe that the administration is committed to providing a quality product. The quality effort should not be added work; it should be integrated into the normal workday. This effort requires resources and staff time (i.e., monetary expenditure). By providing support of this type, the administration demonstrates its commitment. A culture of continuous quality improvement is one in which pathway development is a natural consequence. If it improves quality, it is what is expected and supported.

Physician Participation

Because the ultimate responsibility is with the physician in regards to patient care, the most essential component of the pathway process is physician buy-in. A lack of consistent physician participation and engagement in the development team's effort are problems that will preclude the pathway from achieving the intended goals. A special charge to the physician participants by the senior leaders at the outset can establish clear expectations for the physicians and energize them toward seeing this process through to its successful conclusion.

Resident Staff Participation

In teaching institutions, house staff are generally on the front line in the care of patients; they are often the responsible party for the institution of pathways and compliance with the pathways' orders and interventions. Therefore, enlisting resident participation is vital to the successful implementation of pathways. Strategies to increase the likelihood of house-staff involvement should be considered. At our institution, all incoming residents receive a general introduction to clinical pathways and the expectations related to the clinical pathways are made explicitly clear. Resident participation on pathway teams allows for input from this essential group and communication among the house-staff regarding pathway issues. At the time of implementation of a new pathway, the resident team member participates in the education process of his or her peers. Clear responsibility for resident compliance is delineated, usually through the chief resident. The service chief is responsible for the maintenance of high rates of compliance with pathway usage. If compliance falls or variations rise, and an analysis of the root cause points to resident behavior, the service chief intervenes. The service chief and chief resident introduce new members to the existing clinical pathways at the beginning of each rotation as part of the normal orientation process.

Next Steps

Evaluation of the pathway process is critical to continuous improvement in patient care. The area of long-term patient outcomes has lagged in its development relative to other quality improvement measures. The Rand SF 36 is a long-term, functional health status tool used to measure outcomes at 6month, one-year, and two-year intervals (1). This and other such tools are needed to validate short-term solutions and presumed benefits to patients brought about by the pathway process.

Most clinical pathways focus on an acute episode of care, but this process has potential for a much wider application. Extension of the pathway both before and after the acute hospital episode is possible and frequently desirable. Disease management should be the ultimate goal in our attempts to improve the health of patient populations.

REFERENCES

1. About Rand SF 36: *http://www.mcw.edu/midas.health.*
2. Agency for Health Care Policy and Research: *http://www.ahcpr.gov*
3. Balestracci D: Quality improvement: Practical applications for medical group practice. Center for Research in Ambulatory Health Care Administration, Englewood, 1996, ed 2.
4. Gerteis M, Edgman-Levitan S, Daley J: Through the patient's eyes: Understanding and promoting patient-centered care. San Francisco, Jossey-Bass, 1993.
5. Graham L: Q100 series: Core quality education. Albany, NY, Albany Medical Center, 1996.
6. Jeffrey NA: Paper chase of a cancer patient. *The Wall Street Journal* March 1, 1999:B1.
7. Kaplan R, Norton D: The balanced scorecard measures that drive performance. *Harvard Business Review* XX:75–85, 1992.
8. Kaplan R, Norton D: The balanced scorecard. Boston, Harvard Business Press, 1996:167–189.
9. Langley G, Nolan K, Nolan T: The improvement guide. San Francisco, Jossey-Bass, 1996.
10. Manthey M: Leaders empower staff. Minneapolis, Creative Nursing Management, 1991:35.
11. Merry M: The death of a paradigm. *Inside Case Management* 1:2, 1995.
12. Schibanoff J: Health Care management guidelines: Inpatient and Surgical Care, Milliman and Robertson, 1992.
13. National Institutes of Health: *http://www.nih.gov.*
14. Popp AJ: The neurosurgical workforce: Market effects, public policy, and professional constraints, in Bean JR (ed): *Neurosurgery in Transition, The Socioeconomic Transformation of Neurological Surgery, Concepts in Neurosurgery.* Baltimore, MD, Lippincott, Williams and Wilkins, 1998, 112–132, vol 9.
15. Press Ganey Inc: Patient satisfaction survey results. Albany, NY, Albany Medical Center.
16. Sarkinssian S, Wallace C: Clinical indicators contributing to I.C.U. length of stay in elective craniotomy patients with brain tumor. *Axone* 17:42–45, 1995.
17. Schwarz R: The skilled facilitator. San Francisco, Jossey-Bass, 1994.
18. Taylor W, Thomas N, Wellings J, et al: Timing of postoperative intracranial hematoma. *J Neurosurg* 82: 48–50, 1995.
19. Deleted in proof.
20. United Network of Organ Sharing: *http://www.unos.org.*
21. University Health System Consortium: *http://www.uhc.org.*
22. University Health System Consortium: Benchmark studies: Renal transplant study participation. Oak Brook, IL UHC, 1997.
23. University Health System Consortium (UHC): Process analysis and pathway development. Oak Brook, IL UHC, 1993.
24. Vincenzino J: Trends in medical care costs: Evolving market forces. *Metropolitan Ins Co Bull* 79(3):8–15, 1998.
25. Winslow R, Rundle RL: Aetna reels in wake of $116 million damages verdict. *The Wall Street Journal.* January 22, 1999:B:4.
26. Zander K: Managing outcomes through collaborative care. Chicago, American Hospital Publishing, 1995.

CHAPTER 8

Measuring and Monitoring for Performance Improvement

JEROD M. LOEB, Ph.D., BARBARA I. BRAUN, Ph.D.,
LINDA S. HANOLD, M.H.S.A., AND RICHARD G. KOSS, M.A.

EDITOR'S NOTE: The costs of instituting continuous process improvement are the loss of time involved in pursuing quality improvement team activities and the financial implications of measuring and collecting the data necessary to make real-time, data-based, management decisions. Both are important investments that may temporarily lower productivity over the short-term while greatly enhancing production capability over the long term. It is important to make process measurement as inexpensive and unobtrusive as possible (or the act of measurement will actually disrupt or effect the process itself). It is equally important to choose the correct process measurement probe and measurement probe insertion point within the process. A proper measurement probe requires pilot study validation for measurement reliability and reproducibility. The proper insertion point allows detection of even subtle changes in customer-defined quality characteristics with each empiric attempt at process improvement. If iterations of the plan–do–check–act cycle do not lead to measurable changes in process outcome, the quality improvement team must reexamine the validity of their measurement probe or the appropriateness of their probe insertion point and change their measurement strategy accordingly. Physicians must resist the misguided temptation to act on data simply because they are already measured (no additional cost) and easily available, rather than because they are the most important, relevant, and reliable data for improving the process in question.

KEY CHALLENGES OF QUALITY MEASUREMENT

Arguments about the need for enhanced accountability in health care, although around since early this century, may finally be reaching fruition. Although the faces behind such calls for accountability have surely changed, the overriding intent has not—using the derived information for more appropriate decision making by multiple stakeholders while using the data for quality improvement purposes within health care organizations.

Critical to the notion of accountability in health care is the availability of valid, reliable, and relevant data presented in a manner that enlightens rather than confuses. In health care, these data are derived from the measurement of performance—of individuals, organizations, and systems. This performance may have bearing on clinical outcomes of care, functional health status, patient satisfaction with care, or financial activities within the organization. It has been repeatedly demonstrated that organizations can only improve what they can measure. Performance in health care represents not only an elaboration of what is done within an organization but, because the basis for all measurement is comparative, some estimation of how well the process or outcome of care might fare on a longitudinal basis within the same organization (or perhaps compared with the same process or outcome of care at different organizations).

Measure-related questions can vary, depending on the source of the question. Physicians are usually concerned about how their individual clinical outcomes might compare with the outcomes of other physicians who are in a similar specialty and treating the same types of patients. This type of information can lead to changes in practice patterns, reduce geographic variation in care, and help to implement best practices. Patients are increasingly seeking information on the performance of individual physicians, hospitals, or health plans. Such information can have profound bearing on where or to whom a patient goes to receive health care or medical care. Purchasers are demanding data relating to clinical outcomes, functional health status, patients' perceptions of care quality, and financial performance. From a more teleological perspective, we all are (or should be) concerned about whether limited health care resources are being spent effectively. For example, in the consideration of patients with neurological illnesses, there is considerable interest in defining the mortality rate for a given hospital or surgeon: whether the rate is stable over time and whether the rate is better or worse than in other hospitals. Some of these data are already available in specific regions of the country. As has recently been noted, the era of "scorecard medicine" has arrived (36, 37). However, many complex challenges remain in answering questions with respect to data collection, data analysis, and, ultimately, turning data into useful information for disparate stakeholders.

Everyone wants measurement but no one enjoys being measured. Measurement is rarely a neutral activity. It evokes considerable anxiety and frustration, particularly among those being measured. Consequently, great care must be exerted in assuring that the tools to be used for measurement are scientifically sound. Unfortunately, there is no concordant focus or philosophy that is extant in health care performance measurement today. Some organizations approach measurement from the myopic perspective of identifying the data available and then defining the questions to ask. Others first define the question and then seek data to be used to answer the question. Finally, and perhaps more correctly, others first define the question, then determine whether reliable and valid data are available, and then weigh whether the costs of collecting additional data are reasonable.

Although performance measurement is becoming an expectation within health care, many challenges still remain unsolved; key among these is the question of value. Linking the use of performance measurement to improvements in health care delivery has not been generally demonstrated beyond a number of anecdotal reports. Because the increasing use of performance measurement clearly adds new costs to an already strained health care economy, value must be demonstrated. This demonstration of value should include documentation that the information permits consumers to make better decisions regarding where to go for health care.

This chapter discusses what to consider when choosing performance measures and how to improve performance when opportunities for improvement are identified. Specifically, this chapter describes the purposes of performance measurement, factors to consider when deciding what to measure and at what level of detail, and criteria for evaluating measures. Finally, it presents a structured approach to implementing performance measurement and improvement activities.

ESTABLISHING THE PURPOSES FOR MEASUREMENT

The two most frequently cited purposes for measuring performance are continuous quality improvement (CQI) and demonstrating accountability. CQI in health care involves the application of industrial management techniques with an emphasis on measuring and reducing undesirable process variation (3, 22). Measurement of performance is essential to understand whether a change is an improvement. The principles and tools of CQI are described in detail in other chapters in this book and are not addressed here.

The effectiveness of the CQI movement has been examined, but the results to date have been somewhat equivocal (5, 7). Shortell et al. (34) identified three conditions under which CQI applications are more likely to be effective: (1) when they are carefully focused on areas of real importance to the organization and addressed with clearly formulated interventions; (2) when the organization is ready for change and has prepared itself by appointing capable leadership, creating relationships of trust with physicians, and developing adequate information systems; and (3) when there is a conducive external environment relative to beneficial regulatory, payment policy and competitive factors.

Although it might not be useful to separate measurement for improvement from measurement for the purposes of accountability, such a distinction has been made by a number of authors. Measurement for accountability is based on the premise that external reporting of meaningful data will be useful to purchasers, regulators, and ultimately consumers for choosing the best health care providers (12). Measurement for accountability includes collecting data for use by regulators, purchasers, accreditors, business groups, and consumers or meeting state mandates such as the Pennsylvania Health Care Cost

Containment Council. In theory, purchasers and consumers should use performance measure information to choose the best performing providers at a given cost, thereby driving the market to compete on the basis of quality, which should result in an overall improvement in care. The usefulness of such data for consumers has yet to be demonstrated because of issues related to salience and understandability of individual measures as well as consumers' knowledge of how managed care systems work (16, 33).

In addition to providing information to consumers, public disclosure of performance data can be useful for setting national or regional benchmarks that can also stimulate improvement among health care organizations. In some cases, improvement over time has been demonstrated (15, 25). However, the effectiveness of stimulating improvement through public report cards also remains controversial (see references 9, 13, and 14 for a discussion of value and validity of measurement used in report cards).

Because of its conceptual appeal, the demand for externally reported performance data continues to grow and has spawned several new initiatives designed to standardize the topic areas and measures collected. The need for standardized performance measures is a prominent public policy issue. In the landmark report to President Clinton, the Advisory Commission on Consumer Protection and Quality in the Health Care Industry called for a national effort to develop and implement effective, efficient and coordinated strategies for ensuring the public availability of valid and reliable information on quality (31). Examples of initiatives to standardize measurement include: (1) a performance measurement partnership among the American Medical Association, which addresses performance measurement at the level of the physician; the Joint Commission on Accreditation of Health Care Organizations (JCAHO), which accredited provider health care organizations; and the National Committee for Quality Assurance, which accredits managed health care plans; (2) the National Quality Forum on Health Care Measurement and Reporting, which is a group convened by Vice President Gore to identify a core set of measures, foster investment in data systems, promote dissemination of data, and ensure public access to comparative information, and (3) the Study of Clinically Relevant Indicators of Pharmacologic Therapy (SCRIPT), funded by the Health Care Financing Administration, which is led by the Coalition for Quality in Medication Use comprising 48 public and private sector organizations involved in a medication use and quality improvement project whose goal is to produce a core set of valid and reliable measures related to improving medication use and management.

Performance measurement for improvement and accountability are complementary (30). As mentioned previously, publicly reported performance on selected measures has been improving over time. Though compatible is many ways, these two purposes for measurement can sometimes conflict with regard to the selection of specific performance measures (26). For quality improvement activities, quality improvement leaders may need to develop or customize performance measures that address a specific subject to be measured (e.g., surgical wound infections after craniotomy). Performance measurement for accountability, on the other hand, demands the use of standardized measures that can be risk adjusted, if needed, to facilitate valid comparisons across organizations (12). For example, quality improvement staff in an inpatient facility may suspect an internal problem with postoperative infections in neurosurgery and might wish to launch a longitudinal investigation related to surgical site infections. However, their state requires mandatory data collection and reporting of measures related to cardiovascular surgery, an area in which they have traditionally excelled. Staffing constraints, the costs of additional data collection, and external requirements may prohibit pursuit of the additional initiative. Consequently, the mandated measures may show little use for improving performance in certain circumstances.

Other potential purposes for performance measurement include: to satisfy regulatory or accreditation-related requirements, to make informed judgments about the stability of existing processes (e.g., undesirable process variation), and to identify the need to redesign processes and to determine whether improvements or redesign of processes meet specified objectives. For example, organizations often establish new services, extend product lines, occupy a new facility, or design or redesign functions or systems; performance measurement should be built into new or modified processes to assess whether the processes were designed well.

DETERMINING WHAT TO MEASURE

Determining what to measure is one of the most critical steps in the process of performance measurement. Most performance measurement and improvement projects involve a substantial commitment of staff time and energy, training, and equipment resources, all of which should be directed toward the best return on investment. The decision of what gets measured should be driven not by what data are available but by what needs to be measured. In addition to the broader purposes for measurement described previously, some more immediate reasons for measuring performance include:

1. comparative metrics (i.e., how well a particular process or function compares to others)
2. potential problems requiring investigation
3. external requests by stakeholders
4. quality improvement activities to meet regulatory or accreditation requirements

If carefully considered, it may be possible to achieve multiple objectives or satisfy multiple stakeholders with single or related measurement strategies.

Several criteria or factors should be considered when setting priorities for measurement at the organizational level. These include: (1) the organization's mission, care, and services provided; (2) the expected impact on performance; (3) processes that are high risk, high volume, or problem prone; (4) the relationship of an aspect of care to the dimensions of performance, as described in *Table 8.1*, or to key organizational functions; (5) currently available data; and (6) organizational resources.

The organization's leadership plays a major role in setting priorities for measurement. The Joint Commission definition of health care leaders includes at a minimum the leaders of the governing body, the chief executive officer and other senior managers, department leaders, the elected and appointed leaders of the medical staff and clinical departments, other medical staff members in organizational administrative positions, and the nurse executive and other sen-

TABLE 8.1
Dimensions of Performance

Dimension	Description
Doing the right thing	The **efficacy** of the procedure or treatment in relation to the patient's condition; the degree to which the patient's care and services have been shown to accomplish the desired or projected outcome(s).
	The **appropriateness** of a specific test, procedure, or service to meet the patient's needs; the degree to which the care and services provided are relevant to the patient's clinical needs, given the current state of knowledge.
Doing the right thing well	The **availability** of a needed test, procedure, treatment, or service to the patient or customer who needs it; the degree to which appropriate care and services are available to meet the patient's needs.
	The **timeliness** with which a needed test, procedure, treatment, or service is provided to the patient or customer; the degree to which the care and services are provided to the patient at the most beneficial or necessary time.
	The **effectiveness** with which tests, procedures, treatments, and services are provided; the degree to which the care and services are provided in the correct manner, given the current state of knowledge, to achieve the desired or projected outcome for the patient.
	The **continuity** of the services provided to the patient with respect to other services, practitioners, and providers and over time; the degree to which the patient's care is coordinated among disciplines, among organizations, and over time.
	The **safety** of the patient and others when the services are provided; the degree to which the risk of an intervention and risk in the care environment are reduced for the patient and others, including the health care provider.
	The **efficiency** with which tests, procedures, treatment, and services are provided; the relationship between the outcomes (results of care) and the resources used to deliver patient care and services.
	The **respect and caring** with which care and services are provided; the degree to which those providing care and services do so with sensitivity and respect for the patient's needs, expectations, and individual differences; the degree to which the patient or a designee is involved in his or her own care and service decisions.

ior nursing leaders (2). Several studies have identified the importance of leadership, especially physician leadership, at all stages of the quality improvement–performance measurement process (10, 32). Berwick et al. (3) suggested that barriers to physician involvement may be the most important issue impeding the success of quality improvement in medical care. Weiner et al. (39) studied the effects of top management and board and physician leadership on the extent of clinical involvement in hospital CQI–total quality management (TQM) efforts for a large sample of acute-care community hospitals. They found that active staff physician involvement in governance showed positive, significant relationships with the measures of clinical involvement. On the other hand, physician-at-large involvement in governance showed significant negative relationships.

Several potential sources of information may help inform the decision of what to measure. These include: (1) issues identified in regulatory or accreditation reports, (2) risk-management data, (3) utilization management reports, (4)

Clinical Value Compass Worksheet, Side A

① OUTCOMES ➡ Select a population _____
                                                          (specify patient population)

_____

② AIM ➡ What's the general aim? Given our wish to limit or reduce the illness burden for "this type" of patient, what are the desired results?

_____

_____

TIPS: Path Forward ➡

Worksheet purpose: To identify measures of outcomes/costs that contribute most to the value of care.

1. Select a clinically significant population.

2. Assemble small interdisciplinary team.

3. Use brainstorming or nominal group technique to generate "long" list of measures.

4. Start with west (clinical) on the compass and go clockwise around the compass.

5. Use multivoting to identify "short" list of 4 to 12 key measures of outcomes and costs.

6. Determine what data are needed versus what data can be obtained in real time at affordable cost.

7. Use side B of worksheet to record names and definitions of selected measures of value.

③ VALUE ➡ Select starter set of outcomes/cost measures

Functional   _____
• Physical function   _____
• Mental health   _____
• Social/Role   _____
• Other (eg, pain, health risk) _____
                         _____
                         _____

_____ **Clinical**   **Satisfaction**
_____ • Mortality   • Health care delivery   _____
_____ • Morbidity   • Perceived health benefit _____
• Complications
_____   _____
_____
                    Costs   _____
                    • Direct medical   _____
                    • Indirect social _____
                                       _____

Figure 8.1 Clinical value compass worksheet (side A and side B).

quality improvement activities, (5) staff opinions and needs, (6) outcomes of processes or services, (7) autopsy results, (8) patient/customer demographics and diagnostic information, (9) financial data, (10) infection control surveillance and reporting, and (11) morbidity and mortality conferences. Scientific literature often serves as stimulus for measurement activities by the publication of clinical practice guidelines, external benchmarks, studies that measure compliance with accepted practices, or even knowledge about sentinel events at your or another organization.

Joint Commission standards require that organizations select performance measures for processes that are known to jeopardize the potential safety of the individuals served or are associated with sentinel events in similar health care organizations (20). At a minimum, the processes to be measured include: medication use; operative and other invasive and noninvasive procedures, such as radiotherapy, hyperbaric treatment, CAT scan, and MRI that place the patient at risk; use of blood and blood components; restraint use; seclusion when it is part of the care or services provided; and care or services provided to high-risk populations.

One should thoroughly consider what data are already available internally. Within complex organizations, individuals are often unaware of the various databases, registries, performance measurement systems, research studies, and quality improvement projects in which others are engaged. It may be possible to add data elements or coordinate data collection activities with existing projects.

Another notion to keep in mind is that the focus of measurement activity will receive significantly more attention than areas not selected for measurement. To avoid deterioration in other aspects of a process, it is important to consider including other complementary measures. It is helpful to maintain a "balanced dashboard" that allows you to monitor several aspects of a process simultaneously. Nelson et al. (27), in a series of published tutorials directed at clinicians interested in quality improvement, provided a compass analogy that measures outcomes along four dimensions: clinical (e.g., morbidity and mortality), functional (e.g., health status), satisfaction, and costs. *Figure 8.1* presents a worksheet developed by Nelson et al. that uses the compass framework designed to help clinicians

Clinical Value Compass Worksheet, Side B

④ **SPECIFIC OPERATIONAL DEFINITIONS** ▪ **for key outcome and cost measures**

TIPS: Writing Definitions ➡	Variable name and brief *conceptual* definition	Source of data and *operational* definition
A *conceptual definition* is a brief statement describing a variable of interest. It should tell people <u>what</u> you want to measure and who "owns" it. An *operational definition* is a clearly specified <u>method</u> for reliably sorting, classifying, or measuring a variable. It should be written as an instruction set, or protocol, that would enable two different people to measure the variable, by using the same process and thereby producing the same result. It should explain to people <u>how</u> a variable should be measured.	A. Owner: _____	
	B. Owner: _____	
	C. Owner: _____	
	D. Owner: _____	
	E. Owner: _____	
	F. Owner: _____	
	G. Owner: _____	
	H. Owner: _____	

Figure 8.1   *(continued).*

focus and operationalize their measurement activities (27).

A corollary of the notion of what gets measured gets attention is the fact that the act of measurement often changes the behavior of those being measured, both consciously and unconsciously. The classic example of the observer effect is the "white coat phenomena" in blood pressure measurement (35). In physics, a related concept is the Heisenberg principle, which states that the act of measurement disturbs the object measured (e.g., measuring the position of an electron using photons causes a change in the position of the electron).

DETERMINE SCOPE AND LEVEL OF ANALYSIS

Performance measurement and improvement activities can be approached from several different perspectives: organization or system-wide, key functions, departmental or discipline-specific, or patient-population focused. The majority of improvement activities are focused at the department or discipline-specific (e.g., medicine or nursing) level. Berwick and Nolan (4) described the notion that improvements in health care have traditionally been aimed at trying to perfect the discipline-specific elements of care (i.e., by making doctors better at doctoring, nurses better at nursing, or replacing one drug with a better drug). Modern systems theory, on the other hand, suggests that greater improvements can be made through changing the pattern of interactions and in redesigning the overall flow of work across disciplines or departments (23).

When determining the scope of quality improvement, it is important to remember that narrowing the focus allows organizations to better describe processes related to the area of study, collect data, and identify opportunities for improvement. Nelson et al. (28) recommended the phrase "think big, but start small." Consider establishing goals that relate to long-term outcomes, performance improvement, or cost savings and consider "the complex web of causation." However, rather than developing elaborate study designs or sophisticated protocols to jump start quality improvement activities, Nelson et al. recommended that one strive for simplicity and focus on a limited, manageable, clinically meaningful set of starter measures.

ASSESSING AVAILABLE MEASUREMENT TOOLS

Performance measurement is an evolving science, and the tools, or indicators, used to measure health care processes and outcomes are also evolving. Ten years ago, persons who wanted to use performance measures to monitor health care quality had to develop them de novo. Relatively few measures existed then, and for many health care settings, there were no tools for measuring performance at all. Today, thousands of performance indicators are in use, covering a significant proportion of the health care system. These measurement tools, however, have been designed for a wide variety of purposes and are of uneven quality. Many, perhaps most, have never been tested for scientific integrity.

Performance measures—or indicators—are quantitative tools (e.g., a rate, ratio, index, percentage) that provide an indication of organization or practitioner performance in relation to a specified process or outcome. This section describes the types of measures most useful for performance improvement purposes, identifies the characteristics of good measures, provides guidelines on upholding the scientific integrity of performance measures and measurement processes, discusses the importance of data quality, and offers some guidance on where to find the right measures to meet defined performance measurement goals.

TYPES OF MEASURES

On the basis of insights of Donabedian (11), health care quality monitoring at the level of the organization has focused on structures, processes, and outcomes. The three types of performance measures commonly used to evaluate the quality of health care services correspond to these components.

Structures include such things as staff qualifications and competencies, staffing levels, supervisory practices, documentation and record keeping, equipment, and administrative policies. Structure measures typically evaluate an organization's capability to provide quality care and services. They do not generally reveal direct information about real performance. Structures, however, enable the implementation of key processes, and those processes can produce key clinical outcomes.

A process is an interconnected series of goal-directed steps. Processes include both clinical and nonclinical activities. Clinical processes focus on the way in which different types and intensities of care are provided for different conditions. Patient assessment, diagnosis, care planning, delivery of interventions, and the evaluation of the effectiveness of care are typically evaluated by clinical process measures. Nonclinical processes such as public relations, marketing, and the recruitment of patients, address those administrative activities that are central to conducting the daily business of the organization.

Outcomes result from the unique interaction of the specific process components and may also be clinical or nonclinical. Outcome measures track the achievement of desired outcomes. Unlike structure measures, process and outcome measures usually generate data that describe actual performance. Meaningful performance measurement and significant performance improvement are grounded in the inherent relationship between processes and outcomes. That is why processes and outcomes are allocated the vast majority of resources expended on performance measurement.

Individual performance measures can track desirable events (e.g., number of patients 65 years of age or older receiving a yearly influenza immunization), undesirable events (e.g., surgical procedures complicated by at least one surgical site infection), or events that are desirable within certain parameters but undesirable if they fall outside of those parameters (e.g., patients delivered by cesarean section). In addition, measures differ on the bases of how they are calculated. Some measures are rates, meaning that the numerator, the event being tracked, is a subset of the denominator, the population at risk (e.g., numerator: intrahospital mortality of patients undergoing a percutaneous transluminal coronary angioplasty [PTCA]; denominator: patients undergoing a PTCA). Other measures are ratios in which there is a relationship between two sets of data, but the numerator is not a subset of the denominator (e.g., numerator: ventilated inpatients who develop pneumonia; denominator: inpatient ventilator days). Measures can also be constructed from a continuous variable where the value of a measurement falls along a continuous numerical scale (e.g., trauma patients undergoing selected neurosurgical procedures: time from emergency department or trauma unit admission to procedure).

CHARACTERISTICS OF A GOOD MEASURE

What constitutes a good measure? The answer is multidimensional. On one level, a good measure is consistent with the purpose and intended use of the measurement and is the appropriate tool for achieving the defined measurement goal. Good measures raise important questions about the quality of the health care service provided and identify opportunities for improvement in specific processes and outcomes related to the targeted components of care. In addition, good measures focus on outcomes or processes that are under the control of the health care provider and that are relevant to designated stakeholders such as are patients, consumers, regulators, and purchasers.

At another level, good measures offer a practical and interpretable mechanism for conveying useful information to interested stakeholders. To do so, measures must have a rationale that is clear, focused, and easily understood. Also, to be useful, a measure must capture statistically significant variation in the process or outcome being monitored. Measures that cannot detect variation over time or across settings are of no value to anyone. If the processes or outcomes do not vary, they need not be measured. If a measure cannot detect the variation that does exist, a more sensitive measurement tool is required. Finally, measurement results should be reportable in a manner that is understandable and useful to interested stakeholders.

At a third level, good measures are robust and accurate tools that uphold the scientific integrity of the measurement process by meeting certain criteria. These criteria are generally agreed on across the performance measurement environment. There have been a number of independent efforts by organizations experienced in measuring health care performance, such as the American Academy of Family Physicians (AAFP), the American Medical Association, the Joint Commission, the Foundation on Accountability (FACCT), the National Committee on Quality Assurance (NCQA), and the RAND Corporation, to identify attributes of scientifically sound measurement tools. What is striking about these initiatives is the similarity of the results.

To uphold the scientific integrity of the measurement process, performance measurement tools should possess the following attributes:

- Evidence based;
- Precisely defined and specified;
- Reliable;
- Valid; and
- Risk adjusted (when appropriate).

Evidence Based

The focus and rationale of performance measures should be grounded in science and based on current clinical research and health care knowledge. If scientific evidence is lacking, measures should be based on widespread expert consensus.

Precisely Defined and Specified

To consistently generate meaningful and useful information, data on the same measure must be collected in the same way, every time, across all applicable settings. If the data are not consistently collected in the same way, the ability to generate ''apples to apples'' comparisons will be severely compromised. Consequently, performance measures must be standardized. Standardization requires:

- clear and understandable statements (e.g., numerator, denominator) of what the measurement tool purports to measure;
- rules to identify specific targeted populations (e.g., numerator and denominator);
- defined data elements, corresponding data sources, and allowable values;
- defined sampling procedures (if applicable);
- a specified procedure (algorithm) for calculating the measure value or score; and
- defined and tested risk adjustment specifications (if applicable).

Reliable

Measures are able to consistently identify the events they were designed to identify across multiple health care settings over time. In other words, there should be minimal random error and results should be consistently reproducible wherever the same measurement tools are applied. The same data should always yield the same results regardless of where or when it is collected.

Valid

Validity refers to the extent to which measures have been shown to capture what they were in-tended to measure with respect to the targeted health care construct. The targeted health care construct must also be associated with important health care processes or outcomes. Measures should raise good questions about the quality of health care provided and identify opportunities for improvement.

Risk Adjusted

To generate fair and meaningful comparisons on the performance data, outcome measures are often risk adjusted. That is, the influences of patient factors that differ among groups being compared have been controlled or taken into account. Examples of factors patients might bring to an encounter and for which risk adjustment might be used include complications, comorbidities, health status, and certain demographic characteristics.

DATA QUALITY

The importance of collecting complete and accurate data on performance measures is critical. Because bad data are believed as fervently as good data, inaccurate information can lead to bad decisions and wasted resources by focusing attention in the wrong areas while ignoring real problems and opportunities for quality improvement. In addition, even a small amount of bad data can threaten the credibility of the entire measurement initiative. Once administrators, clinicians, or other stakeholders have reason to question the veracity of the data, successfully initiating changes in structures, processes, or behavior on the basis of measurement findings, is often problematic.

The attributes of good measures outlined above are all directly or indirectly associated with the ability to generate complete and accurate data. Once measures are in place and data collection has begun, it is critical that data quality be carefully and continuously monitored against prespecified standards. Collecting and storing data at the level of individual patients make ongoing quality assessment feasible. Storing measure data at the aggregate level makes it far more difficult to monitor data quality and to identify or investigate anomalies, unless the original data sources are easily accessible.

SOURCES OF MEASURES

There are three primary sources of performance measures. Performance measures can be developed de novo, individual existing measures can be adopted or adapted for use, or a health care organization can contract to participate in an external performance measurement system. Some of the advantages and disadvantages of each approach follow.

De Novo Measure Development

On the bases of the explosion in the number of performance measures appearing in health care over the last 10 years, it is likely that good measures already exist for tracking many important processes and outcomes related to neurologic services (19). However, if suitable measures cannot be found to meet the established measurement goals, they can be constructed. The primary advantage to developing measurement tools de novo is that measures can be precisely configured to meet the defined measurement needs. Nonetheless, developing indicators can be a very complex, resource-intensive endeavor and probably should only be attempted if the predefined measurement goals cannot be met in any other manner.

Measure development usually requires a coordinated, long-term effort that includes measurement experts and clinicians in the targeted area. A well-constructed measure contains the following components:

1. A definition of the measure, including the indicator calculation logic, or algorithm: Typically an indicator is constructed in the form of a rate or proportion consisting of a numerator (the population of interest) and a denominator (the population at risk). This requires constructing rules for identifying the population at risk and the events being tracked, including precise definitions of the populations to be included, and excluded, in the measure. Population inclusions and exclusions could be based on such things as the population upper and lower age limits, certain diagnoses or procedures, a defined time frame before or after a procedure, and so forth. Other measures are ratios in which there is a relationship between two sets of data, but the numerator is not a subset of the denominator. Measures can also consist of a continuous variable in which the value of a measurement falls along a continuous numerical scale.
2. Precisely defined data element definitions: The importance and difficulty of developing

well-defined and well-tested data-element definitions are well documented (21). Data must be collected in the same way on the same measure whenever and wherever the measure is used. Confusing or imprecise data-element definitions will introduce a level of systematic bias into the measurement that will make comparisons over time or across organizations and practitioners uninterpretable. In addition, the more settings in which the measure is expected to be used, the more challenging it will be to construct clearly understood and consistently applied data-element definitions.

3. Recommended data sources: For the same reason of consistency, as mentioned above, it is important that data be derived from the same sources whenever and wherever the measure is used. The most common sources of indicator data are the clinical medical record, administrative databases, and survey data.
4. The development of a risk adjustment strategy so that fair comparisons can be made on the measure: This may require the collection of additional data elements that are not necessary to the calculation of the measure itself. The development of this strategy will probably also necessitate the development of clinically and statistically sophisticated models that we concordant with current scientific and clinical literature, for controlling variation in the measure. For many health care organizations, developing and regularly reassessing these models require a type and level of expertise that are not always readily available (17).
5. The development of data-sampling protocols, if sampling is used: In some circumstances it may not be necessary, or feasible, to collect data on 100% of the patient population addressed by the indicator. In such cases, it may be appropriate, and cheaper, to sample the data. If sampling is used, precise rules for how to implement statistically sound sampling protocols must be developed. Not only do these protocols require statistical grounding, they also need to be consistently applied across all the settings where the measure is used.

Once constructed, new measures must undergo extensive testing to establish that they are reliable (i.e., can consistently and accurately identify the events they were designed to identify) and valid (i.e., useful for identifying opportunities for improvement in the targeted measurement area). Rigorous testing is almost always resource intensive and usually takes several months (it can take years to establish the validity of a measure). If useful indicators are already available, time spent testing new measures might be better spent measuring with existing ones.

Finally, since newly developed measures have never been used before, there is no preexisting database to generate performance comparisons on the measures. This can be a significant disadvantage since all measurement is, fundamentally, about comparison. It will take months, or longer, to establish a database from which statistically sound comparisons may be generated.

Adopting/Adapting Measures

Another source of performance measures is to adopt, or adapt, existing individual indicators. Measures may be adopted without modification. Many well-tested measures are available for adoption, some of them developed by prominent and respected health care entities. Among the better known compendia of performance measures are the Computerized Needs-Oriented Quality Measurement Evaluation System (CONQUEST) from the Agency for Health Care Policy and Research JCAHO's National Library of Health Care Indicators (NLHI) and the American Medical Association's Clinical Process and Outcomes Measurement Directory (1). Sometimes, however, good measures that are designed to function in one environment may need some minor changes to be effective in another setting. In that case, existing measures can be adapted for use by making minor changes in the calculation logic, data-element definitions (included population), or some other specifications.

Measures considered for adoption should not be adopted blindly. When considering an existing measure for use in meeting measurement goals, some investigation may be necessary. For example, have testing and use established the reliability and validity of the indicator? Has the measure identified opportunities for improvement, and is it able to generate fair comparisons? How resource intensive is the measure to collect and use? The standards that apply to measure development also apply to measure adoption. In both cases, the questions are the same. The ad-

vantage when considering measures for adoption is that the answers should already exist.

Adapting measures by making minor modifications in their specifications can be a useful compromise between developing indicators de novo to meet specific measurement goals and adopting measurement tools that were developed and implemented by others to meet their own measurement needs. When adapting measures, it is important to remain alert to the law of unintended consequences. Changes in one component of a measure could result in unanticipated changes in other components, ultimately affecting indicator reliability or validity. If extensive changes are introduced, the measure will require retesting to ensure that its reliability and validity have not been compromised. This is a particular concern if data-element definitions or the indicator calculation logic have been significantly altered.

Performance Measurement Systems

A performance measurement system is an entity that facilitates performance improvement through the collection and dissemination of performance measurement data. Measurement systems generate internal comparisons of performance over time and external comparisons of performance among participants at equivalent times. The advantage to using these entities is that they offer, through an established infrastructure, sets of developed and implemented measures ready for use, along with a populated, comparative database. As a consequence, these systems can provide feedback comparing the performance of an individual participating health care organization with the performance of other organizations collecting data on the same measures. Not all measurement systems are equal, and there are a number of factors that should be taken into consideration when selecting a measurement system to meet defined measurement goals.

1. Measurement system performance measures should meet all of the criteria outlined above, including having established reliability validity. The system should provide clients with details of all defined measure specifications. In addition, the system should have plans in place for maintaining the relevance of their indicators over time through documented procedures for adding, modifying, maintaining, and deleting performance measures.

2. The system should have an operational, automated database. It should also collect and store data at the level of the individual patient; otherwise, data quality cannot be effectively monitored and performance measures cannot be risk adjusted appropriately.
3. The measurement system should monitor the accuracy and completeness of the data it receives from participating organizations. It should also provide ongoing support to participating clients to ensure that data quality is monitored by those organizations as well.
4. The system should risk adjust those measures for which risk adjustment is appropriate. The system should also provide clients with information on how it controls for the influences of confounding patient factors on the measures.
5. The measurement system should make available to its clients, on a timely basis, comparative performance measure–related feedback. This information should be useful in the health care organization's ongoing internal efforts to improve patient care and organizational performance. The system should also provide educational resources to help its clients understand and use the data. If the system uses any external or third-party databases, it is important that the specifications of those databases be shared with the client and the most recent data in them not be more than 12 to 18 months old. The older the data are, the less useful they are for reporting purposes.
6. Finally, it is important to check the size of the comparison groups for those measures that are being used to meet the measurement goals. Statistically valid comparisons may be difficult to generate if the number of organizations collecting data on the same measures is fewer than 30.

PERFORMANCE IMPROVEMENT AND MONITORING

The selection of scientifically sound performance measures plays a key role in performance improvement and in ongoing performance monitoring activities. It is through these processes that health care organizations can continuously identify critical opportunities for improvement—that is, those opportunities that result in either cost savings, improved patient care, or both. This section describes how to translate measurement data into demonstrable improvements in patient care.

Many different performance improvement concepts and approaches are described in this book, such as benchmarking, critical paths, outcomes management, reengineering, CQI, and TQM. These approaches may be dependent on sophisticated computer technologies for data collection and analysis or could, instead, rely on manual check sheets and hand-drawn graphics. Regardless of the name or level of sophistication, a successful approach to performance improvement requires the application of a systematic method, one that ensures that improvement actions are based on sound data and unbiased scientific analyses and that the desired results are achieved.

Many methods have been developed to help organizations plan, test, assess, and implement actions to improve processes. The most well documented of these methods is the plan–do–study–act (PDSA) cycle, or the Shewhart cycle developed by Walter Schewhart and widely disseminated through the teachings of W. Edwards Deming (38). Another well-known process is the FOCUS-PDCA cycle developed by the Hospital Corporation of America (now part of Columbia Health Care Corporation). **FOCUS** stands for **F**ind a process to improve, **O**rganize a team that knows the process, **C**larify current knowledge of the process, **U**nderstand causes of process variation, and **S**elect the process improvement; these steps lead to the plan–do–check–act (PDCA) cycle, which is used to test and implement the process improvement. The Joint Commission developed an approach that incorporates steps that most improvement processes share. It is known as the cycle for improving performance and consists of 4 key activities: design, measure, assess, and improve in addition to a series of major inputs and outputs (see *Fig. 8.2*). Although any of these methods defines an equally effective approach to performance improvement, it is in this context that performance improvement and ongoing monitoring are discussed.

The Design Phase

The design phase involves identifying the objectives for a process and then creating a design that meets those objectives. Key factors

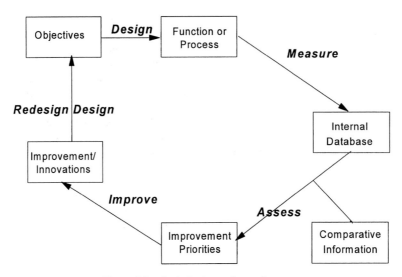

Figure 8.2 Cycle for improving performance.

to be considered during this stage include the following:

- How the process affects patients, staff, and other important groups;
- What expertise and experience within the organization may apply to designing the process;
- What expertise and experience external to the organization may be available and useful to the design process;
- What data are necessary to the design process and how the data will be collected and analyzed; and
- What resources are available and what funds, staff time, equipment, and other resources are required.

Key activities associated with implementing the design phase may include some or all of the following actions.

Organize a Performance Improvement Team

Identify individuals across the organization who are familiar with neurological surgery systems and processes. Identify those who can be most instrumental in recognizing areas for potential improvement and implementing those improvements. To help ensure success, the process improvement team should span staff levels, departments, and disciplines, and, most important, it should include appropriate leadership and medical staff involvement.

Identify Broad Performance Improvement Goals and Objectives

A system or process should be designed/redesigned with a particular purpose(s) in mind, because the outcome of any system is directly dependent on its fundamental design. Thus, if the design of a system is altered, the outcomes will be affected proportionately. For example, if the organization is experiencing a 1% rate of neurological surgery perioperative complications, systems and processes may be perfectly designed to yield a 1% perioperative complication rate.

Improving performance begins with the performance improvement team articulating and defining a series of rational goals for the organization's neurological surgery systems/processes (e.g., to provide high-quality patient care, to maintain or minimize costs, to minimize the risk of surgical complications, justification for additional staff). Develop a list of goals and objectives that includes as many as apply.

Process improvement is often most successful when undertaken in smaller, more circumscribed steps. That is, rather than trying work with the entire system, it may be more effective to define the larger system into a series of complimentary processes and implement assessment and improvement in the smaller units.

Develop a Flowchart of Systems/Processes

A clear understanding of the system/process is essential before opportunities for improvement can be identified. Clarify the organization's neurosurgical processes by using the instructions for flowchart development presented in Chapter 5. The flowchart will help the performance improvement team members see how the process actually works, which is often quite different from how they think it works or how it should work. The team may also want to create a separate flowchart that represents the ideal path of the process and then compare the two charts for discrepancies. As the flowchart steps are analyzed, the team should be able to begin to identify and list potentially vulnerable areas where errors may be introduced.

Organize and Apply Current Knowledge

Organize current information about the process being considered. For example, collect information relative to the neurosurgical complication rate (e.g., the types of complications, the number of occurrences of each of the identified complications, the severity of the occurrence, outcome, costs, source of error), display this information in a matrix, and analyze the distribution of the known complications against the steps/components of the flowcharted system/process (Table 8.2).

Identify those points that appear to be the most vulnerable to error by listing and rank ordering the flowchart steps/components in order of most to least number of associated errors. Put an asterisk beside those complications that resulted in severe consequences (e.g., permanent harm, death, resuscitation, extraordinary costs). Finally, compare the critical flowchart steps/components identified in this step with those speculated during the flowchart analysis. Develop a list of those items that are common to both levels of analysis.

Targeting/Selecting Areas for Improvement

All areas identified through the flowchart analysis and the analysis of current information are important areas to target for improvement.

However, those areas identified as being common to both levels of analysis may be the areas where initial improvement efforts should be focused. Depending on the team's final review and assessment, however, other areas may be identified as having greater priority on the basis of overriding criteria (e.g., those areas where there have been a significant number of occurrences or where consequences have been extremely severe).

Consider the area that has been identified for process improvement and undertake the following activities:

• Define/refine and clarify the intent of the targeted improvement (e.g., to implement improvements that will reduce the possibility of medication administration error).
• Verify that the targeted improvement is under the control or purview of the team or health care organization (e.g., it may be possible to implement improvements that will reduce the possibility of medication administration errors in the operating room; however, if it is determined that most medication administration errors are associated with premedicating the patient and occur on the patient unit, then another team may have to be established or additional members added to the current team).
• Verify that the identified areas for improvement are in need of attention. Determine if current data/information are sufficient, recent, valid, and reliable and support improvement in the identified area; if not, additional data collection may be needed and the following should be considered: define what kind and how much data will be needed; define how the data will be collected; and define who will be responsible for collecting, interpreting, summarizing, and presenting the additional data.
• Conduct a literature review. Do not reinvent the wheel! Search existing literature to determine what work has already been done in the area of the planned improvement. Build on that body of work. Generate a list of key arti-

TABLE 8.2
Example Systems/Processes Matrix

Types of Complications	Number of Occurrences	Severity of Occurrences	Other Considerations (outcomes, costs, etc.)	Source of Error (if known)	Types of Complications
Medication overdose	1	Moderate-required antidote	No harm/cost of antidote ($7.82)	New brand of syringes-unfamiliar calibrations	Medication administration

favorable outcomes. Also, professional societies and expert panels routinely develop scientifically based descriptions of patient care processes. These are good sources of ''best practices'' for a given procedure or treatment. Assessing variation from such established procedures is another good way to identify opportunities for improvement.

The assessment phase will help the performance improvement team validate whether the area selected for improvement is the right area, it will help identify other opportunities for improvement, and it will provide a basis for setting improvement priorities. Because a significant investment of time, effort, and resources is often needed to improve processes, these are key considerations.

The team has already used informal data analysis methods to determine which project should be undertaken. However, once the team has collected data about the identified process, more structured tools for data analysis will be useful. Run charts, control charts, comparison charts, and histograms are all statistical, quantitative tools used to display the process performance data so that one can easily analyze the data and compare them with past performance or to preestablished standards or ideals (see Chapter 5).

Key activities associated with implementing the assessment phase may include the following actions.

Identify Data Analysis Tools

Consider the data that will be generated from your performance improvement project as you review various tools described in Chapter 5 and select the one that is the most appropriate for tracking and presenting your data. Respond to the following questions as the team considers the data analysis approach.

- What data analysis tools will you use for the improvement initiative?
- Will you describe the data that will be displayed? What period of time will be captured in the data display? What will be the defined time segments for data display (e.g., daily, weekly, or monthly data points)?
- What format(s) will be used to report data findings? Is there an ''organizational format'' for reporting performance improvement data? Does your organization have standards for the use of tabular, narrative, or graphic output to communicate performance improvement

information? How can the output be presented to ensure clarity for all users?
- Does the organization have a communication plan? How are other performance improvement initiatives communicated? How often does the team expect to communicate? Is there a central story board? Is the story board communicated in newsletters, departmental meetings, memoranda, and such? Are the data accessible and retrievable for all bona fide users?
- To whom will data/findings be reported?

As mentioned, there are a number of data analysis tools that the team will find useful. The run chart is familiar to health care professionals and one of the simplest tools to construct and use. It can be used during problem identification, data analysis, and results evaluation, or anytime a team needs a simple visual display of performance trends over a specific period of time. Run charts use the plotting of points on a graph to show the levels of performance over time; their purpose is to identify trends and patterns in a process, including movement away from the average. Many other, more rigorous and quantitatively precise data analysis tools may also be useful to you at this stage, including control charts, comparison charts, histograms, scatter diagrams and Pareto charts (see Chapter 5). These tools should satisfy most of your inhouse data analysis needs.

The Improvement Phase

The improvement phase involves implementing improvement actions that are based on the results of measurement and assessment. To improve a process, a team creates, tests, and implements specific innovations, which may involve a redesign of the process or the design of a new process. In general, an improvement effort will involve:

- Selecting an improvement action, which often involves redesigning the process.
- Determining who will implement the action.
- Determining how the action will be implemented.
- Determining how data will be collected to measures the action's effect.
- Implementing the action on a small scale or for a limited time.
- Assessing the effectiveness of the action.
- Implementing the action fully, if the test results warrant it.

Key activities associated with implementing the improvement phase may include all or some of the following actions.

Pilot Testing the Performance Improvement

It is wise to implement the improvement project on a small scale at first and then thoroughly study the results prior to full-scale implementation. This approach allows for validation and refinement of the improvement actions before they are applied across the entire organization. This is of particular importance when the proposed actions require a large investment of organizational resources. Consider the following questions as the team develops pilot test approach and assessment of pilot test results.

- Which area(s) will be used for the pilot test? Why are these areas preferable over other possible areas?
- Do pilot test data indicate that the actions had a positive impact? If so, describe the extent of the change. If not, do the data identify other ways to impact or improve the process? What are they?
- How does the post pilot data compare with the prepilot (baseline) data?
- What other benchmarking databases exist for comparison purposes relative to the this project? Are they internal as well as external databases? Do any professional organizations have this type of comparative data?
- Is the team completely satisfied with the improvement? Has the maximum level of achievement in the identified area been realized? If not, how can the approach be improved before full-scale implementation?
- Are there improvements to be made, on the basis of the pilot test, to increase the efficiency of ongoing monitoring activities (i.e., data collection and data analysis)? Can you decrease monitoring frequency while maintaining the quality of analysis required to maintain the integrity of the project?

Monitoring the Improvement

Once small-scale or pilot testing has been completed and the team is satisfied that the intervention is having the desired impact, the implementation can be expanded to include all relevant areas. Continued monitoring of the process, however, is essential to ensure that the improvement can be sustained over time. Similarly, continued monitoring may help support the identification of other areas for improvement. More intensive measurement in the early stages of improvement implementation is needed to ensure that full-scale implementation is yielding the same results as experienced in the pilot-testing phase. However, once the desired state is achieved across the entire organization, measurement activities can be less intense. Consider the following questions relative to your ongoing monitoring activities:

- According to your performance goals, what percentage of change (e.g., rate of neurological surgical complications) is an acceptable measure of process improvement (now and in the future)?
- Is the change, as measured in outcome benefit, what you expected? If not, why not? What can be done to address the shortfall?
- What monitoring mechanisms will be put in place to ensure that the process is not left to run itself? Is the frequency of monitoring compatible with the frequency of the occurrence for the process being measured? Does this require continuous or intermittent monitoring? Is it automated or manual?
- If multiple locations are affected by the improvement, are there difference in the results among locations? If so, why do you think this has occurred? How will you address this issue?

Finalizing the Process Modification

The final step in the improvement process is to codify the improvement that has been achieved to ensure that it is sustained in the organization. Codification of the improvement may have multiple components, depending on its nature. Consider the following actions and questions when determining what actions are needed to permanently incorporate the improvement into the organization:

- Modify the original process flowchart to incorporate the improvement action(s).
- Do the changes as represented in the updated/revised flowchart require modification of existing organizational policies, procedures, or protocols or the development of new policies, procedures, or protocols? If so, what are they? Who will be responsible for handling this task? What approvals are necessary?
- How will full-scale implementation of this initiative be communicated throughout your

organization? Who needs to know? What communication vehicles will you use? Will communications be varied depending on the audience?

- Is there a need for training relative to the improvement? If so, who should receive training? Who should conduct the training? How will this training be incorporated into routine training activities?
- What kind of training materials will need to be developed? Who will be responsible for this task?

Assessment of Other Areas for Improvement

Successful implementation of one project should lead to the identification of other areas for improvement within the process currently being addressing. In addition, the preliminary work that was done to identify the current area for improvement may have also targeted other critical areas of the system for improvement. Review the findings from the current improvement project and the work done in the design phase to help determine your next focus area. If you wish to look at another process, begin by using the information you already have, but be sure to begin by developing a flowchart of the new process and then selectively moving though the subsequent steps.

CONCLUSION

The guidelines presented in this chapter should help identify performance measurement opportunities and initiate activities to improve organizational performance. The questions and activities are simply a starting point. As you select the process in your system that you wish to address, you will develop more specific questions, customized to your unique situation, and find yourself building on the basics provided here. Familiarize yourself with at least some of the references listed at the end of this chapter, and you will find even more ideas. Like any other system, performance improvement can always be refined.

REFERENCES

1. American Medical Association: Clinical process and outcomes measurement directory. Chicago, American Medical Association, 1999.
2. Berwick DM, Godfrey AB, Roessner J: Curing health care: New strategies for quality improvement. San Francisco, Jossey-Bass, 1990.
3. Berwick DM: Continuous improvement as an ideal in health care [letter]. *N Engl J Med* 320:53–56, 1989.
4. Berwick DM, Nolan TW: Physicians as leaders in improving health care: A new series in *Annals of Internal Medicine. Ann Intern Med* 128:289–292, 1998.
5. Blumenthal D, Kilo CM: A report card on continuous quality improvement. *Milbank Q* 76:625–648, 1998.
6. Carey RG, Lloyd RC: Measuring quality improvement in healthcare: A guide to statistical process control applications. New York, Quality Resources (a division of the Kraus Organization Ltd.), 1995.
7. Chassin MR: Assessing strategies for quality improvement. *Health Aff* 16:151–161, 1997.
8. Chassin MR: Improving the quality of care. *N Engl J Med* 335:1060–1063, 1996.
9. Chassin MR, Hannan EL, DeBuono BA: Benefits and hazards of reporting medical outcomes publicly [letter]. *N Engl J Med* 334:394–398, 1996.
10. Deming WE: Out of the crisis. Cambridge, MA, MIT Press, 1986.
11. Donabedian A: The definition of quality and approaches to its assessment. Ann Arbor, MI, Health Administration Press, 1980.
12. Eddy DM: Performance measurement: Problems and solutions. *Health Aff* 17:7–25, 1998.
13. Edgman-Levitan S, Gerteis M: Measures of quality: What can public reporting accomplish? *Health Care For J* 41:27, 36–37, 61, 1998.
14. Epstein A: Performance reports on quality—Prototypes, problems, and prospects [letter]. *N Engl J Med* 333:57–61, 1995.
15. Hannan EL, Kilburn H Jr, Racz M, Shields E, Chassin MR: Improving the outcomes of coronary artery bypass surgery in New York state. *JAMA* 271:761–766, 1994.
16. Hibbard JH, Jewett JJ: Will quality report cards help consumers? *Health Aff* 16:218–228, 1997.
17. Iezzoni LI: Risk adjustment for measuring health care outcomes. Chicago, Health Administration Press, 1997, ed 2.
18. Joint Commission on Accreditation of Health Care Organizations: A compendium of forms, tables, and charts for use in monitoring and evaluation. Oakbrook Terrace, IL, Joint Commission on Accreditation of Health Care Organizations, 1991.
19. Joint Commission on Accreditation of Health Care Organizations: Development and application of indicators for continuous improvement in surgical and anesthesia care. Oakbrook Terrace, IL, Joint Commission on Accreditation of Health Care Organizations, 1991.
20. Joint Commission on Accreditation of Health Care Organizations: 1999 Hospital accreditation standards. Oakbrook Terrace, IL, Joint Commission on Accreditation of Health Care Organizations, 1999.
21. Koss RG, Turpin RS, Schmaltz S, Sprenger S, McMahill CN: Assessing obstetric care performance measures in healthcare organizations. *New Med* 1:113–119, 1997.
22. Kritchevsky, SB, Simmons BP: Continuous quality improvement: Concepts and applications for physician care. *JAMA* 266:1817–1823, 1991.
23. Leape LL: Error in medicine. *JAMA* 272:1851–1857, 1994.

24. Loeb JM, Nadzam DM: Performance measurement and accreditation, in Seltzer J, Nash D (eds): *Models for Measuring Quality in Managed Care: Analysis and Impact.* New York, Faulkner and Gray, 1997, 79–99.

25. Longo DR, Land G, Schramm W, et al. Consumer reports in health care: Do they make a difference? *JAMA* 278:1579–1584, 1997.

26. Nelson EC, Batalden PB, Plume SK, Mihevc NT, Swartz WG: Report cards or instrument panels: Who needs what? *Joint Comm J Qual Improv* 21:155–166, 1995.

27. Nelson EC, Mohr JJ, Batalden PB, Plume SK: Improving health care, part 1: The clinical value compass. *Joint Comm J Qual Improv* 22:243–258, 1996.

28. Nelson EC, Splaine ME, Batalden PB, Plume SK: Building measurement and data collection into medical practice. *Ann Intern Med* 128:460–466, 1998.

29. Nolan TW: Understanding medical systems. *Ann Intern Med* 128:293–298, 1998.

30. Panzer RJ: Are hospital quality improvement and public accountability compatible? *Joint Comm J Qual Improv* 20:396–401, 1994.

31. President's Advisory Commission on Consumer Protection and Quality in the Health Care Industry: Quality first: Better health care for all americans—Final report to the President of the United States. Washington, DC, President's Advisory Commission on Consumer Protection on Quality in the Health Care Industry, March 1998.

32. Reinertsen JL: Physicians as leaders in the improvement of health care systems. *Ann Intern Med* 128:833–838, 1998.

33. Schneider EC, Epstein AM: Use of public performance reports. *JAMA* 279:1638–1642, 1998.

34. Shortell SM, Bennett CL, Byck GR: Assessing the impact of continuous quality improvement on clinical practice: What it will take to accelerate progress. *Milbank Q* 76:593–624, 1998.

35. Simon JL: Basic research methods in social science. New York, Random House, 1969.

36. Sollis JG, Romano PS: Pennsylvania's focus on heart attack: Grading the scorecard. *N Engl J Med* 338:983–987, 1998.

37. Topol EJ, Califf RM: Scorecard cardiovascular medicine: Its impact and future directions. *Ann Intern Med* 120:65–70, 1994.

38. Walton M: The Deming management method. New York, Perigee, 1986.

39. Weiner BJ, Shortell SM, Alexander J: Promoting clinical involvement in hospital quality improvement efforts: The effects of top management, board, and physician leadership. *Health Serv Res* 32:491–510, 1997.

CHAPTER 9

Patient Satisfaction Surveys: A Start-to-Finish Look

KEN BRODEUR, Ph.D., AND ALEX M. CHEHANSKY

EDITOR'S NOTE: Patient satisfaction surveys are often frustrating for surgeons. In part, this is because of the inherent trust implicit in the patient–physician relationship. Patients want to believe that they will get well, and part of that desire includes a desire to believe that their doctors are the "best." As a result (in the absence of a specific negative experience), most patients consistently rate their physicians as excellent-to-outstanding on professional skill and competency scales, regardless of that physician's actual training, experience, or objective clinical outcomes. In the absence of comparative clinical outcomes data, patient satisfaction most often hinges on cost and timeliness (as it does for any service organization). For health care, for which cost is usually not borne directly by the patient, timeliness becomes the dominant factor for patient-perceived quality. Time to wait for the next available appointment, time spent waiting for the doctor, and time the doctor actually spends with the patient are all components of this perception.

"Perception is reality."

—A fashionable American political axiom

Patient satisfaction is steadily becoming one of the most important aspects of managed health care today. With the advent of renewed interest in the patient–provider relationship, the idea of creating a positive, trusting atmosphere in and around the office has risen to the forefront. Gone are the days of limited competition for health care among providers; instead, we find a patient-dominated realm of numerous providers, all of whom offer quality health care packages. As a result, there is a need to measure the attributes of each individual provider. It is impossible to address problems that we do not even know exist. The easiest way to determine shortfalls in the service industry is to obtain the opinions and views of the people who matter the most to your business: the patient. The only way to accomplish this properly, outside of asking each patient as, he or she leaves the office, is to create a means of accumulating these data over a period of time among a certain cross-section of those who use your services. The means of accumulating data is in the form of a patient satisfaction survey.

During this chapter you will become acquainted with all aspects of the patient satisfaction survey process—from creation of the survey to presenting your facts in an informative way that allows all who work in your business to grasp the importance of the accumulated patient opinions. The current challenge that lies ahead for the service-oriented manager is to enable and sustain a highly proficient service, run and managed by a technically efficient and personable staff, by using the most state-of-the-art technology available. The key is to make the patient the business focus. This, and only this, creates the best scenario for the patient and the business, and allows the business to succeed and continue operating well into the new millennium.

In other words, the provider must see the patient as a valued customer. This must be a two-way relationship that is allowed to grow and nurture over time as visits go by. This is not just an information flow from the provider to the patient, but it is the reverse as well. For example, the organization can use this communication to inform its patients of upcoming changes in services. Sometimes this early warning of future differences in the provided service allows for preplanning on the part of the patient and does not scare them off to seek a new provider. This creates a greater respect for the provider by the patients, and surely enhances their relationship. The positive attributes that emerge from patient satisfaction responsibility do not come easily and take a dedicated effort by the staff and all members of the business to reach fruition. Consider the following pages a guide to initiating, or polishing, your patient satisfaction program. The methods proposed have been well tested in the health care field as well as in many other service industries. When implemented, they create a fully functional workplace with the patient as the focus of your business.

THE QUALITY VALUES

Satisfaction with the patient–supplier relationship is based on a set of indicators called the *quality values.* These quality values have a broad application. This means that you don't have to apply them solely to an organization, you can also apply them to your personal life. You'll see, as we go through this chapter, that quality values are rooted in universal concepts—concepts you can use as founding principles in which to create delight in all customer–supplier relationships: with your husband or wife, employees, coworkers, or the patients you serve, who actually pay for the products and services you provide. Implementation of the quality values ensures market dominance and long-term business viability in the same way that they ensure all relationships last. The first thing that both businesses and individuals want is a long-term relationship. As an individual you don't want your relationships to last a little while and go away, requiring you to develop new ones. The same concept applies to business. You don't want your patients to go away, requiring you to find new ones to replace them. It's hard to stay in business that way. And yet, many businesses function with no understanding of how to create win–win (long-term) relationships.

The second thing we all want as an outcome of our patient–supplier relationship is positive word-of-mouth recommendations. If patients come to see you and get the service they like, and their expectations are exceeded, they're going to tell everyone they know that your company is providing a great product or service. If they don't like your service, or perhaps are only

somewhat satisfied but not delighted, positive word-of-mouth advertising decreases. So if managers interact with their employees using authoritarian and crisis styles of management, negative word of mouth advertising (both within and outside the company) will quickly get around.

Positive world-of-mouth recommendations are at their best when your company is the recognized leader in your particular business or service area. Your company's name becomes synonymous with product and service quality, and your reputation is known as top-notch. If your company practices continuous improvement methods, patients will want your products and services, and will go out of their way to get them. When you're known as the best, this perception ensures marketplace dominance.

Foundation for the Quality Values

During a particularly significant holiday for you and your spouse, you decide that a nice dinner would be a great way to celebrate. You both have a set of internalized requirements that range from elegant ambiance to good-tasting food and wine, and great service to help make your evening special and memorable. You call to make a reservation at a restaurant recommended by some friends. Your babysitter has to leave by 10 PM, so you arrange an earlier reservation to allow ample time to enjoy yourselves. When your meaningful night out arrives, you depart, confidant that it will be an enjoyable experience.

On arrival at the restaurant you discover their parking lot is full, and the valet waves you off, forcing you to park a block down the street. After an arm-in-arm walk with your spouse to stop from slipping in your dress shoes, you make your way to the hostess podium where several other couples are also waiting. You notice a long waiting list in front of the hostess, but stride confidently up to the podium because *you have a reservation.* The hostess informs you that they're running late and the wait time is 40 minutes.

Disappointed, you gather your significant other and head for the bar, determined to wait it out in comfort with a glass of wine. The bar is packed, and no chairs are available. You leave your spouse leaning against a wall and elbow your way toward the bar. One bartender is engaged in a conversation with a customer, packed in at the bar with 20 or so others, all elbow to elbow. You try to get the bartender's attention but it seems he is purposely ignoring you. Approximately 10 minutes go by and finally you're able to place an order for two glasses of wine. He insists on having you pay for the drinks separately, instead of adding them to your dinner tab. You go through an additional 5-minute hassle with your credit card. Someone bumps you as you slink through the crowd and you spill half of one of the glasses.

Your spouse is still leaning against the wall and you commiserate together as you look toward the dining area. Each table seems to be filled with well-settled diners who show no signs of leaving any time soon. You go back to the hostess station to check on your progress on the wait list, but now someone new is there. They give you the dismal news again, "Yes, it's about a 40-minute delay." You ask her to check your name on the list since you've already been waiting for 20 minutes. "Yes, it's a 40-minute delay," she insists.

You calculate how much time you must wait before you get seated. The long walk back to the car dissuades you from leaving to check out another restaurant, so you wait. Finally, your name is called and they seat you at one of the least desirable tables in the establishment. You're in a corner next to the kitchen door, with your back against the wall and your spouse facing the opposite wall, with no view whatsoever, except of each other. You consider asking for another table, but one look around lets you know that there just aren't any available, and besides you might have to go through the tortuous waiting process again just to get a really good table.

You sit there for a little while with your now-empty wineglasses and finally a bus person arrives to fill your water glasses. You try to order another round of wine or even get some menus, but the bus people aren't empowered to talk to the customers. You wait some more. Finally, Jacques, your server, arrives at your table with a flourish. He proceeds to recite the night's diatribe on the specials, what they come with, and all of the excruciating details of each salad dressing and how they're prepared. He hands you some menus and as you ask him to bring you another glass of wine, he says, "I'll give you some time to look at the menus," and departs before you can stop him. You were ready to scan the menu and pick the first thing that looked

good in the interests of time, but it's too late. Jacques is gone. The bus person comes around again and adds a half inch to each of your water glasses. You ask for some bread because you're ready to chew a leg off the table by now and the bus person says, "I'll ask someone." When another waiter comes over and asks who your waiter is, he says he will tell Jacques that you want some bread. Jacques comes back in a few more minutes with your bread, and he asks if you are ready to order. You wonder what happened to the wine you wanted.

We've all had this kind of less than satisfactory experience, whether it's in a restaurant, on an airline, in a hotel, or perhaps with our health care provider. We often wonder, Why does this happen? It seems like these businesses have all the correct ingredients to provide customers with a great experience, but they just can't seem to get it together.

As social scientists, we are engaged in the study of human behavior—specifically, the phenomenon of customer satisfaction. What factors actually make a person satisfied with a product or service? To say, "The Hyatt is a great hotel" or "I'm really excited about buying a Grady White Fishing Boat" isn't exact enough. We want to know what made the hotel experience great, or what exactly it was about the entire boat—purchasing process that made it so satisfying. What do the really good restaurants do that the mediocre ones don't?

At first, studying the phenomenon of customer satisfaction seemed like a daunting task, especially because customer satisfaction has its inseparable opposite—customer dissatisfaction. To understand the nuances of creating satisfaction in each customer–supplier relationship—from buying a 25-cent gumball from a vending machine, to negotiating a government contract, to manufacturing military hardware—seemed impossible. And yet, there were data available. Customer satisfaction is by no means a new concept; in fact, customer satisfaction surveys from customer-focused organizations seem to be everywhere these days. Patient satisfaction surveys happen to be our own area of expertise as well. From designing hundreds of patient satisfaction surveys for many different customer groups, we began to notice that there were patterns in the types of information organizations wanted to elicit from their patients.

The way to start is to begin assembling a library of customer satisfaction surveys from all industries, including health care providers. Categorize the types of questions into the field or construct described. For instance, when a question asked whether the patient's scheduled appointment was timely, this question was put in the Timeliness category. This also included wait times on voice mail or hold, the length of time patients waited in line, and how quickly a patient received lab results. There are hundreds of other situations in which patients have sensitivity toward time.

Questions of reliability; durability; whether it is original, traditional, historical, certified, homegrown, exclusive, and so forth, fall into the Quality construct area. When price is studied for a product or service, there is dizzying array of factors to integrate, such as the quality of health care received, the doctor's ability to communicate with the patient, whether there is no charge when wait times exceed 30 minutes, and on and on. These factors became much clearer to us when the Value construct emerged from our research.

Much has been written about the idea of how mental models can transform thinking and allow new paradigms to emerge. What emerged from our research was 26 predictor constructs of patient satisfaction. Each construct on its own represented a new *mental model*. Instead of requiring abstract levels of study and understanding, these contructs were surprisingly simple and seemed to reflect well the expectations and "gut—level reactions" that every person has as a patient and a customer, and that every supplier endeavors to fulfill to be successful. For the purposes of this book, we defined the 26 predictor constructs as the 10 quality values and 16 quality characteristics (*Table 9.1*).

With the quality values, gut-level feelings of great satisfaction or dissatisfaction can now be recognized, described, and measured in very precise terms. As service providers, you can appreciate that patient satisfaction cannot only be measured it can be examined through the use of detailed analyses, formulas, and matrixes.

How Patient Satisfaction Differs from Customer Satisfaction

Although not entirely different as perceived by the doctor's office, patients derive their overall experience in two forms: patient satisfaction and customer satisfaction. Patient satisfaction is

TABLE 9.1
The 10 Quality Values and the 16 Quality Characteristics

Quality Values	Quality Characteristics
1. Quality	1A. Subject matter expert
	1B. General systems knowledge
	1C. Right the first time
2. Value	
3. Efficiency	
4. Timeliness	4A. On time delivery/being on time
	4B. Only the time required
	4C. All the time required
5. Access	
6. Self-management	6A. Professional appearance
	6B. Self-management
	6C. Service behavior
7. Environment	7A. Plant appearance
	7B. Systems support
	7C. Management support
8. Teamwork	
9. Commitment	9A. Interpersonal relationship
	9B. Information and involvement
	9C. Notification
	9D. Responsibility/accountability
10. Innovation	

the trust built between the doctor and the patient. It is perceived by the patient through the provider's demonstration of human service skills. Human service skills are the demonstration of caring, honest communication, courtesy, friendliness, and compassion. Customer satisfaction deals with the overall experience of the visit and the perceived technical competence of the doctor. Too often, the "generic" term *customer satisfaction* is used to describe the overall experience of the patient, and that detracts from what should be measured—patient satisfaction.

Customer satisfaction is the business aspect of dealing with the doctor. A patient arrives in the doctor's office, signs in, and waits until he is called. After a period of time he is taken to a room, as vital signs are taken, then he waits for the doctor in the exam room. After the exam, the patient leaves. The only measure of how competent the doctor is to the patient may take days, when he finds out whether the pills prescribed to him work. Too long a wait or failure to provide a follow-up appointment may cause some customer dissatisfaction, True satisfaction–patient satisfaction–takes place when the doctor takes the time and gets to know the patient and listens with a genuine respect for the patient and patient's needs.

Patient satisfaction is the *trust* built between the patient and the physician. Human service skills, not technical competence, is the foundation on which trust is built. Patient satisfaction starts with the first impression. If the doctor greets patients with a warm hello and treats them as humans and not as another case, trust starts to build. Patient satisfaction continues throughout the visit, until the patient leaves. If patients leave feeling that their doctor truly listened and knows how they feel, their satisfaction is high.

Patient satisfaction and human service skills should be the doctors focus. When doctors concentrated on being subject matter experts, and view thus as the ultimate way in which patients measure them, they miss what is important to the patient. Although competence is extremely important in health care, trust—built on a demonstration of sincere human service—is the foundation of patient satisfaction.

POWER ANALYSIS: SURVEY SAMPLE SIZE

To maximize the results from any study, it is important to ensure that the data collected are valid and appropriate to the survey. Part of this includes the type of individuals you choose to target and part of this is the amount of people you want your company to survey. These two ''ingredients'' are integral to the success of any fact-finding session. As the definition of integral becomes clearer, both parts must be investigated and researched thoroughly before a decision is made. It is vital that, whatever is decided, the company must follow through with the choices made, or the integrity of the survey is compromised.

In today's business world, deadlines and budgets play a key role. This is why providers are unable to conduct all-inclusive surveys that poll every patient and obtain thoughts from every person that passes through the door. This means that most often a random sample of the targeted audience is taken. By following the appropriate steps, the random sample is representative of your patient base and serves as an accurate basis for your fact-finding foray.

First, let's address the issue of who to target in your survey. Surprisingly, this encompasses more than just ''anyone who uses your services.'' It is key to remember that you must obtain a good cross-section of your target audience.

This allows for greater identification of variation in satisfaction among respondents as well as a more distributed representation of your patient population. It also ensures the validity of your survey, and gives you confidence that your findings were not skewed to indicate a better or worse performance than what truly occurred. Making business decisions and changes to product or service delivery based on inaccurate data is equally or even more dangerous than making decisions without data. If you have already made improvements, inaccurate or incomplete data may not measure the effect of these changes. For example, let's say a professional baseball team is interested in determining the success of a recent promotion that gave all fans entering the game a subscription to Men's Health magazine. The promotions manager for the ball club tells his assistant, ''Only survey the first 1,000 men to come into the stadium. Then you can go and watch the game.'' What is wrong with that line of thinking? The problems with this example are threefold. First, by surveying only men, you lose a target base of all the women who attended the game. Although the magazine is not intended to be read by women, some will still enjoy the promotion and may give it to their significant other as a gift. Second, as explained in the next section, 1,000 surveys are not enough to get an accurate cross-section of the audience you have targeted. Later in this section we present a sample chart of the appropriate sample survey size. Finally, by only using this survey on one night and for the first 1,000 men, you are missing thousands more who were present at a later date. A more appropriate statement by the promotions manager should have been, ''During the next three home games, survey 1,000 men and women a night at various times throughout the game, and ensure that they attended the promotion game.'' You have now set variables for the survey that better allow for data collection and result in a more representative sampling of the target population.

Through statistical analysis we are able to create a table of exactly how many surveys must be completed to achieve the best and most accurate results possible. You can find these tables in many periodicals and source books written on the subject. Another useful table is a *confidence table*. Included is a sample of a chart that was taken from *Measuring and Managing Customer Satisfaction*, by Drs. Steven R. Steiber and Wil-

TABLE 9.2
Approximate Response Rate (Confidence Table)

Sample Size	10%	20%	30%	40%	50%	60%	70%	80%	90%
100	5.9	7.8	9	9.6	9.8	9.6	9	7.8	5.9
200	4.2	5.5	6.4	6.8	6.9	6.8	6.4	5.5	4.2
300	3.4	4.5	5.2	5.5	5.7	5.5	5.2	4.5	3.9
400	2.9	3.9	4.5	4.8	4.9	4.8	4.5	3.9	2.9
500	2.6	3.5	4	4.3	4.4	4.3	4	3.5	2.6
600	2.4	3.2	3.7	3.9	4	3.9	3.7	3.2	2.4

liam J. Krowinski. Their book 13 a comprehensive workbook that they designed to improve survey construction (*Table 9.2*).

Confidence intervals are a function of sample size and the percentage estimate in question. When a sample is drawn from a large group of customers, the intervals are calculated using the confidence interval formula:

$$\text{Confidence interval} = \sqrt{1 - N/M}$$

where N equal is the sample size and M is the total population. This formula will help you to derive additional rows and columns for the confidence table (see *Table 9.2*).

Most often it is impossible to survey all your patients, so a form of random sampling is common in the survey process. A random, nonbiased sample enables the provider to develop confidently a patient care and feedback system.

RELIABILITY AND REPRODUCIBILITY: THE 10 VALUES AND 16 CHARACTERISTICS

The building blocks of the scientific analysis of customer satisfaction are the 10 quality values and the 16 quality characteristics. They represent a highly correlated set of satisfaction indicators that measure the entire spectrum of the customer–supplier relationship. Some quality values stand on their own, whereas others have characteristics and even subelements (see *Table 9.1*). The following paragraphs define quality values and characteristics.

Quality

Quality is the ability to produce consistently the highest standard of error-free products and services.

Characteristics
Subject Matter Expert

Producing quality by having expertise in a given field. Having the ability to produce a consistently high-quality product or service. Having the right mix of talents to obtain the goals of the organization. The ideas and levels of performance excellence of the subject matter expert are used as the benchmark in the industry.

General Systems Knowledge

Knowledge and ability to relate to the mission, vision, goals, values, and guiding principles of the organization. General knowledge of all products and services, including location of materials and services, services offered, pricing availability, hours, and products and services about to be introduced. Use of effective information systems to maximize the communications process and to make general systems knowledge readily available to the customer. Knowledge of the physical plant. Front-line service personnel should have answers to the most commonly asked questions. User-level knowledge of all core services provided as needed.

Right the First Time

Getting the job or service performed right the first time. Customers want an error-free process to occur during delivery of their product or service, without exerting additional time and effort. Especially, they do not want to incur higher costs because the supplier made an error or the product was defective.

Value

Good value for the price compared with the competition. Historically appropriate. Takes into account all variables and conditions. Overall and long-term satisfaction with the deal and with the impression that is formed between the customer and the supplier relative to whether the relationship produced value.

Efficiency

Sequential, logical processes or systems customers can access without redundancy, rework, or waste.

Timeliness

Spending the absolute minimum time necessary for product or service delivery to achieve the desired outcome.

Characteristics

On-Time Delivery/Being on Time

Being at a place at the agreed time or, better yet, being 5 minutes early.

Only the Time Required

Timeliness is based on the customer's concept, not the supplier's. Using efficient, coordinated, and fast-paced delivery systems that convince customers every effort is being made to expedite delivery of the product or service.

All the Time Required

Timeliness based on the nature and function of the process, not some arbitrary number dictated by management. Well-designed, efficient processes performed with precision and energy lead to the fastest turnaround times. Each process seeks its own time to achieve successful completion. Only when tasks are taken to completion are they considered a success. Customers want the sense of completion that comes from knowing the supplier gave the appropriate time and attention to complete the task, and delivered the product in a timely fashion.

Access

Product or service delivery based on the customer's convenience, not necessarily the supplier's, from a facility that is welcoming and open to receiving the customer. One-stop shopping and single points of access are optimal. Customers want to access the system with questions, concerns, and details of their product transactions.

Self-management

Taking responsibility for one's own self. Optimizing one's own talents and abilities for the mutual benefit of self and society.

Characteristics

Professional Appearance

Impressions of dress and physical appearance, appropriate to the standards and norms of the industry as well as to customer expectations, are the initial first-impression quality indicators.

Self-management

Mood-free, positive transactions during which customers interact with respectful suppliers who treat their customers as special people, without personal agendas or negativity. Suppliers must come to the workplace with the desire to provide customers service and to delight them by exceeding their expectations.

Service Behaviors—Courtesy, Friendliness, Enthusiasm, and Attentiveness

Customers want to be treated with respect, and as someone special. Suppliers must demonstrate that customer needs come first and foremost, and suppliers must demonstrate their sincere desire to serve. Customers want the full attention of the supplier during their interaction.

Environment

Factors that support the ability of the worker to produce quality.

Characteristics

Plant Appearance

An environment in which product and service delivery has the comfort of customers in mind, where the atmosphere is pleasant, welcoming, decorated attractively, has adequate seating, and is clean and well organized.

Systems Support

Systems are the enablers of the line supplier. Systems must enable the supplier to achieve quality performance at the front line and at all levels of delivery.

Management Support

Employees are the customers of management in the customer–supplier chain. Managers must create incentives for the worker to produce quality, ensure all resources are in place, provide the training needed, and give workers the responsibility and accountability for exceeding customer expectations, by functioning as suppliers who treat their employees as customers. Managers must lead by example, demonstrating the quality values concepts on a daily basis, so workers feel empowered and supported in the quality culture. Managers must reward quality and innovation on a continual basis to ensure workers feel supported in a quality values culture.

Teamwork

Demonstrated inter- and intraorganizational support, cooperation, coordination, communication, and collaboration. Customers want suppliers who work together internally to create sequential flow without mistakes, redundancy, and rework. Smooth handoffs–for example, between coworkers within a unit or between different departments—are essential. Resource sharing, information sharing, single—access scheduling for customer convenience, and so on, are all good ways that organizations can work more cross-functionally as a team, working within a fully integrated delivery system.

Commitment

The level of dedication to the customer–supplier relationship that ensures the customer seeks no other supplier and always recommends your organization to others.

Characteristics

Interpersonal Relationship

Customers want a relationship with a supplier that based on trust and reliance on one person who they believe has their best interests at heart, and who will take care of their wants, needs, and desires now and in the future. The best supplier demonstrates an unbending desire to achieve— and, if possible, to exceed—the customer's expectations in each and every interaction.

Information and Involvement

A customer wants a supplier who provides all information and constantly solicit customer needs. They ask, ''How are you doing? How can we serve you better?'' Suppliers must be completely honest in disclosing any ''bad news.''

Notification

The customer wants to know up front about terms and conditions, and any anticipated or actual disappointments. This represents openness and integrity, and engenders the quality values. Although bad—news notifications are not what

the customer wants to hear, their disclosure engenders trust, which is the most important factor in any long-lasting customer–supplier relationship.

Responsibility/Accountability

When an outcome is not achieved, the customer wants the supplier to take immediate responsibility and ensure corrective action. This is especially important when one of the quality values has been violated or delivery has not taken place as promised.

Innovation

Constant introduction of state-of-the-art innovations, changes, and improvements to the product or service line. The customer wants the supplier to continue to offer a product line that is one of the best, if not *the* best. Customers want their suppliers to be consistently adaptable to new condition and challenges, and to find new ways to meet their changing requirements.

QUESTIONNAIRE DESIGN
Looking at the Research

The concept of the quality values developed out of an extensive analytical research process. For more than 10 years we have been conducting ongoing studies of organizations through analysis of their employee and external customer satisfaction data. Studies have been performed on more than 160 companies and more than 500,000 population samples. The companies range from state and federal government to private businesses, and deliver all types of products and services. Many studies focused directly on health care populations.

For the last 7 years we have taught courses in the field of customer-focused quality at the university level. Part of the course requirements for each student is to participate in focus groups to identify the key characteristics of customer satisfaction. These students also collect survey instruments from many different organizations, and perform matrix analyses—again, looking for the quality values and characteristics.

These techniques were also applied to organizations in many multidisciplinary focus groups. Doctors of philosophy have served as field advisors for masters' and doctoral students conducting their research in customer satisfaction. The rigorous nature of the academic research requirements validated in every way the lessons we were learning through applied research in the marketplace. The purpose was to get, yet again, another picture of the concepts of quality, what works, what are the constructs, what are the values, and what are the characteristics of quality.

To provide a stronger health care emphasis we formed a number of multidisciplinary focus groups comprised of nurses, doctors, patients, and other representative members of the health care continuum. The team members "benchmarked" all over the country. They collected surveys from every health care industry they could find, and performed matrix analyses (see Chapter 5) of these instruments to identify which of the quality values and characteristics were most pertinent to health care delivery. Design of their survey instruments was based on this analysis. All the surveys that we use today in the survey process are designed based on the quality values and the quality characteristics developed through the research methods presented in this chapter. Not only does this make for good research and survey design it also helps to define on what we should focus to achieve patient satisfaction.

Continuous Improvement Curve

From an organizational perspective, managers want to know why their customers buy, and what will cause them to buy more. What will keep them coming back and make them refer others? Once identified, these factors can be measured and managed to foster continuous improvement.

Human topics of interaction are often about our least common experiences. The best movie, restaurant, shopping mall; a murder, car crash, cancer, heart attack; falling in love, getting a divorce. Customer delight in a customer–supplier relationship is a unique and uncommon experience worthy of telling everyone you know, and then worth reexperiencing. A service experience that is less than delightful is far less worth experiencing or relating. However, a very negative experience with the customer–supplier relationship is also a least common experience, and is worth telling many people how the supplier failed.

When looking at the hotel industry and thinking about how hard the sales department must work to find customers to fill the rooms day in and day out, you may wonder what you could do to make life easier for them. Burnout in sales is high in the hotel industry because people get tired of selling the same old product every day, seeing no change in the average number of hotel rooms booked each week.

But what if you could do one or two things to improve the return-and-recommend rate, with a higher percentage of guests referring someone to the hotel? What if you discovered, for instance, that a change in the way hotel personnel greeted each guest made them feel more welcome in your hotel? What if this simple factor made people feel more comfortable, as if their presence at the hotel was actually valued? What if this was the key factor in changing the customer's perception of the hotel, and that customer then always referred your hotel to at least one other person?

If you were the general manager of the hotel you could track the increase in sales over time, and if you were the salesperson you would see a higher rate of people and groups who didn't have to be "sold" so hard. Slowly, the effect of each guest referring someone else would begin to catch up with your underused capacity.

Now take the continuous improvement curve a step or two further. What if enough demand could be created to keep the hotel full or nearly full for more of the year? Discounts could be eliminated during times of peak demand, and premiums could be charged for even greater profit. You may begin to see the importance of identifying the key strategies for making customer satisfaction happen. This is what the quality values are all about. More importantly, they must fit into what is termed the *basic cycle of improvement*.

The Cycle of Improvement

The basic premise of the cycle of improvement is presented in *Figure 9.1*.

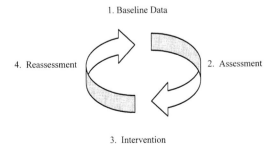

Figure 9.1 The cycle of improvement.

By definition, the cycle of improvement is a continuous process. We start with baseline data to determine where you, as the supplier, are today. This is the official measurement of your starting point and, hopefully, the baseline from which to measure future improvement. This is typically done by surveying your customers and using the quality values as the core set of constructs on which to base your questions.

Some businesses never even get to this most basic stage, or they don't know what they should be measuring. We've taken care of all of that for you. You should measure the quality values, and should apply each of them to your own business. If you aren't a manager of a corporation or don't own your own business, think of some other supplier with whom you have to deal regularly. If you really want to stretch, instead of thinking of a supplier, think of a personal relationship—go for it; it's a healthy process.

For each of the quality values constructs you have an ideal or expected standard of performance. Let's take the quality value of Timeliness as an example. In a bank you should never wait more than 5 minutes in line before you get to the teller or, in submission of your taxes, you shouldn't have to wait more than 30 days to get your tax refund. When you perform an assessment, you compare your baseline data with the ideal. Maybe the average wait at the bank is 11 minutes something needs to be done about that! Maybe, if you're an employee of the Internal Revenue Service, you really want to achieve 30-day tax refunds for everyone, but you're averaging 45 days (or 60 days or . . .)

The assessment is essentially the identification of a gap between actual product or service delivery and an ideal that meets or exceeds the customer's expectations. Some of these types of disparities stand out more than others based on the nature of your business. If you're unlucky enough to have major disparities in each quality value, rank areas of improvement based on what is most critical to your type of business. Implementation of the quality values is a continual process that recognizes the need to improve forever organizational systems and processes. Be thankful that at least you've now become aware of what's really happening, and have successful ways to improve problems. Imagine the companies who lose market share and are not aware of why they are doing so.

Intervention is the exciting part of the continuous improvement process. Our hotel example resulted in a change in greeting policies for employees because it made customers feel welcome—a major part of the Attentiveness quality value, which is also one of the three components of Self-management. The intervention means you are going to analyze the problem, form a hypothesis about what may cure or improve the problem, and implement it. Simple as that. You may now begin to understand the importance of having good data. To make changes in approach, policy, or procedure may be difficult or expensive. Without data you may even be making the wrong changes. But, by using the quality values constructs for your customer satisfaction survey, at least you'll be sure you've got the right problem identified. To complete the cycle of improvement you must remeasure customer satisfaction routinely to determine whether your interventions are working. Give your interventions time to take hold before you remeasure, or you will be disappointed with the fact that the data have not changed. Remember, if what you're doing isn't working, try something else!

Use the tools provided in this chapter to perform your own objective assessment of the current state of your company. Is your company a quality values company? Confer with others to get as many perspectives as possible. What are your company's quality values gaps? Based on this gap analysis, design a survey instrument using the quality values and characteristics to frame your questions. Conduct your survey, analyze the data, and begin to implement your interventions. You are now on your way to creating a quality values organization. Although it is often a good idea to work on the issues that have the most positive impact, it is also good to have some relatively easy improvement wins right off the bat when going through this process in an organization. This gives you some momentum and early feelings of success. Remember to measure the same things, which you set out initially to improve! And don't be afraid to go back to the old way of doing things or trying something different if your new approach doesn't get the results you expect. However, don't hamper your intervention efforts by cutting them short too soon.

When you have realized a measurable improvement from this simple process, you may now join the ranks of companies, suppliers, and individuals on the continuous improvement curve. Take care to repeat this process aggressively in all of the quality values areas to turn that short-term upspike into a continuous improvement curve. As long as you're improving consistently, sooner or later you will achieve improved patient satisfaction.

Guidelines on Questionnaire Design

There are several issues that must be addressed when creating the hard-copy version of the questionnaire to be distributed. The key is to achieve a standardized, reliable survey that measures the parameters of satisfaction effectively within a patient—supplier relationship. As stated earlier, the appropriate sample size is of paramount implied. Your sampling technique (e.g. point of service, mailer, phone survey) should be considered carefully to ensure you collect a sample that truly reflects the target population. You cannot have quality data without a well-designed assessment tool. To help determine which areas of product or service delivery are most important to the patient, and thus should be a part of your survey, a focus group would be beneficial. The following are simple suggestions that will enable you to bypass some of the common mistakes made when designing a survey questionnaire.

First, the questions asked must measure values and must be simple, neutral, and specific. Questions should relate directly to the knowledge desired. To ensure your questions are clear and specific, conduct some pilot testing on co-workers or a small customer sample. If your questions are open to interpretation, your results tend to be less valid.

Second, there must be only one value per question. Two values per question, such as "staff were friendly and helpful" are called *double-barrel questions*. What if the supplier was very friendly but not at all helpful? How does the customer respond accurately to this question? Such ambiguity in survey design forces random answers and is of little help to your business in the long run.

When creating a Likert scale, use standard phrases such as Very Useful somewhat Useful, and Not at All Useful. These are typical responses to which customers can relate making their responses quicker and more appropriate to the question being asked. If you use scales that do not have standard or common definitions, provide some explanation of what each level of

the scale represents. This produces more accurate answers that truly quantify the views of the respondents.

Designing surveys is not a time to show off your power vocabulary. Use terms and words that are common to the English language. Try to be careful with political correctness. What is your gender? is more appropriate than What is your sex? If you have demographic questions in your survey, such as age, education, gender, ethnic background, and so forth, make sure that these are coded categorically (age: 1–25, 26–35, 36–45, 45 +) rather than continuous ("What is your age?"). Make sure the categories do not overlap (e.g., 1–25, 25–35). This saves a lot of work for the analyst when preparing to study the data. We recommend one open-ended question. Make it very broad, such as Do you have any comments? More than one open-ended question results in a great deal of redundancy in responses. Follow these basic guidelines and you have a good chance of developing a useful and informative survey tool.

Data Analysis and Reporting

Many people attempt to design and analyze surveys, and they soon discover that it is much more complicated than it appears on the surface. Data analysis is a particularly scientific process, but it is made much easier through the use of expert systems software programs. Still, analysts must have a theoretical background and must be able to use the software at a level of expertise that allows for application of appropriate statistical models. Good analysis will identify areas in which patient satisfaction is both high and low. It will indicate whether there is statistically significant variation in satisfaction among responding subgroups in the study. The analysis should also provide a prediction model that indicates which satisfaction indicators most influence the patient's desire to return to you for their next product or service requirement, and if or how often they will recommend you to others. Although all of the statistical software programs produce charts, graphs, and tables, the managers in your company will generally not have the software to view the results. It is important, therefore, to choose statistical software that is compatible with your office software. It is very important to display data as information in a presentation format to illustrate the findings. Most managers do not gain much insight from statistical tables and spreadsheets. We highly recommend that you share the patient satisfaction information to enlighten your staff.

Bad questionnaire design, inappropriate analysis, or ineffective informational reporting often result in useless information, wasting all your efforts and resulting in decisions that are not truly data driven. This puts your business in peril of failing to achieve one of its primary missions: patient satisfaction. Remember that data-driven decisions are the best decisions, and patient data are the best data.

Your understanding of how to apply the insights of the quality values is fundamental to your company's continuous improvement curve. Once you understand each construct and its implications, the challenge is to do something positive with it in your own situation.

INTERPRETING THE RESULTS
Complaining for Quality

We believe strongly that everyone has a responsibility to be a *power customer*. This is a challenge for every individual to become part of the quality values revolution. So what are some of the things you can do as power customers? For one, you can give feedback to the supplier. Let's say you are dissatisfied with a front-line service person for rude service. Take the time to talk to the manager. If more of us did that, took that time, it would change the way these companies do business. If more people told them, for example, "I just went over to the lumber department and asked your employee there about electrical issues, and he didn't have a clue, nor did he bother to ask anybody in the store who might have the answer. Your company has failed to give me quality service and I'm not coming back here anymore." Tell somebody who counts, somebody who has a financial investment in the company. You will make a big difference. When you provide the supplier with feedback determine their receptivity. If they're receptive, give them another chance. Don't give them one strike and count them out. Patients, as customers, must help suppliers to improve, but if the suppliers resist and get defensive, then they have neither the opportunity nor the desire to improve. If suppliers do the right thing, and effect the improvement, be a loyal customer to them and give them positive word-mouth advertising. Patients do not need to put up with poor quality, but they must write a letter or file a complaint to let the provider know how they feel. As

a result, we will continue to have better quality, because there's always a supplier out there who's willing to jump over the bar that the patient keeps raising, to rise to the challenge to meet that patient's expectations. Patients as customers are developing suppliers who are more than willing to do whatever it takes to meet their patients' needs. More and more suppliers are receptive. They want to satisfy the patient. They have a customer service attitude that goes a long way toward keeping them in business. They will always be viable. The continuous improvement curve will continue to rise in terms of services requested, as long as suppliers maintain this attitude.

Why Some Customers Don't Complain

Some patients behave like sheep being led to slaughter, but the supplier should not be fooled. Dissatisfied patients who make a decision not to complain are most likely on their way to finding a different supplier. Why don't people complain when they have legitimate grievances? Some of the reasons include

- Pessimism
- Inconvenience
- Discomfort with the role of complainer
- Power of selection (i.e., vote with their feet)

Pessimism

Patients know that the front-line service personnel with whom they are dealing are often quite distant from the actual decision makers who can make a difference. These patients don't believe in their own ability to make an impact, and they don't believe the supplier is especially motivated to meet their needs.

Inconvenience

Patients are in a hurry most of the time and feel they have better things to do than worry about how a provider runs the business. Complaining takes time and energy, and is usually only tapped when a patient is really upset by a particularly bad service experience.

Discomfort With the Role of Complainor

Sharing the shortcomings of a supplier can elicit a defensive reaction that evolves into conflict. Sometimes patients aren't as articulate with their dissatisfaction and may be invalidated by the supplier–a very disempowering experience for the patient.

CHAPTER 10

Patient-Based Assessments in Neurological Surgery

BEVERLY C. WALTERS, M.D., M.SC

EDITOR'S NOTE: Patient satisfaction surveys reflect patient perception. Clinical outcome studies usually measure medical endpoints that may be more important to physicians, for assessing their own professional and technical skill, than for patients, who may only focus on that subset of medical endpoints that impact their own personal life needs and priorities most. Scientifically validated patient assessment instruments such as the Short Form (SF)-36 and the SF-12 go beyond simple subjective, superficial perception to actually measure "wellness" on generic axes that accurately reflect patient health regardless of clinical diagnosis. Combined with objective, diagnosis-specific, clinical outcome measures, these instruments give a more objective indication of the patient outcomes for clinical processes.

"All models are wrong. Some models are useful."

—George Box

Neurosurgeons have come full circle with the current interest in patient-centered outcome measures. In 1904 Harvey Cushing said, "The mere lengthening of a patient's month or years without rendering them more livable is. . .no justification whatsoever of an operative procedure" (7). The delivery of high-quality care is the modern expression of this general sentiment and was articulated some 50 years later by Lembcke, who said, "The best measure of quality is not how well or how frequently a medical service is given, but how closely the result approaches the fundamental objectives of prolonging life, relieving distress, restoring function and preventing disability" (29). Now these goals are combined in outcome measurement that has become a science in itself, involving detailed assessment of a patient's report of well being. The best studied generic measure of patient well being is the Short Form (SF)-36 and its subsets,

the SF-12 and the SF-8 (44). The purpose of this chapter is to explore the general array of outcome measures that are available to clinicians, to examine patient reports as a way of measuring patient outcome, and to suggest ways in which patient well-being measures can be integrated into everyday clinical practice.

OUTCOME MEASUREMENT IN THE PROVISION OF HEALTH SERVICES

The stimulus for careful measurement of outcome in patient care stems from three sources:

- Clinicians, who have always wished to assess the efficacy of their clinical interventions;
- Payers, who need some way of evaluating the outcome of treatment paid for; and
- Patients, who have little interest in measures aside from those demonstrating whether they feel or function better than they did prior to treatment.

Outcome measurement serves multiple functions. For "prognosis," outcome measurement establishes the typical outcome for patients with a given disorder in longitudinal studies of the population at large. In comparative treatment studies, such as randomized controlled trials, outcome measurement serves as the endpoint for effectiveness or efficacy (i.e., therapeutic effectiveness). In everyday practice, it helps to know whether the treatments we are providing are the best quality (as measured by the achievement of desired outcomes) and allows us the opportunity to improve our treatment algorithms (i.e., quality assurance). An international panel of outcome researchers has suggested that there should be standardization of outcome measures, and they cited several advantages (9). These advantages include improving comparability of results of interventions as well as comparing baseline characteristics of patients involved in trials or submitted to treatment. Outcome measurement in turn facilitates the performance of multicenter studies, meta-analyses, and cost-effectiveness studies by providing common accepted measures, which help avoid the perennial problem of "apples and oranges" comparisons. Outcome measurements also, by definition, encourage more complete reporting of relevant outcomes. However, the most important aspect of standardized outcome measures is the potential to significantly improve the medical literature, thereby facilitating the development of meaningful evidence-based practice parameters. The international panel then pointed out factors that should be considered in choosing outcome measures for standardization. These factors include breadth of coverage, demonstrated validity and reproducibility, responsiveness, practicality, importance to patients, and importance to society.

Historically, outcome measures have been primarily clinical, such as those that can be measured by physical examination or imaging studies. However, as health care has become more expensive because of technological advances and increasing demands of an aging population, new outcomes related to usage have become more important. These measures include length of hospital stay, readmission to the emergency department following discharge, use of inhospital reimbursable services, unplanned return to the operating room because of complications from surgery, and so forth. These outcome measures require nothing more than the medical record for generation and are gross measures of the patient's progress through the health care system and the use of health care services. From these data, costs of treatment can be derived or estimated. These measures, however, represent only the first tier of outcome measurement, and most patients would argue that they have little value in establishing whether a given treatment achieves success in alleviating the patient's primary problem or presenting complaint.

As the demand for science in clinical practice has increased, so have the requirements for outcome measurement to be characterized by validity and reproducibility. This means that a simple "How are you doing today?" and replies such as "Fine, thank you," "Not so good," or "So-so," which one hears in the outpatient setting, are not acceptable as legitimate outcome measures. As clinical maneuvers began to vie for leadership as "the best" in any given clinical circumstance, the science of outcomes was born. As endpoints for clinical trials, there had to be concrete evidence that something was measurably different between patients treated in one way over another. The most objective measures were chosen first. These included countable events similar to those described above—days in hospital and returns to the operating room for hemorrhage or infection, deficit, or even death. The next level of assessment involved some sort of objective clinical measure as represented by either the clinical examination or imaging study. Examples of such measures include very formalized measures such as the National Institutes of Health (NIH) Stroke Scale (5) or a less detailed objective measure such as reduction in tumor volume, respectively. To be useful in clinical research, the measures must be studied in the intended clinical circumstance and reliability must be evaluated if different observers are responsible for assessing the patient's clinical performance, or reading and opining on the findings of imaging studies. These objective measures need to be scientifically studied and standardized so that they are reproducible and interpretation is possible in a meaningful way. Although these objective clinical measures might then be satisfactory to clinicians, according to patients and payers, they leave something to be desired, their scientific validity notwithstanding.

Those interest groups, or "stakeholders," are more interested in measures that attempt to assess patient function and quality of life. Functional measures categorize and prioritize the patient's ability to move normally and to carry out usual daily activities. Quality of life involves function but also includes aspects that influence quality of life, such as pain and mental health. The 1948 definition of "health" from the World Health Organization was that "health is a state of complete physical, mental, and social well-being and not merely the absence of disease or infirmity" (46). This definition included all dimensions of health and the full range of being well. The challenge of how to operationalize this definition, or any other definition, has been embraced and met with an elegant refinement of the simple act of asking patients how they are. These measures in general belong to a class of outcomes called patient-based assessments (PBAs).

ATTRIBUTES OF PATIENT-BASED ASSESSMENTS

Quality of life as it relates to health status involves many aspects of a person's life. Because neurosurgical illness occurs in the body, physical aspects of an individual's life are primarily altered. The effect that this alteration in physical status has is often expressed in mental effects as well as bodily function. In addition, changes in the physical and mental aspects of patient abilities lead inevitably to social dysfunction. Therefore, a truly relevant outcome measure will take all of these aspects into consideration and measure them in a scientific, reproducible, and valid way. Such a measure would include both descriptive and evaluative measures. There is an intricate interaction between how a patient functions physically, how he or she feels about this, and his or her evaluation of life in the given dysfunctional circumstance. It is important to remember, however, that there are societal influences (e.g., wealth and education) on quality of life that the health care professional cannot affect with the care provided but that may temper a patient's response to treatment.

To cover fully a patient's response to disease, any health-related quality-of-life measure must sample all the domains of influence. This includes subsets of both mental and physical health.

SF-8, SF-12, SF-18, SF-20, AND SF-36

The generic outcome measure that has been used more than any other, in a variety of diseases and to test a multitude of treatments, is the SF-36 (45). This measure involves surveys of patients at particular points in their treatment as they progress through the health care system. The SF-36 and its antecedents, the SF-18 and SF-20, and their progeny, the SF-12 and SF-8, include assessment of functional ability, well being, and overall health. The entire gamut of function is addressed, including physical functioning, social functioning, role limitations at-

tributed to physical problems, and role limitations attributed to emotional problems. Well being encompasses mental health, pain, energy, and fatigue. Overall health involves the patient's general health perception.

The SF-36 questionnaire is derived from a larger series of questions validated on thousands of patients and initially created to study medical outcomes (38). Normative data from the population at large have been gathered to establish a baseline for health. Although the SF-36 only takes approximately 10 minutes to complete, as a generic measure it is usually used in combination with disease-specific measures, thereby increasing respondent burden and decreasing compliance. As a result, there was a perceived need to shorten the questionnaire further. This led to a study in which regression techniques were used to find a subset of questions that would adequately correlate with the larger survey (44). This gave rise to the SF-12, which is commonly used today in clinical trials and longitudinal studies. Each of the eight conceptual areas sampled by the SF-36 has at least one question in the shorter survey. However, two of the physical health assessment domains (Physical Functioning and Role–Physical) and two of the mental health domains (Mental Health and Role–Emotional) have two questions because of the improvement in precision when they are included. The shorter survey takes only 2 minutes to complete, and entry into a properly constructed database takes as little as an additional 30 seconds. The questions in the SF-12 are listed in *Figure 10.1*. Studies are currently underway to validate an even shorter measure, the SF-8. It is unclear, however, how much shorter the questionnaire needs to be to make it palatable for both clinicians and patients alike.

ADVANTAGES AND DISADVANTAGES OF GENERIC MEASURES

Generic measures such as the SF-36 and SF-12 allow researchers, providers, payers, and patients to use a common language that is based on well-understood concepts in reporting and understanding health. What the generic measures cannot do is to probe the disease-specific dysfunction at which treatment is aimed. For example, patients with epilepsy should have a measure of cognitive function included in their surveillance because a lack of improvement in their

The SF-12™ Health Survey

Instructions for Completing the Questionnaire

Please answer every question. Some questions may look like others, but each
one is different. Please take the time to read and answer each question
carefully by filling in the bubble that best represents your response.

EXAMPLE

This is for your review. Do not answer this question. The questionnaire
begins with the section *Your Health in General* below.

For each question you will be asked to fill in a bubble in each line:

1. How strongly do you agree or disagree with each of the following statements?

		Strongly agree	Agree	Uncertain	Disagree	Strongly disagree
a)	I enjoy listening to music.	○	●	○	○	○
b)	I enjoy reading magazines.	●	○	○	○	○

Please begin answering the questions now.

Your Health in General

1.   In general, would you say your health is:

Excellent	Very good	Good	Fair	Poor
○	○	○	○	○

2.   The following items are about activities you might do during a typical day. Does your
health now limit you in these activities? If so, how much?

		Yes, Limited A Lot	Yes, Limited A Little	No, Not Limited At All
a.	**Moderate activities**, such as moving a table, pushing a vacuum cleaner, bowling, or playing golf	○	○	○
b.	Climbing **several** flights of stairs	○	○	○

Please turn the page to continue.

Figure 10.1   The SF-12 Health Survey. Reprinted with permission from Medical Outcomes Trust and John E. Ware, Jr.

3. During the **past 4 weeks**, have you had any of the following problems with your work or other regular daily activities <u>as a result of your physical health</u>?

	YES	NO
a. **Accomplished less** than you would like	○	○
b. Were limited in the **kind** of work or other activities	○	○

4. During the **past 4 weeks**, have you had any of the following problems with your work or other regular daily activities <u>as a result of any emotional problems</u> (such as feeling depressed or anxious)?

	YES	NO
a. **Accomplished less** than you would like	○	○
b. Didn't do work or other activities as **carefully** as usual	○	○

5. During the **past 4 weeks**, how much did <u>pain</u> interfere with your normal work (including both work outside the home and housework)?

Not at all	A little bit	Moderately	Quite a bit	Extremely
○	○	○	○	○

6. These questions are about how you feel and how things have been with you during the **past 4 weeks**. For each question, please give the one answer that comes closest to the way you have been feeling. How much of the time during the **past 4 weeks** . . .

	All of the Time	Most of the Time	A Good Bit of the Time	Some of the Time	A Little of the Time	None of the Time
a. Have you felt calm and peaceful?	○	○	○	○	○	○
b. Did you have a lot of energy?	○	○	○	○	○	○
c. Have you felt downhearted and blue?	○	○	○	○	○	○

7. During the **past 4 weeks**, how much of the time has your <u>physical health or emotional problems</u> interfered with your social activities (like visiting with friends, relatives, etc.)?

All of the time	Most of the time	Some of the time	A little of the time	None of the time
○	○	○	○	○

THANK YOU FOR COMPLETING THIS QUESTIONNAIRE!

Figure 10.1 *(continued).*

general well being when seizures are controlled may reflect drug side effects or surgical injury. Likewise, patients with Parkinson's disease should have additional measures that assess cognition and communication as part of their health assessment. Patients with traumatic brain injury should have detailed functional assessment done that indicates independence or dependence on others for day-to-day living. These disease entities and others are discussed below.

In spite of the disease-specific limitations of the SF-36 and SF-12, they can easily be used in concert with other measures, are easy to administer and score, and have a wealth of research validating them. For these reasons, they are becoming more widely used in assessment of neurosurgical patients.

EXAMPLES OF PATIENT-BASED ASSESSMENTS IN NEUROLOGICAL SURGERY

The usefulness of patient-based assessments in patients commonly treated by neurosurgeons has been examined in several studies (3, 4, 6, 16–18, 40). These studies and others are reviewed in detail below.

In Parkinson's disease, several studies measuring the ability of the SF-36 to capture adequately the true state of health have been carried out (22, 34). Because of the need for disease specificity in outcome measurement, these studies have usually been investigated as a part of a battery of tests. For example, The Parkinson's Disease Questionnaire (PDQ-39) has been used along with the SF-36, other illness indices (e.g., Sickness Impact Profile, Nottingham Health Profile), and clinical measures (e.g., Hoehn and Yahr Scale, Columbia Scale) (18). Of interest, both the PDQ-39 and the SF-36 correlated more closely with health status and effects of physical dysfunction than did the purely clinical measures. This indicates an inability of the clinical measures (preferred by clinicians) to adequately portray the true health status of patients with Parkinson's disease. The patient-based assessments, on the other hand, appear to be able to reflect the health status appropriately. For this reason, the SF-36 has been recommended as an integral measure of outcome in patients with Parkinson's disease.

In the early 1990s, it was recognized that epilepsy is both a medical diagnosis and a social label (19). With this in mind, Vickrey et al. created a health-related quality-of-life measure for patients with epilepsy, specifically those undergoing surgery (40). These researchers chose the SF-36 as the "generic core" for their Epilepsy Surgery Inventory-55 assessment. In addition, this enlarged and supplemented assessment tool includes disease-specific items: five items assessing cognitive function, eight items measuring role limitations as a result of memory difficulties, four items indicating health perception, and two items assessing a global view of quality of life. This adds up to a total of 55 questions, thus the Epilepsy Surgery Inventory-55, or ESI-55. Vickrey et al.'s (40) studies indicated that the whole assessment tool, which is based primarily on the SF-36, "is reliable, valid, and sensitive to differences in seizure status." In an extensive literature review, Langfitt noted that the ESI-55 captures the "broad impact of epilepsy on quality of life" (28). Other potential assessment tools for epilepsy have also relied on the SF-36 to provide the generic core for general well-being (30, 33, 43). The SF-36 has also been used as a sole measure for general health status (41).

The assessment of outcome in severe traumatic brain injury (TBI) has most commonly been by survival statistics alone. Over the last 20 years, there has been increasing use of a more differentiated outcome measure, the Glasgow Outcome Scale (GOS) (23). This measure divides patients into survival groups on the basis of their general status: good recovery, moderately disabled, severely disabled, or vegetative. However, a quick look at this breakdown reveals that there is not enough differentiation within the groups, although reliability of the measures between the groups may be acceptable. To overcome this, more sophisticated measures such as the SF-12 have been implemented, in conjunction with measures of independence (6). In a study of patients with TBI, researchers showed that, when the primary area of outcome focused on the amount of help or supervision the person required in carrying out daily activities, the Functional Independence Measure (FIM) was superior to the SF-36 (14). This is not surprising, considering that the SF-36 is a more global measure of health status than the FIM. This indicates another circumstance in which additional measures are desirable in specific clinical circumstances.

Patients with cerebrovascular disease have been studied extensively using the SF-36 (1, 10, 24, 37). In a randomized, controlled trial of the SF-36 and the EuroQOL (11), the SF-36 was shown to be equally reliable as an outcome measure in clinical trials, even if answered by a proxy (10). The SF-36 has also been shown to provide good outcomes data for long-term survivors of cerebrovascular accidents (1). Patients with a decline in physical functioning demonstrated a similar decline in mental health (37). Of interest, women with the same physical limitations had higher scores in the mental health and social functioning scores (1). This would not have been elucidated if other outcome measures had been used. Likewise, in a long-term study of young survivors of stroke, the impact on overall quality of life as a result of disability was worse than that reported for their older counterparts (37).

The most common procedures in which neurosurgeons are generally involved include those for diseases of the spine, because this category of illness and dysfunction is a significant health burden to society. Because resolution in symptomatology and improved function are the goals of treatment in spinal disorders, this is one of the most common uses that has been made of patient-based assessments. Whether looking at prognosis (17, 26, 32), therapeutic effectiveness (3, 39), or as screening tools (27), patient-based assessments have been shown to have significant usefulness.

In a study of thoracolumbar burst fractures treated both operatively and nonoperatively, Kraemer et al. noted that there was no correlation between the radiographic presence of kyphosis of the spine and functional outcome using the SF-36 (26). Likewise, Thomas et al. were able to show no correlation between dynamic listhesis postoperatively in patients treated with either laminectomy or laminotomy for spinal stenosis and outcome as measured by the SF-36 (39). In another study, return to work (another popular measure of outcome in spine surgery) did not correlate to degree of physical or social impairment. In fact, more patients had returned to work than would have been predicted by the degree of persistent dysfunction (17). This is additional evidence that the usual outcomes of importance to clinicians may have little relationship to the patients' outcome reports.

The Maine Lumbar Spine study showed a contrast in outcome for patients with sciatica (2) compared with patients with spinal stenosis (3) treated surgically. One of the side benefits of using the SF-36 in this study was that the baseline characteristics of the patients were different, illustrating the difficulty in using nonrandomized comparative studies for determining therapeutic effectiveness.

Whether there needs to be any additional condition- or disease-specific outcome measures added to the SF-36 or SF-12 in treatment of spinal disorders remains unclear. When the commonly used Oswestry Low Back Pain Questionnaire (12) and the Low Back Pain Outcome Score (15) were compared with the SF-36 in assessing outcome, there was significant correlation (16). This begs the question of whether the SF-36 (or, by extension, the SF-12) can stand alone as adequate primary outcome in the treatment of spinal disorders.

Some clinicians are resistant to the notion of burdening patients with lengthy questionnaires to complete and taking valuable time out of the patient encounter to examine the responses, even in the interest of scientific practice. One study has indicated that patients with epilepsy wanted to be asked about their daily lives and their feelings and did not mind completing a questionnaire to provide this information (42). Furthermore, from the clinicians' standpoint, having this information lengthened the patient encounter, but only by about 0.5–4.0 minutes. In addition, the clinicians involved in the study found that, in spite of knowing their patients extremely well or quite well, they gained new information about their patients as a result of the administration of the SF-36. This brought about a change in therapy in approximately 12% of patients. The clinicians in the study indicated that the data obtained from the SF-36 were particularly useful when the quality of life was lowest.

TRACKING PATIENT WELL BEING IN EVERYDAY CLINICAL PRACTICE

The rationale behind rigorous scientific outcome measurement in clinical trials is intuitively obvious. However, understanding the importance of such measurement in daily patient assessment takes a certain commitment to evidence-based practice and the continuous application of clinical science. After that commitment is made, the question then becomes how best to implement such measurement of patient outcome while carrying out an efficient, fiscally viable enterprise. Fortunately, the technological advances in medical informatics and the rapidly improving hardware and software options available to the practitioner make such outcome assessment practical. In practices in which electronic media are used to collect and store patient data, the addition of an outcome measure such as the SF-12 is fairly simple. In one such highly customizable program called Turbo-Doc (Paradise Surgical Associates, Inc., Paradise, CA), a simple template has been inserted to record patient responses to the questionnaire (*Fig. 10.2*). Another clever solution for those without such electronic medical records but with an interest in ongoing outcome measurement is the commercially available

Crosspad (Plexsys Development, Inc., Boston, MA), which has been linked to a new program developed by an independent software firm. In this model, the patient fills out the questionnaire on a clipboard that is linked to a program that collects the information directly, transferring it into computer language and enabling electronic storage and retrieval (*Fig. 10.3*). Likewise, the SF-36 or SF-12 data may be transmitted directly by facsimile or electronically via the Internet and analyzed by the copyright owners of the measure through contractual arrangement. For further information about the above, see the appropriate web pages on the Internet (*www.SF-36.com, www.Turbo-Doc.com*). Using any of these methods, the patient is given the questionnaire at each visit, office personnel enter the data, the physician reviews the data as part of the patient's encounter, and longitudinal studies can be carried out for quality assurance or for more formal

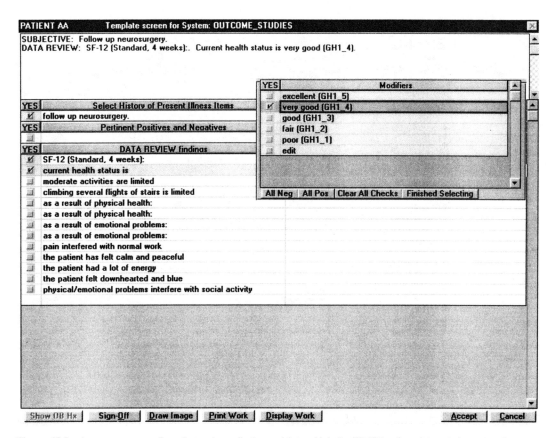

Figure 10.2 A screen capture of an electronic medical record into which the SF-12 has been integrated as a template so that patient responses can be integrated directly into each visit record.

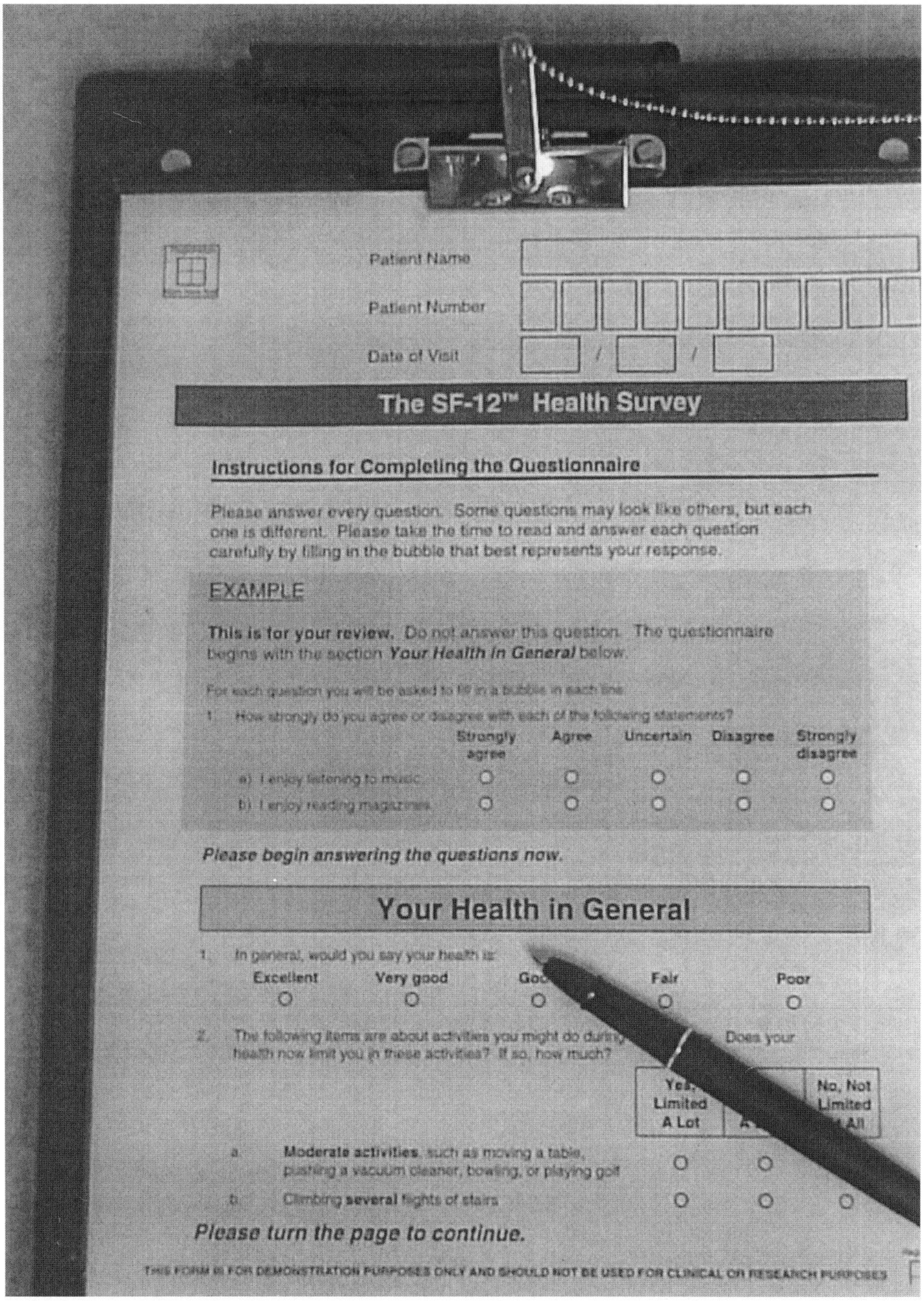

Figure 10.3 An example of the Crosspad device, which is for clinicians who are not using an electronic medical record or who wish to keep their outcomes data in a separate database. The Crosspad can collect the data from the patient and download the information directly into a database.

assessment of prognosis with treatment. Because the SF-12 has been shown to have a high correlation with the SF-36, the shorter questionnaire will most likely increase compliance and be more feasible in clinical practice (21).

PATIENT SATISFACTION

In contrast to the well-studied and scientifically sound measures of well being, another measure from the patient's perspective is satisfaction. Although satisfaction is based on clear principles, namely the patient's feelings about his or her care, the administration and content of questionnaires regarding this area of interest are not well defined. The overall aspect of care being addressed by the questionnaires is whether the outcome that the treatment achieves is worth the experience the patient has had. In spite of urging that patient satisfaction is an integral part of outcomes research and that it should be measured, no real research has gone into the science of patient satisfaction (13). A brief review of some of the neurosurgical entities in which patient satisfaction has been measured reveals a wide variability in how this outcome measurement is carried out.

In skull-base surgery, a comparison of microsurgery and stereotactic radiosurgery for treatment of acoustic neuroma has shown that patient satisfaction is higher with radiosurgery. Patient report of being "very satisfied," "satisfied," or "unsatisfied" determined satisfaction (35) In a later article, the same authors noted that "ninety-three percent of the patients were either very satisfied or satisfied after radiosurgery" (36, p. xx). In a slightly different approach, patients treated with microvascular decompression (MVD) for trigeminal neuralgia and hemifacial spasm were asked, "How satisfied were you with the results of MVD?" and then asked to assign a percentage value (25). Similar to the more general question, this was not standardized in any demonstrable way from person to person. In a similar manner, all patients who underwent orbitozygomatic craniotomy as a means of avoiding disfigurement "were pleased with the cosmetic results of their surgery. . ." (47).

In an effort to determine the effect of "awake" craniotomy on patients with lesions near eloquent cortex, satisfaction was assessed along with any adverse psychological sequelae (8). This was done through two separate but related questions. The first questions was, "Could you please rate your level of satisfaction with the procedure from 0 to 10, where 0 indicates maximum displeasure and 10 indicates maximal satisfaction." The second question was, "If you needed to undergo another craniotomy, would you agree to have it performed under local anesthesia and monitored conscious sedation if it was indicated?" Surprisingly, out of 21 patients who responded, only 3 said that they would not agree to the procedure as performed; of those, 1 patient had a satisfaction rating of 5 (out of 10), and 2 had a satisfaction rating of 10.

Outcome measurement in spine surgery has also attempted to include some form of patient satisfaction. This has ranged from the simple question, "Would you, in retrospect, still choose surgery?" ("yes," "no," "unsure"), in a study of laminectomy for spinal stenosis (20) to the more precise question in a study of dorsal root ganglionectomy for failed back surgery (31). In the latter study, the question was, "Considering the overall pain relief you have experienced after this surgery and considering the hospitalization(s), discomfort, and expense involved, would you go through it all again for the result you have obtained?" ("yes," "no," "unsure"). This is by far the most detailed single question attempting to address patient satisfaction, but it still is nothing more than asking patients if they are satisfied. In no study that I could find was there a comparison of a detailed patient well-being measure with a patient's satisfaction with the treatment undertaken. Until this occurs, patient satisfaction will remain a relatively unscientific outcome measurement.

The responsibilities of care providers in the next century will include scientific outcome measurement from the patient's perspective to demonstrate the effectiveness and efficacy of treatments offered and undertaken. This will include a clear understanding of the tools available, their inferential meaning, and the needs of the patients in this regard. Neurosurgeons will ignore these tools at their collective and individual peril.

REFERENCES

1. Anderson C, Laubscher S, Burns R: Validation of the short form 36 (SF-36) health survey questionnaire among stroke patients. *Stroke* 27:1812–1816, 1996.
2. Atlas SJ, Deyo RA, Keller RB: The Maine Lumbar Spine Study, part II: 1-year outcomes of surgical and nonsurgical treatment of sciatica. *Spine* 21: 1777–1786, 1996.
3. Atlas SJ, Deyo RA, Keller RB, et al: The Maine Lumbar Spine Study, part III. 1-year outcomes of surgical and

CHAPTER 11

Clinical Outcomes Analysis

ROBERT E. HARBAUGH, M.D., F.A.C.S.

EDITOR'S NOTE: The gold standard for objective measurement of diagnosis-specific or procedure-specific or procedure-specific outcomes is clinical outcomes analysis. Without the availability of this critical data for our own practices, patients, managed care organizations, and health care organizations will continue to assess and judge us solely based on cost and timeliness. Outcomes analysis is expensive to perform in terms of time invested to refresh the data continually on a real-time basis. This is a cost that managed care organizations will not likely support, because most do not currently appreciate its usefulness or relevance. To a managed care organization, physician quality is assumed (in the absence of an unexpected number of "sentinel events"), and cost and timeliness are measured (and used to guide managed care decisions). If we are to succeed in bringing empiric science to health care management and clinical patient care, we have to be willing to invest our own time and effort to fill the data void that currently exists for objective and reliable outcomes data. Even if managed care organizations initially turn a blind eye to the availability and relevance of these data, once educated and enlightened in what to look for, patients will insist on knowing these results for making their own health care choices. Managed care organizations will ultimately attach importance to what their primary customers find important.

Outcomes studies have become fashionable, but to many practicing physicians and surgeons, the concept of what constitutes an outcomes study remains nebulous. In this chapter I provide a brief summary of the methodology of outcomes studies and discuss why expert clinicians need to be involved in such studies to ensure their scientific rigor. I also attempt to convince you of the importance of outcomes studies for ensuring quality in neurological surgery, for patient education and for our survival in a very competitive market. After this introduction, I present patients with arteriovenous malformations (AVMs) of the brain as a case study to describe factors that need to be measured to assess treatment outcomes adequately. Finally, the efforts of the Outcomes Committee of the American Association of Neurological Surgeons (AANS) and the Congress of Neurological Surgeons (CNS) to establish an outcomes reporting system are discussed.

REVIEW OF OUTCOMES ANALYSIS

Outcomes analysis has become an increasingly important tool for investigating clinical issues and for determining health care policy. Outcomes research methodology has been employed to identify the relative effectiveness of surgical procedures and other treatment approaches, and to evaluate the cost and benefits of new technology. This type of clinical investigation has also been employed to track and improve health care quality, to study differences in performance among surgeons and hospitals, and to supply patients with meaningful data for making health care decisions. Third-party payers and government agencies are increasingly likely to require some kind of outcomes monitoring for contract purposes and for making policy decisions. Numerous methods, all subsumed under the umbrella term of *outcomes research* (*Table 11.1*), have been and are being used to assess the effectiveness of the care delivered to patients. The outcomes movement has gathered enough momentum that it can legitimately be described as a "revolution in medical care" (25). A brief summary of the various methodologies employed in outcomes research is presented in the following subsections.

Utilization Research

The origin of this area of outcomes research can be traced, in large part, to the seminal research of John Wennberg and his colleagues at

TABLE 11.1
Outcomes Research Methodologies

Category	Examples
Utilization research	Small-area variations
Data synthesis studies	Meta-analysis, decision analysis, cost-effectiveness analysis
Outcomes of treatment	Patient-level analysis, including clinical outcomes, lesional outcomes, functional outcomes, patient satisfaction, and resource utilization
Surgeon or hospital-level analysis	Risk stratification
Population-level analysis	Large database studies
Technology assessment	Any of the above

Dartmouth on the variability of use of health care resources across geographic regions (27, 28). They reported large variations in the rate of surgical procedures and hospital use in small geographic areas, and observed that this variability did not correlate with mortality or other discernible measures of the health of the population (27, 28). Such observations raised many questions regarding the rationale behind many medical decisions and the use of health care resources because the observed variability did not seem to be accounted for by differences in patient populations or rates of illness. Rather, the variability seemed to indicate a more fundamental problem with medical decision making and evaluating the outcome of care. The political climate of the late 1980s and 1990s fueled considerable interest in this type of study. Increasing demand for access to medical care and burgeoning expenditures for care made it imperative for physicians, patients, and third-party payers to evaluate critically the benefit gained from medical intervention. It must be stressed that descriptive analysis of patterns of use does not indicate the "correct" rate of use (18). However, this kind of small-area analysis can be used to indicate procedures in which there is a great deal of imprecision in the indications for surgical intervention.

Data Synthesis Studies

Frequently, outcomes research involves synthesizing the data from multiple studies (3, 17). Even the most elegant and scientifically rigorous

randomized, controlled trial may leave many questions unanswered regarding the effectiveness of care. A single study may not have sufficient numbers of patients to evaluate certain patient subgroups, and such studies often do not take into account important factors such as quality of life and costs. It can be argued that randomized, controlled trials can determine efficacy of treatment, but that outcomes studies methodology is needed to determine effectiveness of treatment. An example may help to clarify this distinction. Postulate a rigorous, randomized, controlled trial of chemotherapeutic agent X for patients with glioblastoma. Assume that this study shows a statistically significant delay in mortality of 6 weeks in the treatment group. This demonstrates the efficacy of the agent, under the constraints of the trial, for achieving this particular clinical end point. However, without data on functional outcomes, quality of life, costs, and other factors it is impossible to say whether the use of agent X is an effective treatment intervention from the standpoint of the patient or society. In other words, would a patient really desire this treatment and is it a reasonable investment of resources? Various data synthesis methodologies, discussed next, could be used to address some of the shortcomings noted in this example.

Meta-analysis

Some of the problems with an individual clinical trial can be circumvented by combining the results of multiple trials. Meta-analysis is a statistical method for evaluating and combining systematically the results of clinical trials to obtain a sample size sufficient for performing subgroup analysis and for determining clinically significant treatment effects (16, 17). This methodology can also be used to explore why individual clinical trials may yield contradictory results. However, meta-analysis still relies on the kind of data collected in the clinical trials, and if patient-oriented outcomes have not been collected, use of this biostatistical tool will not be able to assess adequately the effectiveness of care (6).

Decision Analysis

Decision analysis methodology can also be used for evaluating the effectiveness of treatment alternatives using data generated in clinical trials (1). In decision analysis, competing therapeutic strategies are specified, and clinically relevant outcomes for each strategy are analyzed via a decision tree model. Using data generated from relevant clinical studies, the probabilities of reaching the various clinical outcomes are determined. Each clinical outcome is then assigned a utility (6), such as quality adjusted life years (QALYs). For instance, 1 year of life in perfect health is equal to 1 QALY, death equals 0 QALY. Survival with, for example, a hemiparesis is assigned a utility based on patient perceptions (19). The anticipated value of the various treatment strategies can then be calculated by multiplying the probability of reaching a clinical outcome by its use. The stability of the results can be analyzed further using sensitivity analysis methods whereby the probabilities of reported outcomes are varied according to the range established from various clinical studies (1). Decision analysis can be used to determine the most beneficial treatment approach for an individual patient faced with a difficult treatment decision, or for analyzing the value of various treatment modalities for large populations of patients.

Cost-effectiveness Analysis

Cost-effectiveness analysis is used to determine the relative value of treatments by dividing the cost of a given intervention by the benefit obtained from the intervention (7, 9, 15, 20, 24). As for decision analysis, the benefit of treatment is usually determined by the QALYs to be obtained within a population by application of treatment. Cost-effectiveness is then expressed as dollars invested per QALY. Childhood immunization is often cited as the epitome of a cost-effective procedure: low cost and high benefit. Returning to the example used earlier of chemotherapeutic agent X for glioblastoma, let us assume that the use of this agent costs an additional $10,000 to achieve, on average, an additional 6 weeks of life with a utility of 0.06 QALYs. The cost–benefit of this intervention would be greater than $165,000 per QALY. This kind of analysis can be used to compare the relative values of various interventions and to help make policy decisions about where health care expenditures should be directed.

Outcomes of Treatment

As demonstrated earlier, data synthesis methods differ considerably from more traditional clinical research. This is not the case with other areas of outcomes research. Many outcomes studies resemble traditional clinical research

trials in their goals and study design. First, the goals of this type of outcomes study—determining the effects of treatment and identifying prognostic indicators—are identical to the goals of traditional clinical research. In addition, both outcomes studies and traditional clinical research often employ observational study designs such as case series, case—control studies, cohort studies, or experimental study designs such as randomized trials. There are, however, considerable differences between traditional clinical research and outcomes research in regard to which outcomes are assessed for individual patients and how outcomes rates are analyzed for surgeons and for society.

Patient-level Analysis

Outcomes studies received their name by focusing on treatment outcomes that are patient oriented (4). Although these studies often include traditional measures of treatment such as surgical morbidity and mortality, to qualify as an outcomes study it must be clear that the outcomes being assessed are of importance to the patient.

As is the case with all areas of intellectual endeavor, outcomes research has generated its own jargon. A brief introduction to the taxonomy and vocabulary of outcomes research, with concrete examples, is presented in the following subsection.

Many different kinds of data need to be analyzed to give a complete picture of the effectiveness of medical care, including clinical outcomes, lesional outcomes, functional outcomes, patient satisfaction, and resource utilization. These measures, all legitimate areas of outcomes research, are described briefly here. These categories are not rigid and there is often a good deal of correlation among various categories.

Clinical Outcomes

Surgeons are most familiar with clinical outcomes because these are the measures employed in traditional clinical reasearch. This type of outcomes data deals with the morbidity and mortality of disease processes without treatment (i.e., the natural history) or the morbidity and mortality associated with treatment. Examples include the incidence of hemorrhage from untreated, unruptured aneurysms and the incidence of new neurological deficits after treatment of these aneurysms. Much of the medical literature is composed of observational and experimental studies of varying degrees of sophistication employing these clinical outcomes measures. The best of these studies—prospective, randomized trials—remains the gold standard for determining the efficacy of treatment but, as discussed earlier, often inadequate to determine how effective a given treatment may be (6).

Lesional Outcomes

Lesional outcomes are necessary to determine the effectiveness of treatment in obliterating or correcting a structural or physiological abnormality. To evaluate lesional outcomes, some type of radiological imaging, physiological monitoring, laboratory study, or other means of quantifying a structural or physiological response is needed. For example, the angiographic obliteration rate of intracranial aneurysms after endovascular procedures, or the effect of a dietary regimen on serum cholesterol, are lesional outcomes. This kind of study is well represented in the medical literature and is familiar to practicing physicians and surgeons. However, outcomes methodology places one additional constraint on what is a legitimate lesional outcome. It is necessary that the lesional outcome have a discernible effect on the present or future health of the patient (4, 6). For example, the angiographic obliteration rate of aneurysms after treatment is important only if the risk of future hemorrhage is affected. The patient doesn't care what his angiogram looks like unless it has an effect on his quality or length of life. Similarly, barbiturate coma for control of intracranial pressure in trauma patients is a valid outcome measure only if such control improves patients' survival and ultimate functional health status. If the patients' lives are not saved or improved, control of intracranial pressure is a meaningless measure of the effectiveness of treatment from an outcomes study standpoint.

Of course, there are many times when we do not know whether a lesional outcome will affect patients' lives in the future. For example, will patients with radiological evidence of fusion after spinal instrumentation be more likely to maintain an acceptable quality of life after treatment than patients without such a lesional outcome? In these cases, collection of lesional outcomes data and the correlation of lesional outcomes with functional outcomes over time are necessary to answer these questions.

Functional Outcomes

Functional health status is of obvious importance to our patients. Without knowing whether our interventions improve or preserve the ability of our patients to lead their lives, it is difficult see how a "good outcome" can be determined (4). Nevertheless, many clinical studies uncritically equate low treatment morbidity and mortality with successful treatment. From an outcomes standpoint, this is invalid.

Consider, for example, a series of patients undergoing anterior cervical discectomy and instrumentation for radicular pain that interferes with their jobs and recreational activities. Assume that all patients have meticulous surgery with no residual nerve root compression seen on postoperative imaging studies, excellent radiological fusion rates, and minimal treatment-related morbidity. Although the clinical outcomes (low morbidity) and possibly valid lesional outcomes (good nerve root decompression and high rates of fusion) in this group of patients are excellent, no conclusions regarding the effectiveness of treatment can be drawn without knowing about the functional status of the patients. Traditional clinical end points may be important to the surgeon, but the patient is interested in whether his symptoms will be relieved and how treatment will affect his quality of life. Validated generic instruments such as the SF-12 and SF-36 (*discussed elsewhere in this publication*) are available to assess functional health status after treatment (21). Disease-specific instruments that focus on patient-centered outcomes are also becoming available (21).

Patient Satisfaction

This area of outcomes studies measures the extent to which patients' expectations of medical care are met (2, 12). Numerous environmental factors, many beyond the control of the surgeon, may affect patient satisfaction, and patient satisfaction may not correlate with what we feel are more important clinical, functional, and lesional outcomes (2, 12).

All clinicians have had the experience of dealing with patients who are very happy with their medical care despite what we would consider a less than optimal result and, conversely we have dealt with patients who are not satisfied despite what we might call an excellent result of treatment. Whether a patient is satisfied with his treatment may be the result of many factors in his life that cannot be addressed by his surgical care. Because of this, patient satisfaction measures alone may present a very skewed measure of the effectiveness of care. For instance, one problem with patient satisfaction measures occurs in patients with any disease process that has a relatively benign short-term course. For these disorders, less invasive means of treatment almost always achieve higher patient satisfaction scores if follow-up is brief. This is the case even if the less invasive treatments are largely or wholly ineffective. For instance, a placebo treatment for VIIIth nerve schwannoma may well achieve higher rates of patient satisfaction than an effective alternative, unless the patients were followed long enough to develop symptoms from a slowly enlarging tumor. Patient satisfaction data used in isolation are of very limited value for determining effectiveness of care.

Resource Utilization

The rapidly rising costs of medical care during the last three decades have made it necessary to evaluate our care with regard to the benefits that accrue to the patient per dollar spent to achieve these benefits. Many surgeons react to this as an attempt to ration care, and this is certainly one way in which resource utilization analysis can be used. However, analysis of resource utilization by surgeons can be a very valuable tool to ensure that we are delivering the best possible care at the lowest possible cost. Although resource utilization analysis is more commonly employed in large database studies (see the earlier discussion of cost–benefit analysis), these outcomes measures can also be employed in patient-level outcomes studies. The simplest kind of resource utilization involves tracking measures such as hospital charges and length of stay, and analying these data to determine where we can conserve resources without compromising patient care. More costly is not always better. For example, we found that, by changing our treatment regimen for patients undergoing carotid endarterectomy, we could improve clinical outcomes (fewer complications) and increase patient satisfaction (less invasive monitoring and postoperative discomfort) while at the same time reducing dramatically the cost of care by eliminating intensive care unit monitoring and decreasing the length of hospital stay (11).

Surgeon or Hospital-level Analysis and Risk Stratification

Using patient-oriented outcomes and traditional clinical outcomes, one can explore outcomes rates among various surgeons or hospitals, and can analyze reasons for variation in performance. For this kind of outcomes analysis to be valid, it is necessary to use risk adjustment methods to account for possible differences in patient risk factors from one practice to another. The process of risk stratification or case-mix adjustment is used to separate the effects of treatment from other factors that may have a profound influence on patient-oriented outcomes (14). For example, an 80-year-old patient with a ruptured, 2-cm, basilar apex aneurysm has a much poorer chance of a good functional outcome with surgery than a 40-year-old patient with an unruptured, 1-cm, posterior communicating artery aneurysm, regardless of the knowledge and skill of the surgeon. Numerous patient-specific and lesion-specific factors may need to be assessed to stratify patients properly by risk (14). As discussed later, expert clinician involvement is essential to achieve adequate risk stratification. However, if appropriate risk stratification is done, variations in outcomes among surgeons can be used to determine best practices, to effect appropriate patient referral, and to improve the quality of care for neurosurgical patients.

Population-level Analysis

Many outcomes studies look at the effectiveness of care for a large population of patients rather than at the level of the individual patient, surgeon, or institution (8, 22, 27, 28). Hospital discharge data available from administrative databases such as those maintained by the Health Care Financing Administration or state agencies are used to determine clinical outcomes after various procedures (27, 28). Such large database analyses have particular strengths. Because all patients undergoing a given procedure are included, there is little selection bias in this type of study. Selection bias can produce a very inaccurate picture of the effectiveness of treatment. For example, many experimental and observational clinical studies are restricted to patients cared for at tertiary care centers. It is likely that the outcomes obtained at such centers do not reflect accurately the outcomes obtained at all institutions. In addition, prospective, randomized trials often employ strict patient selection criteria that may not reflect the same risk factors that are found in the population at large. Large database studies avoid this selection bias by looking at all patients who received care over a given period of time.

Large database studies also have potential weaknesses (8). The accuracy of administrative databases in reporting outcomes can be questioned, and they often lack the clinical detail needed to determine risk stratification accurately for the patients involved (13). For these reasons large database studies may reach different conclusions regarding the effectiveness of care than is found in more restricted populations. A good example of this is the much higher mortality found in large database studies of patients undergoing carotid endarterectomy than found in prospective, randomized trials of this procedure (5).

Technology Assessment

There was, and continues to be, a great deal of uncertainty regarding how much added value will accrue to patients from expensive technological innovations. An interest in measuring our ability to deliver effective, efficient, and appropriate health care has begun to replace the blind faith that has often been placed in advanced technology (25). All of the methodologies described earlier can be applied to determine whether investment in technological advances translates into improved health status for our patients.

The Importance of Outcomes Studies

The goal of outcomes studies—to evaluate the effectiveness of medical care—is of obvious importance to our patients, referring physicians, third-party payers, and to society. Nevertheless, many clinicians have questioned the necessity of conducting outcomes research, and have been reluctant to become involved. I believe that this is a mistake. It is vitally important that the clinicians who know the most about the patients and their disease processes take the lead in designing and carrying out reliable outcomes studies. Poorly designed outcomes studies, conducted by people in the insurance industry, government, and academia who often know little or nothing about the disease processes and patients studied, are being performed. The data from these studies will yield a flawed picture of the effectiveness of our care. Unless neurosurgeons generate reliable

outcomes data, our practice will be determined by policies derived from these distorted pictures. As the previous discussion indicates, reliable outcomes studies require great clinical expertise for accurate risk stratification, to interpret patient satisfaction measures, and to determine adequate duration of follow-up. Without the clinical expertise that only we can supply, a very misleading assessment of the effectiveness of neurosurgical care can be produced by outcomes studies that are otherwise methodologically rigorous. In short, outcomes studies will continue to be performed and it is much better for us to do meaningful studies than to have our practice determined by poor studies accomplished by others.

Outcomes Analysis and Quality in Neurosurgery

Currently, assessment is often based on procedural criteria that may have little or no effect on patient outcomes. For instance, health care organizations need to expend a great deal of resources documenting that they have the appropriate processes in place (morbidity and mortality reviews, committee structure, and other bureaucratic requirements) to achieve recognition of quality. *These issues are discussed at length elsewhere in this publication.* It is my belief that we will only be able to assess and improve the quality of neurosurgical care by collecting meticulous outcomes data on patients undergoing neurosurgical procedures, and this cannot be done without the enthusiastic participation of neurosurgeons.

Outcomes Analysis and Patient Education

Without a clear picture of the effectiveness of neurosurgical care, it is impossible for patients to make informed decisions about such care. Patients need to know the options available to them and how their lives are likely to be affected by their decisions for surgical care. When these data are not available, decisions are based on far less reliable information. As more patients have access to medical information of questionable quality through the Internet, this problem will become more acute. Once again, it is only by meticulous tracking of patient-oriented outcomes that we can supply our patients with the information they need to make informed decisions.

Outcomes Analysis and Third-Party Payers

Many third-party payers are now tracking clinical outcomes for use in patient referrals and contracting. It is a concern that these outcomes, usually obtained from administrative databases (see my earlier discussion of large database studies), lack the risk stratification necessary to obtain an accurate picture of the effectiveness of care. For instance, the neurosurgeon who is referred only the most difficult cases because of his particular expertise may be singled out for poor outcomes based on a case mix that is substantially different from other neurosurgeons. Because many lesion-specific and patient-specific factors affect risk adjustment, attempts by third-party payers to adjust the case mix for things like patient age or medical comorbidities may be inadequate. The 50-year-old hypertensive, diabetic patient with a large clivus meningioma and the 50-year-old hypertensive, diabetic patient with a small convexity meningioma are viewed as equivalent patients by all of the methods of risk adjustment used routinely by third-party payers. We recognize that this is invalid. However, without the participation of the expert clinicians in the neurosurgical community, these errors will not be addressed and we will not be able to generate meaningful outcomes data.

CASE STUDY: AVMs OF THE BRAIN

To understand how the methodologies presented earlier can be employed in a particular clinical situation, I next delineate how outcomes studies might be applied to evaluate our treatment of patients with AVMs of the brain.

Risk Stratification of AVM Patients

When planning outcomes studies, various factors that may affect the natural history and risk of treatment of the patients to be studied must be considered. The insight we have gained through our clinical experience, and a critical appraisal of the literature (10, 23), are needed to be sure that the data we collect take such factors into consideration. Accurate risk stratification is one of the reasons why it is essential for those clinicians who know the most about a disease process to be involved in designing outcomes studies. To the clinically naive investigator, all AVMs may be lumped into the same group without considering the vastly different levels of risk that apply to different patients within one diagnostic category.

To the neurosurgeon, it is obvious that the 75-year-old patient with an unruptured 4-cm AVM involving the thalamus has a risk profile, with or without treatment, that differs considerably from the 20-year-old with a 2-cm ruptured AVM of the right frontal lobe. It is equally obvious that to obtain any meaningful outcomes information it is necessary not only to measure such outcomes, but to be aware of factors that stratify patients accurately with regard to their risks with and without treatment. As discussed previously, this process of risk stratification is necessary before any judgments about the effectiveness or appropriateness of care can be made. In short, outcomes studies are essentially meaningless unless appropriate risk stratification has been performed (14).

A critical review of the literature and the clinical experience of those who actually care for these patients suggests which factors to consider when designing a study to collect outcomes data. After the data are collected, multivariate analysis can be used to determine which factors were associated significantly with adverse outcomes. This kind of reevaluation process leads to an increasingly precise understanding of risk factors and increasingly accurate risk stratification. The process of risk stratification must be done with regard to both the natural history of patients with AVMs and to those considering treatment for these lesions.

Risk Stratification for the Natural History of AVMs

The true natural history of an unselected group of AVM patients remains somewhat nebulous. The number of patients with conservatively managed AVMs is relatively small, and the criteria used in the selection of patients for conservative management are often unclear. It is, therefore, difficult to say with certainty whether series that are cited to describe the natural history of patients with central nervous system AVMs are representative of the universal set of such patients. With this caveat in mind, we can use a critical appraisal of the literature and our clinical experience to stratify patients according to their risks. To simplify the process of risk stratification, let's focus on the risk of intracranial hemorrhage from these lesions. This is a reasonable first approximation. Although AVMs may become symptomatic for reasons other than intracranial hemorrhage, it is the risk of AVM rupture that is of greatest importance in assessing the natural history of this lesion.

Based on a review of the literature and our clinical experience, at least six factors have to be taken into consideration for risk stratification of patients with AVMs of the central nervous system. These include patient age, patient comorbidities ("general health"), previous hemorrhage, the location of the AVM, the size of the AVM, and angiographic features of the lesion. Discussion of each of these risk factors is beyond the scope of this chapter, but the importance of a thorough understanding of the disease process being evaluated should be obvious for performing meaningful risk stratification.

Risk Stratification for Treatment/Grading Scales

Currently microneurosurgical excision, neuroendovascular procedures, stereotactic radiation, and combinations thereof are used to treat patients with AVMs. All of the factors discussed earlier that affect the natural history of AVMs need to be considered when stratifying the risk of treatment. Grading scales are familiar examples of how risk stratification can be applied to patients considering treatment for their AVMs. These grading scales attempt to assess the risk involved in the treatment of an individual patient, and allow comparison of results among various series of patients. Lesion-specific and patient-specific factors are important in determining the risks of treatment. Lesion-specific factors include the size of the AVM, the number of feeding vessels, whether the perforating vessels are involved, whether there is a compact or diffuse AVM nidus, the velocity and volume of blood flow through the arteriovenous shunt, the location of the vascular malformation within the brain, and the pattern of venous drainage. Patient-specific factors include the age of the patient, the level of consciousness, the presence of a neurological deficit, and whether a previous hemorrhage has occurred. Grading scales take into account varying numbers of these factor. Currently, no grading system exists that assesses accurately the risk to an individual patient who harbors an AVM that may be treated with various modalities or not treated at all. Good prospective outcomes studies are necessary to allow such a grading scale to be developed. It is almost

certain that a multicenter study is necessary to have a sufficient number of outcome events to evaluate statistically the importance of the factors presented earlier.

Clinical Outcomes After Treatment

Numerous studies exist that document the neurological morbidity and mortality of patients treated with surgical excision, neuroendovascular procedures, radiation, or combination therapy. These clinical outcomes with various treatment modalities can be used in a decision analysis model to determine the most appropriate care for an individual patient with an AVM or to evaluate the relative value of the various treatment modalities for a population of patients.

Lesional Outcomes After Treatment

How best to document lesional outcomes after treatment of patients with central nervous system AVMs is an area of some controversy. The use of magnetic resonance imaging (MRI) and magnetic resonance angiography (MRA) has been advocated as a means by which the obliteration of an AVM after treatment can be ascertained. However, angiography in patients with MRI/MRA evidence of AVM obliteration may reveal the presence of a continued arteriovenous shunt. Because of this, it currently remains necessary that one demonstrate complete obliteration of the AVM via intra-arterial angiography before one can be assured that the lesion has been treated adequately.

We must remember that, in outcomes studies, only lesional outcomes that have a current or potential effect on the patient's health status are valid. I think that in the case of AVMs, the documentation of complete obliteration is valid by this criterion. Although there are those who would argue otherwise, the bulk of the evidence suggests that unless an AVM is obliterated completely, the risk of hemorrhage is not reduced. Therefore, angiography remains the gold standard for determining successful obliteration of central nervous system AVMs, and lesional outcomes based on anything other than this gold standard must be considered highly suspect, regardless of the treatment involved is microsurgical, endovascular, radiosurgical, or a combination thereof.

Functional Outcomes After Treatment

The functional status of patients with AVMs has been evaluated in a number of series. However, the functional outcomes scales used in these analyses are usually quite crude. As we become more sophisticated in evaluating functional outcomes, these areas must receive more attention. The psychological aspects of patients harboring an untreated AVM, and in patients who have undergone treatment for an AVM, also need to be studied in a great deal more detail. The psychological effect of having a potentially lethal, and in some cases untreatable, lesion may be debilitating from a functional standpoint, even if the patient remains neurologically intact.

Patient Satisfaction

As noted earlier, one problem with relying on patient satisfaction measures occurs in patients with AVMs because these lesions have a relatively benign short-term course. For this kind of disease process, less invasive means of treatment almost always achieve higher patient satisfaction scores unless patients are evaluated over a long period of time. This is the case even if the less invasive treatments are often ineffective.

For example, our analysis of the microsurgical versus radiosurgical treatment of AVMs demonstrated a clear superiority of microsurgery for clinical and lesional outcomes (2, 3). This occurs because of immediate obliteration of the AVM in microsurgical patients versus delayed obliteration in a fraction of the radiosurgical patients, and the associated risk of hemorrhage after radiosurgical treatment. Unless patients are clearly aware of the long-term superiority of microsurgery, patient satisfaction data collected shortly after treatment may show a preference for the less invasive treatment.

Resource Utilization for AVM Patients

Resource utilization for patients undergoing treatment of AVMs is also undergoing scrutiny. Once again, this outcomes measure cannot be evaluated in isolation, but needs to be considered in conjunction with the clinical, lesional, and functional outcomes measures noted earlier. Although less invasive forms of treatment may require less resource utilization initially, the long-term cost of such treatments is likely to be higher than early definitive treatment by microsurgical excision (20, 24). This is the case because of continued episodes of hemorrhage in many patients with less invasive therapy (20, 23, 24).

Duration of Follow-up

Much of the preceding discussion documents that to obtain accurate outcomes data on AVM patients, the duration of follow-up needs to be prolonged. Because the short-term morbidity and mortality from an untreated AVM of the central nervous system is relatively low, long-term follow-up is necessary to evaluate factors that affect the natural history of these lesions. In those patients who undergo treatment with stereotactic radiation, a period of several years is necessary to determine whether the AVM is obliterated. During that time, these patients will continue to be at risk for hemorrhage. And in those patients in whom radiation is not effective, the risk persists indefinitely unless further treatment is obtained. In addition, because many of the complications of radiation are delayed, a long period of follow-up is necessary to assess accurately the risks of stereotactic radiation.

Conversely, patients treated with microsurgical excision of their AVMs assume a higher up-front risk of complication in exchange for a lower overall morbidity with time. Clinical outcomes continue to improve after surgery for at least 6 months, and possibly a year (20, 23, 24). Clinical assessment earlier than that may result in inaccurate assessment of the long-term outcome with microsurgical excision.

In short, it is likely that a minimum of 3 years after the last treatment is necessary to determine accurately clinical, lesional, and functional outcomes in patients undergoing treatment for their central nervous system AVMs. Natural history studies assessing factors for risk stratification without treatment require longer periods of time to obtain enough outcomes events to make analysis meaningful, even if a large patient cohort is enrolled and followed meticulously.

Case Study Summary

I hope this case study illustrates the difficulty involved in producing scientifically rigorous outcomes studies of neurosurgical procedures, and how essential it is for neurosurgeons to be involved in designing such studies. Without the expertise of the clinicians who know the most about the disease processes and patients being evaluated, outcomes studies will produce, at best, a very incomplete picture of the effectiveness of neurosurgical care. In the next portion of this chapter I briefly review how the Outcomes Committee and the Committee on the Assessment of Quality of the AANS and CNS are working toward developing reliable outcomes studies.

AANS/CNS OUTCOMES INITIATIVE

The leadership of the AANS and CNS recognized both the threat and the opportunity that outcomes studies posed for organized neurosurgery. The need for organized neurosurgery to develop the infrastructure necessary to perform reliable outcomes studies was appreciated, and in 1997 I was asked to develop this initiative. A strategic plan for developing a neurosurgical outcomes initiative was conceived. The strategic plan included organizing an outcomes committee with expertise in clinical neurosurgery, outcomes methodology, and information technology; initiating educational activities; developing and performing a pilot outcomes study; developing an on-line outcomes reporting system linked to the Neurosurgery On Call (NOC) national neurosurgical Web site, and performing on-line studies using this system.

During the last years we have met these goals. The Outcomes Committee has representatives appointed by the executive committees of each of the clinical neurosurgical sections. The committee also has members with particular expertise in outcomes methodology and information technology. Consultants from Outcome Sciences and the AANS Information Services group add to the ability of the committee to achieve its goals.

Committee members have developed educational materials for the NOC Outcomes Page and have published articles in the AANS Bulletin and in *Neurosurgery*. Outcomes-related topics have been presented at the national neurosurgical annual meetings, at section meetings, and in professional development courses. A separate professional development course in outcomes methodology is being developed. We plan to continue our educational efforts as the rest of the plan develops.

Starting in 1998, our pilot study of the treatment of patients with intracranial aneurysm was begun. The study involves patients being treated for ruptured or unruptured intracranial aneurysms by microsurgical or endovascular approaches. Risk-adjusted, disease-specific data-reporting instruments were developed by Dr. Issam Awad and members of the Cerebrovascular Section Outcomes Committee. Pilot centers include academic medical centers and private practice groups. Clinical, functional, and lesional outcomes are being collected. Patient accrual ended on January 31, 1999, and these patients will be followed for 6 months to determine functional health status after treatment. We plan to analyze the data from the pilot study and to refine the data-reporting instruments, which can then be put on-line to expand the number of neurosurgeons participating in the study.

The committee has also been working to develop a secure, reliable, on-line outcomes reporting system linked to the NOC Web site. We have reached this goal through our collaboration with the AANS Information Services personnel and with outside consultants. Security and confidentiality issues are always of concern when dealing with patient-related data. We have developed a system that is at least as secure as conventional pencil-and-paper documentation of patient outcomes. A full discussion of the security systems developed for this outcomes project can be found on the NOC Outcomes Page (http://www.neurosurgery.org).

Currently there are several on-line studies available to all members of the AANS and CNS:

- Treatment of Carotid Stenosis
- Surgery of Lumbar Disc Herniation
- Treatment of Acute Subdural Hematoma
- Neurosurgical Report Card

The first is a simple, one-page outcomes reporting instrument that can be used for any neurosurgical diagnosis or procedure—the ''Neurosurgical Report Card.'' The report card allows neurosurgeons to track basic outcomes measures such as length of hospital stay, mortality, postoperative infection, and unplanned readmission or return to the operating room by CPT, and ICD-9, codes. Once the database is established, the individual neurosurgeon can compare her data with the overall database.

A more in-depth study of the treatment of patients with carotid artery stenosis is also on-line. This study began in January 1999 to evaluate the clinical, functional, and lesional outcomes of patients with carotid artery stenosis treated by carotid endarterectomy or angioplasty and stenting. The disease-specific reporting instruments were developed by myself and the Cerebrovascular Section Outcomes Committee. The on-line system has worked flawlessly. Data collection forms can be downloaded and printed from the NOC Web site. All data are submitted electronically via the Internet. The system works with any type of computer and does not require the purchase of special software. Pilot sites have been selected for this study but we are encouraging any neurosurgeon involved in treating patients with carotid stenosis to submit patients to the database. It is essential that neurosurgeons submitting data to the study submit data on all the patients they treat. Any member of the AANS or CNS can obtain a user name and password, and gain access to the on-line system by contacting Laurie Singer, at the AANS National Office. Information about the requirements for using the system is also available at the NOC Outcomes Page.

The next study to go on-line will evaluate the treatment of patients with lumbar disc herniation. Dr. Paul McCormick and other members of the AANS/CNS section on Disorders of the Spine and Peripheral Nerves have developed the reporting instruments for this study, which will be on-line by the time this chapter is published. Once again, participation by all AANS and CNS members is being encouraged.

The members of the Outcomes Committee are committed to developing the necessary tools for neurosurgeons to participate in outcomes research in the most cost-effective manner. We are excited about the potential that exists for generating national and international databases, determining best practices, and gaining insight into the value of our neurosurgical interventions. We hope that our neurosurgical colleagues will be as excited as we are, and become involved in this venture.

CONCLUSION

In summary, whether we like it or not, we are living in the era of outcomes studies. Numerous agencies are involved in measuring the outcomes of neurosurgical care, and neurosurgeons are increasingly required to define and document the value of their interventions. Often, those evaluating the outcomes of neurosurgical care have little insight into the issues that arise in the care of our patients and, unfortunately, data from these studies will be used to determine government policy, patient referral, and reimbursement. This is a time of great opportunity. If the neurosurgical community becomes enthusiastically involved in meticulous outcomes studies, we will be able to document the value of our interventions, better inform our patients, and improve the quality of neurosurgical care.

REFERENCES

1. Birkmeyer JD, Welch HG: A reader's guide to surgical decision analysis. *J Am Coll Surg* 184:589–595, 1997.
2. Cleary PD, McNeil BJ: Patient satisfaction as an indicator of quality care. *Inquiry* 25:25–36, 1988.
3. Cook DJ, Mulrow CD, Haynes RB: Systematic reviews: Synthesis of best evidence for clinical decisions. *Ann Intern Med* 126:376–380, 1997.
4. Ellwood P: Shattuck lecture—Outcomes management. A technology of patient experience. *N Engl J Med* 318:1549–1556, 1988.
5. Executive Committee for the Asymptomatic Carotid Atherosclerosis Study: Endarterectomy for asymptomatic carotid artery stenosis. *JAMA* 273:1421–1428, 1995.
6. Feeny DH, Torrance GW: Incorporating utility based quality of life assessment measures in clinical trials. *Med Care* 27(Suppl 3):S190–S204, 1989.
7. Finlayson SRG, Birkmeyer JD: Cost-effectiveness analysis in surgery. *Surgery* 123:151–156, 1998.
8. Fisher ES, Baron JA, Malenka DJ, Barrett J, Bubolz TA: Overcoming potential pitfalls in the use of Medicare data for epidemiological research. *Am J Public Health* 80:1487–1490, 1990.
9. Gold MR, Siegel JE, Russell LB, Weinstein MC: Cost effectiveness in health and medicine. New York, Oxford University Press, 1996.
10. Harbaugh KS, Harbaugh RE: Arteriovenous malformations in elderly patients. *Neurosurgery* 35:579–584, 1994.
11. Harbaugh KS, Pikus HJ, Shumaker GH, Perron AD, Harbaugh RE: Increasing the value of carotid endarterectomy. *J Neurovasc Dis* 1:40–47, 1996.
12. Haslok I: Quality of care and patient satisfaction. *Br J Rheumatol* 35:382–384, 1996.
13. Iezzoni LI: Using administrative diagnostic data to assess the quality of hospital care. *Int J Technol Assess Health Care* 6:272–281, 1990.
14. Iezzoni LI: Risk adjustment for medical outcomes studies, in Grady ML (ed): *Medical Effectiveness Research Data Methods*. Publication Rockford, Agency for Health Care Policy and Research, no. 92–0056. 1992, pp. 83–97.
15. King JT Jr, Glick HA, Mason TJ, Flamm ES: Elective surgery for asymptomatic, unruptured, intracranial aneurysms: A cost-effectiveness analysis. *J Neurosurg* 83:403–412, 1995.
16. L'Abbe KA, Detsky AS, O'Rourke K: Meta-analysis in clinical research. *Ann Intern Med* 107:224–233, 1987.
17. Lau J, Ioannidis JPA, Schmid CH: Quantitative synthesis in systematic reviews. *Ann Intern Med* 127:820–826, 1997.
18. Leape LL, Park RE, Solomon DH, Chassin MR, Kosecoff J, Brook RH: Does inappropriate use explain small-area variations in the use of health care services? *JAMA* 263:669–672, 1990.
19. Nord E: Methods for quality-adjustment of life years. *Soc Sci Med* 34:559–569, 1992.
20. Nussbaum ES, Heros RC, Camarata PJ: Surgical treatment of intracranial arteriovenous malformations with an analysis of cost-effectiveness, in Clinical Neurosurgery: Proceedings of the Congress of Neuro-

logical Surgeons, Baltimore, Williams & Wilkins, 1995, pp 348–369.

21. Patrick DL, Deyo RA: Generic and disease-specific measures in assessing health status and quality of life. *Med Care* 27:217–232, 1989.

22. Paul JE, Weis KA, Epstein RA: Data bases for variations research. *Med Care* 31:96–102, 1993.

23. Pikus HJ, Beach ML, Harbaugh RE: Microsurgical treatment of arteriovenous malformations: Analysis and comparison to stereotactic radiosurgery. *J Neurosurg* 88:64–646, 1998.

24. Porter PJ, Shin AY, Detsky AS, Lefaive L, Wallace MC: Surgery versus stereotactic radiosurgery for small, operable cerebral arteriovenous malformations: A clinical and cost comparison. *Neurosurgery* 41:757–766, 1996.

25. Relman A: Assessment and accountability: The third revolution in medical care. *N Engl J Med* 319:1220–1222, 1988.

26. Deleted in proof.

27. Wennberg JE, Freeman JL, Shelton RM, Bubolz TA: Hospital use and mortality among Medicare beneficiaries in Boston and New Haven. *N Engl J Med* 321:1168–1173, 1989.

28. Wennberg J, Gittelsohn A: Small area variations in health care delivery. *Science* 182:1102–1108, 1973.

CHAPTER 12

The Clinic Dashboard: A Control-Charted Tool to Assess "Real" Change

MICHAEL J. O'LEARY, M.D.

EDITOR'S NOTE: Not all neurosurgical clinical processes are inpatient. Outpatient neurosurgery processes are equally important for the ultimate success of the neurosurgical organization. Some may even suggest that we will not have the luxury of assessing the stability and capability of our inpatient processes if our outpatient processes are not already successful for creating new inpatients. In this chapter, Dr. O'Leary explores the use of statistical process control through control charting and data-based decision making in the outpatient setting, and introduces the concept of a "dashboard" or "instrument panel" as a way of monitoring continually the output of significant processes in real time. Instrument panels or dashboards can also be devised for monitoring inpatient processes such as clinical pathways, or administrative and business processes such as budget management and so forth.

Sweeping changes during the last decade have ushered in the "corporate era" of medicine—a period of mergers and consolidation of the many small, traditional solo practices typifying the profession. Survival among the fierce competitive pressures of the business world requires integration of better *practice metrics*—a new concept to many physician managers. The *Clinic Dashboard* is one such tool, derived from the teachings of W. Edwards Deming, father of continued quality improvement (CQI). The dashboard employs *control charting,* a real-time, statistical measure of the mean and standard deviation of a process, from which out-of-control points can be readily identified (*Fig. 12.1*). These points or trends are beyond those expected statistically for a given process, and as such they have a 99% probability of being distinct from

the normal variation inherent in the process. The key points to learn from this chapter are the following:

- If you're going to measure, do it right.
- To "do it right" you must know the difference between the variation inherent in a given process and true process change.
- How can you know? Control charting!

Before proceeding further, the physician reader must understand that CQI bears no resemblance to most hospital programs described under the various banners of quality assurance, quality improvement, utilization review, and so forth. Generally, these programs have been designed by perhaps well-intentioned nonclinicians, creating time-intensive, often irrelevant tasks that produce little quality improvement while leaving a deep-seated aversion in most busy practitioners to all programs carrying the "quality" label. Unfortunately, few of these "quality managers" have any understanding or training in the Deming concept of "statistically based" quality improvement.

On the positive side, most physicians practicing in the modern era of "scientific" medicine possess a healthy understanding of the statistical method and tests by which two populations may be distinguished. The Clinic Dashboard was designed with the busy clinical practitioner in mind, intuitive enough to be understood without extensive reading of the Deming method, yet powerful enough to provide a metric tool capable of distinguishing the difference between normal variation and true change.

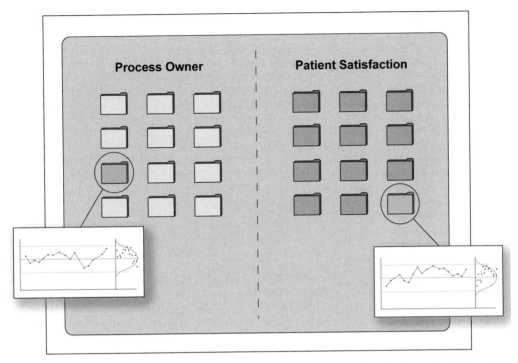

Figure 12.1 Conceptualization of a "dashboard" or "instrument panel" as a way of monitoring continually the output of significant processes in real time.

FOUR SCENARIOS

As an introduction to the dashboard application, consider the following practice vignettes and rank them from worst- to best-case scenario:

Dr. Hangyer Plak: After his 4-year residency and subspecialty fellowship, Dr. Plak opened his private practice, which for the past decade has grown to include a staff of seven and an increasing patient base. During the past 2 years, despite longer hours and greater numbers of patient visits and interventions, the bottom-line return at year's end has decreased by 5% per year. His bookkeeper is a perfectionist beyond reproach, but there are few other methods in place for "measuring" his practice and he has been unable to determine the primary source of the losses. Having surrounded himself with loyal and dedicated employees, he is now faced with laying off one of his veteran staff who has been with the practice since its inception.

Dr. Data Driven: A classmate of Hangyer's, Data has always been a fan of technology,

and since the beginning of his practice he has employed a variety of measuring techniques. He too has noted a decline in receipts during the past 2 years, and he called his staff together to examine the data and determine the primary cause of the losses. His business manager has provided the collections report, which showed a drop in 4 of the last 6 months. Patient survey data for the past 3 months reveals decreased scores in 12 of the 16 questions. The data confirm Dr. Driven's suspicion that the staff are not performing well, and he directs the respective managers of these two centers to "get their act together" by instituting some "sweeping changes" before the next reports come out!

Dr. Nugh Charter: Always the quiet student, Nugh learned about control charting during one of her monthly perusals of the *Harvard Business Review,* and after discussions with her office manager, decided to employ the technique 3 years ago to some of the "key indicators" of her practice's vitality. Results from the last 3 months have indicated a statistically significant fall-off in new patients, prompting a review of her top eight referring practitioners. She discovers two of her most reliable referral sources have switched to another medical center and are now referring to a competing specialist. Taking action, she applies for privileges at the new hospital and also contacts two new practitioners who have just arrived to take the departing physicians' spots at her primary medical center. The control charts for the next 2 months demonstrate significant referral growth.

Dr. Pro Active: A "Renaissance man," Pro has always had a healthy respect for the business aspects of his practice, reflected in the large number of "defined processes," all of which are analyzed through control-charting techniques. He treats his employees like "volunteers" and they have responded by applying their growing knowledge to the enhancement of the practice because they too share directly in its continued clinical and financial success. They are empowered to take corrective actions independently to improve processes in which special causes of variation outside the control limits have been identified. Dr. Active focuses his attention on reducing the common causes of variations—systemic problems that increase the standard deviation surrounding a process. Two months ago the automated Western Electric test analysis regarding patients' assessment of front-desk personnel identified a positive trend that suggested a real statistical improvement in the mean. On investigation, Pro discovered that one of his new employees had changed the check-in process, reducing the wait at the front desk. The new procedure also enhanced the preapproval process, and control charts measuring collections indicated significant gains. The changes were extended to the satellite clinics, which were communicated at the weekly work center lunch. The new employee's innovation improved patient satisfaction and contributed to the bottom line of everyone's paycheck. She was rewarded with her choice from among the four educational opportunities available as incentives for employee self-development.

How would you rank the previous practitioners in terms of desirable practice scenarios? You might intuitively answer 4, 3, 2, 1, but the correct answer is 4, 3, 1, 2, and this is a critical point. When faced with the choice of just trusting the process or collecting data, its better to do the former unless you can determine the difference between true change and variation. Dr. Data Driven could not, and as such he was guilty of the sin of *tampering,* one of the greatest transgressions committed by any manager who is under the stress of external change and feels compelled to act.

TAMPERING

Regardless of whether they are measured, most established practices have a number of processes that are likely stable and are defined readily by the employee in that area (e.g., reception, interventions, billing). In the best-case scenario, a well-intentioned manager, feeling compelled to act by external stressors, misuses data to imply a real change (with usually a negative implication) and then interrupts the process by making changes that are unnecessary and actually detrimental to the output. In the worst-case scenario, the inexperienced manager believes the majority of the problems are "people-related" versus the 90% that should actually be attributed to processes. Arriving with a host of "personal agendas" for which supporting "data" are collected, this manager embarks the organization on an unnecessary effort to change, diverting employees from the work they know how to do and resulting in worse production and increased worker dissatisfaction. All of this was needless because the data simply reflected the normal variation inherent in the particular process. *Data*—a collection of facts—should always be distinguished from *information*—an accurate assessment of facts. *Knowledge* may be defined as an understanding based on the use of information. Knowledge of the difference between the data shifts inherent in normal variation and the reliable information of a true process change is invaluable. *Wisdom* lies in knowledge applied correctly.

THE DEMING METHOD

A comprehensive discussion of W. Edwards Deming is beyond the scope of this chapter, and his admonition applies to me, "teaching of beginners should be done by a master, not by a hack" (2, p. 357). A list of references is provided for those interested in more profound knowledge (3, 4, 6, 8, 9). Instead, our focus is on areas highlighted specifically by the use of dashboard metrics.

While studying for his doctorate in mathematics and physics, which he earned at Yale in 1928, Deming worked summers at the Western Electric Hawthorne plant, where he became familiar with the methods of statistical process control (SPC) developed by Walter A. Shewart (7). These techniques applied the scientific method and statistical sampling to material production, resulting in dramatic improvements. Deming replaced a linear concept of production → inspection → rejection with a cycle of CQI in which tests are applied and the results are used to improve the production process further.

Deming expanded Shewart's concepts into an overall philosophy of *quality management,* applicable to essentially any process. As consultant to the secretary of war during World War II, his method was taught in earnest and played an important role in the massive United States war production effort. Ironically, in the absence of competitive pressures on the United States during the postwar period, most of the methods were dropped at the exact time they were being adopted wholeheartedly in Japan.

Deming was sent to Japan to act as an advisor for the first census taken after the war. Aware of his methods of quality improvement, the Union of Japanese Scientists and Engineers invited him to instruct them. The Plan–Do–Check–Act cycle of CQI became known as the *Deming PDCA cycle* and the field of total quality management (TQM) blossomed in Japanese industry. Key aspects of the *Deming approach* incorporated in the Clinic Dashboard include the following:

- Quality is being "on target" with minimal variation.
- The customer defines quality.
- Quality costs less.

CONTROL CHARTS

Every physician is familiar with the scientific approach integral to modern Western medicine. Statistical sampling techniques determine the characteristics of a population, including mean and standard deviation from the mean. The *probability* that a particular point belongs to the bell-shaped distribution can be calculated (*Fig. 12.2*). In a comparison study examining pain relief in patients given placebo or aspirin, we know that responses using aspirin are *statistically different* from placebo, and thus probably reflect a

shift of the mean in the direction of improved pain relief (*Fig. 12.3*). Control charts work by using similar principles, but in an ongoing versus retrospective fashion (4, 5, 10). The appearance is that of an x–y plot rotated clockwise 90 degrees with three lines from left to right: the mean, the upper control limit, and the lower control limit (*Fig. 12.4*). Control limits reflect the standard deviations from the mean, usually established at three standard deviations (3δ sigma) from the mean. The chance of a point belonging to a population with a mean more than 3δ away is less than 0.27% (27 chances in 10,000 events) (1)! (*Fig. 12.5*).

Variation about the average is ascribed to one of two possible causes. *Special-cause variation* was Deming's term for Shewart's *assignable cause* of variation, which implies a unique person, group, or local condition as the source of the variation. All points outside the upper and lower control limits are defined as special causes and can be detected easily on a control chart. More subtle special-cause variation can also operate within the control limits, and is detected by statistical trend analyses, known as the *Western Electric tests,* which suggest that a pattern is highly unlikely to have occurred from random variation. Ongoing real-time computer analysis of the control charts using these tests defines special causes that would otherwise likely be missed in a process:

- Point outside the control limits
- Series increasing/decreasing
- Multiple points on the same side of the mean
- Alternating points about the mean

Special-cause variation may be of a beneficial or harmful nature. The identification of special-cause variation and its insertion or removal from the process is the *responsibility of the worker.* A particularly slow day in the office might reflect scheduling on a religious holiday, for example. Responsibility for determining the source of the low turnout and for making the correction to the scheduling process in the future belongs to the schedulers, and should not be the primary concern of the physician or practice manager.

A greater source of process variation is derived from problems inherent throughout the system, for which Deming adopted the term *common-cause variation.* When analyzing trou-

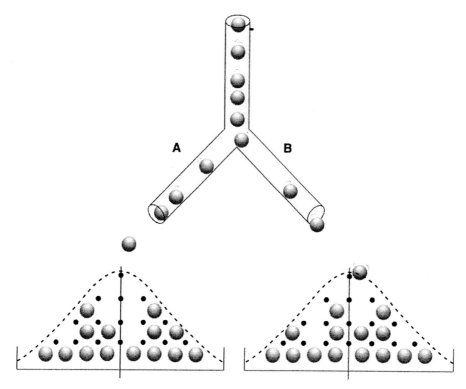

Figure 12.2 Random distributions with means and standard deviations.

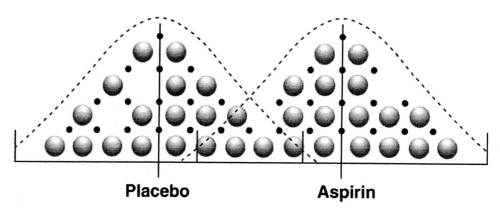

Figure 12.3 Pain relief results comparing placebo with aspirin.

bles in a system, common causes outnumber special causes more than 9:1 (2). Reduction of common-cause variation (and thus improvement in quality) is the *responsibility of management.* Because of its less obvious nature, common-cause variation is often harder to detect, and reflects problems common throughout the process.

An example is the eventual fatigue of machinery or the range of patient arrival times to the clinic. Providing patients with available parking or directions before their appointment may reduce the common-cause variation around the process of arrival times. On the other hand, it might make it worse if the directions are confusing.

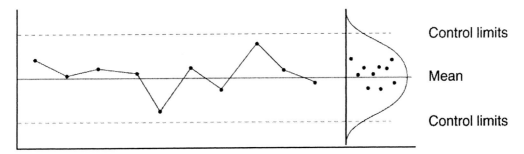

Figure 12.4 Control chart of a process.

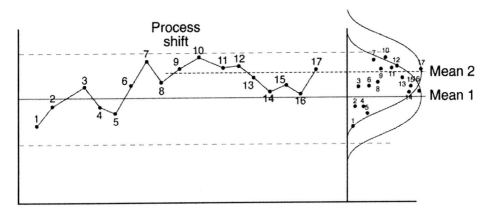

Figure 12.5 A "true" shift in the mean detected by a control chart.

How can you know? "Control chart" your clinical processes.

THE CLINIC DASHBOARD

Most busy clinicians have little time even to define their processes, let alone complete advanced study in TQM. Yet it is the rare physician who is not genuinely interested in improving their clinical practice, knowing its importance. A patient's perception of service quality often influences their sense of professional competence. The Clinic Dashboard was designed with just such a physician in mind. In a manner analogous to the voltmeter in a car, the dashboard indicators provide real-time monitoring of critical practice processes and alert the physician "driver" when a real change has occurred in the process and action is indicated. Calculation of upper and lower control limits allows determination of special-cause variations, which facili-

tates process stabilization. Once stabilized, the computer can apply a series of sophisticated statistical tests to points within the area of common-cause variation that also reliably predict a "real change" in a process mean that otherwise would likely go unnoticed. If the clinical "team" decides that a mean wait of 23 minutes is unsatisfactory, for example, they may institute a series of experiments to improve the process. The success or failure of each intervention will be reflected in the subsequent control charts showing a positive or negative "change," or no change at all from what would be expected by the normal variation of the process. A quality cycle of PDCA has been established.

The Clinic Dashboard opens like a book: The left side reflects the "control-charted" feedback on new patients' perceptions of practice quality (patient satisfaction side), and the right side offers a series of control-charted metrics deemed important by the clinician (the process owner

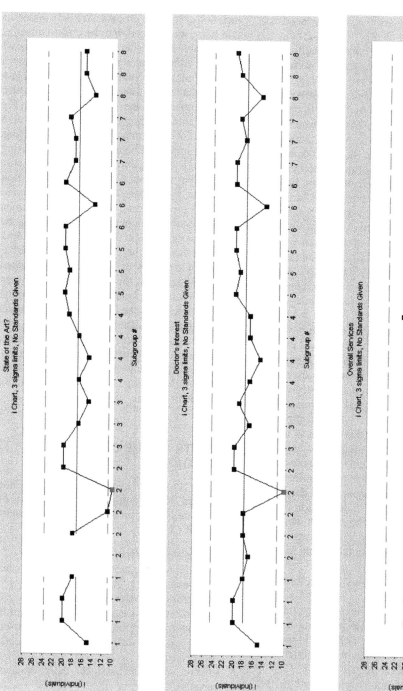
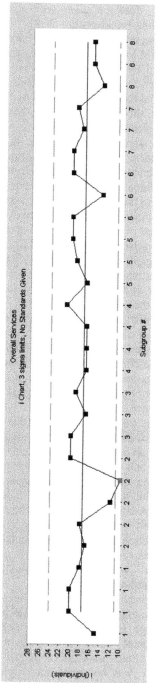

Figure 12.11   Patient satisfaction side. (A) Care perceived as state-of-the-art. (B) Doctor's interest in patient care. (C) Perception of overall services. (D) Overall satisfaction.

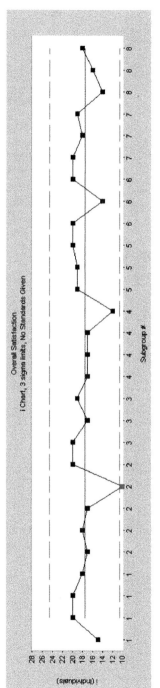

Figure 12.11 *(continued)*.

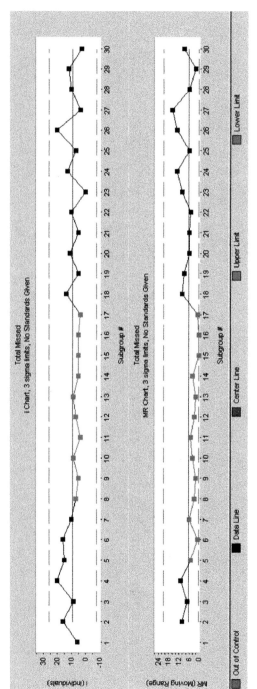

Figure 12.12 Process owner side of the IMR control chart. Total appointments missed.

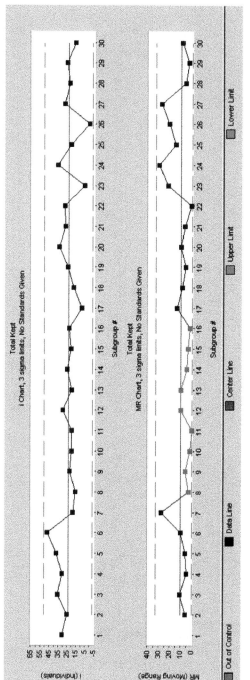

Figure 12.13 Process owner side of the IMR control chart. Total appointments kept.

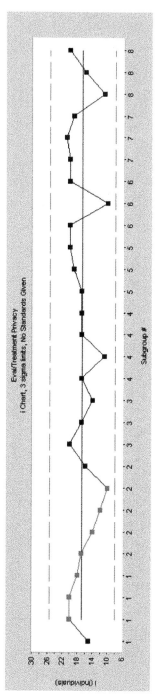

Figure 12.14 Patient satisfaction side. Evaluation/treatment privacy.

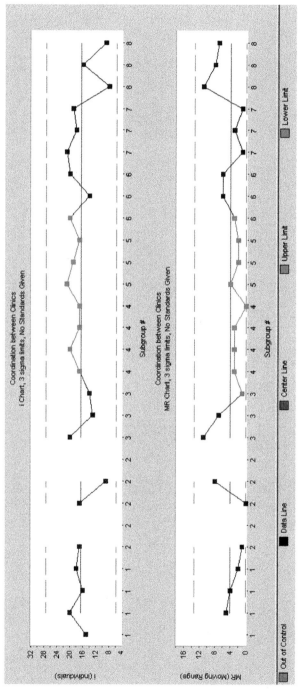

Figure 12.15   Patient satisfaction side. Coordination between Ear, Nose, Throat and Audiology.

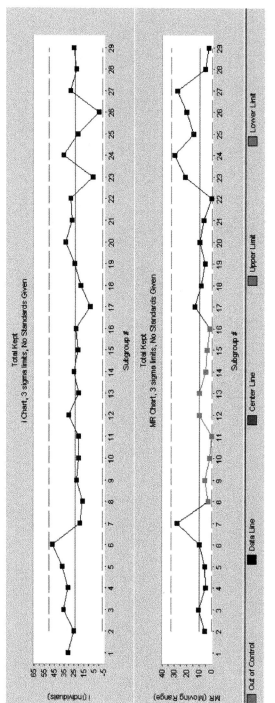

Figure 12.16   Process owner side. Appointments kept.

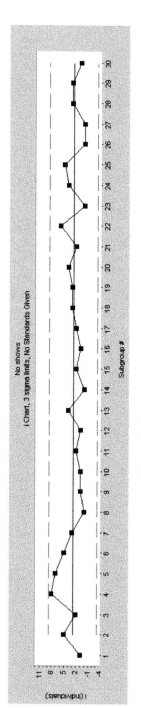

Figure 12.17   Process owner side. No shows.

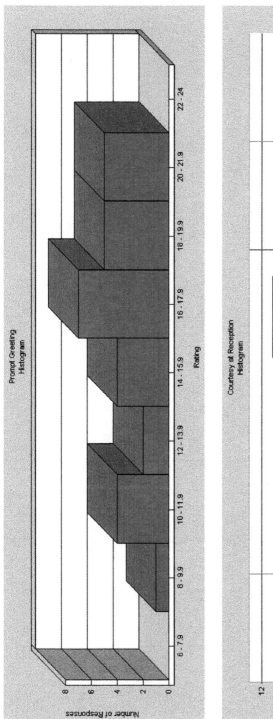

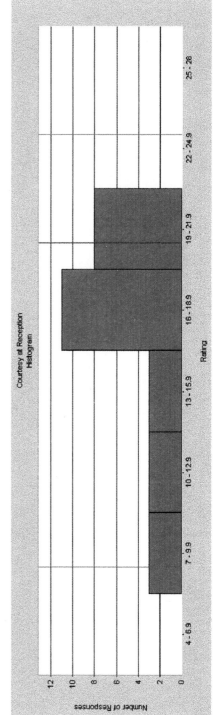

Figure 12.18 Histograms of patient perceptions of the front-desk team (A1–4), the physician (B1–4) and the clinic team (C).

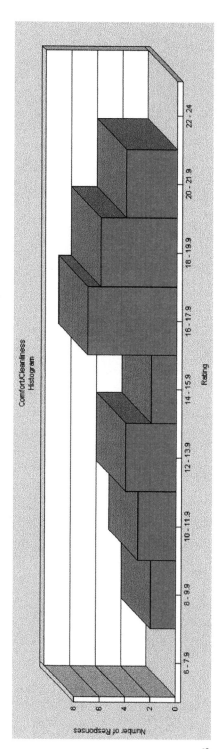

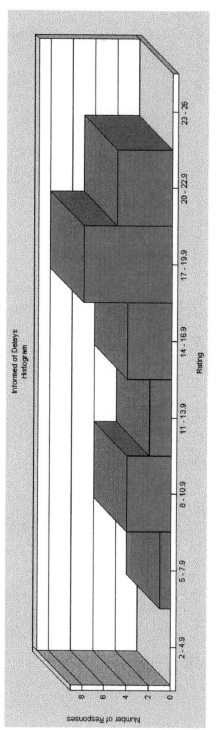

Figure 12.18 *(continued)*.

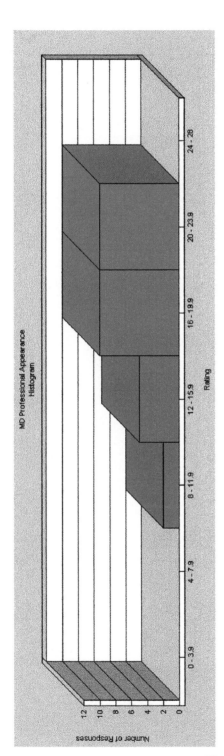

B1

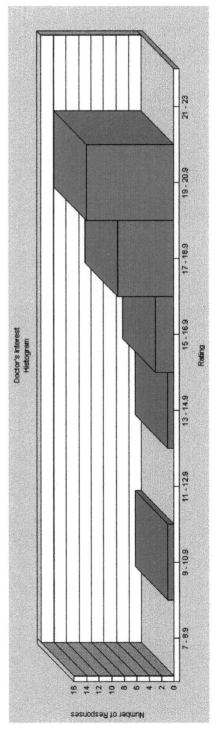

B2

Figure 12.18 *(continued).*

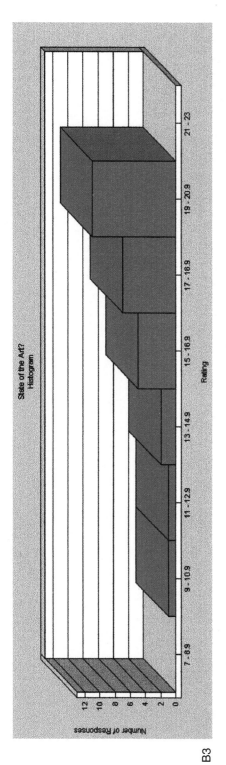

B3

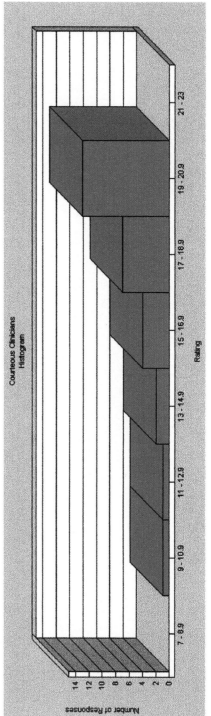

B4

Figure 12.18 *(continued).*

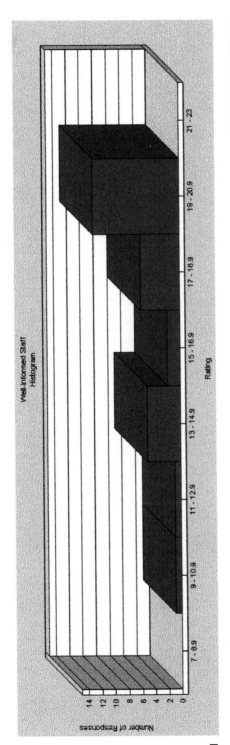

C1

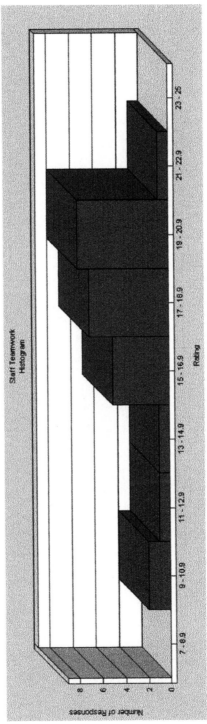

C2

Figure 12.18   (continued).

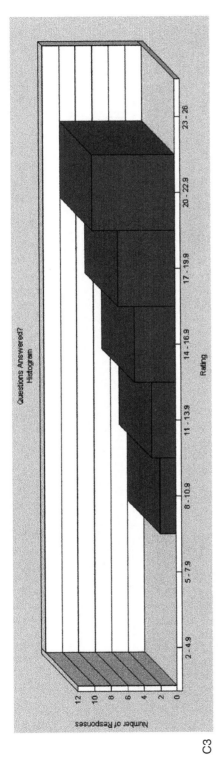

C3

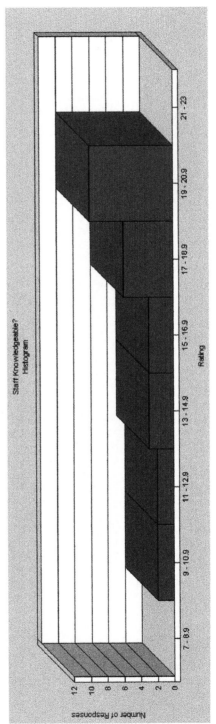

C4

Figure 12.18 (continued).

individual blame in a retroactive fashion. Defining processes becomes everyone's job, because the managers are often too far removed to describe the steps involved. The simple act of measuring enhances production through the Hawthorne effect. Patients seem genuinely surprised to be asked for their opinion, and they have little hesitation in completing the one-page survey while they are waiting. With minimal effort, the physician reasserts responsibility for managing the clinic process—a reflection of personal organization. The clinician is empowered with a real-time software tool that defines the variance in the clinic metrics considered most important, as well as the mean and standard deviation of the patient's perceptions using a customized, reliable satisfaction survey tool. Both sides of the dashboard are amenable to programmable, "seamless" data capture, reducing the need for reentry. Special-cause variation outside the control limits is readily apparent and usually remedied easily by the clinic staff. The software highlights trends within the control limits to define more subtle special causes that would otherwise not be readily apparent. Harmful causes are removed from the process and beneficial ones are discovered, amplified, and incorporated into the process. Together, special-cause variation is reduced, creating stable processes more amenable to the definition and reduction of common-cause variation attributable to the entire system. The responsibility of this more difficult task belongs to the managers, who are freed from the temptation to tamper with the process based on special-cause variation or personal agendas in the absence of real change. Finally, possession of an accurate, ongoing metric positions the clinician to evaluate fully the effects of new changes to the system, such as the introduction of a digital medical record or the addition of physician "extenders." Successful innovations may well define the difference between practice success and failure in light of the progressively shrinking profit margins in health care.

ENTERPRISE ADVANTAGES OF A STANDARDIZED DASHBOARD TOOL

An exponential leap in benefit occurs when the Clinic Dashboard is adopted at an institutional level. Employing relational databases from the individual Clinic Dashboards, a health care entity possesses an instantaneous, real-time

TABLE 12.1
Characteristics Defining the Transformation of Modern Medicine

Characteristic	Modern Medicine	A Deming System
Quality	Costs more	Costs less
The patient	Limited input	Defines quality
Problems	Individual related	Process related
Motivators	Fear and financial reward	Passion and pride of workmanship
Monitors	Retroactive inspection	Prospective control charts
Tampering	Rampant	Minimized
HMO plans	Lowest bidder	Committed to quality
Industry	Intense competition	Improved cooperation

HMO, Health Maintenance Organization.

metric that reflects ongoing patient satisfaction. Opportunities for "best practices" benchmarking are abundant within the institution. A centralized, expert systems process assessment team can be assigned to explore special-cause variations that are not readily apparent at the local level with the potential to contain losses or capitalize rapidly on opportunities presented by real process changes, which would previously have gone unnoticed.

At an even higher level, there exists the opportunity to begin a transformation from the current practice to a "higher form" of medicine based on the principles of CQM (*Table 12.1*). There is almost complete unanimity of opinion among providers and patients that there is an intolerable level of waste in the status quo, leading to a high level of dissatisfaction in both groups. Neither would ideally design a system in which the greatest profit lies in the hands of "corporate middle men," who add no true value to the healthcare provided. Accountability for perceived poor quality in these systems is determined in court with lawyers as the principal beneficiaries.

Adoption of a *process focus* is the first step in transforming the sad state of current affairs. The Clinic Dashboard offers an objective tool to enhance the personal effectiveness and efficiency of a clinical practice. Simply stated, the Clinic Dashboard represents the application of the scientific method to the business of medicine.

REFERENCES

1. AT&T: Statistical quality control handbook. Indianapolis, AT&T, 1956.
2. Deming WE: Out of the crisis. Cambridge, Massachusetts Institute of Technology, 1986, p 357.

3. Gitlow HS, Gitlow SJ: The Deming guide to quality and competitive position. Englewood Cliffs, Prentice Hall, 1987.

4. Gitlow HS, Gitlow S, Oppenheim A, Oppenheim R: Tools and methods for the improvement of quality. Boston, Irwin, 1989.

5. Kume H: Statistical methods for quality improvement. Tokyo, 3A Corporation, 1985.

6. Mizuno S: Management for quality improvement. Cambridge, Productivity Press, 1988.

7. Shewhart WA: Statistical method from the viewpoint of quality. Washington, US Department of Agriculture, 1939.

8. Walton M: The Deming management method. New York, Perigree Books, 1986.

9. Walton M: Deming management at work. New York, Perigree Books, Putnam Publishing Group, 1990.

10. Wheeler DJ, Chambers DS: Understanding statistical process control. Knoxville, SPC Press, 1992.

CHAPTER 13

ISO Registration for Medical Practices and Organizations: The Model for Implementing Total Quality Management

STEVEN F. ISENBERG, M.D.

EDITOR'S NOTE: The International Organization for Standardization (ISO) 9000 is an internationally recognized certification that is based on very strict standards of business practice and management for a wide range of products, services, and systems. Many ISO 9000 companies and organizations make it a practice to do business preferentially with other ISO 9000 firms. ISO 9000 is only beginning to make inroads in medicine. In fact, when beginning the project for this monograph, an informal poll of many of the most savvy and experienced members of our national neurosurgery organizations for practice management and the business aspects of neurosurgery failed to identify a single ISO 9000–certified neurosurgical practice or organization in the United States. We had to go outside the field of neurosurgery to tap first-hand expertise in this area. In this chapter, I share my experience with ISO 9000 in a private otolaryngology practice.

WHAT IS ISO 9000?

The International Organization for Standardization (ISO) is a worldwide federation of national standards' bodies that develops and publishes internationally harmonized standards for a wide range of products, services, and systems. More than 100,000 organizations are registered worldwide with ISO, ranging from legal firms to national utilities and nursing homes. Large amounts of money from industrial ISO organizations such as Ford, Chrysler, and General Motors drive the health care system. If ISO is a mandate within the "Big Three" and their suppliers, it follows that ISO 9000 will ultimately drive health care providers to improve their quality systems.

Standards published by ISO represent a state–of-the-art international consensus on a particular issue. The ISO 9000 series of standards is an extensive family of standards dealing with various quality-system disciplines. ISO 9001, ISO 9002, and ISO 9003 are "requirements standards" that define a minimum framework for the development and implementation of a quality system in any industry sector. As such, they are generic to all nontechnical quality management systems. The requirements specify what must be achieved within the quality system to retain effective management control. They do not specify how to achieve the requirements, thus allowing organizations the freedom to develop or enhance their operations in response to customer needs.

ISO 9000 defines a framework of minimum requirements for the implementation of quality systems to be used in contractual situations. ISO is proof of the medical industry's commitment to quality in the form of independent assessment and certification. The standards have been adopted worldwide as suitable criteria for assessment and registration of companies by independent, accredited, third-party organizations (registrars):

- ISO 9000: Quality management and quality assurance standards.

- ISO 9001: Quality systems—Model for quality assurance in design/development, production, installation, and servicing.
- ISO 9002: Quality Systems—Model for quality assurance in production and installation.
- ISO 9003: Quality Systems—Model for quality assurance in final inspection and test.
- ISO 9004: Generic guidelines for quality management and quality systems.

Although ISO standards should not be compared with the total quality standards, they definitely support the approach by specifying a platform for consistency, continuity, and continuing improvement of managing practices on the basis of the universally accepted plan–implement–check–review (or plan–do–check–act) continuum. Therefore, conformance for ISO requirements often provides an essential and tangible first-step systems approach for organizations wishing to pursue a total quality management (TQM) philosophy. The methods whereby a medical practice goes from being ISO 9000–registered to having a quality system that is based on the principles of TQM are explored later in this chapter. I begin by discussing the actual implementation and subsequent registration of ISO 9000.

POTENTIAL BENEFITS OF ISO 9000 IMPLEMENTATION AND REGISTRATION

The implementation of ISO 9000 can provide a formal, internationally recognized method of quality management to assist medical practitioners and other health care organizations to:

- Operate effectively and economically;
- Respond quickly to changes in the market;
- Improve communication between departments, divisions, and business partners;
- Provide systems that proactively reduce errors; and
- Make quality visible to all users and contributors of the service.

There are also several benefits of ISO 9000 registration:

- Provide confidence to owners, management, customers, and other interested parties that an organization quality system meets an international standard;

- Meet or exceed customer requirements and expectations;
- Define and attain a "milepost" to measure continuing performance;
- Stimulate and motivate employee participation at all levels; and
- Obtain a significant marketing advantage.

GETTING STARTED

To proceed with ISO 9000 registration in a medical practice, it is helpful to proactively anticipate potential implementation problems and overcome the FEAR factor:

- **F**ailure of everyone to understand what ISO registration is and why it is important to them.
- **E**ventual obstacles that will result with any effort to implement change.
- **A**nticipation of delays that will result as a consequence of the schedule interruptions that are indigenous to medical practice.
- **R**esistance to change.

These problems can only be overcome with physician leadership. The FEAR factor is a template that is based on the successful implementation of change with my practice, locally with my peers, and nationally with Project Quality Card™ and the Practice Improvement Program™.

Step 1: Are You a Leader or a Manager?

Both are important, but so is the difference. *Leaders* establish direction by developing a vision of the future along with the strategies needed to achieve the vision. They align people to create the teams that accept the validity of the vision. They motivate and inspire people to overcome barriers.

Managers do the planning and the budgeting. They establish detailed steps and timetables to achieve the needed results. They provide the structure to organize the staffing with policies and procedures and monitoring of implementation. They monitor results, identify outliers, and solve problems.

Most medical offices and physician groups (i.e., medical staffs, local and state medical societies) create structures that permit only management. Leaders must "think outside of the box" to envision change. Leaders must then follow the next steps, and, as I point out later, they must surround themselves with competent managers.

Step 2: Create a Sense of Urgency

Complacency must not be underestimated. Implementing change is often derailed by the leader's failure to assess the level of complacency and surge ahead without the sense of urgency instilled into those who are expected to follow. Do not be fooled by the early commitment of a few followers. Ryan and Gross (12) studied the rate of adoption of a new breed of hybrid seed corn among Iowa farmers. They determined that the epidemiological curve of adoption of the innovator had an S shape, with an early slow phase, involving a few farmers; a rapid middle phase; and a slow third phase, with incomplete penetration to the end. Physician leaders must understand that these early followers, the "cosmopolite," are only a small fraction of the group.

The next subgroup, the "early adapters," represents 13% of the group. They are opinion leaders. They are risk tolerant, well connected socially to the other members of the group, and watched carefully by the "early majority."

The early majority composes one third of the group. The members of this group are very local and pragmatic. The physician leader, to establish a sense of urgency, must assess the willingness to change deep within the early majority. If enough members of the early majority are in step, the "late majority," representing another one third of the group, potentially can be convinced.

The "laggards," representing 15% of the group, compose the final subgroup. The leader must understand that the laggards use the past as their point of reference. They will not follow.

To summarize, the physician leaders must assess and instill the sense of urgency deep into the early majority prior to moving ahead; if they do not, complacency will likely rule the day. To move ahead with ISO, the staff must sense the urgency of establishing the medical practice as a leader in ISO registration. Such a profile provides the staff with job security, methodology to deal with daily common cause variations, and a sense of pride and accomplishment.

Step 3: Creating a Coalition

This step requires the physician leader to identify the talented managers, other leaders, opinion leaders, and team players. These people must have strong position power, broad expertise, and high credibility. They need to work together as a team, and they must have enough power to lead the change. The leader must create trust with open discussions in off-site locations. The coalition must feel the need to develop a common goal that is sensible and appealing.

Step 4: Develop a Vision and Strategy

The guiding coalition and the physician leader need to create a vision to help direct the change effort. At this stage, the leader must chart the course but remain flexible enough to adjust the course to keep the team together. The vision must also be easy to see, beneficial, feasible, focused, and easy to communicate.

Step 5: Communicate the Change Vision

The physician leader must then direct the communication of the change vision. To accomplish this, the leader and the coalition need to keep the vision simple, state it in multiple forums, repeat it over and over, lead by example, allow give and take, and openly address the obvious problems.

Step 6. Empowering Participants to Accomplish Broad-Based Action

In the office, physician leaders or the leader designee needs to empower employees to accomplish the vision. Confrontational supervisors must be controlled by the leader. Within the larger physician community, physicians who compose the early majority and the late majority must be empowered to communicate the vision. The appropriate training and education should be provided.

Step 7: Celebrate Short-Term Wins

A short-term win has three characteristics:

- It is visible to large numbers of people.
- It is unambiguous; few can reasonably argue that it is a "win."
- It is clearly related to the change effort.

Step 8: Consolidating Gains and Producing More Change

The guiding coalition uses the credibility of short-term wins to tackle additional, larger change projects. More help is needed and members of the late majority are recruited. The physician leader must guard against complacency by maintaining clarity of the shared purpose.

Step 9: Anchor Change Into the Culture

Do not expect the alterations to anchor in until the transformation is complete. The new vision must be clearly superior to the old method. Repetitive talking about the value of the change is required. Laggards may need to be removed. Succession must be compatible with the new practices otherwise the old culture will reassert itself.

The physician leader must identify the vision, assess the support, pick a team, become part of the team, encourage the team to become the cheerleader of the shared vision, empower the onlookers, celebrate the wins, create a winning image, and solidify the effort into the recognized history of the culture. The careful implementation of this nine-step process with appropriate recognition of the characteristic acceptance by a group will enable the physician leader to lead change in the office and overcome the FEAR factor, which will lead to the successful implementation of ISO registration in the medical office.

PREPARING TO IMPLEMENT ISO

The objective of an ISO 9001/9002–based quality management system is to decrease the variability (and, therefore, both inefficiency and risk) of managing medical practices. This must be accomplished without removing the organizational freedom and authority that key individuals require to exercise their responsibilities. In most organizations, this does not mean starting from scratch to reinvent the business but requires the formalization and documentation of existing practices so that each may be analyzed for effectiveness and efficiency in conjunction with all the others. It is a misconception that a medical practice needs to only write down what it does. Instead, organizations should consider how each department fits together and documents their system accordingly.

An ISO 9000–compliant quality assurance and quality management system includes up to 20 system elements documented in a pyramid of interconnected policies, procedures, and work instructions. Of the 3 system modules (ISOs 9001, 9002, and 9003), ISO 9001 requires all 20 system elements. The following summary is condensed from the International Standard document ISO 9001, where the official text may be found. "Shall" means a requirement is mandatory.

1. Management responsibility: Shall define, document, and implement a policy for quality that is understood throughout the organization and shall regularly review the system's performance opportunities for improvement.
2. Quality system: Shall establish, document, and maintain a quality system, which includes a quality manual, system procedures, and quality planning.
3. Contract review: Shall establish and maintain documented procedures for contract review to understand clearly the customer's requirements.
4. Design control: Shall establish and maintain documented procedures to control and verify the design of both the product (service) and the service delivery processes to ensure conformance to specified requirements.
5. Document and data control: Shall establish and maintain documented procedures to control all documents and data (including hard copy and electronic media), such as standards and patient records, which are current, appropriate, correct, and accessible.
6. Purchasing: Shall establish and maintain documented procedures to ensure that the purchased product, associated documents, and data conform to requirements. Subcontractors are to be evaluated and selected on their ability to meet subcontract requirements, and the type and extent of control exercised by the supplier over subcontractors is to be defined.
7. Control of customer-supplied product: Shall establish and maintain documented procedures for the control of verification, storage, and maintenance of customer-supplied product provided for incorporation into the supplies or for related activities.
8. Product identification and traceability: Where appropriate, shall establish and maintain documented procedures for identifying the product (service) from receipt or inception and during all stages of production, delivery, and installation.
9. Process control: Shall identify and plan the service and service delivery processes that directly affect quality and shall ensure these processes are carried out under controlled

conditions, the ultimate measure of which is the level of customer satisfaction.

10. Inspection and testing: Shall establish and maintain documented procedures for inspection and testing activities to verify that the specified requirements for the product are met.

11. Control of inspection, measuring, and test equipment: Shall establish and maintain documented procedures to control, calibrate, and maintain inspection, measuring, and test equipment (including test software) used by the supplier to demonstrate the conformance of product to the specified requirements.

12. Inspection and test status: The inspection and test status of product shall be identified and maintained throughout the production, delivery, installation, and servicing of the product to ensure that only a product that has passed the required inspections and tests (or released under an authorized exception) is delivered, used, or installed.

13. Control of nonconforming product: Shall establish and maintain documented procedures to ensure that a product that does not conform to specified requirements is prevented from unintended use or installation.

14. Corrective and preventive action: Shall establish and maintain documented procedures for implementing corrective action in the handling of customer complaints, product nonconformities, and the application of controls to ensure corrective action is taken and that it is effective. Preventive action procedures will detect, analyze, and eliminate potential causes of nonconformities.

15. Handling, storage, packaging, preservation, and delivery: Shall establish and maintain documented procedures to prevent damage or deterioration of product.

16. Control of quality records: Shall establish and maintain documented procedures for identification, collection, indexing, access, filing, storage, maintenance, and disposition of quality records. Quality records shall be maintained to demonstrate conformance to specified requirements and the effective operation of the quality system. They provide internal evidence that requirements are being satisfied and procedures followed and furnish the key to understanding when something goes wrong.

17. Internal quality audits: Shall establish and maintain documented procedures for planning and implementing internal quality audits to verify whether quality activities and related results comply with planned arrangements and to determine the effectiveness of the quality system. These audits are performed on behalf of top management and essential to management review.

18. Training: Shall establish and maintain documented procedures for identifying training needs and shall provide for the training of all personnel who perform activities affecting quality. Appropriate records of training shall be maintained.

19. Servicing: Where servicing is a specified requirement, shall establish and maintain documented procedures for performing, verifying and reporting that the servicing meets the specified requirements.

20. Statistical techniques: Where the supplier identifies the need for statistical techniques required for establishing, controlling, and verifying process capability and product characteristics, shall establish and maintain documented procedures to implement and control their application.

IMPLEMENTING ISO 9000

The implementation of a quality management system conforming to the requirements of ISO 9001 or ISO 9002 requires a commitment from senior management to support the adoption of quality assurance principles of improvement. It requires a review of the effectiveness of the current organizational structure and operational activities and the development of a program with assigned responsibilities. The whole system must be recorded in a way that is easy to understand and that provides for internal and external review and improvement in the future.

It is essential to educate the staff and implement the system in stages. Feedback as to the usefulness of written procedures and documentation must be obtained, and everyone must be involved and their suggestions must be welcomed. The 20 system elements described previously, as specified for medical practice, are compiled in the checklist listed in Appendix A at the end of this chapter. Note that most health care organizations seek an ISO 9002 registration. ISO 9002 eliminates the design and development elements that are usually not needed for health care entities. If, however, your practice wishes to achieve recognition for new procedures or other design and development efforts, ISO 9001 is appropriate. In my case, because we were developing an otolaryngology electronic medical record, we applied for an ISO 9001 registration. The attached checklist was developed for use in organizational assessment or audit, including gap analysis prior to the implementation of an ISO 9000 system. The standard registration process involves an initial contact to a registrar such as SGS International Certification Services, Inc. (Rutherford, NJ; phone: 201-935-1500). An optional preassessment of a quality system can be provided by SGS to assess the medical office's quality system and readiness for registration. If the medical practice desires to hire a consultant, he or she may prepare the practice without a preassessment. SGS, it should be noted, is prohibited from actually helping the practice implement the quality system. Following the preassessment or consultant assistance, SGS reviews the practice's system documentation during the course of the preparation phases to determine that it adequately addresses the requirements of ISO 9001 or ISO 9002. This can be performed on site. Significant omissions are documented in writing and an audit checklist is developed to enable the audit team to reference ISO 9001 or ISO 9002 requirements as well as the practice's documented practices while conducting the initial audit. Checklist development is followed by the initial audit, which comprises on-site evaluation of the practice's implemented quality system as well as ISO 9001 or ISO 9002 requirements. This process usually requires 2 to 2.5 days on site. The on-site auditors interview personnel, and results are reported verbally at the conclusion of the audit. After the on-site initial audit, SGS management reviews everything. When all requirements have been met, a registration certificate is issued. If the practice is registered, its registration remains valid indefinitely, subject to satisfactory results of surveillance and continuation audits. Surveillance audits are usually conducted every 12 months by contract with SGS.

GETTING IT DONE

In our office, we began the initial ISO 9000 registration by obtaining every document we used in the office. We organized all the forms, eliminating the obsolete forms. Next, everyone in the office wrote a list of the jobs that they perform while they flow charted their jobs by job descriptions and work instructions. *Figure 13.1*, for example, documents the "patient care facilitator" position in the office. I followed the checklist in Appendix A and completed all of the elements under management responsibility and quality system. Contract review is particularly important in managed care environments. This required documentation of specific contract requirements for each managed care plan in the office software system. The purchasing of office supplies, evaluation of suppliers, and maintenance of purchasing data fulfilled this element of the assessment checklist. Control of the customer supply product list is particularly important in my practice because of hearing aid dispensing. I evaluated the customer supply product with a survey of my customers seen in my hearing aid business, Physicians Hearing Service (*Fig. 13.2*). Product identification and traceability were accomplished by keeping a log of supplies with the distribution to each of the offices. Process control was accomplished with flow charting (see Chapter 5). Each of the processes in the office, including patient registration, allergy testing, audiometric evaluation, surgery scheduling, office appointment scheduling, and correct control of patient results (lab and radiology), were flow-charted. *Figures 13.3* and *13.4* document the patient call back sheet and telephone response sheet used in my office. Inspection and testing required flow-chart documentation of the interaction of the physician's responsibility and the responsibility of the hospital. The control, inspection measurement, and testing of equipment were necessary for autoclaves, audiometers, brain-stem evoked-response audiometry, electronystagmography, and in vitro allergy testing equipment. Nonconforming products were recorded in a separate file and reviewed for disposition. Corrective and preventative action involves the use of patient incident reports, which are not designed to eliminate the "bad apples" but to improve the processes. The implementation of a nationally based patient satisfaction measurement program through Project Quality Card™ is helpful in the maintenance of patient perceived quality. The published results of Project Quality Card's benchmarked patient satisfaction registration are seen

PATIENT CARE FACILITATOR

PRIMARY RESPONSIBILITIES

1) Patient check out during clinic hours, to include: scheduling of all recommended diagnostic testing and follow up appointments; obtaining surgery information when appropriate; collection of patient copayments when required; providing patients with receipts appropriate.
2) Communication of appointment times for diagnostic tests to patients (or their caregiver), to include providing information to the insured regarding CPT and ICD-9 codes when appropriate.
3) Scheduling of all new patient appointments, including emergency requests from physician offices.
4) Design of clinic schedules to minimize patient wait times, both for the appointments themselves and the waiting area during clinic hours, to include triage of patient waitlisted.
5) Prior authorization of all scheduled diagnostic testing and surgeries when required, including scheduling of observation and in-patient beds when required.
6) Patient phone messages, to include responses.
7) Be a team player!

TIME ALLOTMENT

During Clinic Hours, both East and North:
100%   Patient check out and scheduling, to include emergency visit requests from referring physicians.

During Office Hours:
35%   Patient phone messages to R.N's and M.D.
35%   Maintenance of clinic appointment schedule, chiefly new patient appointments and requests for move-up.
30%   Prior authorization for surgeries and appropriate diagnostic testing.

EMPLOYER'S GOALS

100%   Patients feel they have been treated professionally and courteously.
100%   Patients leave office with clear understanding of follow up care and requirements.
100%   Accurate information recorded on patient superbill, with copayments collected from managed care patients.
100%   Surgeries requiring precertification completed no later than three days prior to surgery.
100%   Bed reservation requests communicated to appropriate facility.
110%   Patient phone messages returned same day or as promised.

PERSONAL GOALS

Divestment of responsibility for surgery precertification and bed reservations.

Figure 13.1   Example of patient care facilitator position flowchart.

I. Please answer as indicated.

1. If possible, please indicate the brand and model of the hearing aid you purchased.

    Brand: Model:

    —— Telex   —— Behind-the-ear

    —— Starkey   —— Full In-the-ear

    —— Microtech   —— Half Size In-the-Canal

    —— Rexton   —— In-the-Canal

    —— Oticon   —— Completely in the Canal

    —— Unitron

    —— Argosy

    —— ReSound

    —— Other (name)

2. When did you get your hearing aid and how much did you pay for it?——

3. Do you feel, comparing our price, service, and product quality to other hearing aid dispensers that you received a good value? (circle one)

    yes   no

4. Do you use your hearing aid? (circle one)

    yes   no

5. If you need a new hearing aid(s) or need service on your current aid, would you see us again? (circle one)

    yes   no

6. How did you hear about us? (check one)

    —— Dr. Isenberg

    —— Friend, relative, "word of mouth"

    —— Hospital

    —— Family Doctor

    —— Walking by

    —— Referred by union/employer

    —— Other

7. Can you buy Pro-line hearing aid batteries cheaper elsewhere? (Our price is $5.00 for a 4-pack.) (circle one)

    yes   no   If yes, what price do you pay?——

8. Andrea and Sherri at PHS have masters degrees in hearing disorders and Dr. Isenberg is a board certified Ear, Nose, and Throat Doctor. Did this matter to you when you decided to purchase your hearing aid from us? (circle one)

    yes   no

II. Please answer each question by placing a check under the most appropriate response.

	poor	fair	good	excellent
1. Rate the quality and performance of the hearing aid your purchased.	—	—	—	—
2. How long you waited to get an appointment.	—	—	—	—
3. Convenience of the location of the office.	—	—	—	—
4. Getting through to the office by phone.	—	—	—	—
5. Length of time waiting at the office.	—	—	—	—
6. Time spent with the person you saw.	—	—	—	—
7. Explanation of what was done for you.	—	—	—	—
8. The technical skills (thoroughness, carefulness, competence) of the person you saw.	—	—	—	—
9. The personal manner (courtesy, respect, sensitivity, friendliness) of the person you saw.	—	—	—	—
10. The visit overall.	—	—	—	—

Figure 13.2   Patient satisfaction survey in the Physician's Hearing Service.

PATIENT TEST CALL SHEET

PATIENT NAME ————————————————————————

TEST PERFORMED ——————————————————— DATE ——————

TESTING CENTER   CDI   CHI   OTHER ————————————————

1) Dr. Isenberg's interpretation: ————————————————————
————————————————————————————————————
————————————————————————————————————
————————————————————————————————————

2) What does Dr. Isenberg feel should be done next?
————————— Call results to patient
————————— RTOff next regular appointment
————————— RTOff in ————— days   weeks   months
————————— Refer to ————————————————————————
————————— Prescription to be called in for patient:
                  ————————————————————————————
                  ————————————————————————————
                  ————————————————————————————

                  Refills ——————————
                  Called in by —————————— Date —————————— Pharmacy# ——————————
————————— Additional testing needed: ————————————————————
                  ————————————————————————————

————————— Other recommendations ————————————————————
                  ————————————————————————————
                  ————————————————————————————

————————— No need to call patient

3) Results sent to PCP from testing facility?   YES   NO
   Results sent/faxed to PCP by ——————— Date ———————

4) Signature of person calling patient ——————————————
   Date and time called ——————————————————

5) Addendum to this form?   YES   NO

FORM 1.9-1

Figure 13.3 Example of patient test call sheet.

Date_____   Time_____

Message Taker_____

PHONE MESSAGE

Patient Name   _____

Person Calling   _____

Chief Complaint   _____

_____

_____

_____

_____

_____

Temperature?_____   ❑ Oral   ❑ Axillary   ❑ Rectal   *(check over)*

❑ Nausea   ❑ Diarrhea   ❑ Vomiting   ❑ How Long? _____

Date last seen by Dr. Isenberg? _____

Family Doctor   _____

Surgery Date _____ Procedure Done _____

Current Medications Being Taken _____

Current Medication Allergies _____

Medication Taken in the Past that Helped _____

Patient:

Home Phone No.   _____

Work Phone No. (if needed)   _____

Pharmacy Phone No.   _____

Dr. Isenberg Recommendations:

Response Called to Patient:

Date _____   Time _____

Initials _____

FORM 1.8-1

Figure 13.4   Example of telephone response sheet.

TABLE 13.1
Percentage of Excellent Ratings by System of Care: Percentage Excellent (95% Confidence Interval)

Criteria	Solo[a] FFS[b]	MSG FFS[b]	HMO[b]	HOI	Project Solo
Technical	75	60[c]	60[c]	53[d]	71
Personal	62	68[c]	68[c]		74
Appointment wait	65	51[c]	40[c]		53
Office location	62	41[c]	40[c]		46
Telephone access	64	42[c]	33[c]		69
Office wait	36	28[c]	29[c]		40
Time spent	56	44[d]	42[c]		55
Explanation	67	53[c]	50[c]		64
Overall	65	50[c]	49[c]		63
	(N = 1677)	(N = 1677)	(N = 6248)		(N = 1858)

FFS, fee for service; MSG, multispecialty group; HMO, health maintenance organization. Sample sizes for other items vary due to differing amounts of missing data: SOLO FFS, 2947-3055; MSG FFS, 882-846; HMO, 3310-3424.
[a] SOLO indicates solo or single specialty.
[b] Data obtained from Ruben et al. [11].
[c] Contrasts different from SOLO FFS at level of $P < 0.001$. Others are not significant at $P > 0.05$.
[d] Data obtained from David Radosevich, Ph.D., Health Outcomes Institute. Primary care physicians only.

TABLE 13.2
Patient Satisfaction Survey Results

	Rank				
Survey Question	Poor (1)	Fair (2)	Good (3)	Very Good (4)	Excellent (5)
Overall visit	0	2.1	15.1	30.8	52.1
Technical skills	0	0.7	7.2	30.3	61.8
Personal manner	0	0.7	7.9	23.2	68.2
Appointment wait	3.3	19.9	26.5	23.2	27.2
Office location	0.7	0.7	20.8	38.3	39.6
Telephone access	0	0.7	14.2	35.5	49.6
Office wait	8.1	18.1	27.5	28.9	17.4
Time spent with person	0	4.0	19.5	34.2	42.3
Explanation	0	1.4	11.5	30.4	56.8

Total number of surveys received as of 12-1-1995 = 152; age range of patients completing survey = 1–82 years; percentage of men/women completing survey = 46.7% men/52.6% women.

in *Table 13.1*. The benchmarking of overall percentage excellence is helpful in management of the office personnel by linking staff bonuses and wages to overall percentage excellence as benchmarked against other practitioners. Each participating physician receives a "report card" of their patient satisfaction results (*Table 13.2*). This program, termed the Patient Assessed Compensation for Employees (P.A.C.E.), is managed by Project Quality Card (website: www.good4docs.com). The handling, storage, packaging, presentation, and delivery of materials include products delivered to the office as well as the "packaging" of patients. Quality records and internal quality audits are maintained by the office manager, and training is accomplished by passing the philosophy of TQM from each member of the staff to trainees. Servicing involves hearing aid warranties by manufacturers, and statistical techniques involve, in addition to the patient satisfaction measurement, the implementation of outcomes of medical treatment. This is accomplished with the use of an on-line clinical outcomes measurement program provided by Outcome Sciences. Costs incurred by the patient at the hospital level are seen in *Figures 13.5* and *13.6*. These figures demonstrate the costs incurred by my patients at the hospital level for the procedures listed. In some situations not demonstrated here, my

HOSPITAL CHARGES

7/92–12/95

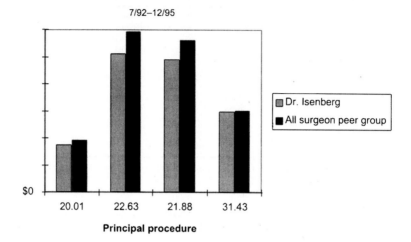

Principal procedure

Procedure	Description	# Cases: Dr. Isenberg
20.01	Myringotomy w/insertion of tube	510
22.63	Ethmoidectomy	198
21.88	Other septoplasty	137
31.43	Closed biopsy of larynx	117

Figure 13.5 Outpatient procedure efficiency, part 1.

patients in-curred greater costs than other physicians did. When this situation occurred, steps were taken to monitor the materials used in surgery and my discharge criteria costs to reduce charges incurred by my patients.

ISO 9000 A MODEL, TQM A PHILOSOPHY

The implementation and subsequent registration of ISO 9000 mean that the medical office now views quality as a system and has that system under control. It does not, however, imply that the practice's quality focus is part of its strategic direction, that it has a strong concern for customer satisfaction, or that it is attempting to improve the working environment for employees so that they will be more effective at facilitating the practice's success. How does the practice go from being merely ISO 9000 registered to having a quality system that is based on the principles of TQM? In this section, I explore how the ISO 9000 compliance quality system and the structures that were put into place to bring it

about are excellent foundations upon which to build a quality system grounded in TQM philosophy.

First, you should know that ISO 9000 is a *model* for quality system. ISO 9000 espouses a certain philosophy which can be partly expressed in the following statements:

- Top management is responsible for the quality system.
- Employees must understand their responsibilities and the authority they are given.
- Employees should have adequate skills and instructions for their job.
- The root cause of the quality system problems must be eliminated.
- The quality system must be reviewed regularly.

TQM is not a *model* but a *philosophy* that can be expressed in the following statements:

- The practice's focus must be on its customers and their requirements.
- Employees should be given increasing levels of responsibility and decision-making ability.

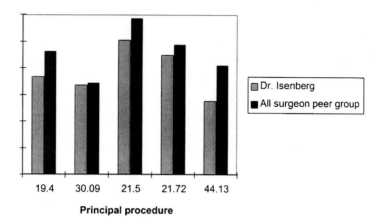

HOSPITAL CHARGES
7/92–12/95

Procedure	Description	# Cases: Dr. Isenberg
19.4	Myringoplasty	75
30.09	Other excision of larynx	50
21.5	Submucous resection of nasal septum	47
21.72	Open reduction of nasal fracture	46
44.13	Other gastroscopy	31

Figure 13.6 Outpatient procedure efficiency, part 2.

• Measurements are central to a fact-based decision making process.
• The practice's processes must be continually improved.

Therefore, ISO 9000 is a model, and TQM is a philosophy that can be expressed through a model such as a Malcolm Baldridge National Quality Awards criteria. What is helpful is that in reviewing and comparing either of the philosophies or the models of ISO 9000 and TQM, they are neither contrary nor mutually exclusive (1, 13). A medical practice can begin its quality journey by becoming compliant to the ISO 9000 standards and continue to deploy the TQM philosophy on that foundation (2, 3). Or they can introduce ISO 9000 compliance into a well-deployed TQM philosophy, such as that of IBM (Rochester, NY), which attained ISO 9000 registration after winning the Baldridge Award.

A normal progression from the medical office that has no quality system at all would be to introduce an ISO 9000 model first and then continue to build the TQM philosophy on that foundation. H. James Harrington, former president of ASQC, confided to *Quality Digest*: "Before you start TQM, you ought to have a quality system. ISO 9000 gets you up to the starting gate. TQM gets you into the winners circle" (10). The remaining portion of this chapter addresses the normal progression from ISO 9000 to TQM.

LEADERSHIP

The ISO 9000 standards require that executive management take responsibility for the quality system, that they develop and deploy the practice's policy for quality, that they ensure the quality policy is communicated and understood by all employees, and that they review the quality system periodically to ensure it continues to be effective. These requirements of the standards can be a basis for coaxing management into deeper levels of executive leadership: setting strategic direction, focusing on aligning work processes to customer satisfaction and performance objectives, and addressing public responsibility.

Executive management's role in TQM is to set the vision for what the medical practice will be to its customers, employees, and community. This vision can be described in a series of value statements. Once the values are set, they must be communicated and deployed throughout the work force by processes and programs. This is similar to what executive management has done with the practice's quality policy. After executive management has accepted and acted on their responsibility to formulate and deploy the practice's quality policy, they have already established the method by which they can formulate and deploy the company's values.

INFORMATION, ANALYSIS, AND BUSINESS RESULTS

The ISO 9000 standards require that the medical practice maintain records of certain activities, for example, employee training and contract reviews. Furthermore, it is expected that during management reviews, practice performance is analyzed and action is taken on the basis of that analysis. These records and reviews can become the cornerstone for the practice to broaden its information base as it expands its ability to make fact-based decisions. Operational data and measurements can be established and reviewed as the practice refines its values and sets goals for improvement. After data are collected, the practice's performance can be compared with that of other medical practices as benchmarking is deployed. This is what is done with the P.A.C.E. system described earlier in the chapter. In this situation, overall customer satisfaction is benchmarked and compared. The results are used to determine employee wages, salaries, and bonuses. Similar benchmarking is available for practice management financial data and clinical outcomes data (*www.outcomesciences.com*). The ISO 9000 requirement to keep and review certain records is a foundation on which to build an increased scope what is collected, analyzed, and reviewed.

STRATEGIC PLANNING

As mentioned previously, the ISO 9000 standards require that executive management set and deploy the quality policy of the medical practice. A quality policy is a rudimentary form of practice values. After a practice has successfully deployed its quality policy, the foundation is laid for formulating and deploying a deeper, richer set of values that address the practice's relationship with its customers, employees, and the public. Within such a value system, the company's culture is defined. Typically, the practice will find that its newly defined values are not the values being acted out everyday, just as its newly defined quality policy was not evident at first either. Rather, management had to overcome the barriers that prevented the quality policy from becoming a reality. In the same manner, management can now overcome the barriers that prevent the practice's values from becoming a reality.

The formulation and deployment of a strategic plan (see Chapter 3) for the medical practice are similar. The mission and vision of the practice and its objectives and goals for the short and long term should align with the stated values and then be deployed throughout the practice. The work done to formulate and deploy the quality policy sets the stage for formulating and deploying the practice's values and strategic plans.

HUMAN RESOURCE DEVELOPMENT AND MANAGEMENT

The ISO 9000 standards require that employees be capable of performing their jobs through properly defined responsibilities and authority, adequate procedural documentation, and thorough employee training. This is no different under a TQM philosophy. As employees' responsibilities and authority increase through empowerment and as they are given more responsibility for improving their work processes, they will need to receive adequate training in team dynamics, problem-solving tools, and so forth. The ISO 9000 concept of giving employees tools and training to be successful on the job will aid the transformation of the work force in a TQM environment. Responsibilities and training needs that were first defined as the ISO 9000 model was deployed will be redefined under the TQM philosophy, but the thought processes that first were exercised in initial deployment will be no different in redeployment.

PROCESS MANAGEMENT

The ISO 9000 standards require that work activities be documented to some degree. They also require that the work processes be audited and corrected when inadequate. Under the TQM philosophy, the practice's work activities need to be continuously improved. The definition of and review of these processes in the ISO 9000 compliant system provide all of the up-front work for continuous improvement efforts. Taking corrective action exercises most of the mechanics of continuous improvement, the main difference being that improvement efforts are initiated even when a process meets its own requirements. Furthermore, the same problem-solving tools (e.g., pareto analysis, cause-and-effect diagrams; see Chapter 5) and training needed to help people take corrective action are applicable to continuous improvement.

The TQM philosophy extends the management of quality outside of a practice upstream to a practice's suppliers, as does the ISO 9000 model. The ISO 9000 standards require that there be control exercised over a supplier's ability to deliver the practice's quality requirements. This attention to the quality of incoming parts and services can be a basis for developing supplier partnerships that work at extending the practice's continuous improvement efforts to its suppliers. It is possible in medical practice to transfer these continuous improvement efforts from the medical practice to the hospital. The practice's quality requirements being extended to the suppliers under the ISO 9000 model can be built on as mutually beneficial partnerships are developed with suppliers under the TQM philosophy.

CUSTOMER FOCUS AND SATISFACTION

The ISO 9000 standards require a certain amount of customer focus in the areas of complaint management (i.e., corrective action), reviewing of contracts to assure that what is promised can be delivered, and reviews of design input to assure that what is designed is what was intended. This initial focus on the customer can be built on to gather a more information (e.g., through customer surveys) and to become more proactive (e.g., customer participation in the design process). Also, the ISO 9000 requirement to define procedures is an excellent beginning for introducing the concept of internal customers and suppliers and moving all employees toward a customer focus.

In my practice, customer focus was integrated with Project Solo/Physicians Information Exchange (PS/PIE). Since its inception PS/PIE has published seminal research on multisite, community-based outcomes research; continuous quality improvement; and practice management (4, 6, 8). Founded in 1994, PS/PIE has grown to include numerous physicians throughout the United States representing most specialties, most states, and many different practice styles (for more information, contact the author.)

Data from customer complaints are typically reviewed in management review meetings. These are always attended by the physician leader. Building on the input during this meeting to include other customer data and on the agenda of this meeting to include strategic planning activities is a way to increase management's focus on the customer. It is also helpful to include "unexpected quality" (9) ideas from the medical office staff during staff meetings. This encourages participation of the staff in the development of practices services, such as review of hospital charges for inaccuracies, soft drinks for patients when the office runs late, and so forth, that separate the practice "from the pack."

LEVERAGING THE ISO 9000 PROJECT STRUCTURES

I have reviewed how the TQM philosophy can be built on the ISO 9000 quality system foundations. Now I address the structures that we put in place to make the quality system ISO 9000 compliant that were then leveraged to further TQM programs and initiatives. I examine three of these structures: the executive management forum, the communication structure, and the implementation team.

As the quality system was being patterned after the ISO 9000 model, there was a forum in which executive management defined the quality policy, approved initiatives, and reviewed the progress of the ISO 9000 registration effort. This may have been a quality steering committee, or the physician and the office manager. Whatever its format, this forum was where the executive staff learned to address quality issues. The forum can continue to be used to address quality issues as the TQM philosophy is implemented. Items such as the initiation of a customer satisfaction survey, an employee satisfaction survey, a recognition system, or an employee suggestion system have a place on this forum's agenda. This is where suggestions for unexpected quality should be entertained.

During the ISO 9000 registration effort, there was a communication structure whereby employees were informed of the quality policy, the ISO 9000 registration effort, the purpose of internal and third-party audits, and other important aspects of the registration effort. The communication structure may have been a newsletter within the office setting, electronic mail messages, employee meetings, or a combination of these. Whatever the structure, people are now familiar with receiving information about the quality effort by some means. That same structure can be used to communicate with employees about elements of the TQM implementation.

Finally, there was a group of people responsible for the ISO 9000 registration. Perhaps this was a cross-functional team whose members had responsibility within their own departments for guiding the effort and collective responsibility to see that the implementation was consistent across the office. This same team can be responsible for TQM implementation.

CONCLUSION

The implementation of an ISO 9000–compliant quality medical office system not only has a system that is under control but one to which the concepts of the TQM philosophy can be easily added. Elements of the ISO 9000 model address at a rudimentary level many of the concepts of the TQM philosophy. By seeing the similarities, a medical practice can expand the rudimentary ISO 9000 concepts to embrace the TQM philosophy. In addition, the structures of ISO 9000 implementation are easily adapted for use in TQM implementation. These facts make a TQM approach a logical enhancement to an ISO 9000–compliant quality system and ISO 9000 registration a logical first step in establishing TQM in a practice where no quality system has previously existed.

There are multiple incentives to pursue ISO 9000 registration. These incentives include improved office efficiency, improved working environment, a quality medical practice that maximizes its potential for patient care and profitability, a distinct marketing advantage, and proactive approach to the inevitable requirement that ISO–registered American businesses will place on their health care suppliers.

APPENDIX

S = Satisfactory IM = Needs Improvement U = Unsatisfactory	N/A = Not Applicable			
	S	IM	U	N/A
4.1　MANAGEMENT RESPONSIBILITY				
4.1.1　Quality Policy				
• How is the quality policy developed and documented?				
• What is top management's role in developing the quality policy?				
• Do the people know the policy?				
• Is policy implemented and maintained at all levels of the organization?				
• Are there any objectives to fulfill policy?				
4.1.2　Organization				
• Is the responsibility and authority of personnel who affect quality defined and documented?				
• Can they control further processing of non-conforming product?				
• Is there an organization chart or equivalent?				
4.1.2.2 Resources				
• How are human resource requirements established?				
• How are people trained?				
• How is the assignment of people accomplished to meet job requirements?				
4.1.2.3 Management Representative				
• Is the management representative appointed by executive management?				
• What are his her responsibilities, authority?				
• Is there evidence that reports of Quality Management System status are given to executive management?				
4.1.3　Management Review				
• How are management reviews accomplished?				
• Who is involved with these reviews?				
• How often are they done?				
• How are these reviews documented?				
4.2　QUALITY SYSTEM				
4.2.1　General				
• Is there a quality manual?				
• Does the manual include a quality management review system?				
• Are the procedures referenced in the manual?				
4.2.2　Quality System Procedures				
• Are there procedures to address the elements of the standard?				
• Are there work instructions?				
• Are other materials referenced?				
• If so, are they appropriate versions?				

S = Satisfactory	IM = Needs Improvement	U = Unsatisfactory	N/A = Not Applicable			
			S	IM	U	N/A
4.2.3 Quality Planning						
• How are quality plans developed?						
• Are Doctors Orders the primary plan?						
• What controls are in the quality plan?						
• Vital signs, etc.						
• How are patient care plans updated as conditions change?						
4.3 CONTRACT REVIEW						
4.3.1 General						
• What constitutes a contract? (e.g., provider agreement, pattern of conduct, schedule)						
• Are there procedures for contract review?						
4.3.2 Review						
• Where is a contract review done?						
• Who does contract review?						
• How are requirements documented?						
• How is capability to meet requirements reviewed?						
4.3.3 Amendment to contract						
• Is there a procedure for amending contracts?						
• How is an amendment communicated to those who need to know?						
4.3.4 Records						
• What records will be maintained of contracts and amendments?						
4.4 DESIGN CONTROL						
• N/A for some organizations. May use if designing care plan for patients.						
• Physician's practices may use because of designing care plan for each patient.						
4.5 DOCUMENT AND DATA CONTROL						
4.5.1 General						
• Is there a procedure for document and data control?						
• How are referenced external documents controlled?						
4.5.2 Document and Data Approval and Issue						
• What documents are controlled?						
• Is there a master list?						
• Who approves documents before issue?						
• How are obsolete documents removed?						
• When obsolete documents are retained, how are they identified?						
• Are the documents readily available to those needing them?						

S = Satisfactory	IM = Needs Improvement	U = Unsatisfactory	N/A = Not Applicable			
			S	IM	U	N/A
4.5.3 Document and Data Changes						
• How are changes to documents reviewed and approved?						
• Are there procedures?						
• Are changes to documents identified? How?						
4.6 PURCHASING						
4.6.1 General						
• Are there procedures for purchasing?						
4.6.2 Evaluation of Subcontractors (Vendors, suppliers, etc.)						
• Are subcontractors evaluated? How?						
• Do you rely on an association to evaluate vendors?						
• Is there evidence of subcontractors evaluation?						
• How are subcontractors added or deleted from approved list?						
4.6.3 Purchasing Data						
• In what form (medium) is the purchase order?						
• Do the purchasing documents clearly describe what is ordered?						
• Does purchasing data relate to quality requirements?						
• Who reviews and approves a purchase order before release?						
4.6.4 Verification of Purchased Product						
4.6.4.1 Supplier Verification at Subcontractor's Premises						
• Do you go to a subcontractor's premises to verify supplies?						
• If so, is there a procedure to handle this?						
4.6.4.2 Customer Verification of Subcontracted Product						
• Do the customers of the practice ever require going to subcontractor's premises?						
• If so, is there a procedure to handle this?						
4.7 CONTROL OF CUSTOMER SUPPLIED PRODUCT						
• What constitutes customer supplied product?						
• Babies, dentures, medications, jewelry, mobility aids, autologous, blood, etc.						
• Clothing and personal items						
• Samples for the lab may or may not be customer supplied product						
• What records are kept of the status?						
• Are there procedures to address this?						
• Are lost damaged or unsuitable items recorded and reported to the customer?						

S = Satisfactory	IM = Needs Improvement	U = Unsatisfactory	N/A = Not Applicable			
			S	IM	U	N/A
4.8 PRODUCT IDENTIFICATION AND TRACEABILITY						
• What requirements are there to identify and trace product or service status?						
• Patient, supplies, prostheses, blood, etc.						
• How is this identification maintained throughout the process?						
• Are sampling lots defined and records maintained for traceability and identification purposes?						
4.9 PROCESS CONTROL						
• How is patient care planned and controlled?						
• Are there procedures to control providing the services and/or products delivered by the practice?						
• Are conditions for providing this service/product controlled?						
• What level of procedure/work instruction is needed?						
• Professionals, licensed, registered, certificated people use their skills?						
• How are suitable equipment or processes defined?						
• What reference standards, codes, regulations, guidelines, etc., are used?						
• How is patient care monitored? What parameters are used?						
• Who approves processes (procedures) and equipment?						
• What are the criteria for workmanship? Protocols?						
• Is equipment maintained as suitable?						
• Many processes may be considered special and rely on skills & training. (such as ultrasound, x-ray nutritionist selecting menus)						
• What records are maintained?						
4.10 INSPECTION AND TESTING						
4.10.1 General						
• What procedures are in place to determine what exams, tests, measurements, assessments will be taken?						
• What records are kept?						
4.10.2 Receiving Inspection And Testing						
• How are patients examined for suitability for treatment/diagnosis?						
• How are supplies and services inspected for conformance?						
• Is the patient, supplies, or service released for further processing before all test results are?						
• If so, is there a procedure for identifying in case a recall is needed?						

S = Satisfactory	IM = Needs Improvement	U = Unsatisfactory	N/A = Not Applicable			
			S	IM	U	N/A
4.10.3 In-Process Inspection and Testing						
• What exams, measurements, tests are used while the patient is in the office?						
• Is there a procedure for establishing this? (Drs. Orders)?						
• Are the tests completed before the patient is moved to next stage of care?						
4.10.4 Final Inspection & Testing						
• What exams, tests, measures, observations are used to determine if a patient is ready for discharge?						
• What inspections, tests, measures are used to verify that supplies or services are conforming and ready for release to the patient?						
• Who authorizes the discharge of the patient?						
4.10.5 Inspection & Test Records						
• What records are kept of exams, tests, measures, etc.?						
• Are there records to indicate the "product" has passed, failed, etc.? See. 4.13						
4.11 CONTROL OF INSPECTION, MEASURING & TEST EQUIPMENT						
4.11.1 General						
• Are there procedures for control of IM & TE?						
• Is the measurement uncertainty known?						
• Is software involved in IM & TE? If so, is it able to be changed?						
• Is software verified in some manner?						
• Is there a list of calibrated IM & TE?						
• What is frequency of calibration checks?						
• If not, what method is used to calibrate?						
4.11.2 Control Procedures						
• Is there a way to determine the selection of IM & TE?						
• Is there a method to identify calibrated IM & TE?						
• Are calibrations to national or international standards?						
• What is the process for calibrating IM & TE? (mfg.'s. instructions)?						
• What happens to "measurements" taken just prior to finding an instrument out of calibration?						
• What records are maintained of IM & TE?						
• Are test lab personal trained and qualified?						
• Is the test lab independently accredited?						
• Are environmental conditions suitable for the device used?						
• How is IM & TE safeguarded, stored, etc.?						

S = Satisfactory	IM = Needs Improvement	U = Unsatisfactory	N/A = Not Applicable			
			S	IM	U	N/A

4.12   INSPECTION AND TEST STATUS

• How is status of a patient identified?				
• How are supplies' inspection status identified?				
• Are "authorized concessions" done? If so, how?				
• Are procedures for the above in place?				

4.13   CONTROL OF NON-CONFORMING PRODUCT

4.13.1 General

• Are there procedures for control of non-conforming product?				
• When are patients non-conforming?				
• How is non-conforming product identified?				
• Are there times when segregation is necessary?				

4.13.2 Review and Disposition of Non-conforming Product

• Who is authorized and responsible for disposing/repair of non-conforming supplies?				
• Who is authorized and responsible for disposing of "non-conforming patients"?				
• What is a non-conforming patient?				
• Are repaired/modified non-conforming items reinspected in accordance with established criteria? Do records reflect this?				
• How is non-conforming product disposed of? How is non-conforming service handled?				

4.14   CORRECTIVE AND PREVENTIVE ACTION

4.14.1 General

• Is there a procedure for corrective and preventive action?				
• Is there a way to determine to what degree corrective and preventive action will be done?				
• If corrective and preventive action requires procedure changes, how is this done?				

4.14.2 Corrective Action

• How are customer (patient and other) complaints handled?				
• Is there customer feedback besides customer complaints?				
• How are service or product non-conformities handled for corrective and preventive action?				
• Is there an investigation of non-conformances?				
• Is there evidence of corrective actions?				
• What controls ensure that corrective and preventive action is effective?				

S = Satisfactory	IM = Needs Improvement	U = Unsatisfactory	N/A = Not Applicable			
			S	IM	U	N/A
4.14.3 Preventive Action						
• What information is used to aid preventive action?						
• Is there evidence of preventive actions?						
• Is there evidence of management reviews of corrective and preventive actions?						
4.15 HANDLING, STORAGE, PACKAGING, PRESERVATION, & DELIVERY						
4.15.1 General						
• Are there procedures for HSPPD?						
• (Several procedures deal with handling patients, not just one.)						
4.15.2 Handling						
• How do patients, supplies and materials get handled?						
4.15.3 Storage						
• How are patients stored (kept so that they are not misplaced, assigned rooms, etc.)?						
• How are supplies stored?						
• Are storage facilities adequate for size and prevention of deterioration?						
• Are stored products identified?						
• Who has authority to receive and issue supplies?						
• Is shelf life a factor? If so, how is this handled?						
4.15.4 Packaging						
• How are patients "packaged" while in the office?						
• How are supplies packaged?						
• Medications?						
• Are the packages critical? If so, what defines appropriate packages?						
4.15.5 Preservation						
• What is done to preserve patients?						
• What is done to preserve supplies?						
• Blood, medications, customer supplied product, sterile packs, etc.						
• Are there procedures for above?						
4.15.6 Delivery						
• How are patients transferred (delivered)?						
• How are supplies delivered?						
• How are services delivered?						
• What about special handling and protection when necessary?						
• Are there procedures for the above?						

S = Satisfactory	IM = Needs Improvement	U = Unsatisfactory	N/A = Not Applicable			
			S	IM	U	N/A
4.16 QUALITY RECORDS						
• Are there procedures for control of quality records?						
• Patient, supplies, documents, forms, etc.						
• How are identification, collection, indexing, access, filling, storage, maintenance, disposition done?						
• Are pertinent subcontractor records maintained?						
• Are records readily available for those who need them?						
• Is there a retention time associated with records?						
• What media are used for various records?						
4.17 INTERNAL QUALITY AUDITS						
• Is there a procedure for internal quality audits?						
• Is there a schedule for doing the audits?						
• Who will audit the Internal audit function?						
• Are the auditors independent?						
• What reports or records are maintained?						
• Is there evidence of timely corrective action?						
• Is there evidence that corrective actions were effective?						
• Are the results documented and reviewed by management?						
4.18 TRAINING						
• Are there procedures for identifying training needs?						
• How are these needs met?						
• What records are maintained verifying training needs are met?						
• Licenses, registrations, certifications, etc.						
4.19 SERVICING						
• What type of servicing is performed?						
• How are customer complaints logged in and evaluated?						
• Are servicing procedures established?						
• Are training needs for servicing identified?						
• Are records kept (products in use, maintenance/repair activities, departmental efficiency)						
4.20 STATISTICAL TECHNIQUES (Relate to 4.10, 4.11, 4.12, 4.13, 4.14)						
• Are there procedures to identify the need for statistics?						
• How is process capability verified?						
• What indicators or "results" (outcomes) are monitored? (patient satisfaction, morbidity rate, infection rates)						
• Are there procedures to implement and control the use of statistics?						

REFERENCES

1. Askey JM, Dale BC: From ISO 9000 series registration to total quality management: An examination. *Qual Management J* 1(4):67–76, 1994.
2. Corrigan JP: Is ISO 9000 the path to TQM? *Quality Progress* 27(May):33–36, 1994.
3. Huyink DS, Westover C: ISO 9000: Motivating the People, Mastering the Process, Achieving Registration! Burr Ridge, IL, Irwin Professional Publishing, 1994.
4. Isenberg SF: Surviving and thriving as an independent practitioner: The search for continuous quality improvement, in *Managed Care, Outcomes and Quality: A Practical Guide*. New York, Thieme, 1997, 203–231.
5. Isenberg SF, Davis C, Keaton S: Project Solo: An independent practitioners initiative for confidential self-assessment of quality. *Amer J Med Qual* 11:214–221, 1996.
6. Isenberg SF, Gliklich RE: Profiting from Quality: Outcomes Strategies for the Medical Practice. San Francisco, Jossey-Bass, 1999.
7. Isenberg SF, Rosenfeld R: Problems and pitfalls in community-based outcomes research. *Otolaryngology-Head Neck Surg* 116:662–665, 1997.
8. Isenberg SF, Stewart M: Utilizing patient satisfaction surveys to assess quality improvement in community-based medical practices. *Amer J Med Qual* 12:188–194, 1998.
9. Kano N, Seraku N, Takahashi F, Tsuji S: Attractive quality and must be quality. *Quality* 14(2):39–48, 1984.
10. Paton SM: Is TQM dead? *Quality Digest* 14(April), 1994.
11. Rubin HR, Gandek B, Rogers WH, et al: Patients' rating of outpatient visits in different practice settings: results from the medical outcomes study. *JAMA* 270:835–840, 1993.
12. Ryan B, Gross NC: The diffusion of hybrid seed corn in two Iowa rural communities. *Rural Sociology* 8:15–24, 1943.
13. Wyble L: ISO 9000 and TQM: Partners in quality. *Circuits Assembly* (January):84, 1994.

CHAPTER 14

Obstacles to Implementing a Quality Philosophy in Neurological Surgery

MARK E. LINSKEY, M.D.

"One of the difficulties in bringing about change in an organization is that you must do so through persons who have been most successful in that organization, no matter how faulty the system or organization is. To such persons, you see, it is the best of all possible organizations, because look who was selected by it and look who succeeded most with it. Yet these are the very people through who we must bring about improvements."

—George Washington (excerpt from second inaugural address as President of the United States)

There are many reasons for individual neurosurgeons, neurosurgical group practices, academic neurosurgical divisions/departments, and national and international neurosurgical organizations to take an active interest in both learning about and applying total quality management (TQM) within their organizations. The most compelling reason is that TQM is the most effective and cost-efficient means yet devised for ensuring predictable excellence for the future, ensuring an optimal level of morale and productivity within an organization and ensuring that an organization will maintain market share and stay in business.

Achieving transformation to a total quality (TQ) approach to neurosurgical practice can be difficult unless it is carefully and proactively planned. The obstacles to be overcome are numerous and varied in terms of origin and motivation. Overcoming these obstacles requires their early identification, a savvy approach to resolution, dogged persistence, and an unswerving constancy of purpose. The purpose of this chapter is to identify many of these obstacles and suggest means for overcoming them.

LEADERSHIP

I cannot over stress that leadership is the single most important ingredient for successfully achieving a quality transformation within an organization. As a result, it is not surprising that failure of leadership or inadequate commitment of leadership is the single most common reason for failure. TQM does not succeed overnight. Implementation requires patience, the commitment and participation of organizational leadership, and a planned program of employee training and education. Leaders themselves must be trained, committed to, adopt, and participate in the transformation. Leaders cannot simply lend their political support and delegate the planning and work of the transformation to others, or the transformation will certainly fail. Lack of, or insufficient genuine leadership "buy in" or delegation of responsibility to others will make TQM a "nonstarter." Leadership training, active involvement, and support are crucial to successful implementation of TQM within a neurosurgical organization.

The same principle holds true for implementing TQM within a neurosurgical service that is part of a larger organization (e.g., a multispecialty group or clinic, hospital, or university). Unless the leadership of the larger organization is participating in, supporting, and leading the overall transformation of the whole organization, attempts at solely transforming the neurosurgical component of the organization will make limited headway and will only achieve limited success at the expense of a large amount of frustration.

Leadership Defined

Leadership is much more than management. *Leadership* is the process of motivating others to take action toward a common goal (6, 7). The job of management is leadership, not supervision. The power to lead comes from three sources: formal authority, personality, and knowledge. The best leaders develop the last two and avoid reliance on the first. Whereas a leader certainly expects results, a good leader empowers subordinates with the resources, training, and authority to live up to those expectations (3). When leadership rapport and subordinate trust have been established, an effective leader is more of a coach or counselor rather than a judge or enforcer.

The characteristics and attributes of a *good* leader are as follows:

- Understands the aims of a system and how the work of the group supports these aims
- Cooperates with all stages toward system optimization
- Understands the differences in people and tries to create joy in work
- Is coach and counsel, not a judge
- Develops knowledge and personality, rather than formal authority, as sources of power

The characteristics and attributes of a *transformational* leader are as follows:

- Identified as an agent for change
- Courageous and outspoken
- Value driven
- Lifelong learner
- Visionary

Not all good leaders are transformational leaders; however, a transformational leader must also be a good leader for the transformation to be successful.

According to W. Edwards Deming (5), "The aim of leadership should be to improve the performance of man and machine, to improve quality, to increase output and simultaneously to bring pride of workmanship to people."

The belief that leaders are born is a romantic myth. Leadership skills can be studied and learned just as any other science or philosophy. The organization with the most experience in the truth and validity of this concept is the military, which relies on successfully training inspirational leaders for its success and existence.

TABLE 14.1
Traditional Manager versus a Quality Leader

Traditional Manager	Quality Leader
Reacts to problems.	Plans for improvements.
"Shoots from the hip"	Makes data-based
Forms crisis management	decisions.
teams.	Pursues continual
Takes a short-term perspective.	improvement.
Blames workers for poor	Takes a long-term
outcomes.	perspective.
Works around the system.	Improves processes.

Leadership training becomes a critical component of an organization's management. With the exception of our "sink-or-swim", trial-and-error experience as chief residents, or our individual personal attempts to emulate our mentors, most neurosurgery training programs provide no formal training in leadership skills or philosophy. The rigorous training crucible we pass through selects for rugged individualists, who jealously guard individual autonomy, are extremely successful individual competitors, and often have not experienced the power and advantages of multidisciplinary "hybrid vigor" as well as group synergy (i.e., effective cooperative support where $1 + 1 > 2$). The characteristics of traditional managers and a transformational leader are compared and contrasted in Table 14.1.

Philosophical Leadership Obstacles

Whereas a private practitioner will be leading nonneurosurgeons (e.g., office staff, P.A.'s, R.N.'s, etc.), private practice groups often function in a similar way to a democracy (if small enough) or a republic (where the senior partners function as a quasi-representative democracy for the neurosurgical associates and other office staff). On the other hand, academic neurosurgery divisions and departments frequently function as an autocracy centered on the division head or department chairperson. Whereas leadership reservations to TQM for solo or group private practices often focus on time and practical relevance issues (see sections on TIME and LACK OF A PROVEN RECORD THAT TQM WORKS IN CLINICAL CARE in this chapter), academic leader concerns have also include power issues.

Power within an autocracy is often maintained

through restriction of information as well as decision-making authority. Only the leader and his or her select designates may be aware of all subordinates' salaries, productivity figures, departmental/divisional financial reserves, and so forth. They may have a visionary agenda for departmental growth and direction but may only share part of that vision with their staff on a periodic, need-to-know basis. If practitioner productivity figures, quality indicator data, and practice cost data are kept at all, they may be only selectively distributed for analysis on a yearly, biannual, or quarterly basis, when the data are too late to be useful for effecting any real-time process change. A fundamental tenant of TQM is involvement of process workers in "real-time" process measurement and analysis with dissemination of critical organizational information to cross-functional teams of process workers and process owners. This can be erroneously perceived as threatening and undesirable to a traditional autocrat.

A traditional autocrat may also confuse the TQM emphasis on consensus within an organization as threatening to his or her authority or as an abdication of responsibility in which leadership is reduced to majority rule, "management by democracy," or "leadership by committee." The reality is that consensus has nothing to do with majority rule. Winning a vote is not the same as achieving consensus. Furthermore, strong leadership and clear leadership vision are major priorities in TQM because they are the most essential prerequisites for TQM implementation success, establishing the proper priorities and direction for TQM efforts, and avoiding suboptimization within an organization. TQM leaders must be secure in themselves and their position, self-confident, knowledgeable, mature, and able to act as visionaries.

Optimization and Suboptimization

Optimization occurs when the goals of the subsystems or parts support the goals of the organization. In a large organization, the subsystems may be individual departments, divisions, or even standing committees (for national organizations). Within a department or group, the subsystems may represent individual neurosurgical practitioners. In a private practice, the subsystems may represent office staff and other allied health professionals employed by the practice. Optimization does not occur naturally

and must be actively managed. In neurosurgical practices, optimization begins during the recruitment process for new staff. There needs to be a mutually beneficial "fit" between the goals and aspirations of the new neurosurgical employee and the goals and needs of the neurosurgical organization that person is joining. As obvious as this may sound, it is amazing how rarely this is actually spelled out in advance or achieved over the long-term.

A new staff member who is recruited with specified goals and aspirations in mind, who later discovers that these goals are not compatible with organizational goals (and thus will not be supported) is destined to be unhappy and disaffected. Similarly, a new staff member who insists on pursuing his or her own professional agenda at the expense of the collective goals of the other members of the neurosurgical organization will create dissention and unrest within the group.

Suboptimization occurs when the goals of the subsystems or parts do not support the goals of the organization and when management fails to lead the organization as a system. The leadership failure may exist within the neurosurgical organization (e.g., senior partner, division/department head) or within the larger organization within which the neurosurgical group practices (e.g., multispecialty clinic, hospital, university, etc.). Achieving optimization within an organization will often require a focused retreat, in which all neurosurgeons within the organization participate, to achieve consensus and the buy in of all neurosurgeons for organizational goals and priorities. This retreat can serve as the platform for beginning strategic planning (see Chapter 3: Strategic Planning).

TIME

Time is the most valuable resource that practitioners have, and the efficient management of time is critical to the success of any neurosurgical organization. This is particularly true for smaller private practice neurosurgical offices, which operate using a very "lean" and cross-trained staff. Time away from actual patient care is potential revenue lost. Time is jealously guarded by most neurosurgeons and daily time allocation usually involves a rigorous triage process in which the most important things each day are attended to, whereas other concerns are either canceled or delayed.

TQM requires regularly scheduled and efficiently organized team meetings (see Chapter 4: Team Procedures for Neurosurgeons). It is the responsibility of organizational leadership to ensure that neurosurgeons and other organizational staff are afforded the time necessary to perform the work. If leadership does not see this use of time as a valuable investment—as important as the patient care it is designed to improve—and important to the survival and improvement of the neurosurgical organization, organizational TQM efforts will fail (see the Leadership section in this chapter).

On the other hand, leadership support is not enough if the staff involved (particularly neurosurgeons) are not personally committed to protecting their TQM time. For this to occur, the involved staff needs to recognize the importance and value of their time commitment to the organization and their patients. Only when that commitment is individually internalized will TQM time commitments appear as priorities on the staff member's ''radar screen'' when they plan their daily schedules. Internalizing this commitment involves an understanding of TQ philosophy and principles and training in TQM tools and methodology and is part of developing organizational ''critical mass'' for achieving a TQ transformation within the organization (see section on CRITICAL MASS).

Stephen Covey uses a time management model in which activities can be divided into four quadrants on the basis of their overall urgency and importance (4) (Table 14.2). The majority of obligations that make it onto a neurosurgeon's daily planner schedule tend to fall into Quadrant I (Urgent and Important). A great deal of these activities involve crisis management and ''putting out fires.'' If a neurosurgeon spends an inordinate percentage of his or her time with Quadrant I activities, the result will be stress and burn out. To achieve personal balance and professional growth, Quadrant I activities must be adequately balanced with Quadrant II activities (Nonurgent but Important). TQM activities fall into Quadrant II. Typical neurosurgeons are so busy that, if they are efficient and organized, most Quadrant III and IV activities never make the cut. If the neurosurgeon in question considers TQM activities to be Quadrant IV activities (Nonurgent and Unimportant), these activities will never make it onto the schedule.

The classic example for failure of these efforts

TABLE 14.2
Time Management Matrix

Importance	Activities	
	Urgent	Not Urgent
Important	Quadrant I	Quadrant II
	Crises	Prevention of crises
	Pressing problems	Expanding
	Deadline-driven	capabilities
	projects	Relationship
	Some meetings	building
	Rare phone calls	Identifying new
	Rare mail	opportunities
		Planning
		Recreation
Not important	Quadrant III	Quadrant IV
	Interruptions	Trivia
	Some phone calls	Busy work
	Some mail	Some phone calls
	Some reports	Some mail
	Some meetings	Time wasters
	Proximate, pressing	Pleasant activities
	matters	
	Popular activities	

Note: This table was adapted from Covey (4).

is when clinical process standardization and stabilization are mandated by hospital or nursing administration without up-front, clinical department leadership and practitioner buy in (see Chapter 6: Defining, Standardizing, Refining, and Stabilizing Processes, and Chapter 7: Establishing Clinical Pathways). A staff neurosurgeon is usually delegated the assigned task of participating in the process as the clinician representative (sometimes by a neurosurgery leader who does not consider the project to be very important for the neurosurgery organization). The assigned neurosurgeon may not recognize the inherent value of the process and is usually the most truant team member in terms of meeting attendance. There will always be clinical patient care issues that can serve as a legitimate excuse for missing an undervalued team meeting. In this scenario, attempts at developing clinical pathways may fail altogether, or even worse, may lead to the institution of onerous, arbitrary, restrictive, and potentially dangerous clinical pathways because of lack of clinician input and leadership.

Time investment into TQM activities thus becomes another critical necessity for successful TQM implementation. Failure to consistently provide the time to do the work of TQM is another major reason for failure to achieve a TQ transformation. It remains the primary responsibility of organizational leadership to ensure that team members have the protected time available to regularly attend the relevant meetings. It is also a leadership responsibility to achieve organizational critical mass by planning and instituting adequate TQM training for personnel as well as achieving staff buy in through organizational strategic planning.

CRITICAL MASS

In the first stage of TQM implementation, top leaders must be trained, committed to, and participate in the transformation. The second priority is to establish a critical mass of personnel within the organization who are trained in TQM principles and techniques and committed to the transformation. The term *critical mass* is taken from nuclear physics, where fission becomes a self-sustaining reaction without the need for infusion of further energy once a critical mass is achieved. The critical mass for TQM is the minimal core of organizational personnel with the necessary position, knowledge, and power within the organization necessary to make the TQ transformation within the organization self-sustaining. Up to the point of achieving critical mass, organizational leadership will need to continuously invest a significant amount of personal time and energy to keep the TQ transformation moving and evolving and to ensure successful TQM implementation. After critical mass is achieved and these individuals start to take joint responsibility for the transformation, leadership can afford to take more of a leadership guidance role, because the energy and motivation will come from the grass roots of the organization.

Employees are often skeptical of new management philosophies until they understand the concepts involved and experience the benefits that can be achieved. They are used to periodic management fads and will usually treat introduction of a new philosophy as yet another management fad unless they are educated and trained in a way that leads to individual understanding and personal internalization of responsibility for the transformation. Ways of assessing whether the philosophy is indeed being adopted include evaluating whether TQ training is ongoing at all organizational levels, as well as assessing whether supervisors are truly focusing on process performance data or are still clinging to a results focus. Unless critical mass can be achieved, any attempt at TQM implementation will simply become an issue treated like a humorous subject for a *Dilbert*® cartoon. Failure to achieve critical mass is another major cause for failure of TQM implementation.

CULTURE

Every organization has its own culture composed of human attitudes, biases, accepted or traditional ways of doing things, regulations, and other formal policies and procedures. Included in this background culture is certain degree of personal comfort and security with the knowledge of the way that things have always been done. As a result, change is unsettling, disruptive, sometimes perceived as threatening, and usually resisted (at least initially).

This resistance to change can arise within people (either individually or collectively) or it may take the form of institutional bureaucratic barriers to change. Individual resistance is most effectively overcome through leadership, constancy of purpose, training and education, and eventual persuasion and recruitment of the involved individuals into the critical mass of the organization. Bureaucratic obstacles can only be reduced by the intervention of organizational leaders who must review their regulations and policies with an eye toward breaking down barriers to change, barriers to interdepartmental cooperation, and barriers to reengineering organizational processes. Certain policies may have to rendered null and void, or be suspended, until such a time as established quality improvement teams can determine whether the policies add value or only cost to the organizational processes in question (see Chapter 6: Defining, Standardizing, Refining, and Stabilizing Processes). It is important for leadership to make it clear that a TQM approach with continuous process improvement (CPI) will be a departure from business as usual and that previous regulations and policies will need to be reviewed along with the processes they affect to determine their future with the organization.

RIGHTEOUS INDIGNATION

Medicine in general and neurosurgery, in particular, are noble professions that are altruistic and contain components of both art and science. In addition, neurosurgeons have invested a significant amount time and effort to master their profession and have very few peers in their sphere of medicine for comparative subject-matter competence. TQM was developed in a production and manufacturing environment and has only relatively recently been applied to service organizations. As a result, the jargon associated with TQM is largely oriented toward production and manufacturing. Many neurosurgeons bristle at the suggestion that their patients should be considered customers or that the practice of neurosurgery can be treated as a production process. To some, this may be a psychological barrier to acceptance of TQM that can only be overcome with patience, education, and demonstration of the usefulness of the approach.

Indignation can also arise over TQM's focus on process standardization and insistence on cross-functional and multidisciplinary input to process improvement. Clinical process standardization can be misinterpreted as infringement of practitioner autonomy unless one realizes that only treatments and interventions with sufficient strength of medical evidence to be considered standards or guidelines are standardized, whereas choices among clinical options remain (see Chapter 6: Defining, Standardizing, Refining, and Stabilizing Processes). Standardization of multidisciplinary clinical pathways that affect neurosurgical care can also be misinterpreted as bureaucratic intrusion "big brother" or unnecessary administrative burden, unless the development of these pathways is instigated or led by neurosurgeons (see Chapter 7: Establishing Clinical Pathways).

WARINESS OF QUASI-RELIGIOUS FANATACISM

The eventual realization of the power and potential of TQM methods can be very exciting, especially in the early stages of training and education. There is some truth to the saying that there is no one more zealous than a recent convert. If newly found enthusiasm comes across as evangelical zeal, it can lead to wariness on the part of neurosurgeons as students of the new philosophy. For this reason, it is extremely important that the education and training that are necessary to achieve critical mass within a neurosurgical organization are taught by knowledgeable experts who are skilled in the science of adult learning (12–15). TQM needs to be taught by experts, especially when the students are neurosurgeons. Unfortunately, courses or seminars led and taught by inexperienced, recently trained, TQM novices can transmit all the negative impressions of a religious revival tent or a political reeducation camp. To avoid this potential "turn off," it is important early during TQM implementation to consider employing experienced external consultants to assist with educating and training the organization's initial critical mass.

PREVIOUS EXPERIENCE WITH WELL-INTENTIONED PRETENDERS

TQM is often confused with past attempts at *quality assurance* (QA) on the part of hospitals and other health care institutions, even though they embody completely different philosophical approaches. Physicians understandably often have a very negative visceral reaction to the mention of QA. Traditional QA commonly targeted physicians for what were usually process deficiencies, undermined the natural cooperative team relationship between physicians and their clinical nursing support, and annoyed and burdened physicians with nonvalue-added additional paperwork. This confusion is often compounded by the frequent hospital practice of entrusting organizational attempts at instituting TQM (i.e., quality improvement or performance improvement) to the same department previously responsible for QA. In many cases, the only real change perceived by physicians is a change in the name on the door of the QA department and a corresponding change in the titles of the personnel within.

Hospitals and other health care institutions are proceeding with implementation of TQM and performance improvement efforts with or without the support and leadership of neurosurgeons. They have no choice in the matter. The Joint Commission on Accreditation of Health Care Organizations (JCAHO) has thoroughly embraced TQM as the optimal way to manage health care organizations, and most of its new indicators used to evaluate hospitals are centered around performance (process) improvement efforts. JCAHO wants proof that clinical processes are being managed in a cross-functional, multidisciplinary manner and that management is monitoring process measures and not managing solely on the basis of results.

JCAHO has so completely internalized the ideas and principles of TQM that they established an Academy of Health Care Quality in 1998. This "academy without walls" is a consortium of five universities with strong TQ faculties (Emory University, Northwestern University, Ohio State University, University of California at Los Angeles, and the University of Pennsylvania) that is governed, managed, and operated by JCAHO. The academy has developed a graduate level teaching curriculum and accelerated learning technologies, is developing a certification examination for certifying health professionals in health care quality, and is scheduled to accept its first students in 2000.

Unfortunately, many of the people assigned to the TQM task do not have the background in science and statistical methodology that is really necessary to perform TQM well. The predictable result is sloppy science. Measurement probes and instruments (including patient satisfaction surveys) may be put into use without prior validation and without ensuring the proper sample size necessary to support generalization of the results obtained. Measurement may mistakenly focus on data that are easily obtained or already available rather than determining the measures that would be most relevant and useful. Administrators and bureaucrats may focus more on cost indicators than valid indicators of quality. Draconian decisions may even have been made on the basis of questionable data in the mistaken belief that they were practicing performance improvement. None of these unfortunate occurrences will persuade neurosurgeons to embrace TQM when they are committed in the name of performance improvement.

FEAR OF COMPETITION

In the past, physicians (including neurosurgeons) have feared and resisted any collection and publication of physician-specific objective outcome data. Much of this fear was legitimate, because only crude data (that could not be adequately adjusted for the medical risk of the patients or the complexity of the actual procedure) were available, and without proper risk and complexity adjustment, "apples could not be compared with apples." Differences noted among physicians might only be apparent differences, and quality judgements that are based on only

apparent differences might lead to unfair competitive advantage. Unfortunately, the lack of participation in improving this process and resistance to any initiative that might lead to physician competition have perpetuated an information vacuum in which patients, hospitals, insurance companies, and managed care organizations have no choice but to judge practitioners predominantly on the basis of cost and timeliness. As a profession, we need to realize that we are already in a competitive situation. Our best chance for fairness lies in getting involved to ensure that the playing field is indeed level and that we are compared on matters that are most important to the actual objective quality of patient care (see Chapters 8–10).

LACK OF A PROVEN RECORD THAT TQM WORKS IN CLINICAL CARE

A certain degree of skepticism is a very scientific and healthy approach for neurosurgeons to take toward any new philosophy or approach to management. It is important to ensure that new changes are not instituted without sufficient promise of success and that TQM does not turn out to be just management fad. Part of the difficulty in obtaining a broader base of support for instituting TQM in neurosurgery is that the approach has its roots deeply grounded in production and manufacturing and has only recently been applied to service organizations. As a result, there is very little track record for TQM in health care to unequivocally demonstrate its advantages and use (1, 2, 8–11, 16, 17, 19). In addition, the earliest introduction of TQM into health care has been through the efforts of health care organization management and administration, and not through the efforts of clinicians.

Administrators have been understandably reluctant to infringe or intrude on clinical care decisions, and as a result, early efforts of TQM in health care have mostly focused upon nonclinical support services, such as administrative and laboratory processes, and not actual patient management processes. Despite excellent theoretical reasons why TQM is the best management strategy for health care, the truth is that we currently have very little objective proof that continuous process improvement actually leads to improvement in the quality of patient care. On the other hand, it is a logical fallacy to conclude that "absence of evidence equates with evidence of absence." The only way to overcome skeptical incredulity is to demonstrate effectiveness, and these efforts are currently underway in many locations.

INSISTENCE ON AN UNREASONABLE DEGREE OF SCIENTIFIC CERTAINTY

Although many neurosurgeons understand, appreciate, and welcome attempts to bring empiric science to the practice of management, we are most used to applying science to epidemiological research, clinical trials, and basic science experimentation. As a result, we sometimes look for more certainty of results and rigor of pilot study design than the real day-to-day world of organizational processes, interpersonal interaction, and patient care services allow. If we will wait until a plan–do–check–act (PDCA) cycle is completed to perfection, we may never get to institute any change at all. It must be kept in mind always that empiric improvement in TQM is continuous. Missteps are allowed and will ultimately be identified by control chart data. Process improvement is like tuning in a radio. You begin by first approximation and then make periodic adjustments (often overshooting in either direction in smaller and smaller increments) until you get the frequency just right. It is not necessary to have perfect empiric experiments each time. What is necessary is to make a start in the right general direction and then continue to assess results through control charting, so that you gradually zero in on your goal.

ACCESS TO KNOWLEDGE AND RESOURCES

Because TQM is relatively new to health care, and even newer to neurosurgery, efforts may fail because of lack of sources for training, tools, resources, and references; however, this obstacle is the easiest to overcome. This monograph represents one resource to assist neurosurgeons and neurosurgical organizations in making a TQM transformation. Many other resources exist and are readily accessible. An incomplete list of professional quality consulting firms that can assist a neurosurgical organization in starting and successfully completing a TQM transformation are listed in Table 14.3

An incomplete list of quality-related web sites is presented in Table 14.4. An incomplete list of available software for quality tools is shown in Table 14.5, and an incomplete list of quality-related peer-review journals is presented in Table 14.6.

TABLE 14.3
An Abbreviated List of Quality Consulting Firms

- Bill Scherkenbach's Quality Management Consulting Company (www.scherkenbach.com)
- Brown-Spath & Associates (www.brownspath.com)
- Computer Sciences Corporation, Health Care Group (www.csc.com)
- Covey Leadership Center (www.franklincovey.com)
- David Butler Associates (www.dbainc.com)
- Executive Learning, Inc. (see Chapter 5) (www.elinc.com)
- GOAL/QPC (www.goalqpc.com)
- The Greely Company (www.opuscomm.com)
- Group Practice Improvement Network (www.gpin.org)
- Gryphon Systems, Inc. (www.strategyroundtable.com)
- Healthcare Engineering, Inc. (www.quality.org/simmons/index.html)
- Heero Hacquebord (www.heero.com)
- Institute for Health Care Improvement (www.ihi.org)
- Joint Commission (JCAHO) National Consulting Services (www.jcwc.com)
- Juran Institute (www.juran.com)
- Oriel, Inc. (formerly Joiner Associates) (see Chapter 4) (www.orielinc.com, www.joiner.com)
- Philip Crosby Associates II, Inc. (www.philipcrosby.com)
- PQ Systems, Inc., Training and Consulting Division (www.pqsystems.com)
- Scholtes Seminars and Consulting (www.pscholtes.com)
- Simmon Dickinson Consulting & Training (www.sdct.com)
- Statistical Process Controls (www.spcress.com)

Note: This list is not intended to be complete or exhaustive. It is presented for general information only. Inclusion on this list is not intended to represent endorsement by the author or the Congress of Neurological Surgeons.

A list of many general and health care quality organizations is provided in Table 14.7. In addition, an extensive bibliography of general and health care–related quality references can be found after the reference section of this chapter. Adequate resources and expertise is readily available and accessible for those with genuine interest in pursuing a TQM program in the future.

DEMING'S SEVEN DEADLY DISEASES AND COMMONLY ENCOUNTERED OBSTACLES

Just as Deming's (5,18) 14 points constitute the fundamental cornerstone approach TQM, he describes seven conditions that will doom any TQM movement. He calls these the ''seven deadly diseases'' (8), and they are the 7 roadblocks that are inherent in most organizations in the western world. The cure for these ''diseases'' requires a complete change in management style. The seven conditions are as follows:

TABLE 14.4
Abbreviated List of Quality-Related Web Sites

General	Health Care
American Productivity and Quality Center (www.apqc.org)	Health Care Financing Administration (www.hcfa.gov)
Benchmarking Exchange (www.benchnet.com)	Institute for Health Care Improvement (www.ihi.com)
Council for Continuous Improvement (www.cci.org)	Joint Commission on Accreditation of Health Care Organizations (JCAHO) (www.jcaho.org)
GOAL/QPC (www.goalqpc.com)	JCAHO, Academy for Health Care Quality (www.jcaho.org)
ISO—International Organization for Standardization (www.iso.ch/welcome.html)	Medical Outcome Trust (www.sf-36.com)
Juran Institute (www.juran.com)	National Association for Health Care Quality (www.hahq.org)
Online Quality (www.curiouscat.com/guides/qlist.htm)	RAND (www.rand.org)
QualiNET—The Internet companion for quality management professionals (www.qualinet.com)	
Quality Function deployment Institute (www.qfdi.org)	
The Quality Junction (www.cris.com/~weterry)	
Quality Management Principles—Forum (www.wineasy.se/qmp)	
Quality On-Line (www.quality.org)	
Quality Resources (www.qualityresources.com)	
Quality Today (www.qualitytoday.com)	
Quality World (www.qualityworld.com)	
Skymark (www.pathmaker.com)	
Statistical Process Controls (www.spcpress.com)	
TQM International (www.tqm-international.co.uk)	
U.S. Navy—Total Quality Leadership Web Site (www.tql-navy.org)	
W. Edward Deming Institute (www.denimg.org)	

Note: This list is not intended to be complete or exhaustive. It is presented for general information only. Inclusion on this list is not intended to represent endorsement by the chapter author or the Congress of Neurological Surgeons.

1. Lack of constancy of purpose to plan products and services that will have a market, keep the organization in business, and provide jobs (Deming's Point #1).
2. Emphasis on short-term goals/profits: short-term thinking that is fed by fear of unfriendly takeover.
3. Performance appraisal systems, merit ratings, or annual reviews, which establish objectives or goals but lack a clear method for meeting the goal, instill fear, and discourage and/or eliminate needed teamwork.
4. Mobility of management; personnel practices that encourage "job hopping" by management and labor.
5. Management with visible figures only.
6. Excessive medical costs in the work force.
7. Excessive costs of warranty and liability, fueled by lawyers that work on contingency fees.

Deming also describes multiple conditions that will impede or impair a TQM program without necessarily dooming it. These he calls "obstacles" (8), because they impede the institutionalization of a TQM program but are curable through the application of the 14 "obligations"

of management (see list below). These obstacles are as follows:

1. Neglecting long-range planning and transformation.
2. Believing that problem solving, automation, gadgets, and new machinery will transform industry.
3. Searching for examples to copy.
4. Offering the excuse "our problems are different!"
5. Relying on quality-control departments.
6. Blaming the work force for problems.
7. Quality by inspection.
8. False starts.
9. The "unmanned computer."
10. Meeting specifications.
11. Inadequate testing of prototypes.
12. Assuming that "anyone who comes to try to help us must understand all about our business."

A detailed discussion of the seven deadly diseases has already been presented in Chapter 1, and the reader is referred to that chapter for additional in-depth review if necessary.

The commonly encountered obstacles listed above and elaborated on below are not as

TABLE 14.5
Abbreviated List of Some Quality Tool Software Resources

Software	Description
allCLEAR™	Windows software package for defining, refining, and standardizing; documenting; and storing from SPSS Inc.
Conquest™ (**CO**mputerized **N**eeds-oriented **QU**ality measurement **E**valuation **S**ys**T**em)	Windows software for measuring and monitoring clinical performance measures from the Agency for Health Care Policy and Research (U.S. government).
FlowMap™	Windows software package for mapping processes and process management from Management-New Style Ltd.
Improvit™	Windows software for constructing control charts from PC Engineering, Inc.
MAP-R™ for Windows	Windows software for constructing and evaluating multi-item scales (e.g., Likert scales) and for monitoring data quality; from Medical Outcomes Trust (applicability includes the SF-12 and SF-36, as well as patient satisfaction surveys)
The Memory Jogger™	Windows software for seven quality-control tools from GOAL/QPC.
The Memory Jogger Plus+™	Windows software for seven management planning tools from GOAL/QPC.
PA Tracker™	Windows Filemaker pro® software for tracking and reporting process-improvement team activities from Creative Software Solutions.
Pathmaker™	Windows software for 21 quality-control and management planning tools from Skymark (see Chapter 5).
PFT™	Windows **P**rocess **F**ocus **T**ools software containing either 9 or 16 quality management tools from Integrated Quality Dynamics, Inc.
Procedure WRITE®	Windows software to assist with defining, refining, and standardizing; documenting; and storing processes from Comprose, Inc.
ProcessID™	Windows Filemaker pro® software for providing structure and tracking of the process of total quality implementation and ongoing organizational total quality management improvement team activities from Creative Software Solutions.
QATS™	Windows **Q**uality **A**ssurance **T**racking **S**ystem software tracking day-to-day quality assurance functions from Progressive Quality Solutions.
QI Analyst 4.0 Enterprise™	Windows software package for charting and relating statistics used in statistical process control from SPSS, Inc.
QMX	Windows ISO 900–compliant package of quality management software from QMX, Inc.
SPC/PI+™	Windows statistical process control and performance improvement software from Qualitran Professional Services, Inc.
Statit Professional QC™	Windows comprehensive software package for continuous process improvement from Statware, Inc.
Strategic Planner™	Windows Filemaker Pro® software for strategic planning from Creative Software Solutions.
Strategy Roundtable™	Windows software for strategic planning from Gryphon Systems, Inc.
TeamFlow® Version 6	Windows process flowchart software designed for use in quality improvement teams from CFM, Inc.
Tool Kit Software Package	Windows software modules for 11 quality-control and management planning tools provided free from the U.S. Navy Total Quality Leadership web site (www.tql-navy.org).
Total Quality Tools® for Windows	Windows software package with 19 quality-control and quality management tools from PQ Systems, Inc.
Winchart™	Windows software for producing control charts from Simmons Dickinson Consulting and Training.

Note: The list is not intend to be complete or exhaustive. It is presented for general information only. Inclusion on this list is not intended to represent endorsement or testing by the author or the Congress of Neurological Surgeons.

"fatal" to an organization as the seven deadly disease. These obstacles represent management practice roadblocks to institutionalizing the quality transformation that are harmful but still "curable" through the application of Deming's 14 obligations of management (i.e., the 14 Points), which are as follows:

1. Create and publish for all employees a statement of the aims and purposes of the com-

TABLE 14.6
An Abbreviated List of Quality Journals, Newsletters, and Magazines

- *American Journal of Medical Quality*
- *Best Practices and Benchmarking in Health Care*
- *Clinical Performance and Quality Health Care*
- *Health Care Forum Journal*
- *International Journal for Quality in Health Care*
- *Joint Commission Journal on Quality Improvement*
- *Journal of Quality Improvement*
- *Journal for Quality and Participation*
- *Journal for Health Care Quality*
- *Quality*
- *Quality Connection* (News from the Institute for Health Care Improvement)
- *Quality Digest*
- *Quality Letters for Health Leaders*
- *Quality Magazine*
- *Quality Management in Health Care*
- *The Quality Observer*
- *Quality Progress*
- *Quality World*
- *QRB—Quality Review Bulletin*
- *Solutions* (the Journal of the Institute of Industrial Engineers)
- *The TQM Magazine*

Note: This list is not intended to be complete or exhaustive. It is presented for general information only. Inclusion on this list is not intended to represent endorsement by the author or the Congress of Neurological Surgeons.

pany or other organization. The management must demonstrate constantly their commitment to this statement.

2. Learn the new philosophy, top management, and everybody.
3. Understand the purpose of inspection, for improvement of processes and reduction of cost.
4. End the practice of awarding business on the basis of price alone.
5. Improve constantly and forever the system of production and service.
6. Institute training (for skills).
7. Teach and institute leadership.
8. Drive out fear. Create trust and a climate for innovation.
9. Optimize toward the aims and purposes of the company the efforts of teams, groups, and staff areas.
10. Eliminate exhortations for the work force.
11. (a) Eliminate numerical quotas for production. Instead learn, and institute methods for improvement.
    (b) Eliminate management by objective. Instead, learn the capabilities of processes and how to improve them.
12. Remove barriers that rob people of pride in their work.

TABLE 14.7
Abbreviated List of Quality Organizations

General	Health Care
American Management Association	American Health Care Quality Alliance
American Society for Quality (ASQ)	American Health Consultants
American Society for Training and Development (ASTD)	American Health Information Management Association
American Statistical Association (ASA)	American Society for Quality (ASQ)—Health Care Division
Association for Quality and Participation	Case Management Society of America
ISO—International Organization for Standardization	Health Care Information and Management Systems Society
Project Management Institute	Health Care Leadership Council
Strategic Leadership Forum (formerly the Planning Forum)	Institute for Health Care Improvement
Union of Japanese Scientists and Engineers (JUSE)	International Society for Quality in Health Care, Inc.
	Joint Commission on Accreditation of Health Care Organizations (JCAHO)
	JCAHO, Academy for Health Care Quality*
	National Association of Health Data Organizations
	National Association for Health Care Quality (NAHQ)*
	National Committee for Quality Assurance†
	National Health Care Cost and Quality Association
	Society for Health Systems
	Society for Health Care Epidemiology of America

Note: This list is not intended to be complete or exhaustive. It is presented for general information only. Inclusion on this list is not intended to represent endorsement or by the author or the Congress of Neurological Surgeons.
*Provides certification (or will soon provide certification per JCAHO-AHQ) for health professionals.
†Provides accreditation for managed organizations.

13. Encourage education and self-improvement for everyone.
14. Take action to accomplish the transformation.
(Please see Chapter 1 for an in-depth discussion of Deming's 14 Points.)

Neglect of Long-Range Planning and Transformation

Quadrant I (Table 14.2) activities, including crises and so-called "emergencies", can dominate leadership time commitment to the point that long-range planning never occurs. Long-range planning is one of the most important responsibilities of leadership, with tremendous ramifications for the future existence, health, and prosperity of the organization. As the major Quadrant II activity of leadership, long-range planning should assume a central position and primacy in leadership time management and scheduling priority.

Belief That Problem Solving, Automation, Gadgets, and New Machinery Will Transform Industry

It is seductive to think that significant improvements in the quality of neurosurgery can come about simply through acquisition of new technology (both hardware and software). The truth is that performance improvement is more a function of improving processes, personnel training, and personnel interaction than the acquisition of new devices or technological capabilities. New hardware and software are fashionable and sexy, and a bare minimum to satisfy capability is necessary. However, the hard work of CP requires more than trappings and gadgets.

The Search for Examples to Copy

Benchmarking is useful as a starting point for organizations that are so lost and adrift that they do not know where to begin with TQM. However, benchmarking alone is naïve. Each organization is different in terms of environmental causes and strength and training of personnel. Benchmarking is reasonable as a starting point for CPI, as long as CPI is performed to fine tune an individual organization's processes to their own circumstances. As a quality "end-in-itself", benchmarking is an abject failure in terms of TQM. As W. Edwards Deming (18) said, "[there is no] instant pudding."

Offering the Excuse "Our Problems Are Different!"

Each organization has unique environmental circumstances and personnel capabilities. However, this does not mean that the problems faced by an organization, the goals it aspires to achieve, or the customers that it serves are unique. Many of the basic principles and philosophies to be applied to successful CPI apply to all organizations regardless of their circumstances. Other principles and philosophies simply require minor modifications to be applicable. It is a mistake to assume that a professional TQM consultant cannot assist and facilitate your organization toward a TQ transformation, simply because they are outsiders and do not appreciate all of your specific individual circumstances.

Reliance on Quality-Control Departments

Quality belongs in the hands of management, supervisors, and production workers. Adding another layer of bureaucracy that is separate from these individuals, to handle quality improvement, completely misses the point. The striving toward quality needs to be part of whatever process is necessary for organizational survival, not external to it. Quality needs to be internalized into every worker within the process, not regulated or mandated from outside.

Blaming the Work Force for Problems

It has been estimated that workers within a production process are accountable for about 15% of problems with process outcomes. The other 85% of problems arise as a result of problems with the process itself (8). Workers work within the system, but management creates the system. System problems are the responsibility of management and not the workers.

Quality by Inspection

Inspections are too late, unreliable, and ineffective. Managers that rely on inspection to guarantee quality will never improve quality. The focus must shift to process improvement (PI).

False Starts

Beginning and publicizing a move toward TQM without the commitment of leadership, time, and resources are the most common types of false start. Starting informal management participation groups for workers or informal "quality circles" provides short-term employee comfort that something is being done, but it contributes to long-term employee disillusionment and is usually an attempt by management to temporarily rid themselves of the problems of people. TQ efforts can only thrive if management is committed to acting on the recommendations of quality improvement teams.

The "Unmanned Computer"

Starting databases and collecting process-measurement data are useful and important. However, these steps are only useful if the data are distributed to process workers in real time, so that processes can be stabilized and improved as a result of data feedback. Collecting data that are never analyzed or used, or analyzed and distributed too late to be of any use, is a waste of time and resources.

Meeting Specifications

Meeting specifications are the currently accepted way of doing business in the United States. Quality is assumed in the absence of complaints or obvious defects. As a result, comparisons can only be made on the basis of cost and timeliness. A process that produces outputs within specification limits can still be improved by continually reducing output variation within these limits. The result is further improvements in quality and lower costs.

Inadequate Testing of Prototypes

PDCA cycles should be performed on a small-scale, trial basis before general adoption of the tested changes. Sometimes, changes that seem reasonable and promising do not empirically turn out to be advantageous in real-world application. An organization needs to know this before wasting time, energy, and other resources on a large process change that will lead to disillusionment among process workers and process owners.

The Assumption That "Anyone Who Comes to Try to Help Us Must Understand All About Our Business"

W. Edward Deming said "It is possible to know everything about a business except how to improve it" (18) and "Help toward improvement can only come from some other type of knowledge" (5). As neurosurgeons, if we already knew everything there was to know about neurosur-

gery, we would not have needed a neurosurgery residency training program. If we knew everything there was to know about CPI, we would not need outside professional consultants. We need to be willing to solicit, and be open to, the recommendations of outside expert consultants.

CONCLUSION

Instituting a TQM transformation within a neurosurgical organization is not be easy; however, nothing worthwhile ever is easy. I hope that this monograph provides the necessary background, explanation, and resources to start you on your road to TQM. It is a beginning, but it is not sufficient. Individual training through outside expert consultants, as well as further individual study, is necessary. Ultimately, the presence or absence of skilled and dedicated leadership determines whether the effort succeeds or fails. The rewards of success are virtually limitless.

REFERENCES

1. Bingham J: The magic valley experience in health care quality improvement, in Goldfield N, Pine M, Pine J (eds): *Measuring and Managing Health Care Quality.* Gaithersburg, MD, Aspen Publishers, 1993, 531–535.
2. Blumenthal D: Total quality management and clinicians clinical decisions. *JAMA* 269:2775–2778, 1993.
3. Byham WC, Cox J: Zappl: The lightening of empowerment. New York, Harmony Books, 1988.
4. Covey SR: The seven habits of highly effective people: Powerful lessons in personal change. New York, Simon and Schuster, 1989.
5. Deming WE: Out of the crisis. Cambridge, MA, Massachusetts Institute of Technology, Center for Advanced Engineering Studies, 1986.
6. Department of the Navy: Fundamentals of total quality leadership, Publication No. CIN P-500-0012. Washington, D.C. Department of the Navy, Total Quality Leadership Office, November 1992.
7. Department of the Navy: Total quality leadership glossary, Publication No. 94–01. Washington, D.C. Department of the Navy, Total Quality Leadership Office, March 1994.
8. Guinane CS, Sikes JI, Wilson RK: Using the PDSA cycle to standardize a quality assurance program in a quality improvement-driven environment. *Jt Comm J Qual Improv* 20:696–705, 1994.
9. Hallum A, Schiff L: Quality comes to life: Stories in obstetrics. *Qual Manage Health Care* [special issue] 49: 1993, December.
10. James BC: Quality management for healthcare delivery. Chicago, Hospital Research and Educational Trust, 1989.
11. Kibbe DC, Bentz E, McLaughlin CP: Continuous quality improvement for continuity of care. *J Fam Pract* 36:304–308, 1993.

12. Knowles MS, Malcom S: The adult learner: A neglected species. Houston, Gulf Publishing Co., 1984, 3rd ed.
13. Knowles MS, Malcom S, eds: Handbook of adult education in the United States. Washington, Adult Education Association of the U.S.A., 1960.
14. Knowles MS, Malcom S: The modern practice of adult education: Andragogy versus pedagogy. New York, Associated Press, 1970.
15. Knowles MS, Malcom S: Using learning contracts: Approaches to individualizing and structuring learning. San Francisco, Jossey-Bass Publishers, 1986.
16. McEachern JE, Makens PK, Buchanan ED, Schiff L: Quality improvement: An imperative for medical care. *J Occup Med* 33:364–373, 1991.
17. Pachciarz JA, Abbott MI, Gorman B, Henneman CE, Kuhl M. Continuous quality improvement of Pap smears in an ambulatory care facility. *Qual Rev Bull* 18:229–235, 1992.
18. Walton M: The Deming management method. New York, Putnam Publishing Group, 1986.
19. Zimmerman MR, Weston CB: Quality comes to life: Stories in obstetrics. *Qual Manage Health Care* [special issue] 49: 1993.

BIBLIOGRAPHY

GENERAL QUALITY BIBLIOGRAPHY

1. Ackoff R: Creating the corporate future: Plan or be planned for. New York, Wiley, 1981.
2. Aguayo R: Dr. Deming: The American who taught the Japanese about quality. New York, Lyle Stuart, 1990.
3. Albrecht K, Zemke R: Service America! Doing business in the new economy. Homewood, IL, Dow Jones-Irwin, 1985.
4. Akoa Y, ed: Quality function deployment: Integrating customer requirements into product design. Cambridge, MA, Productivity Press, 1990.
5. Amsden RT, Butler HE, Amsden DM: SPC simplified: Practical steps to quality. White Plains, NY, Quality Resources, 1989.
6. Argyris C: Integrating the individual and the organization. New York, John Wiley & Sons, 1964.
7. Asaka T, Ozeki K, eds: Handbook of quality tools: The Japanese approach (lesson 6). Cambridge, MA, Productivity Press, 1990.
8. Askey JM, Dale BC: From ISO 9000 series registration to total quality management: An examination. *Qual Management J* 1(4):67–76, 1994.
9. Atkinson JW: An introduction to motivation. Princeton, NJ, Van Nostrand, 1964. Reprinted in Kohn A: No contest: The case against competition. Boston, Houghton Mifflin, 1986.
10. AT&T Quality Steering Committee: Process quality management & improvement guidelines, Issue 1.1 Indianapolis, IN, AT&T Quality Steering Committee, 1988.
11. AT&T: Statistical quality control handbook. Indianapolis, IN, AT&T, 1956.
12. Barker J: Discovering the future: The business of paradigms. Tape, 38 minutes, stock No. 0120-LF-020-8900. Joel Barker, Films Inc., 1-800-323-4222, extension 44.
13. Barker JA: Paradigms: The business of discovering the future. New York, NY, Harper Business of Harper Collins Publishers, 1992.
14. Bennis W: The planning of change. New York, Holt, Rhinehart, and Winston, 1976, 3rd ed.
15. Bennis W, Nanus B: Leaders: The strategies for taking charge. San Francisco, Harper-Row, 1985.
16. Bowditch JL, Buono AF: A primer on organizational behavior. New York, Wiley, 1990.
17. Brache AP, Rummler GA: The three levels of quality. *Quality Progress* 21:46–51, 1988.
18. Brassard, M: The memory jogger plus +. Methuen, MA, GOAL/QPC, 1989.
19. Burchill G, Brodie CB: Voices into choices: Acting on the voice of the customer. Madison, WI, Oriel Incorporated, 1997.
20. Byham WC, Cox J: Zappl: The lightening of empowerment. New York, Harmony Books, 1988.
21. Caldwell C: Mentoring: The evolving role of senior leaders in a TQM environment. *Qual Management Health Care* 1:13–21, 1993.
22. Cannie JK: Keeping customers for life. New York, AMACOM, 1991.
23. Collins JC, Porras JI: Built to last: Successful habits of visionary companies. New York, Harper Business, 1994.
24. Collins JC, Porras JI: Building your company's vision. *Harvard Business Review* 74:65–77, 1996.
25. Conway WE: Leadership—The catalyst for continuous improvement [newsletter]. Conway Quality, Inc. 1:1–2, 1991.
26. Corrigan JP. Is ISO 9000 the path to TQM? *Qual Prog* 27(May):33–36, 1994.
27. Covey SR: The seven habits of highly effective people: Powerful lessons in personal change. New York, Simon and Schuster, 1989.
28. Covey SR. Principle-centered leadership. New York, Simon and Schuster, 1991.
29. Covey SR, Gulledge K: Total quality leadership. Provo, UT, Covey Leadership Center, Inc., 1993.
30. Covey SR, Gulledge K: Seven habits and Deming's 14 points. Provo, UT, Covey Leadership Center, Inc., 1993.
31. Cowles M: Statistics in psychology: An historical perspective. Hillsdale, NJ, Lawrence Earlbaum Associates, 1989.
32. Crawford-Mason C, Dobyns L: The Deming library [videotapes, volumes I–XX]. Washington, CC-M Productions, 1989, 1990, and 1991.
33. Creech W: The five pillars of TQM. New York, Truman Talley Books, 1994.
34. Crosby PB: The art of getting your own sweet way. New York, McGraw-Hill, 1972.
35. Crosby PB: The eternally successful organization. New York, McGraw-Hill, 1988.
36. Crosby PB: Leading. New York, McGraw-Hill, 1990.
37. Crosby PB: Let's talk quality. New York, McGraw-Hill, 1989.
38. Crosby PB: Quality is free. New York, McGraw-Hill, 1979.
39. Crosby PB: Quality Process Improvement Management College [course materials]. San Jose, CA, Philip Crosby Associates, Inc., 1987.
40. Crosby PB: Quality without tears: The art of hassle-free management. New York, McGraw-Hill, 1984.
41. Crosby PB: Running things: The art of making things happen. New York, McGraw-Hill, 1986.
42. Delbecq AL, Van de Ven AH: A group process model

for identification and program planning. *J Appl Beh Sci* 7:466–492, 1971.

43. Delbecq AL, Van de Ven AH, Gustafson DH. Group techniques for program planning, a guide to nominal group technique and Delphi processes. Scott Foreman, 1975.

44. Deming WE: The new economics for industry, government, education. Cambridge, MA, Massachusetts Institute of Technology Press, 1993.

45. Deming WE: Out of the crisis. Cambridge, MA, Massachusetts Institute of Technology, Center for Advanced Engineering Studies, 1986.

46. Deming WE: Quality, productivity and competitive position. Cambridge, MA, Massachusetts Institute of Technology, Center for Advanced Engineering Studies, 1982.

47. Deming WE: Sample design in business research. New York, John Wiley, 1961.

48. Deming WE: Statistical adjustment of data. New York, John Wiley, 1943 and 1964.

49. Deming WE: Theory of sampling. New York, John Wiley, 1950.

50. Department of the Navy: Fundamentals of total quality leadership. Publication No. CIN P-500-0012. Washington, D.C. Department of the Navy, Total Quality Leadership Office, November 1992.

51. Department of the Navy: Introduction to total quality leadership. Washington, D.C. Total Quality Leadership Office, November 1992.

52. Department of the Navy: Methods of managing quality. Washington, D.C. Total Quality Leadership Office, December 1996.

53. Department of the Navy: Systems approach to process improvement, (Publication No. CIN P-500-0004), Washington, D.C. Total Quality Leadership Office, February 1997.

54. Department of the Navy: Team skills and concepts. (Publication No. CIN P-500-0014). Washington, D.C. Total Quality Leadership Office, October 1995.

55. Department of the Navy: Total quality leadership glossary. Publication No. 94–01. Washington, D.C. Department of the Navy, Total Quality Leadership Office, March 1994.

56. Deutsch M: The resolution of conflict. New Haven, CT, Yale University Press, 1973.

57. Donnell A, Dellinger M: Analyzing business process data: The looking glass. AT&T Bell Laboratories Technical Publications Center, 1990.

58. Drucker P: The practice of management. New York, Harper and Row, 1954.

59. Duncan AJ: Quality control and industrial statistics. Homewood, II, Irwin, 1986.

60. Ernst & Young Quality Improvement Consulting Group, Huge EC, ed: Total quality: An executive's guide for the 1990s. Homewood, IL, Richard D. Irwin, Inc., 1990.

61. Finn L, Kramer T, Reynard S: Design of experiments: Shifting quality improvement into high gear. Madison, WI, Joiner Associates, Inc., 1987.

62. Fisher R, Ury W: Getting to yes. Boston, MA, Houghton-Mifflin Co., 1991.

63. Fuller FT: Eliminating complexity from work: Improving productivity by enhancing quality. *National Productivity Review* Autumn:327–344, 1985.

64. Gabarro JJ, Kotter JP: Managing your boss. *Harvard Bus Rev* May–June: 150–157, 1993.

65. Gabor A: The man who discovered quality. New York, Times Books, 1990.

66. Garvin DA: What does "product quality" really mean? *Sloan Management Rev* 26:25–43, 1984.

67. Garvin DA, March A: A note on quality: The views of Deming, Juran, and Crosby. Boston, MA, Harvard Business School, 1986.

68. Gibson JL, Ivancevich JM, Donnelly JH Jr: Organizations: Behavior, structure, processes. Dallas, TX, Business Publications, 1976.

69. Gitlow HS: Planning for quality, productivity, and competitive position (lesson 6). Homewood, II, Richard D. Irwin, Inc., 1990.

70. Gitlow H, Gitlow S: The Deming guide to quality and competitive position. Englewood Cliffs, NJ, Prentice-Hall, 1987.

71. Gitlow HS, Gitlow S, Oppenheim A, Oppenheim R: Tools and methods for the improvement of quality. Homewood, IL, Richard D. Irwin, Inc., 1989.

72. Glass GV, Stanley JC: Statistical methods in education and psychology. Englewood Cliffs, NJ, Prentice-Hall, 1970.

73. GOAL/QPC: The memory jogger: A pocket guide of tools for continuous improvement. Methuen, MA, GOAL/QPC, 1988.

74. GOAL/QPC Research Committee: 1990 Research report: Total quality management master plan. An implementation strategy. Methuen, MA, Goal/QPC, 1990.

75. GOAL/QPC Research Committee: 1991 Research report: Benchmarking. Methuen, MA, GOAL/QPC, 1991.

76. Goldratt EM, Cox J: The goal. Croton-on-Hudson, NY, North River Press, 1986.

77. Gordon JR: A diagnostic approach to organizational behavior. Boston, MA, Allyn and Bacon, Inc., 1987.

78. Gordon T: Leader effectiveness training: L.E.T. New York, Bantam Books, 1977.

79. Gunter B: A perspective on the Taguchi methods. *Qual Prog* 20:44–52, 1987.

80. Hamel G, Prahalad CK: Competing for the future. *Harvard Bus Rev* 72:122–128, 1994.

81. Hammer M, Champy J: Reengineering the corporation: A manifesto for business revolution. New York, Harper Collins, 1993.

82. Hersey P, Blanchard KH: Management of organizational behavior: Utilizing human resources. Englewood Cliffs, NJ, Prentice-Hall, 1988.

83. Hosotani K: Japanese quality concepts: An overview. White Plains, NY, Quality Resources, 1992.

84. Hunter WG: Mapping our way to economic success: Two untapped resources. Report No. 4. Madison, WI, Center for Quality and Productivity Improvement, 1986.

85. Huyink DS, Westover C: ISO 9000: Motivating the people, mastering the process, achieving registration! Burr Ridge, II, Irwin Professional Publishing, 1994.

86. Imai M: Kaizen: The key to Japan's competitive success. New York, Random House, 1986.

87. Ishikawa K: Guide to quality concepts. White Plains, NY, Quality Resources, 1991.

88. Ishikawa K: Guide to quality control. White Plains, NY, UNIPUB-Kraus International, 1982.

89. Ishikawa K, Lu D: What is total quality control? Englewood Cliffs, NJ, Prentice-Hall, 1985.

90. Joiner B: Total quality leadership versus management

by result. Madison, WI, Joiner Associates, Inc., 1985.

91. Joiner BL: Fourth generation management. New York, McGraw-Hill, Inc., 1994.

92. Joiner BL: The key role of statisticians in the transformation of North American industry. *Amer Stat* 39: 224–227, 1985.

93. Joiner B, Scholtes P: The quality manager's new job. *Qual Prog* 52–56, October 1988.

94. Juran JM: Bureaucracy: A challenge to better management. Harper and Brothers, 1944.

95. Juran JM: Management of inspection and quality control. Harper and Brothers, 1945.

96. Juran JM: Case studies in industrial management. New York, McGraw-Hill, 1955.

97. Juran JM: Managerial breakthrough. New York, McGraw-Hill, 1964.

98. Juran JM: Management of quality [course materials]. Wilton, CT: Juran Institute, Inc., 1981.

99. Juran JM: The quality trilogy: A universal approach to managing for quality. *Qual Prog* 19:19–24, 1986.

100. Juran JM: Juran on planning for quality. New York, Free Press, 1988.

101. Juran JM, Gryna FM (eds): Quality control handbook. New York, McGraw-Hill, 1988, ed 4.

102. Juran JM: Juran on leadership for quality: An executive handbook. New York: The Free Press, 1989.

103. Kano N, Seraku N, Takahashi F, Tsuji S: Attractive quality and must be quality. *Quality* 14(2):39–48, 1984.

104. Kanter RM: The change masters. New York, Simon & Schuster, 1983.

105. Kaplan RS, Norton DP: The balanced scorecard—Measures that drive performance. *Harv Bus Rev*: 71–79, January–February 1992.

106. Kaplan RS, Norton DP: Putting the balanced scorecard to work. *Harv Bus Rev*: 134–137, September–October 1993.

107. Katner RM: The change masters. New York, Simon and Schuster, 1983.

108. Katzenbach JR, Smith DK: The wisdom of teams: Creating the high-performance organization. Boston, Harvard Business School Press, 1993.

109. Kauffman DL Jr: Systems one: An introduction to systems thinking. Minneapolis, Future Systems, Inc., 1980.

110. Keirsey D, Bates M: Please understand me: Character and temperament types. Del Mar, CA, Prometheus Nemesis Book Company, 1984.

111. Kepner CH, Benjamin BT: The new rational manager. Princeton, NJ, Princeton Research Press, 1981.

112. Kepner CH, Benjamin BT: The rational manager. New York, McGraw-Hill, 1965.

113. Kilian CS: The world of W. Edwards Deming. Knoxville, TN, SPC Press, 1990.

114. King R: Better designs in half the time. Methuen, MA, GOAL/QPC, 1987.

115. Knowles MS, Malcom S: The adult learner: A neglected species. Houston, Gulf Publishing, Co., 1984, ed 3.

116. Knowles MS, Malcom S (eds): Handbook of adult education in the United States. Washington, DC, Adult Education Association of the U.S.A., 1960.

117. Knowles MS, Malcom S: The modern practice of adult education: Andragogy versus pedagogy. New York, Associated Press, 1970.

118. Knowles MS, Malcom S: Using learning contracts: Approaches to individualizing and structuring learning. San Francisco, Jossey-Bass Publishers, 1986.

119. Kohn A: No contest: The case against competition. Boston, Houghton Mifflin, 1986.

120. Koontz H, O'Donnell C: Principles of management: An analysis of managerial functions. New York, McGraw-Hill, 1972.

121. Kotter JP: What leaders really do. *Harv Bus Rev* 103–110, May–June 1990.

122. Kroeger O, Thuesen J: Type talk. New York, Dell Publishing, 1988.

123. Kroeger O, Thuesen J: Type talk at work. New York, Dell Publishing, 1992.

124. Kume H. Statistical methods for quality improvement. White Plains, NY, UNIPUB-Kraus International, 1985.

125. Latzko W: Quality and productivity for bankers and financial managers. Milwaukee, American Society for Quality Control, 1986.

126. Lele MM, Sheth JN: The customer is key. New York, John Wiley & Sons, 1991.

127. Likert R: New patterns of management. New York, McGraw-Hill, 1961.

128. Lipnack J, Stamps J: Virtual teams. New York, John Wiley & Sons, 1997.

129. Lippincott S: Meetings: Do's, don'ts and donuts. Pittsburgh, Lightouse Point Press, 1993.

130. Logan FA: Fundamentals of learning and motivation. Dubuque, IA, William C. Brown, 1970.

131. Lowe TA, McBean GM: Honesty without fear. *Qual Prog* 22:30–34, 1989.

132. Lowe TA, Mazzeo JM: Three preachers, one religion. *Quality* 25:22–25, 1986.

133. Mann, N: Keys to excellence: The story of the Deming philosophy. Santa Monica, CA, Prestwick Books, 1985.

134. Markova D. The art of the possible. Conari Press, 1991.

135. Maslow AH: Motivation and personality. New York, Harper and Row, 1954.

136. Mawhinney TC: Total quality management and organizational behavior management: An integration for continual improvement. *J Appl Beh Anal* 1992.

137. Mayo E: The social problems of an industrial civilization. Andover, MA: Andover Press, 1945.

138. McConnell J: Analysis and control of variation. Dee Why, Australia, Delaware Books, 1987.

139. McConnell J: Safer than a known way. Dee Why, Australia, Delaware Books, 1988.

140. McGregor D: The human side of enterprise. New York, McGraw-Hill, 1960.

141. Metz EJ: Managing change: Implementing productivity and quality improvements. *Nat Prod Rev* 3: 303–314, 1984.

142. Meyer C: How the right measures help teams excel. *Harv Bus Rev* 95–103, May–June 1994.

143. Miller GL, LaRue LK: The whats, whys, and hows of quality improvement. Milwaukee, ASQC Quality Press, 1992.

144. Miller LM, Howard J: Managing quality through teams. Atlanta, The Miller Consulting Group, 1991.

145. Mizuno S, (ed). Management for quality improvement: The seven new OC tools. Cambridge, MA, Productivity Press, 1988.

146. Moen RD, Nolan TW: Process improvement: A step-

by-step approach to analyzing and improving a process. *Qual Prog* 20:62–68, 1987.

147. Moen RD, Nolan TW, Provost LP: Improving quality through planned experimentation. New York, McGraw-Hill, 1991.

148. Moosbruker J: Developing a productive team: Making groups at work. Team building: Blueprints for productivity and satisfaction. Alexandria, VA, NTL Institute for Applied Behavioral Science, 1988.

149. Naisbitt J: Megatrends: Ten new directions transforming our lives. New York, Warner Books, 1982.

150. NBC, Producer. If Japan can . . . why can't we? New York, NBC White Paper, 1980 (2 videotapes, 80 minutes total).

151. Neave HR: The Deming dimension. Knoxville, TN, SPC Press, 1990.

152. Nolan TW, Provost LP: Understanding variation. *Qual Prog* 23:70–78, 1990.

153. Oriel Incorporated: Plain & simple learning and application guides. Madison, WI, Oriel Incorporated, 1995.

154. Oriel Incorporated: The team trail guide, (CD-ROM). Madison, WI, Oriel Incorporated, 1998.

155. Paton SM: Is TQM Dead? *Qual Dig* 14: (April), 1994.

156. Pearce JA II: Corporate mission statements: The bottom line. *Executive* 1:109–116, 1987.

157. Peters T: Thriving on chaos: Handbook for management revolution. New York, Harper & Row, 1987.

158. Peters TJ, Waterman RH Jr: In search of excellence: Modules from America's best run companies. New York, Harper & Row, 1982.

159. Plsek PE: Tutorial: Quality improvement project models. *Qual Manag Health Care* 1:69–81, 1993.

160. Pruitt D, Rubin J: Social conflict. New York, McGraw-Hill, 1993.

161. Reddy B: Intervention skills, process consultation for small groups and teams. San Diego, CA, Pfeiffer & Company, 1994.

162. Reilly L: Deming WE: A lesson learned from the master? *Washington Tech* 6:23, 1991.

163. Roberts W: Leadership secrets of Attila the Hun. New York, Warner Books, 1987.

164. Ross PJ: The role of Taguchi methods and design of experiments in QFD. *Qual Prog* 21:41–47, 1988.

165. Rummler GA, Brache AP: Managing the white space. *Training* 28:55–70, 1991.

166. Ryan KD, Oestreich DK: Driving out fear in the workplace. San Francisco, Jossey-Bass, 1991.

167. Satir V: Peoplemaking. Palo Alto, CA, Science and Behavior Books, Inc., 1972.

168. Schein EH: Organizational culture. *Amer Psych* 45: 109–119, 1990.

169. Schein E: Organizational culture and leadership. San Francisco, Jossey-Bass, 1985.

170. Scherkenbach WW: Deming's road to continual improvement. Knoxville, TN, SPC Press, 1991.

171. Scherkenbach WW: The Deming route to quality and productivity: Roadmaps and roadblocks. Rockville, MD, Mercury Press, 1987.

172. Scholtes PR: An elaboration on Deming's teachings on performance appraisal. Madison, WI, Joiner Associates, Inc., 1987.

173. Scholtes PR, Hacquebord H: Beginning the quality transformation, Part I. *Qual Prog* 21:28–33, 1988.

174. Scholtes PR, Hacquebord H: Six strategies for beginning the quality transformation, Part II. *Qual Prog* 21:44–48, 1988.

175. Scholtes PR, Joiner B, Braswell B, et al: The team handbook. Madison, WI: Joiner and Associates, 1988.

176. Scholtes P, Joiner B, Streibel B: The team handbook, second edition. Madison, WI, Oriel Incorporated, 1996.

177. Schultz LE: An introduction to the new management philosophy. Cambridge, MA, Center for Advanced Engineering Study, Massachusetts Institute of Technology, 1988.

178. Schwartz RM: The skilled facilitator. San Francisco, Jossey-Bass, 1994.

179. Shafritz JM: Dictionary of personnel management and labor relations. Oak Park, IL, Moore, 1980.

180. Shewhart WA: Economic control of quality of manufactured product. New York, Van Nostrand, 1932.

181. Shewhart WA: Statistical method from the viewpoint of quality. Washington, DC, U.S. Department of Agriculture, 1939.

182. Shingo, S: Zero quality control: Source inspection and the Poka-Yoke system. Stamford, CT, Productivity Press, 1986.

183. Sink DS, Tuttle TC: Planning and measurement in your organization of the future. Norcross, GA, Industrial Engineering and Management Press, 1989.

184. Snee R: In pursuit of total quality. *Qual Prog* 19: 25–31, 1986.

185. Stone D, Patton B, Heen S: Difficult conversations: How to discuss what matters most. New York, NY, Viking, 1999.

186. Suarez JG: Managing fear in the workplace. (Publication No. 93-01). Washington, D.C. Department of the Navy, Total Quality Leadership Office, January 1993.

187. Suarez JG: Three experts on quality management: Philip B. Crosby, W. Edwards Deming, Joseph M. Duran (Publication No. 92-02). Washington, D.C. Department of the Navy, Total Quality Leadership Office, July 1992.

188. Sullivan LP: Quality function deployment. *Qual Prog* 16:1983.

189. Sullivan LP: The seven stages in company-wide quality control. *Qual Prog* 19:77–83, 1986.

190. Tague NR: The quality toolbox. Milwaukee, ASQC Quality Press, 1995.

191. Satir V: Making contact. Millbrae, CA, Celestial Arts, 1976.

192. Tichy NM, Devanna MA: The transformational leader. New York, Wiley, 1986.

193. Tjosvold D, Johnson D: Productive conflict management. Coon Rapids, MN, Team Media, 1989.

194. Townsend P: Commit to quality. New York, Wiley & Sons, 1986.

195. Tribus M: The application of quality management principles in industrial research and development. From selected papers on quality and productivity improvement. Washington, DC, American Quality and Productivity Institute, 1988.

196. Tribus M: Deming's redefinition of management. From selected papers on quality and productivity improvement. Washington, DC, American Quality and Productivity Institute, 1988.

197. Tribus M: Deming's way. From selected papers on

quality and productivity improvement. Washington, DC, American Quality and Productivity Institute, 1988.

198. Tribus M: Reducing Deming's 14 points to practice. From selected papers on quality and productivity improvement. Washington, DC, American Quality and Productivity Institute, 1988.

199. Tribus M, Tsuda Y: Creating the quality company. Cambridge, MA, Center for Advanced Engineering Study, Massachusetts Institute of Technology, 1983.

200. Tuckman BW: Development sequence in small groups. *Psychol Bull* 63–93, 1965.

201. Tuckman BW, Jensen MAC: Stages of small group development revisited. *Group Org Studies* 2:1977.

202. Walton M: Deming management at work. New York, G. P. Putnam's Sons, 1990.

203. Walton M: The Deming management method. New York, Dodd Mead, 1986.

204. Wanous JP, Reicheri AE, Malik SD: Organizational socialization and group development: Toward an integrative perspective. *Acad Manag Rev* 9:1984.

205. Wheeler DJ: Charts done right (Manuscript no. 56). Knoxville, TN, Statistical Process Controls, Inc., 1991.

206. Wheeler DJ: Shewhart's charts: Myths, facts, and competitors. Milwaukee, WI, ASQC Quality Progress Congress Transactions, 1991.

207. Wheeler DJ: Understanding variation: The key to managing chaos. Knoxville, TN, SPC Press, Inc., 1993.

208. Wheeler DJ, Chambers DS: Advanced topics in statistical process control. Knoxville, TN, SPC Press, 1995.

209. Wheeler DJ, Chambers DS: Understanding statistical process control. Knoxville, TN, SPC Press, 1992.

210. Wilson L, Edmondson A: Deming's elusive eighth point: Why you can never drive fear out of the organization and what to do about it. Minneapolis, St. Paul, Pecos River Learning Centers, 1991.

211. Wyble L: ISO 9000 and TQM: Partners in quality. *Circ Assem* 84:1994.

212. Zeithhaml VA, Parasuraman A, Berry LL: Delivering quality service. New York, The Free Press, 1990.

HEALTH CARE QUALITY BIBLIOGRAPHY

1. Abbott WM: The operations improvement program at Massachusetts General Hospital: A paradigm for change. *J Vasc Surg* 28:381–383, 1998.

2. Agency for Health Care Policy and Research: Using clinical practice guidelines to evaluate quality of care: Volume 2: Methods. Rockville, MD, U.S. Department of Health and Human Services, 1995.

3. Al-Assaf AF, Schmele JA: Textbook of total quality in healthcare. Elray Beach, I, Dlucie Press, 1993.

4. American Medical Association: Clinical process and outcomes measurement directory. Chicago, American Medical Association, 1999.

5. Anderson C, Laubscher S, Burns R: Validation of the short form 36 (SF-36) health survey questionnaire among stroke patients. *Stroke* 27:1812–1816, 1996.

6. Arvantes JC: Using TQM to forge customer-driven strategic planning. *Qual Letter Health Care Leaders* 5:2–12, 1993.

7. Ashton CM, Kuykendall DH, Johnson ML, et al: A method of developing and weighting explicit process of care criteria for quality assessment. *Med Care* 32:755–770, 1994.

8. Babakus E, Mangold WG: Adapting the SERVQUAL scale to the health care environment, in Bloom P, et al (eds): *Enhancing Knowledge development in marketing*. Chicago, American Marketing Association, 1989.

9. Babakus E, Mangold WG: Adapting the SERVQUAL scale to hospital services: An empirical investigation. *Health Serv Res* 26:767–786, 1992.

10. Baker JG, Granger CV, Ottenbacher KJ: Validity of a brief outpatient functional assessment measure. *Amer Physic Med Rehabil* 75:356–363, 1999.

11. Batalden PB, Mohr JJ, Nelson EC, Plume SK: Improving health care, part 4: Concepts for improving any clinical process. *Joint Comm J Qual Improv* 22: 651–659, 1996.

12. Batalden PB, Nolan TW: Knowledge for the leadership of continual improvement in healthcare, in Taylor RJ (ed):: *Manual of Health Services Management*. Gaithersburg, MD, Aspen Publishers, 1993.

13. Batalden PB, Stoltz PK: A framework for the continual improvement of healthcare: Building and applying professional and improvement knowledge to test changes in daily work. *Joint Comm J Qual Improv* 19:424–447, 1993.

14. Bernstein S, Hilborne LE: Clinical indicators: The road to quality care? *Joint Comm J Qual Improv* 19: 501–509, 1993.

15. Berwick DM: Continuous quality improvement as an ideal in health care. *N Engl J Med* 320:53–56, 1989. [see comments].

16. Berwick DM: Peer review and quality management: Are they compatible? *Qual Rev Bull* 16:246–251, 1990.

17. Berwick DM: Controlling variation in health care: A consultation from Walter Shewhart. *Med Care* 29: 1212–1215, 1991.

18. Berwick DM: The double edge of knowledge. *JAMA* 266:841–842, 1991.

19. Berwick DM: Seeking systemness. *Health Care Forum J* 35:22–28, 1992.

20. Berwick DM: The clinical process and the quality process. *Qual Man Health Care* 1:1–8, 1992.

21. Berwick DM: Quality of health care: Part 5. Payment by capitation and the quality of care. *N Engl J Med* 335:1227–1231, 1996. [Comments and discussion. *N Engl J Med* 1997;336:805–807].

22. Berwick DM, Enthoven A, Bunker JP: Quality management in the NHS, II: The doctor's role. *Br Med J* 304:304–308, 1992.

23. Berwick DM, Godfrey AB, Roessner J: Curing health care: New strategies for quality improvement. San Francisco, Jossey-Bassey, 1991.

24. Berwick DM, Howard HH: Who pays. *N Engl J Med* 321:541–542, 1989.

25. Berwick DM, Nolan TW: Physicians as leaders in improving health care: A new series in *Annals of Internal Medicine*. *Ann Intern Med* 128:289–292, 1998.

26. Bingham J: The magic valley experience in health care quality improvement, in Goldfield N, Pine M, Pine J (eds): *Measuring and Managing Health Care Quality*. Gaithersburg, MD, Aspen Publishers, 1993, 531–535.

27. Blumenthal D: Total quality management and clinicians clinical decisions. *JAMA* 269:2775–2778, 1993.

28. Blumenthal D: Part I: Quality of care—What is it? *N Engl J Med* 335:891–894, 1996. [Comments and discussion. N Engl J Med 1996;335:891–894].

29. Blumenthal D: Quality of health care: Part 4: The origins of the quality-of-care debate. *N Engl J Med* 335:1146–1149, 1996. [Comments and discussion N Engl J Med 1997;336:804–806].

30. Blumenthal D: The future of quality measurement and management in a transforming healthcare system. *JAMA* 278:1622–1625, 1997.

31. Blumental D, Epstein AM: Quality of health care: Part 6. The role of physicians in the future of quality management. *N Engl J Med* 335:1328–1331, 1996. [Comments & discussion N Engl J Med 1996;336:805–806].

32. Blumenthal D, Kilo CM: A report card on continuous quality improvement. *Milbank Q* 76:625–648, 1998.

33. Bolster CJ: Quality research initiatives. *Top Health Care Financ* 18:7–11, 1991.

34. Bowers MR, Swan JE, Koehler WF: What attributes determine quality and satisfaction with health care delivery. *Health Care Manage Rev* 19:49–55, 1994.

35. Brook RH: Quality of care: Do we care? *Ann Int Med* 115:486–490, 1991.

36. Brook RH: Health care reform is on the way. Do we want to compete on quality? *Ann Intern Med* 120: 84–86, 1994.

37. Brook RH, Appel FA: Quality of care assessment: Choosing a method for peer review. *N Engl J Med* 288:1323–1329, 1973.

38. Brook RH, Chassin MR, Fink A, et al: A method for the detailed assessment of the appropriateness of medical technologies. *Int J Technol Assess* 2:53–63, 1986.

39. Brook RH, Davies-Avery A, Greenfield A, et al: Assessing the quality of medical care using outcome measures: An overview of the method. *Med Care* 15(suppl):1–165, 1977.

40. Brook RH, McGlynn EA, Cleary PD: Quality of health care: Part 2. Measuring quality of care. *N Engl J Med* 335:966–970, 1996. [Comments and discussion. N Engl J Med 1997;336:804–807].

41. Brothers TE, Robison JG, Elliot BM: Relevance of quality improvement methods to surgical practice: Prospective assessment of carotid endarterectomy. *Amer Surgeon* 63:213–219, 1997.

42. Brott T, Adams HP, Olinger CP, et al: Measurements of acute cerebral infarction: A clinical examination scale. *Stroke* 20:864–870, 1989.

43. Caldwell C: What healthcare can learn from TQM's past. *Health Care Exec* 8:26–28, 1993.

44. Carey RG, Lloyd RC: Measuring quality improvement in healthcare: A guide to statistical process control applications. New York, Quality Resources (a division of the Kraus Organization Ltd.), 1995.

45. Carey RG, Seibert JH: A patient survey system to measure quality improvement: Questionnaire reliability and validity. *Med Care* 9:834–845, 1993.

46. Chassin MR: Assessing strategies for quality improvement. *Health Aff* 16:151–161, 1997.

47. Chassin MR: Quality of health care: Part 3. Improving the quality of care. *N Engl J Med* 335:1060–1063, 1996.

48. Chassin MR, Hannan EL, DeBuono BA: Benefits and hazards of reporting medical outcomes publicly [Letter]. *N Engl J Med* 334:394–398, 1996.

49. Ciccone KR, Lord JT: IQA-2: Continuous performance improvement through integrated quality assessment. Chicago, American Hospital Publishing, Inc., 1989.

50. Claery PD, McNeil BJ: Patient satisfaction as an indicator of quality of care. *Inquiry* 25:25–36, 1988.

51. Cohen E, Anderson-Miles E. Benchmarking: A management tool for academic medical centers. *Best Prac Benchmarking Health Care* 1:57–61, 1996.

52. Cook DJ, Mulrow CD, Haynes RB: Systematic reviews: Synthesis of best evidence for clinical decisions. *Ann Intern Med* 126:376–380, 1997.

53. Corrigan JD, Smith-Knapp K, Granger CV: Validity of the functional independence measure for persons with traumatic brain injury. *Arch Phys Med Rehabil* 78:828–834, 1997.

54. Dans P, Weiner J, Ottr S: Peer review organizations: Promises and potential pitfalls. *N Engl J Med* 313: 1131–1137, 1985.

55. Demos MP: What every physician should know about the National Practitioner Data Bank. *Arch Intern Med* 151:1708–1711, 1991.

56. Deyo RA, Battie M, Beurskens AJHM, et al: Outcome measures for low back pain research. *Spine* 23: 2003–2013, 1998.

57. Donabedian A: Evaluating the quality of medical care. *Milbank Mem Fund Q* 44:166–206, 1966.

58. Donabedian A: The definition of quality and approaches to its assessment. Ann Arbor, MI, Health Administration Press, 1980.

59. Donabedian A: Criteria, norms and standards of quality: What do they mean? *Am J Pub Health Admin Med* 71:409–412, 1981.

60. Donabedian A: The criteria and standards of quality. Ann Arbor, MI, Health Administration Press, 1982.

61. Donabedian A: The methods and findings of quality assessment and monitoring: An illustrated analysis. Ann Arbor, MI, Health Administration Press, 1985.

62. Donabedian A: Quality assessment and assurance: Unity of purpose, diversity of means. *Inquiry* 25: 173–192, 1988.

63. Dorman P, Slattery J, Farrell B, Dennis M, Sandercock P: Qualitative comparison of the reliability of health status assessments with the EuroQol and SF-36 questionnaires after stroke. *Stroke* 29:63–68, 1998.

64. Dorman P, Waddell F, Slattery J, Dennis M: Is the EuroQOL a valid measure of health-related quality of life after stroke? *Stroke* 28:1876–1882, 1997.

65. Durbin S, Haglund C, Dowling W: Integrating strategic planning and quality management in a multi-institutional system. *Qual Management Health Care* 1: 24–34, 1993.

66. Eddy DM: Performance measurement: Problems and solutions. *Health Aff* 17(4):7–25, 1998.

67. Edgman-Levitan S, Gerteis M: Measures of quality: What can public reporting accomplish? *Health Care For J* 41:27, 36–37, 61, 1998.

68. Ellrodt AG: Introduction of total quality management (TQM) into an internal medicine residency. *Acad Med* 68:817–823, 1993.

69. Ellwood P: Shattuck lecture—Outcomes management. A technology of patient experience. *N Engl J Med* 318:1549–1556, 1998.

70. Epstein A: Performance reports on quality—Proto-

types, problems, and prospects. *N Engl J Med* 333: 57–61, 1995.

71. Fairbank JC, Couper J, Davis JP, O'Brien JP: The Oswestry low back pain disability questionnaire. *Physiotherapy* 66:271–273, 1980.

72. Feeny DH, Torrance GW: Incorporating utility based quality of life assessment measures in clinical trials. *Med Care* 27(suppl 3):S190–S204, 1989.

73. Fischer LR, Solberg LI, Kottke TE: Quality improvement in primary care clinics. *Joint Comm J Qual Improv* 24:361–370, 1998.

74. Flexner A: Medical education in the United States and Canada: Report to the Carnegie Foundation for Advancement of Teaching. New York, Merry-Mount Press, 1910.

75. Gagel BJ: Health care quality improvement program: A new approach. *Health Care Financ Rev* 16:15–23, 1995.

76. General Accounting Office: Report cards: A useful concept but significant issues need to be addressed. Washington, DC, U.S. Government Printing Office, 1994.

77. Gerard JC, Arnold FL: Performance improvement with a hybrid FOCUS-PDCA methodology. *Joint Comm J Qual Improv* 22:660–672, 1996.

78. Gerszten PC: Outcomes research: A review. *Neurosurg* 43:1146–1155, 1998.

79. Gift RG, Kinney CF: Overcoming barriers to benchmarking in healthcare organizations. *Best Prac Benchmarking Health Care* 1:3–9, 1996.

80. Goldberg HI, Wagner EH, Fihn SD, et al: A randomized controlled trial of CQI teams and academic detailing: Can they alter compliance with guidelines? *Joint Comm J Qual Improv* 24:130–142, 1998.

81. Goldman EF, Nolan KC: Strategic planning in health care: A guide for board members. Chicago, American Hospital Publishing, 1994.

82. Goldstone J: The role of quality assurance versus continuous quality improvement. *J Vasc Surg* 28: 378–380, 1998.

83. Gosfield AG: Who is holding whom accountable for quality? *Health Affairs* 16(3):26–40, 1997.

84. Granger CV, Cotter AC, Hamilton BB, Fiedler RC, Hens MM: Functional assessment scales: A study of persons with multiple sclerosis. *Arch Phys Med Rehabil* 71:870–875, 1990.

85. Greenough CG, Fraser RD: Assessment of outcome in patients with low-back pain. *Spine* 17:36–41, 1992.

86. Grevitt MP, Khazim R, Webb J, Mulholland RC, Shepperd J: The short form-36 health survey questionnaire in spine surgery. *J Bone Joint Surg* 79(B): 48–52, 1997.

87. Guinane CS, Sikes JI, Wilson RK: Using the PDSA cycle to standardize a quality assurance program in a quality improvement-driven environment. *Joint Comm J Qual Improv* 20:696–705, 1994.

88. Hallum A, Schiff L: Quality comes to life: Stories in obstetrics. *Qual Manage Health Care* (special December issue) 49, 1993.

89. Hannan EL, Kilburn H Jr, Racz M, Shields E, Chassin MR: Improving the outcomes of coronary artery bypass surgery in New York state. *JAMA* 271: 761–766, 1994.

90. Haslok I: Quality of care and patient satisfaction. *Br J Rheumatol* 35:382–384, 1996.

91. Headrick LA, Neuhauser D: Quality health care. *JAMA* 271:1711–1712, 1994.

92. Hibbard JH, Jewett JJ: Will quality report cards help consumers? *Health Aff* 16:218–228, 1997.

93. Hobson JP, Meara RJ: Is the SF-36 health survey questionnaire suitable as a self-report measure of the health status of older adults with Parkinson's disease? *Qual Life Res* 6:213–216, 1997.

94. Horak BJ: Strategic planning in healthcare: Building a quality-based plan step by step. New York, Quality Resources, 1997.

95. Horowitz CR, Goldberg HI, Martin DP, et al: Conducting a randomized controlled trial of CQI and academic detailing to implement clinical guidelines. *Joint Comm J Qual Improv* 22:734–750, 1996.

96. Hungate RW: Whither quality? *Health Aff* 15: 111–113, 1996.

97. Iezzoni LI: Risk adjustment for medical outcome studies, in Grady ML (ed): *Medical Effectiveness Research Data Methods* Publication no. 92-0056. Rockville, MD, Agency for Health Care Policy and Research. 83–87.

98. Iezzoni LI: Risk adjustment for measuring health care outcomes. Chicago, Health Administration Press, 1997, ed 2.

99. Iezzoni LI: Using administrative diagnostic data to assess the quality of health care. *Int J Tech Assess Health Care* 6:272–281, 1990.

100. Iglehart JK: Competition and the pursuit of quality: A conversation with Walter McClure. *Health Aff (Millwood)* 7:79–90, 1988.

101. Isenberg, SF: Surviving and thriving as an independent practitioner: The search for continuous quality improvement: Managed care, outcomes and quality. A practical guide. New York, Thieme, 1997.

102. Isenberg SF, Davis C, Keaton S: Project Solo: An independent practitioners initiative for confidential self-assessment of quality. *Amer J Med Qual* 11: 214–221, 1996.

103. Isenberg SF, Gliklich RE, Reinhardt U, Cheng MTM: Profiting from quality: Outcomes strategies for medical practice. San Francisco, Jossey-Bass, 1999.

104. Isenberg SF, Rosenfeld R: Problems and pitfalls in community-based outcomes research. *Otolaryn Head Neck Surg* 116:662–665, 1997.

105. Isenberg SF, Stewart M: Utilizing patient satisfaction surveys to assess quality improvement in community-based medical practices. *Amer J Med Qual* 12: 188–194, 1998.

106. Institute of Medicine: Clinical practice guidelines: Directions for a new program, in Field MJ, Lohr KN (eds): *Committee to Advise the Public Health Service on Clinical Practice Guidelines.* Washington DC, National Academy Press, 1990.

107. James BC: Quality management for healthcare delivery. Chicago, Hospital Research and Educational Trust, 1989.

108. David MJ, Hadar EJ: Long-term follow-up review of patients who underwent laminectomy for lumbar stenosis: a prospective study. *J Neurosurg* 89:1–7, 1998.

109. Jencks SF: Measuring quality of care under Medicare and Medicaid. *Health Care Finance Rev* 16:39–54, 1995.

110. Jencks SF, Wilensky G: The health care quality im-

provement initiative—A new approach to quality assurance in Medicare. *JAMA* 268:900–903, 1992.

111. Jenkinson C, Layte R, Jenkinson D, et al: A shorter form health survey: Can the SF-12 replicate results from the SF-36 in longitudinal studies? *J Publ Health* 19:179–186, 1997.

112. Jenkinson C, Peto V, Fitzpatrick R, Greenhall R, Hyman N: Self-reported functioning and well being in patients with Parkinson's disease: Comparison of the short-form health survey (SF-36) and the Parkinson's disease questionnaire (PDQ-39). *Age Aging* 24:505–509, 1995.

113. Joint Commission on Accreditation of Health Care Organizations: A compendium of forms, tables, and charts for use in monitoring and evaluation. Oakbrook Terrace, IL, Joint Commission on Accreditation of Health Care Organizations, 1991.

114. Joint Commission on Accreditation of Health Care Organizations: Development and application of indicators for continuous improvement in surgical and anesthesia care. Oakbrook Terrace, IL, Joint Commission on Accreditation of Health Care Organizations, 1991.

115. Joint Commission on Accreditation of Health Care Organizations: Exploring quality improvement principles: A hospital leader's guide. Oakbrook Terrace, IL, Joint Commission on Accreditation of Health Care Organizations, 1993.

116. Joint Commission on Accreditation of Health Care Organizations: Implementing quality improvement: A hospital leader's guide. Oakbrook Terrace, IL, Joint Commission on Accreditation of Health Care, Organizations, 1993.

117. Joint Commission on Accreditation of Health Care Organizations: 1999 Hospital accreditation standards. Oakbrook Terrace, IL, Joint Commission on Accreditation of Health Care Organizations, 1999.

118. Joint Commission on Accreditation of Health Care Organizations: Striving towards improvement: Six hospitals in search of quality. Oakbrook, Terrace, IL, Joint Commission on Accreditation of Health Care Organizations, 1992.

119. Joint Commission on Accreditation of Health Care Organizations: Using quality improvement tools in a health care setting. Oakbrook Terrace, IL, Joint Commission on Accreditation of Health Care Organizations, 1992.

120. Kassirer JP: The quality of care and the quality of measuring it. *N Engl J Med* 329:1263–1265, 1993.

121. Kassirer JP: The use and abuse of practice profiles. *N Engl J Med* 330:634–636, 1994.

122. Kenagy JW, Berwick DM, Shore MF: Service quality in health care. *JAMA* 281:661–665, 1999.

123. Kennedy MP: Implementation of quality improvement methodology and the medical profession. *J Qual Clin Prac* 18:143–150, 1998.

124. Kibbe DC, Bentz E, McLaughlin CP: Continuous quality improvement for continuity of care. *J Fam Pract* 36:304–308, 1993.

125. Kilo CM, Kabcenell A, Berwick DM: Beyond survival: Toward continuous improvement in medical care. *New Horizons* 6:3–11, 1998.

126. Koss RG, Turpin RS, Schmaltz S, Sprenger S, McMahill CN: Assessing obstetric care performance measures in healthcare organizations. *New Med* 1:113–119, 1997.

127. Kritchevsky SB, Simmons BP: Continuous quality improvement. Concepts and applications for physician care. *JAMA* 266:1817–1823, 1991.

128. Kuperman G, James B, Jacobsen J, Gardner RM: Continuous quality improvement applied to medical care: Experiences at LDS hospital. *Med Decision Making* 11 (suppl 4):S60–65, 1991.

129. L'Abbe KA, Detsky AS, O'Rourke K: Meta-analysis in clinical research. *Ann Int Med* 107:224–233, 1987.

130. Laiben GR: Putting quality improvement into (your) practice. *Missouri Med* 94:73–75, 1997.

131. Laiben GR: Putting quality improvement into (your) practice: Part two. *Missouri Med* 94:177–179, 1997.

132. Laiben GR: Putting quality improvement into (your) practice. Part three. *Missouri Med* 94:228–230, 1997.

133. Laffel G, Berwick DM: Quality in health care. *JAMA* 268:407–409, 1992.

134. Laffel G, Blumenthal D: The case for using industrial quality management science in healthcare organizations. *JAMA* 262:2869–2873, 1989.

135. Langfitt JT: Comparison of the psychometric characteristics of three quality of life measures in intractable epilepsy. *Qual Life Res* 4:101–114, 1995.

136. Langlais RJ: Recognizing organizational impediments to the total quality management process. *Best Practices & Benchmarking in Health Care* 1:16–20, 1996.

137. Lansky D: The new responsibility: Measuring and reporting on quality. *Joint Comm J Qual Improv* 19:545–551, 1993.

138. Leape LL: Error in medicine. *JAMA* 272:1851–1857, 1994.

139. Leebov W: The quality quest: A briefing for healthcare professionals. Chicago, American Hospital Publishing, Inc., 1991.

140. Lembcke P: Evolution of the medical audit. *JAMA* 199:111–118, 1967.

141. Loeb JM, Nadzam DM: Performance measurement and accreditation, in Seltzer J, Nash D (ed): *Models For Measuring Quality in Managed Care: Analysis and Impact.* New York, Faulkner and Gray, Inc., 1997, 79–99.

142. Lohr, KN: How do we measure quality? *Health Aff* 16(3):22–25, 1997.

143. Lohr KN (ed): Medicare: A strategy for quality assurance, vol. 1. Washington, DC, Washington National Academy Press, 1990.

144. Lohr K (ed): Quality assurance for medicare. Washington, DC, National Academy of Science, 1990.

145. Lohr K, Schroeder S: A strategy for quality assurance in Medicare. *N Engl J Med* 322:707–712, 1990.

146. Longo DR, Daugird AJ: Measuring the quality of care: Reforming the health care system. *Am J Med Qual* 9:104–115, 1994.

147. Longo DR, Land G, Schramm W, et al: Consumer reports in health care: Do they make a difference? *JAMA* 278:1579–1584, 1997.

148. Luce JM, Bindman AB, Lee PR: A brief history of health care quality assessment and improvement in the United States. *West J Med* 160:263–268, 1994.

149. Marszalek-Gaucher E, Coffey RJ: Transforming

healthcare organizations: How to achieve and sustain organizational excellence. San Francisco, Jossey-Bass, 1990.

150. Mayer-Oakes SA, Barnes C: Developing indicators for the Medicare Quality Indicator System (MQIS): Challenges and lessons learned. *J Qual Improv* 23: 381–390, 1997.

151. McEachern JE, Makens PK, Buchanan ED, Schiff L. Quality improvement: An imperative for medical care. *J Occup Med* 33:364–373, 1991.

152. McGlynn EA: Six challenges in measuring the quality of health care. *Health Aff* 16(3):7–25, 1997.

153. McHorney CA, Ware JE, Rogers W, et al. The validity and relative precision of MOS short- and long-form health status scales and Dartmouth COOP charts: Results from the medical outcomes study. *Med Care* 30:MS253–MS265, 1992.

154. Merry MD: Physician leadership for the 21st century. *Qual Management Health Care* 1:31–41, 1993.

155. Merry MD: Total quality management for physicians: Translating the new paradigm. *Qual Rev Bull* 16: 101–105, 1990.

156. Messner K: Barriers to implementing a quality improvement program. *Nurs Management* 29:32–35, 1998.

157. Mohr JJ, Mahoney CC, Nelson EC, Batalden PB, Plume SK. Improving health care, Part 3: Clinical benchmarking for best patient care. *Joint Comm J Qual Improv* 22:599–616, 1996.

158. Mullan F, Politzer RM, Lewis CT, et al: The National Practitioner Data Bank: Report from the first year. *JAMA* 268:73–79, 1992.

159. Nadzam DM, Turpin R, Hanold LS, White RE: Data-driven performance improvement in healthcare: The Joint Commission's Indicator Measurement System (IMSystem). *J Qual Improv* 19:492–500, 1993.

160. National Committee for Quality Assurance: A roadmap for information systems: Evolving systems to support performance measurement, HEDIS 3.0/ 1998, vol. 4 Washington, DC, National Committee for Quality Assurance, 1997.

161. Nelson CW: Patient satisfaction surveys: An opportunity for total quality improvement. *Hosp Health Serv Admin* 35:409–427, 1990.

162. Nelson EC, Batalden PB, Plume SK, Miheve NT, Swartz WG: Report cards or instrument panels: Who needs what? *Joint Comm J Qual Improv* 21: 155–166, 1995.

163. Nelson EC, Batalden PB, Plume SK, Mohr JJ: Improving health care, Part 2: A clinical improvement worksheet and users' manual. *Joint Comm J Qual Improv* 22:531–548, 1996.

164. Nelson EC, Berwick DM: The measurement of health status in clinical practice. *Med Care* 27:577–590, 1989.

165. Nelson EC, Mohr JJ, Batalden PB, Plume SK: Improving health care, Part 1: The clinical value compass. *Joint Comm J Qual Improv* 22:243–258, 1996.

166. Nelson EC, Splaine ME, Batalden PB, Plume SK: Building measurement and data collection into medical practice. *Ann Internal Med* 128:460–466, 1998.

167. Newman JA Jr: Lessons in quality from other industry experiences. *Top Health Care Financ* 18:1–6, 1991.

168. Nolan TW: Understanding medical systems. *Ann Intern Med* 128:293–298, 1998.

169. Office of Program Development, Agency for Health Care Policy and Research: Design of a survey to monitor consumers' access to care, use of health services health outcomes, and patient satisfaction. Washington, D.C., Office of Program Development, Agency for Health Care Policy and Research, Department of Health and Human Services, 1995.

170. O'Leary D: Moving healthcare toward CQI. The Joint Commission's plans for the future. *Qual Lett Health Leaders* 3:12–16, 1991.

171. O'Leary DS: Performance measures. How are they developed, validated, and used? *Med Care* 33: JS13–JS17, 1995.

172. Pachciarz JA, Abbott MI, Gorman B, Henneman CE, Kuhl M: Continuous quality improvement of Pap smears in an ambulatory care facility. *Qual Rev Bull* 18:229–235, 1992.

173. Palmer RH: Quality health care. *JAMA* 275: 1851–1852, 1996.

174. Palmer RH: Quality of care. *JAMA* 277:1896–1897, 1997.

175. Panzer RJ: Are hospital quality improvement and public accountability compatible? *Joint Comm J Qual Improv* 20:396–401, 1994.

176. Patrick DL, Deyo RA: Generic and disease-specific measures in assessing health status and quality of life. *Med Care* 27:217–232, 1989.

177. Paul JE, Weis KA, Epstein RA: Data bases for variations research. *Med Care* 31:96–102, 1993.

178. Perrine KR: A new quality-of-life inventory for epilepsy patients: Interim results. *Epilepsia* 34(4): S28–S33, 1993.

179. Peto V, Jenkinson C, Fitzpatrick R, Greenhall R: The development and validation of a short measure of functioning and well being for individuals with Parkinson's disease. *Qual Life Res* 4:241–248, 1995.

180. President's Advisory Commission on Consumer Protection and Quality in the Health Care Industry: Quality first: Better health care for all Americans. Final report to the President of the United States. Washington, DC, President's Advisory Commission on Consumer Protection and Quality in the Health Care Industry, March 1998.

181. Reinertsen JL: Physicians as leaders in the improvement of health care systems. *Ann Intern Med* 128: 833–838, 1998.

182. Relman AC: Assessment and accountability: The third revolution in medical care. *N Engl J Med* 319: 1220–1222, 1988.

183. Report Card Pilot Project: Key findings and lessons learned: 21 plans' performance profiles. Washington, DC, National Committee for Quality Assurance, 1995.

184. Roberts J, Coale J, Redman R: A history of the Joint Commission on Accreditation of Hospitals. *JAMA* 258:936–940, 1987.

185. Rubin HR: Can patients evaluate the quality of hospital care? *Med Care Rev* 47:265, 1990.

186. Rubin HR, Ware JE Jr, Nelson EC, Meterk M: The patient judgements of hospital quality (PJHQ) questionnaire in patient judgements of hospital quality: Report of a pilot study. *Med Care* 28(suppl): 517–522, 1990.

187. Rubin HR, Rogers WH, Kahn KL, Rubinstein LV, Brook RH: Watching the doctor watchers: How well

do peer review organization methods detect hospital care quality problems? *JAMA* 267:2349–2354, 1992.

188. Sampson E, Marthas M: Group process for the health professions. Albany, NY, Delmar Publishers, Inc., 1990.

189. Scheckler WE: Continuous quality improvement in a hospital system: Implications for hospital epidemiology. *Infect Control Hosp Epidemiol* 13:288–292, 1992.

190. Schneider EC, Epstein AM: Use of public performance reports. *JAMA* 279:1638–1642, 1998.

191. Schoenbaum S, Murrey K: Impact of profiles on medical practice. Conference on Profiling. Washington, DC, Agency for Health Care Policy and Research, 1992, 92–102.

192. Schwartz JS: Measuring quality: Where are we? Where are we going? And how will we know when we get there? *Ann NY Acad Sci* 729:150–158, 170–174, 1994.

193. Segal ME, Schnall RR: Determining functional/health status and its relation to disability in stroke survivors. *Stroke* 25:2391–2397, 1994.

194. Sellick JA Jr: The use of statistical process control charts in hospital epidemiology. *Infect Control Hosp Epidemiol* 14:649–656, 1993.

195. Shine KI: Quality of health and health care. *JAMA* 273:244–245, 1995.

196. Shortell SM, Bennett CL, Byck GR: Assessing the impact of continuous quality improvement on clinical practice: What it will take to accelerate progress. *Milbank Q* 76:593–624, 1998.

197. Shulkin DJ: Quality management in an academic integrated delivery system: The case of the University of Pennsylvania Health System. *Int J Qual Health Care* 9:171–176, 1997.

198. Simon JL: Basic research methods in social science. New York, Random House, 1969.

199. Smits H: The PSRO in perspective. *N Engl J Med* 305:253–259, 1981.

200. Sollis JG, Romano PS: Pennsylvania's focus on heart attack: Grading the scorecard. *N Engl J Med* 338:983–987, 1998.

201. Solodky C, Chen H, Jones PK, Katcher W, Neuhauser D: Patients as partners in clinical research: A proposal for applying quality improvement methods to patient care. *Med Care* 36(suppl):AS13–AS20, 1998.

202. Steiber SR, Krowinski WJ: Measuring and managing patient satisfaction. American Hospital Publishing, Inc., 1990.

203. Strasser S, Davis RM: Measuring patient satisfaction for improved patient services. Ann Harbor, MI, Health Administration Press, 1991.

204. Takahashi T: The paradox of Japan: What about CQI in healthcare? *Joint Comm J Qual Improv* 23:60–64, 1997.

205. Tarlov AR, Ware JE Jr., Greenfield S, et al: The medical outcomes study: An application of methods for monitoring the results of medical care. *JAMA* 262:925–930, 1989.

206. Tilley BC, Lyden PD, Brott TG, et al: Total quality improvement for reduction of delays between emergency department admission and treatment of acute ischemic stroke. The National Institute of Neurological Disorders and Stroke rt-PA Stroke Study Group. *Arch Neurol* 54:1466–1474, 1997.

207. Topol EJ, Califf RM: Scorecard cardiovascular medicine: Its impact and future directions. *Ann Intern Med* 120:65–70, 1994.

208. Tunick PA, Etkins S, Horrocks A, et al: Re-engineering a cardiovascular service. *Joint Comm J Qual Improv* 23:203–216, 1997.

209. Vickrey BG, Hays RD, Graber J, et al: A health-related quality of life instrument for patients evaluated for epilepsy surgery. *Med Care* 30:299–319, 1992.

210. Wagner AK, Ehrenberg BL, Tran TA, et al: Patient-based health status measurement in clinical practice: A study of its impact on epilepsy patients' care. *Qual Life Res* 6:329–341, 1997.

211. Wagner AK, Keller SD, Kosinski M, et al: Advances in methods for assessing the impact of epilepsy and antiepileptic drug therapy on patients' health-related quality of life. *Qual Life Res* 4:115–134, 1995.

212. Ware JE Jr, Kosinski M, Keller SD: A 12-item short-form health survey: Construction of scales and preliminary tests of reliability and validity. *Med Care* 34:220–233, 1996.

213. Ware JE Jr, Sherbourne CD: The MOS 36-item short-form health survey (SF-36). *Med Care* 30:473–483, 1992.

214. Ware JE Jr, Sherbourne CD: The MOS 36-item short-form health survey (SF-36) I. Conceptual framework and item selection. *Med Care* 30:473–483, 1992.

215. Ware JE, Snyder MK, Wright WR: Development and validation of scales to measure patient satisfaction with health care services: Volume 1. Final report. Part A: Review of the literature, overview of methods, and results of construction of scales. Carbondale, Il, Southern Illinois University School of Medicine, 1976.

216. Weed LW: Knowledge coupling: New premises and tools for medical care and education. New York, Springer-Verlag, 1991.

217. Weiner BJ, Shortell SM, Alexander J: Promoting clinical involvement in hospital quality improvement efforts: The effects of top management, board, and physician leadership. *Health Serv Res* 32:491–510, 1997.

218. Weingart SN: House officer education and organizational obstacles to quality improvement. *Joint Comm J Qual Improv* 22:640–646, 1996.

219. Weingart SN: A house officer-sponsored quality improvement initiative: Leadership lessons and liabilities. *Joint Comm J Qual Improv* 24:371–378, 1998.

220. Wilson A, McDonald P: Comparison of patient questionnaire, medical record, & audio tape in assessment of health promotion in general practice consultations. *Br Med J* 309:1483–1485, 1994.

221. Wyszewianski L, Kratochwill EW: Changing clinicians' behaviors in an academic medical center: Does institutional commitment to total quality management matter? *Am J Med Quality* 12:3–10, 1997.

222. Zimmerman MR, Weston CB: Quality comes to life: Stories in obstetrics. *Qual Manage Health Care* (special issue), 1993.

223. Zuckerman A: Health Care strategic planning: Approaches for the 21st century. Chicago, Health Administration Press, 1998.

PART II

Cost in Neurological Surgery

CHAPTER 15

Cost Effectiveness Analysis: Theory, Basis, and Methods

MICHAEL J. RUTIGLIANO, M.D., M.B.A.

Because of the rapid rise of health care costs over the past 25 years medical treatments and technologies are now evaluated with regard to both medical efficacy and economic efficiency. The United States spends more than $1 trillion dollars annually on health care for its citizens, which represents between 13–15% of its Gross Domestic Product (GDP). While one can argue whether this amount is too much or too little to spend, there is little debate that such an enormous expenditure must be spent as cost-effectively as possible. When this chapter was first published in Neurosurgery *in 1995 the neurosurgical literature was practically devoid of articles primarily concerned with the cost-effectiveness of treatment strategies. However, articles now exist addressing the cost-effectiveness of treatments of a wide range of neurosurgical conditions from cerebral metastasis, to arteriovenous malformation, to un-ruptured cerebral aneurysms, to name but a few. The increase of such data in our literature underscores the importance of understanding the theoretical basis and methods underlying cost-effectiveness analysis. As with any analytical method the results, conclusions, and implications of these studies can only be properly understood with a firm appreciation of the method employed to derive them.*

GENERAL CONSIDERATIONS

Cost-Effectiveness Analysis (CEA) measures the cost of medical technology per unit of some defined health output. By measuring both the cost and the effectiveness of a program, CEA is able to provide a means of comparison between technologies that are designed to produce similar end results. CEA can also be used to compare a treatment strategy with a baseline, such as observation alone, in a disease with a well-established natural history. For example, one could compare stereotactic radiosurgery with microsurgery for Grades 1 through 3 arteriovenous malformations and compare both with the disease's natural history. CEA is a popular methodology for policy makers, because it can be applied to a range of technologies and subjected to a budget constraint to generate a list of medical technologies that can be ranked in order of most to least cost effective. Theoretically, one would then fund programs in this order until all resources in the budget constraint are exhausted. It is imperative to understand that CEA is primarily concerned with the efficiency with which resources are used to obtain a given health care result and provides only a gross measure of value judgments regarding risks (manifested by complications) and patient preferences. For example, a CEA concerning microsurgery and stereotactic radiosurgery for arteriovenous malformations would not reflect a patient's individual preference for the immediate risk and benefit offered by microsurgical resection versus the delayed risk (of subsequent hemorrhage awaiting obliteration) and benefit of stereotactic radiosurgery. Unless an issue of concern can be expressed as an economic cost or manifest itself by changing the output measure (e.g., by reducing the quality of survival added), then the issue will go largely ignored in such an analysis.

CEA is designed to compare the economic efficiency of treatments for a particular disease. It is not designed to determine whether a treatment is "too expensive" or "a good buy," and no absolute level of cost effectiveness exists for any given treatment or program. The results of any CEA should be viewed as a part of a larger data set that includes all of the other variables of importance in allocating health resource.

The general form of CEA is shown in Equation 1.

$$\frac{(C_1 + C_2 + ..) - (S_1 + S_2 + ..)}{\text{Unit Effectiveness}} \quad (1)$$

C_n represent various costs, S_n represents various savings, and the denominator represents some defined effect of the procedure under evaluation. The denominator may be measured in life years added (usually adjusted for quality), disease-free years added, pain-free years added, or a similar quantifiable outcome often subject to some qualitative description. For example, years of life added may be adjusted for quality of life by developing an index for various disabilities such that years of normal health are multiplied by 1.0, years survived with a minor disability are multiplied by 0.8, years survived with a moderate disability are multiplied by 0.5, and so on. By using such a method, one arrives at a unit of effectiveness known as quality-adjusted life years (QALYs), a popular method of measuring survival in CEA. CEA is generally used to assess the efficiency of various health care technologies to produce a health output (effect) within the constraint of limited resources. This is to be contrasted with other analytical techniques used to assess various economic parameters of medical care, such as cost benefit analysis (CBA) and decision analysis.

CBA is similar to CEA in that it measures the cost of a given technology and compares it with the benefits derived. The general form of CBA is shown in Equation 2.

$$(C_1 + C_2 + ..) - (B_1 + B_2 + ..) \text{ or } C_n \div B_n \tag{2}$$

C_n represents costs, and B_n represents benefits derived. The major difference between CBA and CEA is that everything in the CBA equation is expressed in monetary terms. Health care outcomes are converted to monetary units by a variety of techniques (6, 11), most of which attempt to measure future wage levels or some indicator of the economic productivity of the patients being treated. Because of the obvious econometric difficulty with such measurements and the complete lack of consideration for nonmonetary aspects of human life, CBA has found little use in medical economics.

Decision analysis is a term that represents a broad range of methodologies designed to use computer models to aid in complex decision making (1, 8, 15, 24, 25). Such analyses will often be designed to determine dominant treatment strategies when one or more medically acceptable options exist for a particular disease. Factors such as complications, effectiveness rates, costs, and patient preferences can be assigned probabilities consistent with the known literature to drive various modeling programs. Decision analysis can be particularly helpful when many treatment options exist that have nearly equal efficacy but that carry with them different complications occurring at various rates (8). If costs are of concern, they can be used as a decision variable to help determine the dominant strategy or they can be applied to the analysis after a dominant strategy has been determined without prior consideration of cost.

MEASUREMENT OF COSTS

A firm understanding of the concept of cost definition and measurement is central to the correct interpretation of CEAs. Most economists define cost as the amount of resources consumed for a given purpose. Further, total cost must include a measure of benefits foregone by not using such resources for the next best alternative (opportunity cost). For the purposes of CEA, we must be able to place a monetary value on all costs in the analysis. Because the measurement of opportunity costs is highly subjective and open to value judgments, it is often not included in the analysis. However, the importance of this concept for resource allocation decisions should not be lost because eventually all allocations are subject to some budget constraint.

When considering cost determination for CEA, it is important to remember that health care charges (physician fees, hospital bills, drug prices) are not necessarily equated with costs (12, 14). Because the internal accounting systems of most health care providers (including physicians and hospitals) are designed to maximize reimbursement rather than define and recover costs of various services, the actual charge for a service often is not reflective of its true cost. Therefore, care must be exercised when interpreting CEAs that use actual hospital and physician charges to drive the cost determination.

The determination of cost also depends heavily on the point of view of the analysis (discussed below). For example, from the point of view of an entire society, cost is represented by the monetary value of the actual resources used; from a third-party payer's point of view, it is the amount of money paid out for health care; from a hospital's point of view, it is the monetary value of the actual resources used to provide care; and from a patient's point of view, it is often only the out-of-pocket expense for the care they receive. Given this, costs can generally be divided into direct health care costs, direct personal costs, direct non-health care costs, and indirect costs. Not all of these cost categories are used for every viewpoint.

The most important of the costs to be considered is the direct health care cost. This cost category is the one with which the physician usually has the most experience. This cost is a net amount that represents the costs, less any savings, of the treatment and its consequences. This category of cost is usually the dominant one in most CEAs and is often the only one considered. This is especially true when a national health system viewpoint is considered (discussed below). The general form of the direct cost is shown in Equation 3.

$$C_D = (C_{Rx} + C_{AdRx} + C_{Morb} + C_{RxLE}) \quad (3)$$
$$- (C_{SvRx} + C_{SvMorb})$$

C_D represents direct cost; C_{Rx} represents direct costs of the program/treatment; C_{AdRx} represents direct costs of additional treatment/studies based on results/information of first treatment/study; C_{SvRx} represents savings from avoiding additional treatment/studies based on results/information from first treatment/study; C_{Morb} represents direct costs of morbidity attributable to program; C_{SvMorb} represents savings of morbidity avoided because of program; and C_{RxLE} represents cost of additional health problems occurring in the years of life added by the program.

As can be seen from the equation above, the direct cost is a net amount that reflects the difference in resources expended ($C_{Rx} + C_{AdRx} + C_{Morb} + C_{RxLE}$) less savings generated by the technology under evaluation ($C_{SvRx} + C_{SvMorb}$). The direct cost (or savings) for each variable represents the cost of the equipment, supplies, personnel (including physician fees), and overhead attributable to that variable. For example, the total direct cost of a screening test for carotid occlusive vascular disease, such as duplex ultrasound, would include the costs directly attributable to the test itself (C_{Rx}), the costs of any additional tests (C_{AdRx}) that were indicated (e.g., angiography) as the result of information derived from the first test, the costs of treatment for morbidity directly related to the test or subsequent tests (C_{Morb}) done on the basis of the information of the first test, and the costs of additional health care required (C_{RxLE}) for other medical conditions a person might incur in the years of life expectancy added by the test. From this, one would subtract any savings in health care expenditures by avoiding further tests (C_{SvRx}) because of the information derived from the first test and the savings from morbidity averted (C_{SvMorb}) as the result of information from the test.

Although most of the variables discussed above seem to have a logical place in the calculation of total direct costs, some argue that the future medical costs of illnesses unrelated to the treatment or test addressed by the CEA should be excluded (2). They consider medical cost equivalent with other consumption costs that arise in years of added life expectancy, such as food, shelter, transportation, and so on. However, it can be countered that from the perspective of the health care system, future medical costs that arise out of increased life expectancy are relevant because they affect the total health care budget (18, 28, 29). Other costs of living would not directly affect this budget constraint and, thus, can be ignored. The difficulty of determining C_{RxLE} varies directly with the amount of survival added by the treatment in question. Therefore, it is much easier to determine C_{RxLE} for a procedure that adds a relatively small amount of life expectancy on average, such as surgery and/or radiation therapy for glioblastoma multiforme, than for a procedure on a newborn that may add a lifetime, such as the repair of a congenital heart defect.

The remaining costs are more difficult to measure and depend more on value assumptions than do direct medical costs. Direct personal costs represent such items as transportation to and from health care providers, home services required because of health concerns, cost of ancillary programs, such as fitness clubs, and so on. These costs take on importance in the analysis only when considered from the patient's point of view.

Direct non-health care costs are generally used when the broad societal point of view is considered in a CEA. These are the costs or savings that are not directly related to health services but that can be indirectly attributable, for example, reductions in property damage resulting from fewer alcohol-related accidents as the result of an educational program aimed at preventing alcohol abuse. Indirect costs and savings are more controversial. They represent the changes in the productive use of time, gains in productivity, and the opportunity costs of receiving health care for patients. Because these activities require strong value assumptions to place monetary amounts on them, one can make a strong argument for excluding them from the numerator in a CEA. By including them, characteristics of a CBA are introduced into the analysis (28). At any rate, the improved (or reduced) quality of life that many of these items affect should be represented in the denominator of the CEA equation as represented by QALYs. Because of this, indirect costs are usually excluded from monetary consideration in the numerator.

VIEWPOINT

The major determinant of cost and savings is the viewpoint of the analysis. As stated above, different segments of the health care system will be affected by costs and savings in very different manners and thus will recognize them in different ways. It is usually appropriate to use the point of view of the actual decision maker, but it can be helpful to carry out the analysis from many points of view. If similar conclusions are derived from many different viewpoints, then the conclusion of such a CEA would be more powerful, especially as it pertains to policy making. Most CEA studies in the medical literature will use a national health care system viewpoint. Other viewpoints are briefly described for the sake of completeness. All of the viewpoints have basic assumptions and constraints, described below.

Societal Viewpoint

The basic assumption underlying CEA from the societal point of view is that society wants to maximize the total health benefit aggregate within some given resource constraint and to minimize the cost of obtaining this goal. From the societal perspective, the resource constraint equals the GDP of that nation. Therefore, the cost of a program is equal to its net economic burden on the GDP. Economic costs (savings) to health care providers, government, individuals, employers, and producers of goods and services are all included, regardless of who bears the cost or enjoys the savings. An assumption that a highly centralized decision-making process for resource allocation exists or that noncentralized

decision makers (physicians, administrators, etc.) incorporate knowledge of societal cost effectiveness into their decision making is implicit from this viewpoint.

Once these conditions are met, a list of available medical technologies can be formulated that is ranked from the most to the least cost effective. Preference to the funding of these programs would be ordered, by rank, to obtain the most health output for the least amount of resources until the budget constraint is exhausted. Of course, programs that create both costs savings and health benefits would always be included, because they would only add to the resource pool available. Note two things when considering this point of view: 1) the use of a given technology is based only on its cost effectiveness today, which ignores any possible future contributions of the technology that might eventually result in more cost-effective methods, and 2) the costs in such an analysis are not monetary payouts but rather are the monetary value of the resources consumed to provide health care that are thus unavailable for other uses (opportunity costs), which, strictly speaking, may be items other than medical care.

National Health Care System Perspective (NHCS)

The NHCS perspective is the most often used for CEA and is probably the most useful for policy makers. The constraint in this analysis is the national health care budget or national health care expenditure target. The overall goal is to obtain maximal health care benefit within the resource constraint.

A major difference between the NHCS viewpoint and that of the broader society is that costs and savings not directly affecting the use of health care resources are not considered in the calculation of costs (i.e., the numerator) (28). Therefore, nonhealth direct and indirect costs (savings) are not included in the numerator because they do not directly affect the relevant budget constraint. As stated above, both variables give a measure of quality of life and, therefore, continue to be reflected in the denominator (QALYs). Indirect costs or savings may directly affect the budget when one considers that losses or gains in productivity can be reflected in taxable income that would contribute to the NHCS budget. However, it is difficult to measure this in the aggregate and the amount of tax revenue that goes to the NHCS budget is dependent on much more than increases and decreases in national productivity.

Third-party Payers

From the third-party payer perspective, costs are generally equal to the amount paid out for health care claims and savings are represented by payments that were avoided. Therefore, some procedures can have an infinite cost effectiveness to third-party payers simply because they do not offer payment for an effective procedure, and therefore, cost is shifted either to the patient or to society at large. The constraint for this viewpoint is not fixed, because premiums and payouts are greatly controlled by the third-party payer and can be adjusted to meet costs and provide profit.

Hospitals

Resource usage in a hospital setting should represent the cost of the resources used to provide a given service, including the appropriate allocation of the various fixed costs required for that service. Because most cost accounting systems in use in the hospital setting are designed to maximize reimbursement rather than account for accurate cost bases, this task is much more difficult than it may at first seem (12). Charges are based on the same premise and differ significantly from the true cost of the service plus some margin to provide for future expansion. The constraint under which a hospital operates is dependent on how the hospital views its primary objective (28). If the hospital believes that the delivery of health care is its primary objective, then revenues (including donations, payments, etc.) serve as the constraint. However, the hospital may view income as its primary objective (as an indicator of future growth) and the ability to deliver "quality" care as the constraint. Either way, the major difficulty lies in determining accurate cost bases for procedures in the hospital setting.

Patients

The cost to the patient is almost always the out-of-pocket expense of the procedure in question. In addition, direct non-health care costs take on an increasingly important role because the patient directly bears the burden of these costs, such as transportation, missed wages, and so on. The constraint from this viewpoint obviously varies widely because of great variations

in personal wealth, current and future income, and age. Further, because of the myriad of health insurance plans in the United States, the out-of-pocket expense for a given procedure varies widely.

DISCOUNTING

Once the viewpoint has been selected and the appropriate costs and outcome effectiveness have been determined, the results must be discounted to account for the effects of time. A common misperception is that discounting is used to account for inflation. Inflation is corrected for by adjusting all monetary values to a given base year, which is, by convention, 1987. Discounting, on the other hand, is used to reflect the fact that money (and benefits) held today is worth more, in absolute terms, than at any time in the future.

It is a widely held economic tenant that a dollar today is worth more than a dollar tomorrow or at any future time (time value of money). This is so not because of the erosive effects of inflation but rather because X dollars held today can be invested at some rate (r) to yield $X(1 + r)$ dollars tomorrow. More generally, X dollars today will be worth $X(1 + r)^1$ t years from now, assuming a constant rate. Therefore, X dollars received t years from now have a present value of $\$X/(1 + r)$, given a discount rate, r. Thus, future costs require discounting because money spent on care some time in the future is clearly worth less in terms of present value than if the same absolute amount was spent today.

Although discounting future benefits has been more controversial in the past, it now is standard practice (4, 5, 19, 28, 29). The rationale for this practice is multifactorial. First, effects need to be discounted because they are being compared with dollars that are discounted. Failure to do so greatly overstates the cost effectiveness of the program under question. The numerator declines as the result of discounting, and the denominator remains constant (at least in terms of base units). Second, it can be argued that from the patient's perspective, people are short term oriented. One would, in general, rather enjoy a year of good health now than a year of good health 10 years from now. Further, if one is forced to wait 10 years for the benefit of that year, one would demand more than a year to compensate him or her for the delayed benefit. Third, discounting

TABLE 15.2
Demonstration of Marginal Cost Effectiveness of Sequential Stool Guaiac Testing for the Detection of Colon Cancer[a]

No. of Tests	No. of Cases	Incremental Gain	Total Cost ($)	Incremental Cost ($)	Marginal Cost ($)	Average Cost ($)
1	65.9469	65.9469	77511	77511	1175	1175
2	71.4424	5.4956	107690	30179	5492	1507
3	71.9004	0.4580	130199	22509	49150	1810
4	71.9385	0.0382	148116	17917	469534	2059
5	71.9417	0.0032	163141	15024	4724695	2268
6	71.9420	0.0003	176331	13190	47107214	2451

[a] Calculations: 1. Incremental Gain = No. of Cases Detected $Test_{n+1}$ − No. of Cases Detected $Test_n$; 2. Incremental Cost = Total Cost $Test_{n+1}$ − Total Cost $Test_n$; 3. Marginal Cost = Incremental Cost/Incremental Gain; 4. Average Cost = Total Cost/No. of Cases. Discrepancies in calculations are the result of the authors' numerical rounding practices. Reprinted by permission of *The New England Journal of Medicine* (26).

comparing one strategy with the next most expensive or intensive option (9, 10, 19). This is done by measuring the differences between the net costs and effectiveness of two options in ratio form, as shown in Equation 4.

$$\frac{C_2 - C_1}{E_2 - E_1} \qquad (4)$$

This ratio provides a measure of extra cost per extra unit of outcome when comparing two different options. Incremental CEA seeks to answer the question, "If Option 2 is better than Option 1, then at what price?" This differs from marginal cost effectiveness, which determines the additional cost and effectiveness of one additional unit of service of the same option. As an example, consider a study that compared different screening strategies for left main coronary artery disease (19). The screening options consisted of observation alone, various thresholds of ST segment depression on exercise electrocardiography as an indication to proceed to coronary angiography, and angiography for all patients (not discussed for our purposes). Costs included the costs of screening, angiography, and coronary artery bypass surgery, and effects were measured in expected life years gained as a result of the surgery. *Table 15.3* illustrates the results of the analysis. Note the difference between the cost effectiveness ratios for the various screening options. There appears to be little difference between observation alone ($275/expected life years added) and the most aggressive criteria for proceeding to coronary angiography (1-mm ST depression on exercise electrocar-

diography) at $471/expected life years added. However, because more than one option is available to produce the same end result (expected life years added), the correct comparison is between the differential costs and effects of one screening option and the next most expensive strategy. When we do this, we see that using 1 mm of ST depression instead of the 2 mm criterion results in the addition of life expectancy at a cost of $196,250/QALY gained. The additional expected life years (0.004 yr) that would not be realized by use of the 2 mm criterion come at a cost of $196,250 each or 417 times the cost effectiveness of the 1 mm criterion when considered alone. To simplify the illustration of incremental CEA, discounting practices have been excluded from the above data. Correct discounting practices were used in the original study (19).

Incremental CEA is a critically important part of any CEA in which different treatments or programs are able to produce similar end results. With the emergence of several seemingly competing technologies in neurosurgery, incremental CEA may prove helpful, at least as an economic measure of the value added by a given procedure. Comparisons of stereotactic radiosurgery and microsurgery for a number of diseases, instrumentation and no instrumentation for fusion rates, and malignant glioma treatment strategies (fractionated radiotherapy + surgery ± chemotherapy, etc.) are but a few examples in which importance of the CEA will lie in the differential cost and effectiveness of different treatment strategies.

TABLE 15.3
Incremental Cost Effectiveness of Various Screening Strategies for Left Main Coronary Artery Disease[a]

Treatment Options	Life Expectancy (yr)	Cost per Patient ($)	Cost Effectiveness Ratio ($/yr)	Incremental Cost Effectiveness Ratio ($/yr)
1. Observe	14.862	4086	275	
2. 3-mm ST ⇓	15.133	5468	363	5100
3. 2-mm ST ⇓	15.214	6378	419	11235
4. 1-mm ST ⇓	15.218	7163	471	196250

[a] Example calculations:

1. $\text{Cost Effectiveness Ratio} = \dfrac{\text{Program 3 Cost}}{\text{Life Expectancy}} = \dfrac{\$6378}{15.214} = \$419/\text{quality-adjusted life year added};$

2. $\text{Incremental Cost Effectiveness Ratio} = \dfrac{(\text{Program 3 Cost} - \text{Program 2 Cost})}{(\text{Life Expectancy 3} - \text{Life Expectancy 2})} = \dfrac{(\$6378 - \$7163)}{(15.214 - 15.133)} = \$11,235/$ quality-adjusted life-years added by using 2-mm ST depression threshold for coronary angiography compared with 3-mm ST depression.

The above data ignore discounting practices to simplify the illustration of incremental cost effectiveness analysis. The original study used proper discounting practices (19).

SUMMARY

Medical practices are increasingly subjected to economic evaluations. CEA is a reasonable method, because it measures the cost per unit of health output without having to put a value on the health output in monetary terms. CEA is highly dependent on the viewpoint of the analysis, the method of cost determinations, and the assumptions and assigned probabilities that drive the analysis. All costs and benefits in the analysis must be subjected to the appropriate discounting procedures, and sensitivity analysis should always be included to test the robustness of the outcome. Marginal CEA examines the cost per unit of health output of one additional unit of the treatment under consideration. Incremental CEA is useful to compare the cost per unit output of treatments of different intensities or methods with the same general aim.

It is important to remember that CEA, by itself, does not determine whether a treatment or program is too costly. Cost effectiveness data are of little value when they stand alone. The usefulness of the analysis is derived from comparing competing treatments with each other or with a well-established baseline, such as the observation of a disease with a well-documented natural history. As neurosurgeons, we must consider the inclusion of methods designed to measure the costs and resource expenditures of procedures that we evaluate in clinical trials and prospective series. Given that there does exist a limit to what we can spend on health care and that many of the diseases we treat have more than one effective treatment option, the collection of accurate cost data becomes increasingly important to help assure the correct allocation of resources. However, it is equally important to remember that the cost effectiveness of any given treatment should be considered as only another datum point, understanding the limitations of the method, in any decision about health care policy.

REFERENCES

1. Auger RG, Wiebers DO: Management of unruptured intracranial arteriovenous malformations: A decision analysis. Neurosurgery 30:561–569, 1992.
2. Avorn J: Benefit and cost analysis in geriatric care: Turning age discrimination into health policy. N Engl J Med 310:1294–1301, 1984.
3. Beck JR, Kassirer JP, Pauker SG: A convenient approximation of life expectancy (the "DEALE"): I—Validation of the method. Am J Med 73:883–888, 1982.
4. Beck JR, Pauker SG, Gottlieb JE, Klein K, Kassirer JP: A convenient approximation of life expectancy (the "DEALE"): II—Use in medical decision making. Am J Med 73:889–897, 1982.
5. Bowie RD: Health economics: A framework for health service decision-making. N Z Med J 104:99–102, 1991.
6. Bulpitt CJ, Fletcher AE: Economic assessments in randomized controlled trials. Med J Aust 153[Suppl]: S16–S19, 1990.
7. Burner ST, Waldo DR, McKusick DR: National health expenditures projections through 2030. Health Care Financing Rev 14:1–29, 1992.
8. Disch DL, Greenberg ML, Holzberger PT, Malenka DJ,

Birkmeyer JD: Managing chronic atrial fibrillation: A Markov decision analysis comparing warfarin, quinidine, and low dose amiodarone. Ann Intern Med 120:449–457, 1994.

9. Eddy DM: *Screening for Cancer: Theory, Analysis, and Design.* Englewood Cliffs, Princeton-Hall, 1980.

10. Eisenberg JM: Clinical economics: A guide to the economic analysis of clinical practices. JAMA 262: 2879–2886, 1989.

11. Emery DD, Schneiderman LJ: Cost effectiveness analysis in health care. Hastings Center Rep July/August: 8–13, 1989.

12. Evans DB: Principles involved in costing. Med J Aust 153[Suppl]:S10–S12, 1990.

13. Evans DB: What is cost effectiveness? Med J Aust 153[Suppl]:S7–S9, 1990.

14. Finkler SA: The distinction between costs and charges. Ann Intern Med 96:102–109, 1982.

15. Fisher WS III: Decision analysis: A tool of the future—An application to unruptured arteriovenous malformations. Neurosurgery 24:129–134, 1989.

16. Hudgins WR: Patients' attitude about outcomes and the role of gamma knife radiosurgery in the treatment of vestibular schwannomas. Neurosurgery 34:459–465, 1994.

17. Hurley S: A review of cost effectiveness analysis. Med J Aust 153[Suppl]:S20–S23, 1990.

18. Keeler EB, Cretin S: Discounting of life-saving and other nonmonetary effects. Management Sci 29: 300–306, 1983.

19. Lee TH, Fukui T, Weinstein MC, Tostenson ANA, Goldman L: Cost effectiveness of screening strategies for left main coronary artery disease in patients with stable angina. Med Decis Making 8:268–278, 1988.

20. Letsch SW, Lazenby HC, Levit KR, Cowan CA: National health expenditures, 1991. Health Care Financing Rev 14:1–30, 1992.

21. Martens L, van Doorslaer E: Dealing with discounting: An application to the cost effectiveness of intracoronary thrombolysis with streptokinase. Int J Tech Assess Health Care 6:139–145, 1990.

22. McCallum JE, Turbeville D: Cost and outcome in a series of shunted premature infants with intraventricular hemorrhage. Pediatr Neurosurg 20:63–67, 1994.

23. McNeil BJ, Varady PD, Burrows BA, Adelstein SJ: Measures of clinical efficacy: Cost-effectiveness calculations in the diagnosis and treatment of hypertensive renovascular disease. N Engl J Med 293: 216–221, 1975.

24. Michaels JA, Galland RB: Management of asymptomatic popliteal aneurysms: The use of a Markov decision tree to determine the criteria for a conservative approach. Eur J Vasc Surg 7:136–143, 1993.

25. Munro AJ, Warde PR: The use of a Markov process to simulate and assess follow-up policies for patients with malignant disease: Surveillance for stage I nonseminomatous tumors of the testes. Med Decis Making 11:131–139, 1991.

26. Neuhauser D, Lewicki AM: What do we gain from the sixth stool guaiac? N Engl J Med 293:226–229, 1975.

27. Penar PL, Wilson JT: Cost and survival analysis of metastatic cerebral tumors treated by resection and radiation. Neurosurgery 34:888–894, 1994.

28. Weinstein MC: Principles of cost-effective resource allocation in health care organizations. Int J Tech Assess Health Care 6:93–103, 1990.

29. Weinstein MC, Stason WB: Foundations of cost effectiveness analysis for health and medical practices. N Engl J Med 296:716–721, 1977.

The Socioeconomic Implications of Neurosurgical Diseases

PETER C. GERSZTEN, M.D., M.P.H.

As a result of the rising costs of health care during the 1970s and 1980s, great emphasis has been placed on controlling health care costs. From a societal perspective, this emphasis impacts a diverse range of concerns, from the effects on global economic competitiveness to the determination of the amount of resources that should be reasonably dedicated to health care. To begin to understand the impact of neurosurgery on health care expenditure, one first has to determine the socioeconomic impact of the common diseases that we treat as a specialty. In this chapter, I provide the reader with a survey of common neurosurgical diseases and an estimation of their socioeconomic impact. The paucity of specific data regarding expenditures, outcomes analysis, and cost-effectiveness data relating to these diseases and their treatments highlights the necessity for future work in this area.

Over the past decade, an increasing focus has been placed on socioeconomic issues related to neurosurgery. In his 1994 presidential address to the American Association of Neurological Surgeons, Julian T. Hoff, M.D., described how the organization was originally supported by the three roles of research, teaching, and patient care. However, over time, socioeconomic issues have formed a fourth "leg" on which organized neurosurgery is founded. He stated that neurosurgery "needs to have a comprehensive socioeconomic base to establish goals and objectives that are consistent with its other more traditional activities including science, education, and patient care" (11).

This chapter addresses the socioeconomic implications of neurosurgical diseases. A variety of neurosurgical diseases are surveyed and information is presented regarding the socioeco-nomic impact of disease management and treatment. Data about incidence, prevalence, and expenditures are included. To understand the socioeconomic implications of the specialty of neurosurgery, it is first essential to understand the place of neurosurgical disease processes as part of the health care arena (19).

During the 20th century, communicable rather than noncommunicable diseases became predominant health problems. Evidence has grown that people's behavior largely determines the time and disease mechanisms of death. The Public Health Service has estimated that half of the premature deaths in the Unites States are due to the choices that people make in their everyday activities (41). *Table 16.1* shows that 46% of all deaths per year in the United States are attributed to self-induced behavior that is based on lifestyle choices (28). Almost 40% of deaths are attributable to tobacco, diet, and activity patterns, or alcohol alone. It is important to put such numbers into context when examining the implications of neurosurgical disease processes on the overall health of the population. Neurosurgical diseases have a relatively insignificant impact on the overall medical as well as economic health of society in relation to these other conditions.

The major costs to society of neurosurgical disease processes are due to the economic devastation produced by the disease state rather than the direct costs of diagnosis and treatment. Although there has been an explosion in medical technology for the management of neurosurgical problems, these costs pale when compared with the medical or nonsurgical costs associated with the management of patients with neurosurgical

TABLE 16.1
Actual Causes of Death in the United States

Cause of Death	Estimated Number of Deaths	% of Total Deaths
Tobacco	400,000	19
Diet/activity patterns	300,000	14
Alcohol	100,000	5
Toxic agents	60,000	3
Firearms	35,000	2
Sexual behavior	30,000	1
Motor vehicles	25,000	1
Illicit use of drugs	20,000	1
Total	970,000	46

disorders (44). The latter costs include the costs of medical treatment and the costs associated with disablement, which has three components: impairment, disability, and handicap. Any discussion of the impact of neurosurgery on health care must include an explanation these terms. Both the medical costs as well as the indirect costs of care are far greater than the direct surgical costs for the majority of neurosurgical diseases. Unfortunately, data regarding these costs are also much more difficult to obtain.

Impairment refers to any loss or abnormality of psychological, physiological, or anatomical structure or function and occurs at the organ level (50). The major costs for this component are engendered during acute care and in rehabilitation settings (44). *Disability* occurs at the level of the person and relates to the loss of personal activity or function as a result of the impairment (50). The major costs for this component are found in rehabilitation and in early attempts to reintegrate the patient into the community (50). The last component of disablement, *handicap*, involves the ability of the patient to function in the community and to achieve economic self-sufficiency. The costs here are associated with the loss of economic potential produced by the injury and the accommodations society must make for the individual's disablement (44).

Another dimension of the socioeconomic implications of neurosurgical disease processes is understanding different types of costs (32). The direct medical costs of care usually are associated with monetary transactions and represent costs that are incurred in providing care. Examples include payments for physicians' fees, purchase of a pharmaceutical product, or purchasing a diagnostic test. However, monetary transactions that are undertaken as a result of illness or

health care are not limited to direct medical costs alone. Direct nonmedical costs are those that are incurred because of illness or the need to seek medical care. The costs include the cost of transportation to the hospital or physician's office, cost of special clothing needed because of the illness, the cost of hotel stays for receiving medical treatment at a distant medical facility, and the cost of modification of a home to accommodate an ill individual. These costs are generally paid out of pocket by patients and their families.

Indirect costs, in contrast to direct costs, do not stem from transactions of goods or services. Instead, they represent the cost of morbidity (e.g., time lost from work) or mortality (e.g., premature death leading to removal from the work force). Indirect costs include those of loss of earnings and of workforce participation (44). As expected, data on such costs are notoriously difficult to obtain. Finally, intangible costs are those related to pain, suffering, and grief. These costs result from the medical illness itself and from the medical care services used to treat the illness. These costs are difficult to measure as part of a clinical economics study, although they are clearly considered by clinicians and patients in deciding among treatment alternatives.

Direct costs are relatively easy to obtain. These include costs of the hospital and physician, acute medical care, and rehabilitation. Those indirect costs that can be relatively easy to calculate include transportation for medical care, personal assistance, adaptive equipment, nonprescription drugs and supplies, housing modifications, and lifetime care. Very difficult to calculate are the other indirect costs, which consist primarily of wages, opportunities lost, and the impact of altered participation in the labor force on family earnings. These costs are variously obtained by estimations after a determination has been made of the impact of the disease state on workforce participation. Unfortunately, previous attempts to measure such costs for different neurosurgical disease processes are almost nonexistent. Such data are for the most part simply not available for presentation in this chapter.

One final concept that must be addressed to understand the socioeconomic implications of neurosurgery is small-area variations in treatment patterns. In 1982, a landmark study was published that revealed that the amount and types of medical care people receive vary substantially, depending on the local hospital market area and the region of the country in which they live (47). The usage rates of almost all kinds of medical care were strikingly different. Moreover, the variations seemed to be almost exclusively the result of differences in beliefs among physicians regarding the best way to treat certain conditions. These researchers developed the concept of ''small-area analysis,'' which, for the first time, allowed for the calculation of population-based rates of medical care usage by patients, hospitals, and health care providers. Before the implementation of this methodology, only overall numbers of procedures, treatments, and tests could be ascertained (17).

Before this type of analysis was conducted, most physicians thought that after adjustments for age, sex, and other potential variables were made, rates of usage for a procedure should be similar and consistent across regions. Contrary to this belief, the practice of medicine and surgery in the United States and other countries were found to be characterized by a remarkable degree of inconsistency (17, 42). Along these lines, there are large differences in the rates of spinal procedures among the four large geographic regions of the United States (northeast, Midwest, south, and west). The probability of being treated with a spinal arthrodesis in the western United States is nearly nine times that in the northeast (7). Likewise, there are statistically significant differences with respect to use rate of spinal operations among states (16). Finally, there are marked differences even within states. The likelihood of a resident of the Washington state being treated by a spinal operation varies by a factor of 15, depending on the county of residence (42, 43).

Similar variations have been seen for many medical procedures and conditions in every location in which they have been studied. The major reasons for such variations in medical decision making seem to relate to lack of agreement among physicians regarding the most appropriate form of treatment for certain conditions. A major factor in the lack of consensus is a paucity of knowledge regarding the outcomes of many types of medical and operative interventions (17). It will only be with further research into the outcomes of neurosurgical interventions that such consensus will be reached. The significance of an understanding of the exis-

tence of small-area variations in neurosurgery is an appreciation for the confounding effects that such variation has when attempting to measure the socioeconomic implications of most neurosurgical interventions.

TRAUMATIC BRAIN INJURY

Large variation is found in the estimates of the number of persons suffering brain injury, as a result of substantial differences in definitions of terms, inclusion and exclusion criteria, and specific details of the research designs (21). In the United States, traumatic brain injury (TBI) accounts for nearly 40% of all deaths from acute injuries. In addition, 200,000 persons with head injuries require hospitalization each year (40). Another 1.74 million people suffer a mild TBI that results in a physician visit or temporary disability of at least one day (45). The loss of potential income, the cost of acute care, and the continued expenses of rehabilitation and medical care are enormous. Each year, about 80,000 survivors of TBI will have some disability or require increased medical care, which will lead to annual direct medical costs of an estimated $48.3 billion (including the costs of acute-care hospitalization and the costs of various rehabilitation services) (12).

Approximately 1.9 million persons in the United States suffer a skull fracture or intracranial injury annually, half of which restrict activity (45). This number represents approximately 1% of all injuries. In 1994, intracranial injuries accounted for approximately 1% of nearly 93 million emergency department visits that year (37). Only 16% of all head injuries result in hospital admission (8). Incidence rates for TBI vary from 132 to 367 per 1000,000 persons (18, 26). It is possible to estimate an average rate of fatal plus nonfatal hospitalized brain injury of about 237 per 100,000 persons per year (21).

Few studies have addressed the prevalence of TBI because the majority of cases are not fatal, and many patients with mild TBI are not hospitalized (40). Few data are available concerning the prevalence of head injury in the population as a whole. One investigator estimated the disability rate on the basis of hospital admissions and survival rates (20). On the basis of a residual deficit rate of 10% for patients with mild injuries, 67% for those with moderate TBI, and

100% for severely injured patients, a disability rate of 33 per 100,000 was calculated for the entire population of patients with TBI. Thus, approximately 100,000 persons in the United States are estimated to have disabilities resulting from TBI.

In 1990, 150,000 persons died of acute traumatic injury, accounting for 8% of all deaths in the United States. The exact percentage of deaths involving significant brain injury is not known, but approximately 52,000 deaths in the United States are attributed to head injury each year. The reported mortality rate from TBI varies from 14 to 30 persons per 100,000 each year. This range of rates probably reflects a lack of specificity of diagnosis on some death certificates (21).

For the population as a whole, men are approximately twice as likely as women to sustain a TBI. For TBI of certain causes, the discrepancy between the male and female incidence may be even greater in the pediatric population than in adults. In children, 80% of assaults and motorcycle/bicycle injures involve male victims. However, this ratio decreases to near equivalency in elderly individuals, most likely because the most common cause of TBI in this age group is falls, for which both sexes are at similar risk. The risk for TBI peaks between the ages of 15 and 30 years (40). The peak age for men and women is similar. Similarly, the rates of mortality from TBI are highest for those 15 to 24 years of age (40). The significance of this age distribution is that TBI affects individuals during their most productive years of life. This adds greatly to the indirect socioeconomic costs of TBI.

Racial and ethnic differences in brain injury rates have not been determined accurately, although some studies show a higher brain injury incidence in nonwhite individual compared with white individuals (21). There is justifiable concern over the quality of the data used to determine these rates. However, multiple studies have shown that the risk of TBI is highest in persons with the lowest income levels (4).

Reported changes in TBI-related morbidity and mortality rates over the past 50 years vary to some extent, most likely because of differences in methods of case ascertainment as well as changes in the causes of TBI and in the management of victims. One study found that mortality rates from head injuries fell 22% from 1979 through 1992 (33). The decline was most pronounced in the early 1980s and was similar for both men and women.

TRAUMATIC SPINAL CORD INJURIES

There are approximately 11,000 new cases of acute spinal cord injuries per year, or 4 per 100,000 persons (10). The estimated prevalence of persons living with spinal cord injuries is between 300,000 and 500,000 cases. An increased prevalence during the past decade has been attributed mainly to enhanced longevity of spine-injured patients (34). Increased survivorship as well as improvements in neurological outcome have been attributed to enhanced medical, surgical, and prehospital care (34). Spinal cord injury is most common in young adult men. It is estimated that 63% of new traumatic injuries occur in individuals between the ages of 16 and 30 years, with a 4:1 male:female ratio (35).

There are very few accurate data on the total cost of spinal cord injuries. The estimated annual cost to support and treat all patients with a spinal cord injury is over $4 billion (36). As expected, the initial hospitalization costs (including acute care and rehabilitation) and the annual follow-up expenses vary tremendously depending on the level of the injury (44). In one study, researchers found that costs of acute and rehabilitation care vary from $67,950 in the low-level paraplegic patient to $426,592 in the respirator-dependent, high-quadriplegic patient (44). Similarly, these researchers noted that annual follow-up expenses for the low-level paraplegic patient were $10,109 compared with $141,238 for the respirator-dependent, high-quadriplegic patient. Regarding economic opportunities lost, lifetime foregone earnings vary from $141,253 in the patient who is incompletely paraplegic to $308,054 in the completely quadriplegic patient (6).

NONTRAUMATIC SPINAL DISORDERS

Although several quality studies have been performed on the socioeconomic impact of both closed head injuries and traumatic spinal cord injuries, this has not been the case with nontraumatic spinal disorders such as those of neoplastic, vascular, or congenital etiology. Most research has focused on the impact of benign low-back pain, and that information is presented here.

Aside from the common cold, no condition afflicts the U.S. population with greater incidence and prevalence than low-back pain. Over 10 million people are disabled because of low-back pain, with over 250 million workdays lost per year (22). Over $50 billion is expended on the management of low-back pain each year (9), with approximately $11 billion of that in the worker's compensation system (46). Two thirds of Americans suffer an incapacitating episode of low-back pain at least once in their lives, one third are suffering at any one time, and over one tenth are seeking medical care. An estimated 25% of American workers will experience some low-back pain each year, with 50% to 60% experiencing some disabling pain during their working career (44).

The total cost of low-back pain is distributed in the following manner: 45% for permanent disability payments, 22% for temporary disability payments, and 33% for medical expenses. Medical costs are distributed as follows: 33% for physicians, 33% for hospital bills, 7% for drugs, 5% for appliances, 9% for physical therapy, and 12% for diagnostic tests (44). In one study that examined over 5,000 individuals who reported their first incidence of low-back pain in 1988, it was noted that only 243 (or 0.45%) underwent surgery (5). Thus, surgical intervention involves only a small fraction of the total socioeconomic impact of this disease process.

CARPAL TUNNEL SYNDROME

Carpal tunnel syndrome (CTS) has an estimated incidence of 0.1% and self-reported prevalence of 1.5% (38). One recent study determined the incidence to be 346 cases per 100,000 person years (29). This incidence is 3.5 times higher than the rate 20 years ago. This rate difference is believed to have resulted from a rise in the incidence of the disease as well as newer diagnostic tests, different case definitions and case reporting sources, and different exposure to risk factors (29).

Of those persons who develop CTS, most are 40 to 60 years old, 70% are women, 70% undergo carpal tunnel release surgery, and 45% receive some form of workers' compensation (15). Over 200,000 surgical procedures are performed each year for CTS (3). The total direct medical costs for the treatment of CTS per year in the United States is almost $1 billion.

CTS is known to occur more commonly in occupations involving repetitive or forceful wrist and hand activities. Work disability that is due to CTS is often prolonged, and workers with CTS frequently change occupations, even if they are treated surgically. Twenty-three percent of workers who undergo carpal tunnel release remain out of work because of CTS at 6 months following surgery (15). One study found that 45% of patients changed jobs or were absent from work for prolonged periods during a 30-month follow-up period after carpal tunnel surgery (15). Therefore, CTS affects the working population mainly during their most productive years. It is also often associated with an inability to continue employment at the same job, leading to direct financial losses. This translates into an enormous indirect cost to society.

CENTRAL NERVOUS SYSTEM TUMORS

Approximately 13,100 new cases of central nervous system (CNS) tumors were expected during 1999 (23). The overall incidence of primary spinal cord tumors is approximately 15% of that of brain tumors. The combined incidence of all CNS tumors is between 2 and 19 cases per 100,000 persons per year depending on age. There is an early peak (3.1 per 100,000) between 0 and 4 years, a trough (1.8 per 100,000) between 15 and 24 years, and then a steady rise in incidence that reaches a plateau (17.9–18.7 per 100,000) between 65 and 79 years of age. CNS tumors are the most prevalent solid neoplasms of childhood, the second-leading cancer-related cause of death in children younger than 15 years of age, and the third-leading cancer-related cause of death in adolescents and adults between the ages of 15 and 34 years.

Less than 2% of the 550,000 cancer deaths per year are attributed to CNS tumors. Deaths from CNS tumors were the fifth leading cause of cancer deaths in men aged 40–59 years and women aged 20–39 years. The five-year relative survival rates for most CNS tumors have not changed significantly since 1974 except in the pediatric population.

Several factors have led to a lack of data regarding the socioeconomic implications of CNS tumors. Given their relative rarity compared with other more common forms of cancer such as lung, breast, and prostate, such data have simply not been collected. In addition, this is an extremely diverse group of patients, with a diversity in both pathologies and ages. The high incidence of CNS tumors in children argues for an uncalculated loss of lifetime productivity and societal contribution that makes the indirect costs enormous. Placing a dollar amount on such indirect costs requires a multitude of assumptions that are both difficult and inexact. On the other end of the spectrum, high-grade glial neoplasms in very elderly individuals with extremely short lengths of survival have much lower indirect costs.

CEREBRAL ANEURYSMS

The incidence of subarachnoid hemorrhage from cerebral aneurysms is 6–10 cases per 100,000 individuals and has remained constant over the past 30 years (31). There are approximately 25,000 new cases of ruptured aneurysms per year in the United States, and cerebral aneurysms produce death or disability in approximately 18,000 persons per year (31, 39).

The prevalence of intracranial aneurysms is difficult to calculate. The frequency of both ruptured and unruptured aneurysms discovered at autopsy is approximately 1%–2% of cases (49). The prevalence of unruptured intracranial aneurysms is between 0.3% and 5% (1, 27). Overall, there is a 1.6:1 female:male ratio with cerebral aneurysms (14). This ratio increases dramatically with age to 4.16:1 for those individuals who are 70 years or older.

It is estimated that 10% of patients die immediately and without warning and another 25% are disabled or die as a result of the initial hemorrhage. Therefore, only 65% of subarachnoid hemorrhage patients are eligible for some type of intervention (2, 13). Mortality rates at 1 month are reported to be as high as 60% (24). This translates to a mortality rate of 2.7 deaths per 100,000 individuals.

Of the those surviving a ruptured aneurysm, the likelihood of disability is quite high. Only 60% of those who undergo intervention enjoy a strong recovery (14). However, even among this group, there may be significant cognitive deficits. One study found that only 17% of patients had no or mild cognitive impairment (25). Another study found that only 23% of patients with a good neurological outcome were employed 1 year after a subarachnoid hemorrhage compared with 50% employed prior to the event (30).

In regards to the cost of aneurysms, the detection of an aneurysm prior to rupture not only profoundly affects the patient's health but also may result in saving health care dollars (24). Wiebers et al. (48) estimated the lifetime cost for patients with unruptured aneurysms who are hospitalized and treated as $5.225 million per year in the United States. This is compared with a $1.7556 billion per year lifetime cost for patients suffering from a subarachnoid hemorrhage (48).

CONCLUSION

The socioeconomic impact of neurosurgical disease processes is difficult to quantify. Although the incidence and prevalence of the more common disorders can be ascertained, little data exist on both their direct and indirect costs. *Table 16.2* lists the incidence of a variety of neurosurgical disease states. As overall mortality from other causes decreases and longevity increases, the incidence of many neurological diseases, such as CNS tumors (both primary and metastatic) and degenerative spine disorders, increases. Therefore, the impact of neurosurgical disease processes on the health of society and the overall cost of medical care should increase. The problem of variations in the management of these disorders confounds the process of data collection. There is an urgent need to begin acquiring accurate data that show the costs to society of these diseases as well as the outcomes of neurosurgical interventions. The specialty of neurosurgery will increasingly rely on such information to compete for both research dollars as well as third-party-payer reimbursement. In the future, it will be more important than ever

TABLE 16.2
Incidence of Several Neurosurgical Disease States

Diagnosis	Incidence per 100,000 Persons
Low-back pain	30,000
Carpal tunnel syndrome	2,800
Traumatic brain injury	150
Occlusive cerebral vascular disease	96
Intracerebral/intracranial hemorrhage	30
Malignant neoplasm of brain	12
Subarachnoid hemorrhage (nontraumatic)	8
Traumatic spinal cord injury	4

for neurosurgeons to direct our energies toward obtaining this elusive yet vital information.

REFERENCES

1. Bannerman RM, Ingall GB, Graf CJ: The familial occurrence of intracranial aneurysms. *Neurology* 20: 282–292, 1970.
2. Bonita R, Thomson S: Subarachnoid hemorrhage: Epidemiology, diagnosis, management, and outcome. *Stroke* 16:591–594, 1985.
3. Chung KC, Walters MR, Greenfield MLVH, Chernew ME: Endoscopic versus open carpal tunnel release: A cost-effectiveness analysis. *Plastic Reconstructive Surg* 102:1089–1099, 1998.
4. Collins JG: Types of injuries by selected characteristics: United States, 1985–1987. *Vital Health Stat* 10:175, 1990.
5. Conrad DA: Low back pain: Economic analysis of its impact on the U.S. non-elderly population, in Bigos S (ed): *Report of the Low Back Pain Guidelines Panel to the Office of the Forum of the Agency for Health Care Policy and Research*. Washington, DC, Department of Health and Human Services, 1993.
6. DeVivo MJ: The cost of spinal cord injury: A growing national dilemma, in Apple DF Jr, Hudson LM (eds): *Spinal Cord Injury: The Model, Proceedings of the National Consensus Conference on Catastrophic Illness and Injury*. Atlanta, 1989, 109–113.
7. Deyo RA: Non-surgical care of low back pain. *Neurosurg Clin N Am* 2:851–862, 1991.
8. Fife D: Head injury with and without hospital admission: Comparisons of incidence and short-term disability. *Am J Public Health* 77:810–812, 1987.
9. Frymoyer JW, Cats-Baril WL: An overview of the incidences and costs of low back pain. *Orthop Clin N Am* 22:263–271, 1991.
10. Gerhart KA: Spinal cord injury outcomes in a population-based sample. *J Trauma* 31:1529–1535, 1991.
11. Hoff JT: Towards better balance. The 1994 presidential address. *J Neurosurg* 81:651–655, 1994.
12. Johnston MV: The economics of brain injury: a preface, in Miner ME, Wagner KA (eds): *Neurotrauma. Treatment, Rehabilitation and Related Issues*. Boston, Butterworths, 1989, 163–186.
13. Kassell NF, Drake CG: Timing of aneurysm surgery. *Neurosurgery* 10:514–519, 1982.
14. Kassell NF, Torner JC, Haley EC Jr, et al: The International Cooperative Study on the Timing of Aneurysm Surgery: Part 1. Overall management results. *J Neurosurg* 73:18–36, 1990.
15. Katz JN, Lew RA, Bessett L, et al: Prevalence and predictors of long-term work disability due to carpal tunnel syndrome. *Am J Industrial Medicine* 33:543–550, 1998.
16. Keller RB, Rudicel SA, Liang MH: Outcomes research in orthopaedics. *Instr Course Lect* 43:599–611, 1994.
17. Keller RB, Soule DN, Wennberg JE, Hanley DF: Dealing with geographic variations in the use of hospitals: The experience of the Main Medical Assessment Foundation Orthopaedic Study Group. *J Bone Join Surg Am* 72:1286–1293, 1990.
18. Klauber MR, Marshall LF, Luersson TG, et al: Determinants of head injury mortality: Importance of the low risk patients. *Neurosurgery* 24:31–36, 1989.
19. Knickman JR, Thorpe KE: Financing for health care, in Kovner AR (ed): *Health Care Delivery in the United States*. New York, Springer, 1997, 267–293.
20. Kraus JF: Epidemiology of head injury, in Cooper PR (ed): *Head Injury*. Baltimore, Williams & Wilkins, 1993, 1–26.
21. Kraus JF, McArthur DL, Silverman TA, Jayaraman M: Epidemiology of brain injury, in Narayan RK, Wilberger JE Jr, Povlishock JT (eds): *Neurotrauma*. New York, McGraw-Hill, 1996, 13–30.
22. Kriegler JS: Medical management of chronic low back pain, in Hardy RW Jr (ed): *Lumbar Disc Disease*. New York, Raven Press, 1993, 293–298, 2nd ed.
23. Landis SH, Murry T, Bolden S, Wingo PA: Cancer statistics, 1999. CA *Cancer J Clin* 49:8–31, 1999.
24. Lindley JG, Wirth FP: Epidemiology of cerebral aneurysms, in Ratcheson RA, Wirth FP (eds): *Ruptured Cerebral Aneurysms: Perioperative Management. Volume 6: Concepts in Neurosurgery*. Baltimore, Williams & Wilkins, 1994, 15–22.
25. Ljunggren B, Sonesson B Saveland H, et al.: Cognitive impairment and adjustment in patients without neurological deficits after aneurysmal SAH and early operation. *J Neurosurg* 62:673–679, 1985.
26. MacKenzie EJ, Edelstein SL, Flynn JP: Hospitalized head-injured patients in Maryland: Incidence and severity of injuries. *Maryland Med J* 38:725, 1989.
27. McCormick WF: Intracranial arterial aneurysm: A pathologist's view. *Curr Concepts Cerebrovasc Dis Stroke* 8:15–19, 1973.
28. McGinnis JM, Foege WH: Actual causes of death in the United States. *JAMA* 270:2208, 1993.
29. Nordstrom DL, DeStefano F, Vierkant RA, Layde PM: Incidence of diagnosed carpal tunnel syndrome in a general population. *Epidemiology* 9:342–345, 1998.
30. Ogden JA, Mee EW, Henning M: A prospective study of impairment of cognition and memory and recovery after subarachnoid hemorrhage. *Neurosurgery* 33: 572–587, 1993.
31. Sahs AL, Nibbelink DW, Torner JC, eds: Intracranial Aneurysms and Subarachnoid Hemorrhage: A Cooperative Study. Baltimore, Urban and Schwarzenberg, 1981.
32. Schulman KA, Glick HA, Yabroff KR, Eisenberg JM: Introduction to clinical economics: Assessment of cancer therapies. *Monogr Natl Cancer Inst* 19:1–9, 1995.
33. Sosin DM, Sniezek JE, Waxweiler RJ: Trends in death associated with traumatic brain injury, 1979 through 1992. Success and failure. *JAMA* 273:1778–1780, 1992.
34. Stillerman CB, Roy RS, Weiss MH: Cervical spine injuries: Diagnosis and management, in Wilkins RH, Rengachary SS (eds): *Neurosurgery*. New York, McGraw-Hill, 1996, 2875–2904, 2nd ed.
35. Stover SL, Fine PR: Spinal Cord Injury: The Facts and Figures. Birmingham, AL, University of Alabama Press, 1986.
36. Stripling TE: The cost of economic consequences of traumatic spinal cord injury. *Paraplegia News* August:50–54, 1990.
37. Strussman BJ: National Ambulatory Medical Care Survey. 1994 Emergency Department Summary. *Advance Data from Vital and Health Statistics of the*

Centers for Disease Control and Prevention/National Center for Health Statistics 275:1–17, 1996.

38. Tanaka S, Wild DK, Seligman PJ, et al: The US prevalence of self-reported carpal tunnel syndrome: 1988 National Health Interview Survey data. *Am J Public Health* 84:1846–1848, 1994.

39. Taylor CL, Zhong Y, Selman WR, Ratcheson RA, Rimm AA: Mortality rates, hospital length of stay, and the cost of treating subarachnoid hemorrhage in older patients: institutional and geographic differences. *J Neurosurg* 86:583–588, 1977.

40. Torner JC, Choi S, Barnes TY: Epidemiology of head injuries, in Marion DW (ed): *Traumatic Brain Injury.* New York, Thieme, 1999, 9–25.

41. U.S. Department of Health and Human Services, Public Health Service: For a Healthy Nation: Returns on Investment in Public Health. Washington, DC, U.S. Government Printing Office, 1994.

42. Volinn E, Diehr P, Ciol MA, Loeser JD: Why does geographic variation in health care practice matter? *Spine* 19:2092S–2100S, 1994.

43. Volinn E, Mayer J, Diehr P, et al: Small area analysis of surgery for low back pain. *Spine* 17:575–581, 1992.

44. Watts C, Esser GB III: Economic overview of spinal disorders, in Menezes AH, Sonntag VK (eds): *Principles of Spinal Surgery.* New York, McGraw-Hill, 1996, 25–36.

45. Waxweiler RJ, Thurman D, Sniezek J, et al: Monitoring the impact of traumatic brain injury: A review and update. *J Neurotrauma* 12:509–516, 1995.

46. Webster BS, Snook SH: The cost of compensable low back pain. *J Occup Med* 32:13–15, 1990.

47. Wennberg JE, Gittelsohn A: Variations in medical care among small areas. *Sci Am* 246:120–134, 1982.

48. Wiebers DO, Torner JC, Meissner I: Impact of unruptured intracranial aneurysms on public health in the United States. *Stroke* 23:1416–1419, 1992.

49. Winn HR, Almaani WS, Berga SL, Jane JA, Richardson AE: The long-term outcome in patients with multiple aneurysms. Incidence of late hemorrhage and implications for treatment of incidental aneurysms. *J Neurosurg* 59:642–651, 1983.

50. World Health Organization: International Classification of Impairments, Disabilities, and Handicaps. Geneva, Switzerland, World Health Organization, 1980.

CHAPTER 17

Cost Considerations from a Societal Prospective: The Oregon Health Plan—Design and Implementation of a Novel Method of Health Care Delivery to Individuals Living in Poverty

ANDREW GLASS, M.D.

Editor's Note: Consideration of health care costs from a societal prospective is an extremely complex matter. For policymakers, opportunity costs (paying for one item at the expense of another) becomes a very real issue that must be reconciled within a fiscal, political, and medically ethical context. In 1989, the state of Oregon attempted to address these issues in a systematic manner that would attempt to expand the availability of their Medicaid program by covering only medical conditions and procedures that met certain criteria of effectiveness and economic efficiency. In this chapter, I provide the reader with insight into the foundations, development, and implementation of the Oregon Health Plan. The issues discussed provide valuable information on the process of implementing large-scale changes in publicly funded health care toward more broader coverage of individuals at the expense of breadth of coverage for individual medical conditions.

In the late 1980s, Oregon, like the rest of the United States, found that a large fraction of its poorer citizens lacked insurance to cover basic health care. Poor persons tended to use emergency room facilities when crises arose but otherwise avoided the medical system for routine or preventive care. Conversely, the insured population could obtain whatever care they desired, but at considerable cost. Hospitals and all medical providers recognized that the care delivered to uninsured persons was paid by shifting costs from poor individuals to those who could pay, inevitably driving up the costs of health insurance. The causes of inadequate or unavailable medical insurance are complex and beyond the scope of this discussion. However, the solutions offered must be examined within the intricate framework of federal and state programs that both pay for the care of the poor and contribute to its structure and function with an elaborate system of targeted programs and regulations to manage them.

Oregon sought its own unique solution to this problem in the innovative program now known as the Oregon Health Plan (OHP). OHP was a relatively complex amalgam of initiatives that each attacked a specific defect in the system of funding medical care for the poor. Priority setting has become the most well-known aspect of the OHP as it became an explicit attack on the manner in which physicians, hospitals, and health plans distribute finite resources to a population that is increasingly demanding more and more medical care. The Health Services Commission of Oregon developed a prioritized list of health services in a public forum with significant citizen input. Such a process was very political at the start and has remained so to the present day, often leaving its purer roots in the world of cost-effectiveness analysis for the world of the public forum, state legislature, and federal bureaucracy.

MEDICAL INSURANCE IN THE 1990S

As seen in *Table 17.1*, the majority of Americans are privately insured (7). Overwhelmingly, insurance comes with employment, often as a considerable tax benefit that is usually paid for by pretax dollars. Unfortunately, such coverage only accrues to those individuals who are in better paying positions, because low-paying jobs often come with no benefits. Medicare for practical purposes covers individuals over age 65 with a few others also included because of disability, and so forth.

The Medicare and Medicaid programs were passed into law in 1965 to address concerns about the inadequacy of health insurance for elderly and poor persons, respectively. Although Medicare is fully funded by the federal government, Medicaid is paid for with both state and federal monies, with the federal contribution fixed at between 50% and 83% of the total expenditure. This amount is calculated by comparing a state's average per capita income with the national average. States with a higher per capita income receive a higher federal contribution. In recent times, the range of federal contribution has ranged from 50% (13 states) to 77.2% (Mississippi) and averages 57% (8).

TABLE 17.1
Patterns of Health Insurance in the United States

Insurance	Population (millions)	Percentage
Private Insurance	167	59.6%
Medicare	37	13.3%
Medicaid	36	12.8%
Uninsured	40	14.3%
Total (U.S. population)	280	100%

Note. Data are condensed from information on the Health Care Financing Administration's Web site at http://www.heca.gov.

MEDICAID

Under Medicaid law, each state pays a portion of the costs incurred by Medicaid with the remainder contributed by the federal government. Thus, to get any federal money, each state has to allocate and spend state funds for their Medicaid program. Each state determines the amount of money it is willing to spend on its Medicaid program. The formulas used and the complex calculations that they involve are beyond my understanding. What follows is an oversimplification of the process followed by each state.

First, it is important to remember that states generally have to spend some of their own money to get federal matching funds. Furthermore, the rules governing which individuals are covered by federal programs, on the basis of a "categorical" eligibility (i.e., blind, disabled, pregnant and poor, child and poor, etc), vary considerably. For some programs, states are required to provide coverage (i.e., spend their own money) and for some, there are options that they can exercise by enrolling more or fewer individuals.

Second, individual and family eligibility for Medicaid is complex and reflects the effects of a series of targeted initiatives over the years. These laws attempted to address inadequate coverage of one group or another, but the layering on of one after another special group has made the assessment of who is or is not eligible exceedingly difficult. In the Medicaid program, individuals may be eligible for benefits only if their income falls below a certain fraction (e.g., 100%, 133%, etc.) of the federal poverty level (FPL) and they meet certain other conditions. The Health Care Financing Administration (HCFA) defines these categories of eligibility, which are summarized in the list below (9):

- Individuals are generally eligible for Medicaid if they meet the requirements for the AFDC [XXXXXXXXXXXXXXXXXXXXXX] program that were in effect in their state on July 16, 1996, or—at state option—more liberal criteria;
- Children under age six whose family income is at or below 133% of the federal poverty level (FPL);
- Pregnant women whose family income is below 133% of the FPL (services to women are limited to those related to pregnancy, com-

plications of pregnancy, delivery, and postpartum care);

- SSI [Social Security Insurance] recipients in most states (some states use more restrictive Medicaid eligibility requirements that predate SSI);
- Recipients of adoption or foster care assistance under Title IV of the Social Security Act;
- Special protected groups (typically individuals who lose their cash assistance due to earnings from work or from increased Social Security benefits, but who may keep Medicaid for a period of time);
- All children born after September 30, 1983, who are under age 19, in families with incomes at or below the FPL (this phases in coverage, so that by the year 2002, all such poor children under age 19 will be covered); and
- Certain Medicare beneficiaries.

Additional optional categories include the following:

- Infants up to age 1 and pregnant women not covered under the mandatory whose family income is no more than 185% of the FPL (the percentage amount is set by each state);
- Children under age 21 who meet what were the AFDC income and resources requirements in effect in their state on July 16, 1996 (even though they do not meet the mandatory eligibility requirements);
- Institutionalized individuals eligible under a "special income level" (this set by each state—up to 300% of the SSI federal benefits rate);
- Individuals who would be eligible if institutionalized but who are receiving care under home and community-based services waivers;
- Certain aged, blind, or disabled adults who have incomes above those requiring mandatory coverage, but below the FPL;
- Recipients of state supplementary income payments;
- Certain working and disabled persons with family income less than 250% of FPL who would qualify for SSI if they did not work;
- TB-infected persons who would be financially eligible for Medicaid at the SSI income level if they were within a Medicaid-covered category (however, coverage is limited to TB-related ambulatory services and TB drugs);
- "Optional targeted low-income children" included within the Children's Health Insurance

Program (CHIP) established by the Balanced Budget Act of 1997 (BBA); and
- "Medically needy" persons (described below).

The categories are diverse but generally concentrate on mothers and children living in poverty, with additions from a number of other groups who represent individuals who are medically indigent. In no circumstance is poverty by itself adequate to obtain Medicaid. "Medicaid does not provide medical assistance for all poor persons. Even under the broadest provisions of the federal statute, Medicaid does *not* provide health care services even for very poor persons *unless* they are in one of the groups designated below. And low income is only one test for Medicaid eligibility for those within these groups; their resources also are tested against threshold levels (as determined by each state within federal guidelines)" (9, p. xxx).

As stated above, an individual must satisfy an income criterion to qualify for Medicaid. This is usually expressed as a function of the FPL, which is a level of annual income set by HCFA for different-sized families. An added complexity to Medicaid is the significant variation among the states in setting eligibility criteria related to the FPL. "Within broad national guidelines established by federal statutes, regulations and policies, each state: 1) establishes its own eligibility standards; 2) determines the type, amount, duration, and scope of services; 3) sets the rate of payment for services; and 4) administers its own program" (9, p. xxx). Given this broad policy, Medicaid policies for eligibility, services, and payment are complex and vary considerably even among similar-sized and/or adjacent states. Thus, a person who is eligible for Medicaid in one state might not be eligible in another state. Furthermore, the services provided by one state may differ considerably in amount, duration, or scope from services provided in a similar or neighboring state. In addition, Medicaid eligibility and/or services within a state can change during the year. Once covered by Medicaid, an individual is eligible to receive the full complement of medical care, as the benefits outlined by HCFA are generous; only access to the program is limited The below list details the scope of Medicaid services.

Required basic services:

- Inpatient hospital services,
- Outpatient hospital services,

- Prenatal care,
- Vaccines for children;
- Physician services,
- Nursing facility services for persons ages 21 or older,
- Family planning services and supplies,
- Rural health clinic services,
- Home health care for persons eligible for skilled-nursing services,
- Laboratory and x-ray services,
- Pediatric and family nurse practitioner services,
- Nurse-midwife services,
- Federally qualified health-center (FQHC) services, and ambulatory services of an FQHC that would be available in other settings, and
- Early and periodic screening, diagnostic, and treatment (EPSDT) services for children under age 21.

Most common of the 34 currently approved optional Medicaid services:

- Diagnostic services,
- Clinic services,
- Intermediate-care facilities for the mentally retarded (ICFs/MR),
- Prescribed drugs and prosthetic devices,
- Optometrist services and eyeglasses,
- Nursing facility services for children under age 21,
- Transportation services,
- Rehabilitation and physical therapy services, and
- Home and community-based care to certain persons with chronic impairments.

Note that Title XIX of the Social Security Act (the Medicaid program) allows considerable flexibility within the states' Medicaid plans. However, some federal requirements are mandatory if federal matching funds are to be received. A state's Medicaid program must offer medical assistance for certain basic services to most categorically needy populations. Other funding may be available for approved optional services (9).

Uninsured Americans that qualify for none of the programs listed above number approximately 40 million. They either have jobs that do not provide health insurance, do not qualify for one or another Medicaid program, or are not old enough for Medicare. Mostly they are the "working poor," individuals who earn enough to exceed Medicaid levels of family income but not enough to afford individual health insurance

policies. Across the United States, these individuals represent about 14% of the population. Most states have no program for the uninsured and rely entirely on the charitable care delivered by individual health care providers and hospitals when faced by the patient and family who cannot pay for needed care. The uninsured typically are cared for by city, county, and state inpatient facilities and only at the time of acute illness or accident, with routine care and any preventive activities being essentially unknown.

The Medicaid program allows states to apply for waivers of one or another provision of the law to implement a local program designed either to improve access, deliver new services, or to try an innovative health care delivery system. In recent years, these waivers have been commonly applied for and granted with about half of the states involved in one program or another. One type, the Section 1115 waiver, is directed toward research and development and includes the most significant departures from the usual way of doing things as described above. These waivers are customarily granted for 3–4 years, during which time annual reports are required and monitored by the federal government. If states exceed the mandate of their waivers, they may be required to modify their programs by HCFA.

Some of the waivers granted by HCFA have been designed to expand the Medicaid program to the uninsured population, and several states, including Oregon, have used this method to expand coverage to the uninsured who meet no federal guideline except that of income below the FPL.

GENERAL ORGANIZATION OF OHP

In 1989, approximately 18% of Oregon residents lacked health insurance. The Oregon Medicaid program, using the funds allocated to it by the state legislature, insured some 250,000 individuals whose incomes fell below approximately 57% of the FPL. There were at least 100,000 individuals whose incomes fell below the FPL but who had no health insurance. Emergency room and other acute-care visits among the uninsured population constituted their entire contact with the medical care system. Hospitals and medical care providers were plagued by high rates of unpaid care, and insurance rates were rising rapidly in a broad pattern of cost shifting from those unable to pay to those with health insurance (14).

The overall intent of OHP was to expand care of the uninsured and, in so doing, address the problems noted above. The method was multifaceted and included a set of bills in the legislature to address different aspects of the problem, the development of the "Prioritized List of Health Services," a Section 1115 waiver from HCFA, and a broad reorganization of the delivery of care to poor persons.

Oregon's solution involved a comprehensive reform that addressed three parts of the problem:

- The inability of certain individuals to obtain health insurance because of a preexisting medical condition,
- The lack of employment-related insurance for workers in many small businesses, minimum-wage jobs, and temporary positions, and
- Uncontrolled expenditures for costly and ineffective therapies for the few at the expense of routine and preventive therapy for the many.

Three pieces of legislation were drawn up and passed in the development of the OHP to address the goal of health insurance for every Oregon resident. Although all bills passed in 1989–1990, only two came into force and remain in place to this day (14). The defeat of the third bill ultimately prevented the full scope of health insurance reform that had originally been contemplated and stymied the move to universal insurance.

The first bill to be implemented, in July 1990, was the authorization of the Oregon Medical Insurance Pool to ensure reasonably priced coverage for individuals who had been denied insurance because of a number of preexisting medical conditions. This legislation has continued in force until the present, but it has affected relatively few individuals—about 5,000 at any one time and 40,000 different individuals in the 1990–1998 period.

The second bill was the employer mandate to require all employers either to offer group health insurance for their "permanent" employees (defined as those who worked over 17.5 hours per week and were neither seasonal nor temporary) or to pay into a statewide insurance pool through a payroll tax. This mandate was to be phased in over four years, with an implementation date of July 1995. Unfortunately, this law never came into effect through a combination of factors. The

law required a waiver from the federal Employee Retirement Income Security Act (ERISA) and was written by state legislators to automatically "sunset" by January 2, 1996, if the waiver had not been received by that date. The waiver never was received, and the law never came into effect.

The third bill, and the centerpiece of the legislation for the OHP, was a bill that, (a) authorized the Health Services Commission (HSC), (b) outlined its charge to develop a prioritized list of health services that would govern the care delivered to poor persons, and (c) mandated a novel method of payment of medical costs. The entire charge to the Commission is contained in two sentences of this landmark bill. "The commission shall report to the Governor a list of health services ranked by priority, from the most important to the least important, representing the comparative benefits of each service to the entire population to be served. The recommendation shall be accompanied by a report of an independent actuary retained for the commission to determine rates necessary to cover the costs of the services" (16, p. xxx).

The Commission would develop a list, each line of which would consist of a health service and its accompanying treatment(s). Then the Commission would rank these procedures by importance and report that list to the governor. An actuary would analyze the list, item by item, take into account the population of the state, and project the cost of each line. The actuary would then total these projected costs, starting at the "most important" line and accumulate the costs down to the "least important" line. In this way, the legislators would know the projected costs of any set of health services simply by totaling the dollar amounts for each line within that set of services. If the Commission could develop a prioritized list of services that was termed *essential* (called the Basic Health Care Package [BHCP]), it could easily be priced as the sum of the lines within that package. From such a calculation, the legislature could determine the dollars needed to fund a set of health benefits for a given population of Medicaid beneficiaries.

In a different approach, if the legislature set a dollar amount that it was willing to spend on the Medicaid program, the prioritized list could be used to specify which diagnoses and treatments would be covered. Specifically, one could examine the list from the top down and identify that line where the budgeted money ran out.

And, from the point of view of health care policy, one could also examine the list of services to see the entire range of what was and was not covered above the line to determine if the budgeted amount was adequate to fund the agreed-on BHCP.

Prior to the OHP, only those individuals in the state with incomes below 57% of the FPL and a categorically specified need could receive benefits. This situation, as pointed out above, was exceedingly complex, inequitable, and produced considerable turmoil in budgets of the state, local hospitals, and medical providers. The principal idea of the OHP was to broaden the coverage to everyone below the FPL but to restrict the benefits to the BHCP as noted above. Underlying this plan was the belief that health services that ranked "low on the list" were often discretionary and unnecessary to the BHCP yet still costly enough that their elimination would free up enough funds to cover a large number of presently uninsured Oregon residents.

The changes may more easily be understood when contrasted to the Medicaid program before passage of these laws. In Oregon, and in other states, Medicaid programs managed their budgets by controlling the number of enrollees allowed into their health care system. This was usually accomplished by expanding or restricting eligibility criteria of one or another categorical program. A frequently used technique was to lower the eligible income level so that only individuals and families below, for example, 60% of the FPL could be enrolled in Medicaid. The OHP changed this system so that everyone below 100% of the FPL was eligible for Medicaid, but the services for which they were covered were limited to those "above the line," as determined by the funding allocated by the legislature. In other words, the Medicaid question changed from "who is covered" to "what is covered."

THE PRIORITIZATION PROCESS

The Health Services Commission was charged by Oregon Senate Bill 27 to devise a prioritized list of health services. The membership of the Commission was specified to include five physicians (including one doctor of osteopathy) with expertise in obstetrics, neonatology, pediatrics, adult medicine, geriatrics or public health, a public health nurse, a social services worker, and "four consumers of health care." Appointments would be made by the governor and confirmed by the state senate and would be for a renewable term of four years. The Commission was to ". . . actively solicit public involvement in a community meeting process to build a consensus on the values to be used to guide health resource allocation decisions" (16, p. xxxx).

There were few precedents for such a process. In 1983–1984, Oregon Health Decisions, a private citizen's group formed to influence health policy, had conducted a wide-ranging survey of 5,000 Oregon residents at large and small meetings across the state to learn of their views regarding health care (6). There was significant support for five main items:

- Better protection for the dignity and autonomy of sick and dying patients,
- More emphasis on disease prevention and health promotion,
- Universal access to an adequate level of health care,
- Control of health care costs, and
- Fair and open decisions about the rationing and allocation of resources.

A grant from a local foundation funded "The Oregon Medicaid Priority-Setting Project" in 1988–1989. This project convened a number of focus groups of health care professionals from various disciplines to "first, describe the elements of care necessary for their particular patient populations: and second, to assign ranks to these services in light of available outcomes and effectiveness research"(6, p. xxx). These focus groups were followed by a two-day intensive meeting to assign ordinal values from 1 to 10, from the lowest to the highest priority, to "broad areas of services necessary to any Medicaid program" (p. xxx). There was little variation across the scores, with 82% having a score of 10 and 90% being above 7. Taken together, this project gave little guidance to the Commission in their task of development of the prioritized list. It did demonstrate that such decisions could be developed in a public forum and that there existed broad support for the process of ranking health services in the order of their importance.

Not withstanding the work described above, the Health Services Commission needed to meet for many hours in multiple sites across Oregon for approximately a year. The meetings were all public and there was much public testimony from a broad spectrum of citizens, health care professionals, business leaders, politicians, and academics. A minority of voices disagreed with the basic premise that health care services could or should be prioritized. Their criticisms fell into two broad categories, the ethical and the practical.

The ethical criticism pointed out that the reforms being undertaken were only in programs that covered poor individuals, and only poor persons were being asked to accept a lesser range of health services (4). Some items that were presently covered by Medicaid would certainly not be covered by the OHP. More penetrating was the concern expressed by some that a partial solution to the health care problems of poor persons might impede a more definitive complete solution, largely by producing some minimal improvements that would lessen the pressure to find a definitive solution (4).

The Commission grappled with the ethical issue and came to the conclusion that the funding and practice of medical care under the Medicaid system was as unethical as anything they might be able to devise. Priority setting and rationing were apparent everywhere, and a large block of poor persons were getting no care whatsoever. There was also no evidence that a reduced package of benefits would lead to less care. Indeed, the Commission felt that the more rational care embodied in the BHCP was likely to deliver more and better coverage by its elimination of useless and unproven procedures and promotion of routine and preventive care. Finally, the Commission agreed that the OHP was imperfect but that it was likely to be improved in the future (5). It seemed unlikely, and history has borne this out, that there would be a national health insurance program for everyone anytime soon. Without such a program, it was better to move toward wider and better access to health care than to wait for a final solution that might not come for years, if ever.

The practical criticism raised the nettlesome issue of inadequate data to prioritize health services. There have been few studies and even fewer randomized trials that evaluated the effectiveness of treatments for the majority of diseases. Evidence-based medicine may be the future gold standard for the evaluation of therapies for all diseases, however in the early 1990s, there were few studies that the Commission

would be able to use to make the list. Moreover, there were a number of competing methodologies that had been suggested and used in smaller efforts to evaluate the effectiveness of treatments but no standard method to compare every diagnosis–treatment pair and to develop a rank-ordered prioritized list.

The Commissioners grappled with this issue for a number of months, reviewing and ultimately modifying or rejecting a number of suggested methods. They received testimony from scores of panels of physicians who were asked to make judgments about the effectiveness of various treatments in helping to restore patients with certain conditions to health as well as estimates of the costs of providing the treatments. They received testimony from more than 1,000 citizens at public forums across the state. These forums in particular served to crystallize for the Commission and for the state the public values about health care that would prove particularly important in the final prioritization process. The Commission produced its first prioritized list in mid-1990, using a mathematical approach and the Quality of Well-Being Scale of Kaplan (12). There were many anomalies on that list, with condition–treatment pairs clearly out of place, largely because of the inadequate and incomplete data available for such a model.

An alternative methodology was developed by Commissioners that grouped the pairs into 17 categories of health problems ranging from acute, potentially fatal conditions that could be treated to restore full function to conditions that were unaffected by current treatment. There were categories for conditions that were self-limited and for which treatment was unnecessary and categories for preventive care. Commissioners used their expert panels, literature reviews, and their own clinical judgment to assign all diagnosis–treatment pairs to 1 of 17 categories. Each item was further ranked ". . . according to 13 criteria including life expectancy, quality of life, the cost effectiveness of a treatment, and whether it would benefit many people. Treatments that prevent death and lead to full recovery were ranked first, maternity care was ranked second, and treatments that prevent death without full recovery were ranked third. Treatments that result in minimal or no improvement in the quality of life were ranked last. The diagnosis and treatment items were then prioritized within the categories on the basis of outcomes data, a scale for the quality of well-being, and a consideration of the reasonableness of the rankings'' (1, p. xxx).

The Medicaid program required a waiver of some of its rules for the implementation of the OHP. The prioritized list was submitted to the HCFA in 1991 for such a waiver but was rejected in the following year as violating sections of the Americans With Disabilities Act. The objectionable part of the process to President Bush's administration was the use of measures of ''quality of life'' by nondisabled persons in judging the ability of a treatment to restore an individual to his or her prior state. The opinion said that such valuations on their face discriminated against disabled individuals who might have different views of their physical state than nondisabled persons. Denying them a particular therapy on the grounds that it might not lead to a full restoration to ''normal'' could be discriminatory (1).

The state had no practical recourse but to reexamine the prioritized list, which it did in the next few months, simplifying its methodology to avoid any consideration of quality of life before or after treatment. The only factors considered were as follows: (a) The condition–treatment pairs were ranked according to the likelihood that treatment would prevent death, (b) those remaining condition–treatment pairs whose treatments have an equivalent ability to prevent death or whose conditions have no risk of mortality were rank ordered by the average lifetime cost of treatment, from the least expensive to the most expensive, and (c) any condition–treatment pairs not separable by both of these measurements were sorted alphabetically by diagnosis (11).

The Commission then reviewed the initial sort line by line to determine whether the data resulted in an appropriate relative ranking of the line item. It was at this point that the subjective criteria (*Table 17.2*) came into play. These val-

TABLE 17.2
Subjective Criteria in Development of the Oregon Health Plan

Criteria	Description
General preventive services	This judgment determines the placement of three lines: children, adult, and dental preventive services.
Comfort care	This judgment determines the placement of one line.
Maternity care	This judgment considers the placement of services required from conception through the first 28 days of life. Examples are pregnancy care and neonatal services.
Family planning services	This judgment determines the placement of services for preventing pregnancy or planning families. There were four lines involved and this is a high priority for the federal government.
Prevent a condition before treatment	This judgment considers the importance of interceding early in the process before the condition develops. An example is placing the treatment for dysplasia of the cervix before the treatment of cervical cancer.
Medical ineffectiveness	This judgment considers the fact that the specified treatment for the condition does not achieve its objective in the majority of the cases. An example is the dental services that provide only marginal improvement.
Prevent additional complications	This judgment considers the importance of interceding to stabilize or to prevent deterioration of a condition. An example is the treatment of glaucoma.
Prevent future costs	This judgment considers the importance of interceding early before resources must be spent in crisis. An example is the treatment of insulin-dependent diabetes.
Cosmetic services	This judgment reflects the fact that cosmetic services are not a covered benefit for Medicaid in Oregon.
Self-limiting conditions	This judgment considers the fact that these conditions will run their course without, or in spite of, medical intervention. An example is the treatment of acute upper respiratory infections.
Congruent conditions	This judgment considers the fact that the organ system and/or etiology of the conditions are similar to that of another condition/treatment pair elsewhere on the list or that the outcomes of the condition/treatment pairs are congruent.
Public health risk	This judgment reflected the fact that prevention of communicable diseases is a high priority for the state and federal government. An example is the treatment of syphilis.

ues had been developed at the public meetings, forums, and surveys described above. In a process they labeled "hand adjustment," the Commissioners moved a few lines that appeared out of their logical position, using their own medical judgment and their interpretation of the values elicited from the state's citizens. When completed in 1992, the new prioritized list looked essentially like the previously rejected 1991 list. A change in administrations in Washington, DC, occurred after the election of 1992, and the new Secretary of Health and Human Services approved the waiver and allowed the OHP to enroll its first member in early 1994. Over 100,000 individuals enrolled in the first year, boosting the Medicaid rolls from 250,000 to nearly 370,000 at their peak.

THE PRIORITIZED LIST

The prioritized list has been issued every two years, most recently in 1999 (15). It initially consisted of 743 lines, each 1 of which included one or more International Classification of Disease—Ninth Revision—Clinical Modification (ICD-9-CM) diagnoses and accompanying treatments listed for each line by Current Procedural Terminology—Fourth Edition (CPT-4) codes. When there was more than one ICD-9-CM code, they were grouped by logical medical categories and identified by a single phrase to capture the sense of that line. The CPT-4 codes that identi-

fied the particular treatments available for that diagnosis were meant to identify all the treatment that could be used for that particular condition. Diagnostic maneuvers of any type were not included in the prioritized list, as they were and are still routinely covered by Medicaid. Thus, physicians seeking a diagnosis are routinely reimbursed for any tests they may order in that search.

The items presented in the accompanying tables are from the most recent iteration of the prioritized list (1999). There have been a few changes in the list as noted below, but there has been no change in its basic structure and very little change in the order of diagnoses and their treatments since its first implemented version in 1994. *Tables 17.3, 17.4, and 17.5* are abstracted from the prioritized list. The short diagnostic description typically includes more than one ICD-9-CM code but is described here by a shorter description for ease of reference. Similarly, medical and/or surgical treatment may involve many CPT-4 codes and are too numerous to display here. *Table 17.3* lists the first 15 lines, *Table 17.4* lists the 15 lines just above the funded area that ends at line 578, and *Table 17.5* lists the bottom 15 lines. The governor's current proposal includes a request to HCFA to move the funded line up to line 567 or 568. Such a move would leave everything below this point unfunded.

TABLE 17.3
Prioritized List for the Oregon Health Plan, Lines 1–15

Line	Diagnosis	Treatment
1	Severe/moderate head injury	Medical and surgical
2	Insulin-dependent diabetes mellitus	Medical
3	Peritonitis	Medical and surgical
4	Acute glomerolunephritis	Medical, including dialysis
5	Pneumothorax and hemothorax	Tube thoracostomy/thoracotomy, medical
6	Hernia w/obstruction	Surgical
7	Addison's disease	Medical
8	Flail chest	Medical and surgical
9	Appendicitis	Appendectomy
10	Ruptured spleen	Repair/splenectomy
11	Tuberculosis	Medical
12	Deep open wound of neck	Repair
13	Croup, epiglotitis	Medical, intubation, tracheostomy
14	Pneumococcal pneumonia	Medical
15	Whooping cough	Medical

Note. See text for details.

such entities. Dental services have been offered to OHP members since 1994 when the initial enrollment began.

In the first year of operation, Medicaid enrollment grew by over 100,000 members, expanding the number of Oregon residents receiving medical care under this program by nearly 40%. From 1990 to 1996, the proportion of Oregon residents without health insurance fell from 18% to 11% (13). This was a time of excellent growth for the entire economy of Oregon—a time for significant job creation and economic prosperity. In the last two years, however, the economy has cooled perceptibly and the number of Oregon residents on the OHP has declined by a few percentage points. The causes of this decline are much debated, as the mandate to enroll all individuals below the FPL remains. Some critics blame the legislature, which cut appropriated funds to the OHP, which led OMAP, the administrator of the program, to institute a number of cost-saving measures, including stricter eligibility rulings (e.g., a three-month period of low income rather than the previously mandated single-month period), restriction of coverage for some college students, and premiums of $6–$28 monthly depending on income and family size.

Others have pointed to the rising economy and the greater number of employed citizens who earn more than the FPL. This has been further confounded by Oregon's enactment of a minimum wage that is significantly higher than the federal minimum wage. Paradoxically, such a situation allows Oregon residents to earn more money but lifts them above the FPL and out of Medicaid health insurance. The Employer Mandate legislation of 1989–1990 would have addressed this population; however, the lack of a federal ERISA waiver caused the law to expire without implementation on January 2, 1996.

New programs from HCFA have further confused the situation to the point that it has become difficult to disentangle the effect of federal programs on the rates of the uninsured from the effects of the OHP. An example of this is CHIP, which mandates state coverage, and a big federal match, for the enrollment of poor children in a categorical program meant expressly for them. This program has probably significantly contributed to a decline in the number of children lacking health insurance to not more than 8%. Yet in many other states, enrollment in this program has been considerably less than projected, perhaps because of the significant state contribution required or because of other unrealized factors (2,3).

When the legislature initially passed the OHP, they assumed that they would have some autonomy from federal oversight and some responsibility for OHP structure and function. The basic idea of OHP operation was embodied in the idea of a moveable funding line. The prioritized list ordered health services in such a way that the BHCP was located well within the funded services, perhaps within the first 350–400 lines. Indeed, there has been little disagreement about the value of diagnoses and treatments in that area of the list and probably for another 100 lines either in Oregon or in other evaluations (17). Likewise, there has been little disagreement about services that fall at the bottom of the list. The debates, as they should, have concerned items in the middle, perhaps from lines 500 to 650, where there was demand for service, much of which could be considered elective treatment, if funds were available. The full implementation of the prioritized list required that the funding line could be moved at the discretion of the legislature in response to exigencies of the state budget. Thus, in prosperous times, more diagnoses and treatments could be funded, and in tight times, fewer could be funded. But at all times the BHCP was deemed safe, as it resided well up the list.

Two years after the implementation, in response to a perceived shortage of state funds, the line was moved from 606 to 581. In 1997, Oregon requested that the line be moved to 574, but HCFA only allowed a move to 578 and stated that they believed significant compromises in care of the Medicaid members were threatened by any further restriction of benefits. HCFA administrators have stated that they will not allow further moves to the line though the governor has proposed a further 10-line move in his most recent budget proposal. Legislators have reacted angrily to HCFA's veto of line movement, as they see a lack of cooperation in implementation of OHP rules from their federal partners. HCFA, for its part, sees the OHP as an experiment and is entirely willing to exercise its authority if it perceives any compromise of medical care for Medicaid members (10).

In this setting, legislators have reverted to the same remedies as used in other states, limiting access to Medicaid and restricting enrollment in the program so as to limit their expenses. Needless to say, this runs counter to the underlying philosophy of the OHP but may be the only remedy available to them. There has been much negotiation and conversation between the legislature, OMAP and the Health Services Commission about this situation in a continuing dialogue.

CONCLUSION

Medicaid, and health care for poor persons in general, has become an intensely political process. New designs of health care delivery like the OHP must meet the reality of funding by state legislatures and the forces of the intensely competitive and complex medical marketplace. Every design, whether novel or traditional, must develop a constituency and work effectively in the public arena. Fortunately, the OHP continues to experience high levels of customer satisfaction, a great deal of public good will, and grudging acceptance by the medical community as a better way to care for poor individuals. Explicit priority setting is new in the United States. It replaces the older practice of implicit, hidden priority setting by the medical and insurance community that restricted access to care for many, that forced the insured to pay for the uninsured without admitting that it was doing so, and that was unsatisfactory to both the patient and the provider communities. The very public process used in the development of the OHP in a series of meetings and the implementation of the OHP served to clear the air about many of these issues, clarified the debate, and helped to develop a program that has delivered decent medical care to a large fraction of poor persons in the state.

REFERENCES

1. Bodenheimer T: The Oregon Health Plan—Lessons for the nation, *N England J Med* 337:651–655,720–723, 1997.
2. "Child Health Plan Enrollment Lags." *Montgomery Advertiser*, p. xx, May 1, 1998.
3. "Child Health Program Gets Off to Slow Start." *The Washington Post*, pp. xx, xx, April 13, 1999.
4. Daniels N: Is the Oregon rationing plan fair? *JAMA* 1991,265:2232–2235.
5. Garland MJ: Justice, politics and community: Expanding access and rationing health services in Oregon. *Law, Medicine Health Care*, 20:67–80, 1992.
6. Golenski JD, Thompson SM: A history of Oregon's Basic Health Services Act: An insider's account. *QRB* XX;:144–149, 1991.
7. Health Care Financing Administration: Web site: *http://www.hcfa.gov*.
8. Health Care Financing Administration: Web site: *http://www.hcfa.gov/medicaid*.
9. Health Care Financing Administration: Web site: *http://www.hcfa.gov/medicaid*/ormedmed.htm.
10. Health Care Financing Administration: Letter to OMAP, 1998.
11. Kaplan RM: Value judgment in the Oregon Medicaid experiment, *Med Care* 32:975–988, 19xx.
12. Kaplan RM, Anderson JP: A general health policy model: Update and applications. *Health Services Res* 23:203–235, 1988.
13. Office for Oregon Health Plan Policy and Research: Effects of the Oregon Health Plan: A report prepared by the Office for Oregon Health Plan Policy and Research, City, OR, 1998.
14. Oregon Health Services Commission, Prioritization of Health Services: A Report to the Governor and the Legislature, Salem, OR, 1991.
15. Oregon Health Services Commission, Prioritization of Health Services: A Report to the Governor and the Legislature, Salem, OR, 1999.
16. Oregon state Senate, Senate Bill 27.
17. Last name, XX: Acceptability of Oregon prioritization list among Finnish medical doctors, Ryynanen O-P, 2nd International Conference on Priorities in Health Care, London, October 8–10, 1998.

CHAPTER 18

Quantifying Neurosurgical Outcomes: How Do We Measure the Effectiveness in Cost-Effectiveness Analysis?

JOSEPH T. KING, JR., M.D., M.S.C.E.

The comparison of medical treatments based on economic efficiency is an inescapable reality of modern medical practice. Although the tabulation of treatment costs can often be straight forward, the determination of treatment effectiveness is more elusive. Because simple outcome measures, such as survival, are inadequate for use in sophisticated economic analysis, more in-depth techniques have been developed to quantify outcome measures. Dr. King describes several techniques that are used to determine utility in medical treatment outcomes. Both the theoretical basis, as well as methodology, is explained, providing a valuable resource for the clinician to better understand the increasing number of cost-effectiveness studies in the medical literature.

Quantification of outcomes for any medical intervention, including neurosurgery, is a difficult and elusive problem. Considerable effort has been expended in this area, because quantified outcomes are increasingly in demand by patients, physicians, hospitals, third party payors, and the government. One powerful application of quantified outcomes data is cost-effectiveness analysis. Cost-effectiveness analysis combines clinical and economic outcomes into a unified metric, the cost-effectiveness ratio (10). The cost-effectiveness ratio can be used to inform patient, physician, hospital, third party payor, and societal decision-making. This chapter will focus on the quantification of clinical outcomes for use in cost-effectiveness analysis.

MEASURING OUTCOMES IN COST-EFFECTIVENESS ANALYSIS

A variety of clinical outcomes measures have been used in cost-effectiveness analyses. These include survival [e.g., ''life years'' or ''years of life saved'' (YOLS) (7, 19, 31, 38)], survival with good or bad vision [i.e., ''sight years'' (8)], survival with visual impairment [i.e., ''quality-adjusted years of vision'' (20)], and duration and quality of survival [i.e., ''quality-adjusted life years'' (6, 9, 13, 28–30, 42, 54, 55)]. The use of survival as an outcomes measure, expressed as life years or YOLS, has a certain appeal. It is readily understood, easily measured, and a prerequisite for more sophisticated assessments. Unfortunately, analyses that use only length of survival fail to incorporate patient quality of life. This is particularly problematic in neurosurgery, where neurosurgical diseases and treatments often impact significantly on patient quality of life. Consistent with this realization, most contemporary cost-effectiveness analyses incorporate patient quality of life. Of note, the Public Health Service (PHS) Panel on Cost-effectiveness in Health and Medicine recommends the incorporation of patient quality of life in cost-effectiveness analyses (18).

Measuring Quality of Life

The methodology of cost-effectiveness analysis requires valuations of health states on a standardized scale. The valuations must be derived from patient preferences and they should be measured on an interval scale. The interval scale should range from 0.0 (the value of death) to 1.0 (the value of optimal health) (18). Techniques have also been developed for measuring the utility of states worse than death (34). Most popular quality of life measurement instruments do not meet these requirements, and thus cannot be used in cost-effectiveness analyses. These instruments have the virtue of ease of administration–they are usually paper and pencil questionnaires that can be self-administered by patients. For example, the Medical Outcomes Study Short-Form General Health Survey (SF-36) is a generic 36 item patient-completed questionnaire that can be used in patients with any disease (43, 53). The SF-36 measures patient well being in each of eight domains: physical functioning, role functioning, bodily pain, general health, vitality, social functioning, role emotional, and mental health. The SF-36 has been validated across numerous diseases and is sensitive to changes in disease status. In neurosurgical and neurological diseases, the SF-36 has been applied to stroke (2), back problems (43), lumbar laminectomy (1), and hyperhidrosis (37). Unfortunately, the SF-36 cannot be used in cost-effectiveness analyses. The instrument does not produce a single quality of life value with interval scaling bounded by death = 0.0 and optimal health = 1.0.

Generic quality of life measurements (e.g., SF-36) can be used to measure quality of life in any health state. These instruments may not accurately measure quality of life in some disease states or may fail to document when there is a change in disease status. Several disease-specific quality of life instruments have been developed to address these difficulties. One such instrument is the Epilepsy Surgery Inventory (ESI)-55, which was developed to assess epilepsy surgery patients (51). The ESI-55 measures patient quality of life in 11 domains: health perceptions, energy, overall quality of life, social function, emotional well-being, cognitive function, physical function, pain, emotional role limitations, physical role limitations, and memory-related role limitations. Similar to the SF-36, the ESI-55 does not produce an interval scaled quality of life value bounded by death = 0.0 and optimal health = 1.0. Thus, it cannot be used to measure patient preferences for use in cost-effectiveness analyses.

Researchers have developed several methods for measuring quality of life that have the characteristics required for cost-effectiveness analyses. These methods allow the determination of the value of health states by measuring patient preferences for the health states. Patient preferences are also known as utilities. In distinction to its use in the philosophy of utilitarianism, economists and quality of life researchers define utility as the strength of an individual's preference (47). The concept of utility is derived from modern economic utility theory formulated by Von Neumann and Morgenstern (52). Economic utility theory and psychological scaling methods are the two theoretical traditions from which spring the three methods that are commonly used to measure preferences for health states: (a) the standard gamble, (b) the time trade-off, and (c) rating scales. The standard gamble and time trade-off are implicit techniques that are derived from expected utility theory; they ask the subject to perform certain tasks and infer utility based on the results. Rating scales are direct techniques based on psychological scaling methods; they ask the subject to directly value health states. A more complex method, multiattribute utility theory, applies these measurement techniques to derive the utilities for a wide array of health states in generic preference-weighted health state classification systems (27).

Standard Gamble

Von Neumann and Morgenstern (52) first described the standard gamble as a means of measuring utility. The standard gamble is considered by many investigators to be the gold standard for assessing patient preferences. The standard gamble involves asking subjects to make quantitative decisions based on consideration of a health state and then calculates the utility for the health state. The health state may be one that the subject is experiencing presently (e.g., a stroke patient may be asked to make decisions based on their present stroke symptoms). The health state may be one with which the subject is familiar (e.g., the spouse of a stroke patient may be tested on stroke health states). Alternatively, naïve subjects may be tested on health states that are detailed in a written scenario. The scenario describes several attributes of the health state. These scenarios are developed after consultation with health providers, patients with the diseases, and caretakers (21).

Whether the subject is aware of the particulars of the health state from direct experience (e.g., stroke patient), close familiarity (e.g., stroke patient spouse, health care provider), or a written health state scenario, the testing protocol is the same. The subject is asked to consider a hypothetical choice between two options: (a) continuing in the less-than-perfect health state that is under consideration with certainty, or (b) accepting the results of a gamble. Losing the gamble results in immediate death, whereas winning the gamble immediately restores the subject to optimal health. The choice contrasts the certainty of a less than perfect state (e.g., major stroke) to the uncertainty of either optimal health or death. A sample scenario for major stroke from the work of Gage et al. (17) is presented in Figure 18.1. We use the stroke scenario to illustrate administering the standard gamble and calculating the utility for a health state. Table 18.1 details how the probability of winning the gamble is systematically varied until the respondent cannot choose between the certainty of continuing life with a neurologic deficit (stroke health state) and the gamble between death and optimal health.

This point of indifference is then used to calculate the utility of the stroke health state. At the indifference point, the patient cannot choose between the health state and the gamble because they are of equal value. The value of the gamble can be determined by calculating the expected value. The expected value is calculated by summing the products of the probability of each outcome and its corresponding value. In the stroke example, a gamble with a 30% chance of dying and a 70% chance of living with optimal health has an expected value of 0.70 (recall that the value for death = 0.0 and the value of optimal health = 1.0). The details of the calculation follow:

$$
\begin{aligned}
\text{Expected} &= (\text{probability of death} \\
\text{value} &\quad \times \text{ value of death}) \\
&\quad + (\text{probability of optimal health} \\
&\quad \times \text{ value of optimal health}) \\
&= (0.30 \times 0.00) + (0.70 \times 1.00) \\
&= (0.00) + (0.70) \\
&= 0.70
\end{aligned}
$$

Thus, the utility for major stroke as measured in this patient is 0.70.

Visual aids, such as a color probability wheel, have been used to assist patients in their considerations of probability (46). With the availability of personal computers with powerful graphics capabilities, dedicated software can be used to administer the standard gamble (e.g., U-Maker, Frank Sonenberg, © 1992). These programs provide a depiction of the gamble using graphics. During testing, as the gamble probabilities are varied, the graphic changes to represent the different probabilities of winning the gamble. Once the subject has reached an indifference point, the software calculates the utility as detailed above.

Time Trade-Off

The time trade-off method was developed as an alternative to the standard gamble (50). The

The right side of your body is totally limp (paralyzed from the stroke);

the right side of your face droops

- You cannot bathe or get dressed without help

- You cannot walk at all; you spend all of your time either in bed or in a wheelchair

- You can feed yourself with difficulty

- You can think clearly

- You find it hard to write

- Your speech is slurred and some people cannot understand what you are saying

- You can have sex, but with some difficulty

Figure 18.1   Sample of a written health state scenario for major stroke from Gage et al. (17) describing the impact of the health state on various daily activities.

TABLE 18.1
Sample Stroke Health State Utility Measurement Using the Standard Gamble

Standard Gamble Probability Presented to Subject	Subject Preference: Stroke Health State or Results of Standard Gamble	Comments
100% chance of death, 0% chance of optimal health	Stroke	Subject prefers stroke health state when the outcome of the gamble is certain death.
0% chance of death, 100% chance of optimal health	Standard Gamble	Subject prefers gamble with a 100% chance of optimal health to the stroke health state.
50% chance of death, 50% chance of optimal health	Stroke	Subject is unwilling to risk 50% chance of death for 50% chance of optimal health. Subject prefers to live in the stroke health state.
10% chance of death, 90% chance of optimal health	Standard Gamble	Subject is willing to risk 10% chance of death for 90% chance of optimal health. Subject prefers this uncertain outcome to the certainty of continuing to live in the stroke health state.
40% chance of death, 60% chance of optimal health	Stroke	Subject is unwilling to risk 40% chance of death for 60% chance of optimal health. Subject prefers to live in the stroke health state.
20% chance of death, 80% chance of optimal health	Standard Gamble	Subject is willing to risk 20% chance of death for 80% chance of optimal health. Subject prefers this uncertain outcome to the certainty of continuing to live in the stroke health state.
30% chance of death, 70% chance of optimal health	Unable to choose (i.e., indifferent)	Subject cannot choose between the gamble and the stroke health state. Both options have equal value. The value of the stroke health state is calculated at 0.70.

standard gamble requires subjects to choose between suboptimal quality of life and a chance for death or optimal health. The time trade-off requires subjects to exchange years of life for optimal health. Some patients find the time trade-off easier to understand and perform than the standard gamble. As with the standard gamble, subjects are asked to make hypothetical decisions based on the consideration of a health state. The subject may be living in the health state (e.g., stroke patient), familiar with the health state (e.g., stroke patient spouse), or naïve to the health state (e.g., written scenario).

Subjects are provided with an estimate of their life expectancy based on their age and the health state under consideration. After considering the health state, the subject is offered the option of immediate optimal health in exchange for a reduced life expectancy. The respondent must choose between continuing the remainder of their life in the health state under study or accepting a shorter life span and restored to optimal health. In effect, they are deciding on a trade-off between *quantity of life* and *quality of life*. Visual aids are used to depict the choice (46). The decreased life span is varied systematically until the subject is indifferent between a full life span in the suboptimal health state under study and a decreased life span in perfect health

(Table 18.2). Utility is then calculated by dividing the duration of optimal health by the full life span in the health state under study. For example, a subject with a 20-year life expectancy is willing to trade-off 6 years of life in exchange for immediate optimal health. The utility is calculated as follows:

$$\begin{aligned} \text{Utility} &= (\text{duration of optimal health})/ \\ &\quad (\text{life expectancy}) \\ &= (\text{life expectancy} - \text{no. of yr willing} \\ &\quad \text{to trade-off})/(\text{life expectancy}) \\ &= (20 \text{ yr} - 6 \text{ yr})/(20 \text{ yr}) \\ &= (14 \text{ yr})/(20 \text{ yr}) \\ &= 0.70 \end{aligned}$$

Rating Scales

Rating scale techniques are derived from the psychophysical tradition of measuring preference (44). The two most commonly used methods are the visual analogue scale and categorical scaling. For the visual analogue method, the subject is presented with a linear scale that is anchored at one end by 0, which represents death, and at the other end by 1, which represents optimal health (Fig. 18.2). The subject indicates the value of the health state under consideration by selecting a point on the line that corresponds to the quality of life associated with the health state. Often the scale is printed on paper, and the

TABLE 18.2
Sample Stroke Health State Utility Measurement Using the Time Trade-Off

Years of Life Expectancy Traded for Optimal Health (baseline life expectancy = 20 years)	Subject Preference: Time Trade-off versus Continuing in Stroke State	Comments
19 years, 364 days (19.997 years)	Stroke	Subject prefers the stroke health state for 20 years rather than trade-off all of their remaining life span, except 1 day, in exchange for 1 day of optimal health, followed by death.
1 day (0.003 years)	Time Trade-off	Subject will trade-off 1 day of life expectancy in the stroke state in exchange for optimal health for 19 years, 364 days, followed by death.
10 years	Stroke	Subject is unwilling to trade-off 10 years of their remaining 20-year life span in the stroke state in exchange for optimal health for 10 years, followed by death.
2 years	Time Trade-off	Subject will trade-off 2 years of their 20-year life expectancy in the stroke state in exchange for optimal health for 18 years, followed by death.
8 years	Stroke	Subject is unwilling to trade-off 8 years of their remaining 20-year life span in the stroke state in exchange for optimal health for 12 years, followed by death.
4 years	Time Trade-off	Subject will trade-off 4 years of their remaining 20-year life span in the stroke state in exchange for optimal health for 16 years, followed by death.
6 years	Unable to choose (i.e., indifferent)	Subject cannot choose between living 20 years with the stroke and trading 6 years of their 20-year life expectancy in exchange for optimal health for 14 years, followed by death. Both options have equal value. The value of the stroke health is calculated at 0.70.

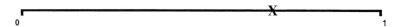

Figure 18.2   Visual analogue scale used to measure utility. One extreme of the scale is labeled 0, which corresponds to the value of death. The opposite end of the scale is labeled 1, which corresponds to optimal health. The subject undergoing utility testing is instructed to place a mark on the scale that corresponds to their preference for the health state under consideration. X represents the mark. Measuring the location of the mark in relation to the end points provides the utility value for the health state. In this example, the value for the health state is 0.70.

subject conveys a valuation by placing a written mark on the scale. Multiple health states can be rated on the same scale by making unique marks for each state. Alternatively, visual aids, such as a feeling thermometer felt board with movable pointers, can be used (48). Utility is determined by direct measurement of the mark in relationship to the endpoints of 0 and 1.

Categorical scaling is a variation of this method, in which the scale is divided into multiple equal segments, one of which must be chosen for the valuation (Fig. 18.3). A line is divided into 11 equal segments labeled from 0 to 10. The subject expresses their valuation of the health state that is under consideration by placing a mark in one of the 11 categories on the

scale. The integer value that corresponds to the selected category is divided by 10 to convert the valuation to a standardized utility valuation ranging from 0.0 to 1.0.

Multiattribute Utility Assessment

Multiattribute utility theory, an extension of von Neumann-Morgenstern utility theory, allows the calculation of utilities for health states as a function of each of the utilities of several attributes considered individually (27). Each health state can be defined in terms of several attributes, the utilities of which can be assessed by the measurement techniques that are described above. These values are combined using a function to arrive at a utility for each of the

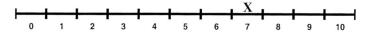

Figure 18.3 Category scale used to measure utility. The scale is divided into 11 categories, ranging from 0 (death) to 10 (optimal health). The subject undergoing utility testing is instructed to place a mark in one of the 11 categories that corresponds to their preference for the health state under consideration. X represents the mark. The value of the category is divided by 10, which converts the valuation to a standardized utility score. In this example, the value for the health state is 0.70.

specific health states. The technique allows the determination of the utility of a large number of health states without having to measure the utility of each state. The challenge is in determining the appropriate mathematical function for combining the utilities from a small number of constituent attributes. Several generic preference-weighted health state classifications systems have been developed by using the tenets of multiattribute utility theory, including the EuroQol (12), the Health Utilities Index (HUI:3) (14), the Quality of Life and Health Questionnaire (QLHQ) (22), and the Quality of Well-Being Scale (QWB) (26).

WHICH MEASUREMENT TECHNIQUE IS BEST?

Convincing arguments have been made on behalf of each of the techniques that are described above. The standard gamble is firmly grounded in utility theory, and many consider it the gold standard for utility measurement. In addition, it may be particularly suited to health states that involve surgical treatment. Proponents argue that the standard gamble reflects actual decisions patients make when considering surgical interventions, where uncertain outcomes of the intervention (i.e., cure and death) are weighed against the current health state (4, 15, 49). Critics of this view argue that the standard gamble does not reflect actual health-related decisions, because there are often outcomes other than death or optimal health that may result from interventions, such as disability (35). Another criticism of the standard gamble is that patients can find it difficult to understand and implement decisions based on chance and probability (45). In addition, most patients are risk adverse and will go to great lengths to avoid a chance of death (25). This results in higher values for utilities that are measured with the standard gamble compared with other techniques.

The time trade-off is not without its critics. It lacks the theoretical foundation of the standard gamble, and the time trade-off has been criticized for confounding preferences for health states with preference for time (24). Rating scales are easy to administer and readily understood by subjects, but their results are not as reliable or valid as the standard gamble or the time trade-off. The PHS Panel on Cost-effectiveness in Health and Medicine notes the ongoing controversy regarding selecting the most appropriate utility measurement method and recommends choosing the approach that most closely resembles the clinical problem (18). In studies of neurosurgical diseases or interventions where there is inherent risk to the patient from both the disease and the treatment, the standard gamble is probably the preferred methodology, with the time trade-off a reasonable alternative.

WHOSE PREFERENCES SHOULD BE MEASURED?

Values that are obtained for health states depend on the population in which they are measured. In general, individuals more familiar with a health state will give higher values than naïve individuals. The appropriate population in which to measure preferences is a matter of some debate. Investigators have used patients who are experienced with the health state that is under investigation, patient surrogates, health professionals, and members of the community. Differences in utilities associated with a health state are often seen when different populations are used to assess preferences (5, 11, 32, 36, 40). For example, Boyd et al. (5) used the standard gamble, category rating, and a questionnaire to measure utilities for colostomy in rectal cancer patients with colostomies, surgeons and oncologists, rectal cancer patients without colostomies, and healthy volunteers. Utility values were inversely proportional to the subject's familiarity with colostomies. The highest utility values were measured in patients with colostomies, followed by physicians; patients without colostomies had the lowest values.

The appropriate population to measure utility depends on the perspective of the cost-effectiveness analysis. Most utility data published on neurosurgical or neurological disease has been measured in either effected patients or in populations at risk for the disease. These include utilities for stroke in patients with atrial fibrillation (16, 17), arteriovenous malformations (39), suspected carotid artery disease (41), a history of thrombophlebitis (33), and in general medical patients (33). Stroke utilities have also been measured in health care providers (3). The PHS Panel on Cost-Effectiveness in Health and Medicine recommends that a societal perspective is most appropriate when making policy decisions about resource allocation (18). Based on this recommendation, a cost-effectiveness analysis from the societal perspective should be based on utility values that are derived from an informed cross section of the general public. None of the utility measurements on neurosurgical disease published to date meet this criterion. An analysis from the perspective of the patient might reasonably use the utilities measured in actual patients. The correct answer to the ''whose preferences?'' question depends on the perspective of the cost-effectiveness analysis, which in turn is determined by the questioner.

APPLICATION OF UTILITY MEASUREMENT TECHNIQUES IN NEUROSURGERY

Among neurosurgical disease states, cerebrovascular disease has attracted virtually all of the utility measurement research. Although this body of work is impressive, the balance of neurosurgical and neurological diseases have received little or no scrutiny by investigators interested in measuring patient preferences. Shin et al. (39) used the standard gamble to measure utilities for major and minor strokes in cerebral arteriovenous malformation patients. Sixty-one percent of patients had permanent deficits from prior strokes. The patients were presented with scenarios that described a major stroke (dominant hemiplegia) and a minor stroke (dominant arm and hand numbness). The mean utility was 0.45 for major stoke and 0.81 for minor stroke. O'Meara et al. (33) used the standard gamble to measure preference in general medical patients. Major stroke had a utility of 0.29 in this population. Gage et al. (16) used the time trade-off to

measure utility in patients with atrial fibrillation at risk for stroke. The mean utility was 0.39 for major stroke and 0.75 for minor stroke. In a second study that employed both the standard gamble and the time trade-off (17), major stroke had a value of 0.0, moderate stroke was 0.07, and mild stroke was 0.94. Solomon et al. (41) used rating scales to measure utilities for patients without stroke. The mean utility was 0.36 for major stroke and 0.92 for minor stroke. Aoki et al. (3) used the standard gamble to measure utilities associated with health states that are defined in a modified Glasgow Outcome Scale (23). The investigators assessed utilities by using the standard gamble in Japanese health care providers–utilities for various stroke states ranged from 0.08 to 0.85.

CONCLUSIONS

Cost-effectiveness analysis requires the measurement of patient quality of life outcomes. A variety of techniques have been developed for the quantification of quality of life. Three of these techniques are capable of generating quality of life measurements that can be incorporated into cost-effectiveness analyses: the standard gamble, the time trade-off, and rating scales. The standard gamble may be the most appropriate technique for neurosurgical investigations. Researchers are beginning to apply these methodologies to neurosurgical and neurological diseases, particularly cerebrovascular disease. The growing demand from patients, physicians, hospitals, third party payors, and the government for quantitative outcomes will require the measurement of patient preferences across the broad spectrum of neurosurgical and neurological diseases.

REFERENCES

1. Albert TJ, Mesa JJ, Eng K, McIntosh TC, Balderston RA: Health outcome assessment before and after lumbar laminectomy for radiculopathy. *Spine* 21: 960–962, 1996.
2. Anderson C, Laubscher S, Burns R: Validation of the short form 36 (SF-36) health survey questionnaire among stroke patients. *Stroke* 27:1812–1816, 1996.
3. Aoki N, Kitahara T, Fukui T, et al: Management of unruptured intracranial aneurysms in Japan: A Markovian decision analysis with utility measurements based on Glasgow Outcome Scale. *Med Decis Making* 18:357–364, 1998.
4. Ben-Zion U, Gafni A: Evaluation of public investment in health care. Is risk irrelevant? *J Health Econ* 2: 161–165, 1983.

5. Boyd NF, Sutherland HJ, Heasman KZ, Tritchler DL, Cummings BJ: Whose utilities for decision analysis? *Med Decis Making* 10:67, 1990.

6. Chang RW, Pellissier JM, Hazen GB: A cost-effectiveness analysis of total hip arthroplasty for osteoarthritis of the hip. *JAMA* 275:858–865, 1996.

7. Curchill DN, Lemon BC, Torrance GW: A cost-effectiveness analysis of continuous ambulatory peritoneal dialysis and hospital hemodialysis. *Med Decis Making* 4:489–500, 1984.

8. Dasbach E, Fryback DG, Newcomb PA, Klein R, Klein BEK: Cost-effectiveness of strategies for detecting diabetic retinopathy. *Med Care* 29:20–39, 1991.

9. Derdeyn CP, Powers WJ: Cost-effectiveness of screening for asymptomatic carotid atherosclerotic disease. *Stroke* 27:1944–1950, 1996.

10. Drummond MF, Stoddard GL, Torrance GW: *Methods for the Economic Evaluation of Health Care Programmes*. Oxford, Oxford University Press, 1987.

11. Epstein AM, Hall JA, Tognetti J, Son LH, Conant L: Using proxies to evaluate quality of life. *Med Care* 27[suppl]:S91–S98, 1989.

12. Essink-Bot ML, Stouthard ME, Bonsel GJ: Generalizability of valuations on health states collected with EuroQol questionnaire. *Health Econ* 2:237–246, 1993.

13. Etchason J, Petz L, Keeler E, et al: The cost-effectiveness of preoperative autologous blood donations. *N Eng J Med* 332:719–724, 1995.

14. Feeny D, Furlong W, Boyle M, Torrance GW: Multi-attribute health status classification systems: Health utilities index. *PharmacoEconomics* 7:490–502, 1995.

15. Gafni A, Birch S: Preferences for outcomes in economic evaluation: An economic approach to addressing economic problems. *J Health Econ* 11:325–339, 1995.

16. Gage BF, Cardinalli AB, Albers GW, Owens DK: Cost-effectiveness of warfarin and aspirin for prophylaxis of stroke in patients with nonvalvular atrial fibrillation. *JAMA* 274:1839–1845, 1995.

17. Gage BF, Cardinalli AB, Owens DK: The effect of stroke and stroke prophylaxis with aspirin or warfarin on quality of life. *Arch Intern Med* 156:1829–1836, 1996.

18. Gold MR, Siegel JE, Russell LB, Weinstein MC: *Cost-effectiveness in Health and Medicine*. New York, Oxford University Press, 1996.

19. Goldman L: Cost-effectiveness perspectives in coronary heart disease. *Am Heart J* 119:733–740, 1990.

20. Gottlieb LK, Schwartz B, Pauker SG: Glaucoma screening: A cost-effectiveness analysis. *Surv Ophthalmol* 28:206–226, 1983.

21. Groome PA, Hutchinson TA, Tousignant P: Content of a decision analysis for treatment choice in end-stage renal disease: Who should be consulted? *Med Decis Making* 14:91–97, 1994.

22. Hadorn DC, Sorenson J, Holte J: Large-scale outcome evaluation: How should quality of life be measured? Part II: Questionnaire validation in a cohort of patients with advanced cancer. *J Clin Epidemiol* 48:619–629, 1995.

23. Jennett B, Bond M: Assessment of outcome after severe brain damage: A practical scale. *Lancet* 1:480–484, 1975.

24. Johannesson M, Pliskin JS, Weinstein MC: A note on QALYs, time tradeoff, and discounting. *Med Decis Making* 14:188–193, 1994.

25. Kahneman D, Tversky A: Choices, values, and frames. *Am Psychol* 39:341–350, 1983.

26. Kaplan RM, Anderson JP: A general health policy model: Update and applications. *Health Serv Res* 23:203–235, 1988.

27. Keeney RL, Raiffa H: *Decisions with Multiple Objectives: Preferences and Value Tradeoffs*. New York, Wiley, 1976.

28. King JT Jr, Glick HA, Mason TJ, Flamm ES: Elective surgery for asymptomatic, unruptured, intracranial aneurysms: A cost-effectiveness analysis. *J Neurosurg* 83:403–412, 1995.

29. King JT Jr, Justice AC, Aron DC: Management of incidental pituitary microadenomas: A cost-effectiveness analysis. *J Clin Endocrinol Metab* 82:3625–3632, 1997.

30. King JT Jr, Sperling MR, Justice AC, O'Connor MJ: A cost-effectiveness analysis of anterior temporal lobectomy for intractable temporal lobe epilepsy. *J Neurosurg* 87:20–28, 1997.

31. Kinosian BP, Eisenberg JM: Cutting into cholesterol: Cost-effective alternatives for treating hypercholesterolemia. *JAMA* 259:2249–2254, 1988.

32. Najman J, Levine S: Evaluating the impact of medical care and technologies on the quality of life: A review and critique. *Soc Sci Med* 15F:105–115, 1981.

33. O'Meara JJ III, McNutt RA, Evans AT, Moore SW, Downs SM: A decision analysis of streptokinase plus heparin as compared with heparin alone for deep-vein thrombosis. *N Eng J Med* 330:1864–1869, 1994.

34. Patrick DL, Starks HE, Cain KC, Uhlmann RF, Pearlman RA: Measuring preferences for health states worse than death. *Med Decis Making* 14:9–18, 1994.

35. Richardson J: Cost utility analysis: What should be measured? *Soc Sci Med* 39:7–21, 1994.

36. Sackett DL, Torrance GW: The utility of different health states as perceived by the general public. *J Chronic Disord* 31:697–704, 1978.

37. Sayeed RA, Nyamekye I, Ghauri AS, Poskitt KR: Quality of life after transthoracic endoscopic sympathectomy for upper limb hyperhidrosis. *Eur J Surg Suppl* 580:39–42, 1998.

38. Schulman KA, Lynn LA, Glick HA, Eisenberg JM: Cost-effectiveness of low-dose zidovudine therapy for asymptomatic patients with human immunodeficiency virus (HIV) infection. *Ann Intern Med* 114:798–802, 1991.

39. Shin AY, Porter PJ, Wallace MC, Naglie G: Quality of life of stroke in younger individuals: Utility assessment in patients with arteriovenous malformations. *Stroke* 28:2395–2399, 1997.

40. Slevin ML, Stubbs L, Plant HJ, et al: Attitudes to chemotherapy: Comparing views of patients with cancer with those of doctors, nurses, and general public. *BMJ* 300:1458–1460, 1990.

41. Solomon NA, Glick HA, Russo CJ, Lee J, Schulman KA: Patient preferences for stroke outcomes. *Stroke* 25:1721–1725, 1994.

42. Stason WB, Weinstein MC: Allocation of resources to manage hypertension. *N Eng J Med* 296:732–739, 1977.

43. Stewart AL, Greenfield S, Hays RD, et al: Functional status and well-being of patients with chronic condi-

tions: Results from the Medical Outcomes Study. *JAMA* 262:907–913, 1989.

44. Streiner DL, Norman GR: *Health Measurement Scales: A practical guide to their development and use.* New York, Oxford University Press, 1989.

45. Torrance GW: Social preference for health states. *Socio-Econ Plann Sci* 10:129–136, 1976.

46. Torrance GW: Measurement of health state utilities for economic appraisal: A review. *J Health Econ* 5:1–30, 1986.

47. Torrance GW: Utility approach to measuring health-related quality of life. *J Chronic Dis* 40:593–600, 1987.

48. Torrance GW, Boyle MH, Horwood SP: Application of multi-attribute theory to measure social preference for health states. *Operations Res* 30:1043–1069, 1982.

49. Torrance GW, Furlong WJ, Feeny D, Boyle MH: Multi-attribute preference functions: Health utilities index. *PharmacoEconomics* 7:503–520, 1995.

50. Torrance GW, Thomas WH, Sackett DL: A utility maximization model for evaluation of health care programs. *Health Serv Res* 7:118–133, 1972.

51. Vickrey BG, Hays RD, Graber J, Rausch R, Engel J Jr, Brook RH: A health-related quality of life instrument for patients evaluated with epilepsy surgery. *Med Care* 30:299–319, 1992.

52. von Neumann J, Morgenstern O: *Theory of Games and Economic Behavior.* New York, Wiley, 1953.

53. Ware JE, Sherbourne DC: The MOS 36-item short-form health survey. *Med Care* 30:473–483, 1992.

54. Weinstein MC, Stason WB: Cost-effectiveness of coronary artery bypass surgery. *Circulation* 66(suppl 3): III56–III65, 1982.

55. Williams A: Economics of coronary artery bypass grafting. *Br Med J* 291:326–329, 1985.

CHAPTER 19

Cost-Accounting Issues in Medical Practice: The Need for Activity-Based Costing

YUHCHANG HWANG, Ph.D., AND ALISON J. KIRBY, Ph.D.

Understanding the cost of production for a given product or service is the basis for profit generation in any business enterprise. The service sector, particularly medicine, has traditionally placed less emphasis on cost accounting than has manufacturing with its large capital equipment, labor, and raw material costs. However, with the advent of managed care, capitation, and risk-sharing contracts, it is now imperative that medical practices have an accurate knowledge of what it costs to provide medical care for a given population of patients. Drs. Hwang and Kirby discuss the dangers of simplistic traditional cost-accounting methods and introduce us to a more appropriate cost-accounting tool, activity-based costing, which is better suited to allow medical practices to face the challenges of assuming more financial risk for the care that they provide to their patients.

In this chapter, we describe why it is important for today's physicians to accurately determine the costs of the services that they perform. We first introduce a traditional approach to computing costs often utilized in an indemnity or fee-for-service setting. However, in the modern era of managed care, capitation, and risk-sharing contracts, traditional cost-accounting systems can lead to inaccuracies when calculating the true costs of providing medical services. Such information may result in economically disadvantageous consequences for physicians as they make decisions, such as setting contract rates with insurers. Second, we describe an alternative cost accounting approach, activity-based costing (ABC), which is likely to provide a much clearer picture of the true costs that are associated with the different services provided by physicians. This clearer picture provides a more reliable cost information, which results in better decision-making and cost control.

RELEVANCE OF ACCURATE COSTS OF SERVICES

Consider a neurosurgeon in a group practice. The physician is probably aware of the clinic's most recent year's profit, because it determines the payout available to the partners. However, does the physician know what an office consultation costs? Does the physician know the cost of performing a procedure, such as a revision shunt valve or distal catheter? The response to these questions may be: "Why would a physician want to know?"

There were times when knowing these costs was of little relevance. When the majority of patients were covered by indemnity plans, detailed cost information had minimal impact on a clinic's profitability. However, as third party payers have moved to managed care, capitation, and risk-sharing programs, knowing and managing costs has become essential to guaranteeing practice profitability. Knowing the cost of providing different services enables physicians to make better decisions when negotiating contracts with third party payers and when deciding on venues for expansion or consolidation of their practices.

The accurate measurement of the cost of performing a specific procedure or service is often complicated, difficult, and expensive. The first step in measurement is to understand the costs. Costs can be defined as those resources consumed by activities that result in services or products to patients. In this setting, resources include tangible and intangible medical supplies and support or services available at a clinic. Tangible resources are the medical equipment, facility, and hardware, whereas intangible resources include the physician's knowledge and expertise. All resources have their constraints and limitations. Equipment generally has a useful life, and physicians have a limited amount of time available per day. Putting it in simpler terms, a costing procedure is a systematic way of assigning dollar amounts to each patient or procedure to track the resources consumed for serviced provided. Thus, for a clinic, the resources consumed would include the physician's time, medical supplies, malpractice insurance, salaries and benefits for reception secretaries, medical-record staffs, nurses, scheduling clerk, insurance claim processing clerk, expenses for space, and other management fees. Resources consumed would also include costs related to X-ray equipment, computers, office software, transcription, space expenses, and management fees. The activities furnished by the consumption of resources include performing operations, maintaining patient records, in-office visits, hospital visits, insurance authorization, billing, collection of claims, and resolving collection disputes. The services provided to patients (i.e., products) are surgical procedures (including the pre-surgery visit, surgery, follow-up office visits), and/or office consultations. Figure 19.1 depicts the flow and relationships among resources, activities, and services. The goal of a good costing

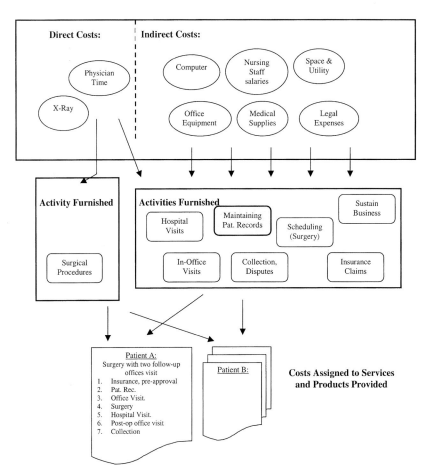

Figure 19.1 Schematic depicting various direct and indirect costs, activities supported, and assignment scenarios based on services provided.

system is to causally assign and trace all the expenditures or resources incurred to the final products and services consumed by the patients.

DISTINCTION BETWEEN DIRECT AND INDIRECT COSTS

In Figure 19.1, a dashed line separates the resources incurred into two categories, direct and indirect costs. Direct costs are resources that are clearly and directly consumed by a specific cost object (in this example, a specific patient). In contrast, indirect costs are resources that are consumed jointly by all patients, thus being difficult to trace back to a specific patient. For example, salary and fringe benefits paid to medical record staff would be an indirect cost, because it is difficult or impractical to trace the portion of costs that are attributable to patient A, who has visited the office three times during the past month. Unfortunately, most expenses incurred in a clinic are indirect costs. Indirect costs are also often referred to as support expenses (see Fig. 19.1).

PITFALLS OF TRADITIONAL COST ALLOCATION APPROACHES

If these indirect costs cannot be traced to individual patients, how should one assign them when computing an overall cost for each patient? Traditionally, indirect costs are grouped by functions or departments and spread evenly to various cost objects or patients. This traditional cost allocation process conjures up an image of evenly spreading peanut butter on a sandwich! For example, the clinic may combine all the indirect resources into one big cost pool and divide those costs by a simple denominator, such as the number of patient visits. The set of indirect costs is then presented as support expenses per visit–the peanut-butter spreading approach.

The difficulty with this traditional costing method is that it may potentially cause severe cross-subsidization of costs among patients, that is, some patients are assigned more costs than they cause the clinic to incur and others are assigned less. Patients that require simple, but frequent, consultations are likely to have excess costs allocated, whereas patients that visit less frequently but use special equipment or require long consultations would be considered less costly than in reality. If all patient services were reimbursed, either based on reported costs or cost-plus reimbursement, then such inaccurate cost data would be of little concern for physicians. However, such inaccuracies can have severe financial consequences to a medical practice when contracting with many third party payers with different reimbursement rates and coverage allowances.

The following example will be used to illustrate the difficulty with traditional cost-accounting methods. Consider Tables 19.1 to 19.4, which represent patient groups, number of visits, office expenses, and a variety of reimbursement scenarios. All cost information was derived using traditional costing methods. Table 19.1 represents a reimbursement scenario where payments are guaranteed at 110% of costs.

Total annual support costs amount to $54,000 with an average cost per visit of $16.40. Assigning costs to the two patient groups on the basis of the number of visits results in allocated costs of $49,200 and $4,920 for HMO-A and HMO-B patients, respectively. If reimbursement is assured at charges of 110% of cost, then profits

TABLE 19.1
Cost Allocation and Cost-plus Reimbursement

	Avg. No. of Visits	No. of Patients	Sum of Visits	Actual Support Expenses	Cost Allocated No. of Visits	Reimbursement (10% above cost)	Profit
Patient HMO-A	10	300	3,000	$45,240*	$49,200	$54,120	$4,920
Patient HMO-B	3	100	300	8,880*	4,920	5,412	492
Total		400	3,300	$54,120	$54,120	$59,532	$5,412
Average Cost Per Visit				$54,120/3,300 = $16.40			

* Costs would not available using a traditional cost-accounting system.

TABLE 19.2
Cost Allocation and Fixed Rate Reimbursement

	Avg. No. of Visits	No. of Patients	Sum of Visits	Actual Support Expenses	Cost Allocated No. of Visits	Reimbursement A: $17.10 B: $27.44	Profit
Patient HMO-A	10	300	3,000	$45,240*	$49,200	$51,300	$2,100
Patient HMO-B	3	100	300	8,880*	4,920	8,232	3,312
Total		400	3,300	$54,120	$54,120	$59,532	$5,412
Average Cost Per Visit				$54,120/3,300 = $16.40			

* Costs would not available using a traditional cost-accounting system.

TABLE 19.3
Cost Allocation, Fixed Rate Reimbursement—Adding Patients from HMO-C

	Avg. No. of Visits	No. of Patients	Sum of Visits	Actual Support Expenses	Cost Allocated (No. of Visits)	Reimbursement A: $17.10 B: $27.44 C: $27.44	Profit
Patient HMO-A	10	300	3,000	$45,240*	$52,500	$51,300	($1,200)
Patient HMO-B	3	100	300	8,880*	5,250	8,232	2,982
Patient HMO-C	3	100	300	8,880*	5,250	8,232	2,982
Total		500	3,600	$63,000	$63,000	$67,764	$4,764
Average Cost Per Visit				$63,000/3,600 = $17.5			

* Costs would not available using a traditional cost-accounting system.

TABLE 19.4
Cost Allocation, Fixed Rate Reimbursement—Reduce Patients from HMO-A

	Avg. No. of Visits	No. of Patients	Sum of Visits	Actual Support Expenses	Cost Allocated (No. of Visits)	Reimbursement A: $17.10 B: $27.44 C: $27.44	Profit
Patient HMO-A	10	248	2,480	$37,398*	$44,413	$42,408	($2,005)
Patient HMO-B	3	100	300	8,880*	5,372.5	8,232	2,859.5
Patient HMO-C	3	100	300	8,880*	5,372.5	8,232	2,859.5
Total		440	3,080	$55,158	$55,158	$58,872	$3,714
Average Cost Per Visit				$55,158/3,080 = $17.91			

* Costs would not available using a traditional cost-accounting system.

are $5,412. Furthermore, regardless of whether the number of visits or some other basis is used to allocate the costs to the two groups, the total profit will be $5,412. In this setting, profits are both guaranteed and limited to be 10% of costs. There is no way to enhance the profit rate either by cost saving measures or by changing the mix of patient population. Consequently, there is no potential return for investing in better under-standing of the costs of different patient types; therefore, inaccurate costing of patient types causes no negative consequences to the clinic.

INACCURATE COST DATA AND DECISION MAKING

Table 19.2 considers a more realistic scenario in which physicians are paid a fixed rate per visit. HMO-A pays a fixed rate of $17.10 per visit, whereas HMO-B pays $27.44 per visit. Now the clinic has the ability to alter its insurer mix and control costs, thus affecting profitability. Currently, the clinic's traditional cost system indicates an overall profit of $5,412. Both patient groups appear profitable, in particular the HMO-B patients with their apparent profitability rate of 40%.

The clinic is considering signing a new contract with HMO-C for 300 patients. The new patients are believed to be similar to those from HMO-B and the per-visit rate proposed by HMO-C is also $27.44. The clinic compares the per-visit cost of $16.40 with the fixed reimbursement rate offered by HMO-C. It anticipates a total increase in operating expenses of $4,920 ($16.40 × 300) and increases in revenues of $8,232 ($27.44 × 300). Based on its cost data, the clinic anticipates that the new patients will generate $3,312 in additional profits, increasing profits from $5,412 to $8,724. It eagerly accepts the new patients.

However, during the ensuing year the added patient pool causes additional traffic in the front office and medical records room, and it results in more frequent logging of over-time and greater use of temporary employees. At year-end, the physicians examine the year's financial results and are mystified to find that profits were actually $4,764, a decrease of $648 from the previous year and $3,960 below budget, as illustrated in Table 19.3. Although revenues increased exactly as expected ($8,232), support expenses jumped by $8,880 instead of the predicted $4,920.

Upset about the apparent lack of control of support expenses, the physicians were ready to look for a new office manager. From their traditional cost-accounting data, they noted that patients from HMO-A were generating only $17.10 per visit reimbursement but apparently costing $17.50 per visit. The clinic projected that if it dropped 52 of these low margin patients it would cut operating expenses by $9,100 ($17.5 × 52 patients × 10 visits per patient), assuming that the actual support expenses associated with HMO-A patients decrease proportionally with the number of visits. (In reality, due to fixed expenses, the amount of cost reduction (savings) is likely to be less than $9,000. Thus, the actual outcome could be far more severe than those presented in Table 19.3.) Consequently, a profit increase of $208 was expected.

To their surprise, the physicians again discovered that after dropping some of the supposedly unprofitable patients, the clinic's net profit had actually decreased by $1,050. The clinic was now completely at a loss in deciding how to manage its support expenses, and how to negotiate successfully with insurance companies.

The root of the problem in the above example was not poor decision making or an irresponsible office manager; rather, it was the cost system itself. The traditional cost system provided misleading indications of cost, therefore, prompting the clinic to make incorrect decisions, choices that decreased rather than increased profits. Why was the cost system providing misleading cost numbers? The cost allocation process assumed that all support expenses increased in proportion with the number of visits. In reality, many indirect or support expenses relate to activities that are not driven by the volume of visits. Although it is clear that medical record activities and insurance claims processing increase with increasing patient visits, other costs depend on issues that are independent of patient visit volume, such as the number of insurance carriers a clinic deals with. Understanding and predicting these hidden costs of providing additional services is almost impossible if one has to rely on a traditional costing system. As a result, poor decisions are frequently made.

To find out the true cost of adding an additional HMO to the existing patient pool or the true savings of dropping a group of patients, one needs a more sophisticated cost system than the traditional one described above. With more accurate cost data provided by a more sophisticated cost system, physicians are much more likely to make profit-enhancing choices.

ACTIVITY-BASED COSTING–A BETTER WAY FOR COST FINDING

Unlike traditional costing methods, ABC attempts to first identify the activities that drive the demand for support resources (3). It then explores the patterns of how various products and services consume those activities. In searching for cause and effect, the ABC method focuses on activities that drive resource consumption and costs (1). In Figure 19.1, the activities furnished section denotes the types of activities incurred in clinics or hospital practices. Table

TABLE 19.5
Summary of Cost Activities

Set of Activities
Establishing initial record, pre-approval
Routine insurance verification, approval
Maintaining patient medical records
Surgical procedures
Hospital visits
Office visits
Insurance claims
Collections and disputes

19.5 shows a typical list of activities, which are encountered on a daily basis by a typical physician's office, that acts to drive the cost-structure of a practice. Almost all of the patients seen by a physician consume at least some or all these activities. More importantly, all the resources (direct or indirect) incurred at the clinic are for the purpose of providing these activities. Most of these activities are value adding, in the sense of being part of the service provided to patients. In contrast, some of the activities may be viewed critically, because they do not contribute to the service provided by the clinic. Activities, such as resolving billing disputes, are not considered value adding with regard to patient care (the product). However, one cannot deny the fact that all these activities cost money. Understanding the costs of all these activities helps isolate the activities that are excessively costly relative to the value that they generate, and therefore, the activities that should best be streamlined.

Tracing Resources to Activities Pools

Identifying all resources related to each specific activity is the next task in tracing costs to services using ABC. Consider the third activity listed above, maintaining patient medical records. Resources consumed in maintaining medical records are shown in Figure 19.2. The percentages indicate the portion of each resource used by the patient record keeping activity. The cost of the maintaining patient medical records activity is then an aggregate of computer and software costs, office equipment and supplies costs, and staff salaries and fringe benefits. This total cost may be divided into costs of two sub-activities, the cost of initial record setup and the cost of routine record keeping, based on the estimated relative time spent on each. This may be necessary, because the practice probably sees

many patients for just a single visit and many other patients on an ongoing basis. In contrast, in primary care practices this extra split in costs might be unnecessary if one assumes that most patients will visit on an ongoing basis.

Defining the Services and Products

Current Procedural Terminology (CPT) coding and International Classification of Diseases (ICD) coding are familiar examples of defined sets of services. Although CPT coding serves as a basis for most third party reimbursement, it does not necessarily reflect the full range of services. There could be hundreds of codes for a typical clinic. A costing system that gives detailed costs for each individual CPT code would be impractical and senseless. For costing purposes, one needs to regroup various CPT codes or ICD procedures into manageable and meaningful processes or products. If practice support expenses tend to be fairly similar across different types of surgical patients, then for simplicity, one might even use just two categories of services: surgical patients and consultation only patients. Depending on the use of the cost information (whether for identifying streamlining opportunities or for contracting support) and the type of third party payers, with whom the clinic deals, the grouping process could be further refined. For example, if a third party payer pays either a capitated rate or a rate based on completing a specific episode of procedure or treatment, then the definition of product or services related to surgical patients can be grouped according to the number of follow-up visits.

Identifying the Cost Driver

The cost driver provides the final linkage between the activities defined and the product or services provided by a clinic. The cost driver reflects the cause of activity; it defines the measurement unit for the demand on the activity generated by the products or services. Continuing with the activity of maintaining patient medical records, assume that a surgical procedure (e.g., CPT 61700) is performed on a specific patient. What is the cost of maintaining patient medical records assigned to this specific patient? To answer this question, one needs to know what generates the need for maintaining patient medical records. First, what generates the demand for routine record keeping? Second, what generates the demand for initial record setup?

Indirect Resources

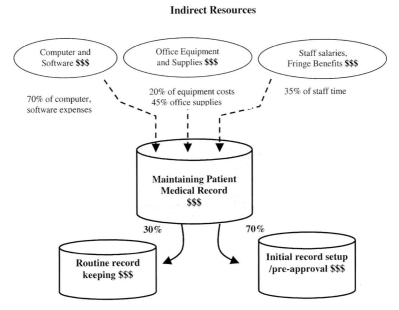

Figure 19.2 Activity-based costing scheme for determining an accurate cost of maintaining patient records for both established and new patients.

Does the number of patients drive the costs in the routine record keeping activity, or do the number of visits and the number of operations cause this activity and its costs to increase? Consider the details of this activity. Each time a patient visits the clinic, a staff member pulls the medical record, adds a new form for the visit, and delivers the record to an exam room for the physician. Later, lab reports need to be attached to the record, transcripts of the new visit will be keyed into the computer, and finally, a staff member will file the patient's record. An almost identical process is followed if a patient has surgery. Therefore, because each visit and each operation generates demand for the routine record keeping activity, a cost driver for this cost pool would be the sum of the number of visits (both in-hospital and clinic) and operations performed in a given period. This is appropriate, because the effort of record keeping performed by the staff and computer is virtually independent of the medical complexity of the visit or surgery. Thus, for costs associated with regular visits, an appropriate cost driver would be the number of visits or operations.

The number of visits, however, will probably not be an appropriate driver of the cost of estab-

lishing new patient records and acquiring pre-approval for treatments. This is because the time staff members spend on setting up a record and obtaining pre-approval from an insurance company would be unrelated to the number of visits. All patients may require the service, but the amount of service is likely to be unrelated to the number of visits. Thus, the number of patients might be a better driver for allocating the expenses of these startup, medical record activity costs.

To complete the example, assume that annual spending on computers (including depreciation), software, consulting, and system maintenance is estimated at $80,000. Cost of office equipment, such as depreciation of file cabinets, desks, and furniture in the reception area is estimated at $60,000 and spending on office supplies at $40,000. Two staff members share the responsibility of medical records and insurance claims with annual salaries and benefits of $90,000. Furthermore, suppose that the estimated number of in-clinic visits per year is 12,000, that each of the four surgeons in the group performs about 250 operations, and there are 2,500 in-hospital visits per year. The number of new patients is about 600. Figure 19.3 illustrates a simple esti-

The federal government did not seriously become a third party until the Social Security Amendment of 1965 in Title XVIII (Medicare) and Title XIX (Medicaid). With it, the government planted the seeds for what was to become an entitlement mentality for health care services in the general population. With both government funding and the creation of an entitlement mentality, it was not long before health care costs began to climb rapidly. Over this time, too, employers became increasingly accountable for funding the health insurance needs of their employees. Few physicians are unaware of the almost logarithmic increase in medical care costs that followed. The increase in care costs resulted with the development of concerns about overutilization of medical services and the appropriateness of service delivery. The development of Professional Standards Review Organizations, as a result of Senator Wallace Bennett's amendment in 1972, further paved the way for direct government oversight in physician patient care activity. These organizations evolved into the peer review organizations, which were created in the 1970s and continue today, as established organizations seeking to review the appropriateness of physician care.

Thus, a utilization management infrastructure in this country developed from mechanisms to fund medical care by third party payers. An entitlement mentality, third party payment, and provider oversupply resulted in skyrocketing costs during the 1960s, 1970s, and early 1980s, which at times reached double digit percentage annual increases (7, 19). These new payers of services became concerned with the unbridled rising costs and sought to create management infrastructures to better control the business. During this time, the movement of physician practices from a cottage industry of independent practitioners to increasingly larger aggregated business units added to the complexity. Rich endowments resulted in unparalleled expansion of medical research and the development of effective, but expensive, technologies. As systems became bigger and bureaucracies became more complex, consumers simultaneously demanded better access, higher quality, and lower costs.

FORCES SHAPING THIRD PARTY PAYER AND HEALTH DELIVERY SYSTEMS

Significant increases in healthcare costs have strained governmental coffers, made businesses less profitable and competitive, and created worry in individuals struggling to afford access to insurance. These are very potent forces much bigger than a local insurer or managed care company. As economic forces are applied to an enlarging medical bureaucracy, the increasing complexity of administering medical care is as problematic for third party payers as it is for physicians.

The historical changes in care cost increases and administrative bureaucracy have been accompanied by a variety of other related activities including:

- Evolution of governmental and pseudo-governmental compliance organizations.
- Multilevel concerns regarding fraud and abuse.
- Extension of Occupation Safety & Health Agency (OSHA) activities to include physician practices.
- Stark I and II amendments addressing physician self-referral.
- New methodologies for developing payment to physicians.
- New, sometimes expensive, technologies for diagnosing and treating patients.
- Dramatic advances in pharmaceutical sciences.
- Further evolution of provider organization, including group practices, Physician-Hospital Organizations (PHOs).

The increasing complexity and sophistication of the system dealing with physicians has led to considerable professional anxiety and concern in the rapidly changing practice of medicine. In addition to facing rapidly expanding clinical requirements, physicians are also burdened with concerns regarding government reporting, accreditation standards, employer needs, OSHA, marketplace demands and competition, running a complex business, and a large number of additional challenges not addressed in earlier medical school curricula.

Thus, not only is the current medical environment continuously evolving, its evolution is driven by public non-professional needs and desires, economics, and politics. This integrated "big picture" is a critically important concept for physicians to understand as they seek to deal with managed care and integrated delivery systems.

It is also the case that medical directors for

third party payers are not in the same power position that they are in hospitals, medical schools, and medical professional activities. Community based physicians are often surprised to learn that their suggestions to a managed care organization medical director are not implemented on the weight of logic alone. (Internally, we refer to this process as magical thinking.) To a physician working within a third party payer environment, it is not unlike trying to effect change in their high school class. In high school, physicians were often high achievers with high grades who also had to interact with popular students, less intelligent students, and students with different orientations, such as business and art. This wide diversity and level of skills are present in any large corporation. Frequently, the formation of a policy involves the interaction of many of these types of individuals working as a team in which the physician medical director receives a single vote. Like the political process, organizations make mistakes, realize them, and correct them through time but not before the targets of those activities (patients, physicians) have perceived, often-substantial, changes in the way care is delivered. It is an ongoing challenge for physician executives to acquire power and influence in organizations that did not originally include them in senior positions and in which they are viewed cautiously by non-clinically trained managers (9).

Generally, from the perspective of third party payer, neurosurgery and neurosurgeons have been relatively non-problematic. It is actually quite striking how little information on third party payers, managed care, and insurance company issues are in the neurosurgical literature. For the most part, there is not a serious oversupply of neurosurgeons, given the difficult and long training period necessary. Additionally, with the possible exception of spinal surgery, which has been recently reviewed extensively, there are comparatively few neurosurgical procedures that can be open to question on the grounds of medical necessity. Generally, one does not allow someone to perform surgery on his or her central nervous system without a fairly apparent reason. (i.e., medical necessity is self-evident.) The gastroenterologist "scoping for dollars" has no neurosurgical equivalent.

The principal issues for neurosurgeons with respect to third party payers include changes in the organizational structure of how medicine is practiced, methodologies by which payment for services is administered, and the impact of medical management strategies on professional autonomy for physicians who previously were in a relatively unregulated environment. Physicians must prepare to operate in an uncertain future where multiple options are appearing on a daily basis (6).

INFRASTRUCTURE AND SYSTEMS TO PROVIDE CARE

Third party involvement in the delivery of health care has been principally structured around the overall management of medical care costs. One can view the benefit structure of health plan offerings as a continuum between highly managed and non-managed oversight of medical care delivery (Fig. 20.1). Physicians often tend to see this spectrum of organizational control as multiple attempts by third party payers to extract a profit by controlling their professional lives and the market. On the contrary, these programs were historically developed in response to market pressures largely based on the perception of rising health-care costs in the absence of measurable improvement and quality. Products offered are, in fact, a response continuum of control and benefit structures that subtly exchange varying amounts of freedom and control for lowered health care costs. In our region, it is the business community that has been most influential in precipitating the development of health maintenance organization (HMO), point of service (POS), and preferred provider organization (PPO) programs. While these are developed and administered by third party payers, it is clearly the case that they are in fact

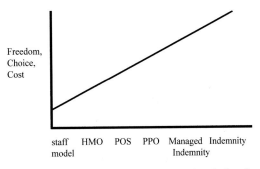

Figure 20.1 Managed care spectrum showing the benefit structure of health plan offerings.

responding with products demanded by the larger marketplace. The difference between the unmanaged indemnity programs and more restrictive HMOs can be $400 to $500 per member per month in costs, so the differences are quite palpable.

Major classes and characteristics of various managed care products are as follows:

1. Unmanaged Indemnity: In these types of programs, claims are paid as they are received. Historically, cost controls might be limited to co-pay or coinsurance amounts, which have been proven to reduce medical demand (31). Controls in this category are largely limited to simple descriptions of benefit limits.

2. Managed Indemnity: Managed indemnity was introduced among the first means of controlling spiraling health-care costs. Early on, a second surgical opinion was a meaningful method for controlling costs. However, by the mid-1980s, it was only infrequently that the second surgeon did not agree with the first. Thus, this modification probably added costs at the end of its useful product cycle. During this period, intensified case management was also introduced by the industry. Early in my career, medical directors were frequently called when patients exceeded certain percentiles for length of stay. Large actuarial firms such as Milliman and Robertson compiled statistical tables describing percentile ranks for various lengths of stay and for various disease conditions (8). In this still largely inspection technology, interventions started after the patient had exceeded a length of stay cutoff to create a more intensified discharged planning program. Managed indemnity programs also introduced the concept of precertification and preauthorization, the so-called ''Mother may I'' approach to determining medical necessity. The effectiveness of this tool has been called into question on a number of occasions but probably had some chilling effect on over-utilization (2, 10, 21, 23, 24, 27–30, 36). Historically, a number of medical management tools developed during the period where managed indemnity was (and regionally still is) in effect (Fig. 20.2).

3. Preferred Provider Organizations: PPOs represent the next step in attempting to control costs. Preferred providers were approached by insurers to create networks. The deal from the third party to these physicians was to increase patient flow to their offices in exchange for a slightly lower fee schedule. Often, various features of managed indemnity or HMOs are also added. Cost savings here accrued from identifying more cost-effective providers and reducing their fees. In an era when physician over-supply began to manifest itself, this was (and is) a reasonable approach to selectively controlling costs and improving quality. Downsizing the physician workforce cannot be easily accomplished from a policy perspective; narrowed networks represent a management approach to this issue (22).

4. Health Maintenance Organization: At a further extreme of the control continuum, HMOs identify a network of physicians who can be more tightly controlled and managed. Early HMOs were frequently composed principally of staff physicians (a staff model), who were actual employees of the HMO and who provided care to patients on a capitated or salary basis. This type of arrangement is impractical for an organization seeking to expand outside the limits of a metropolitan area or defined region. To expand, HMOs found that they needed additional contract providers and expanded to the larger independent practice association (IPA) model. Geographical expansion has also resulted in practical alterations to closed panel networks, where members could only see certain practitioners for coverage, with less limited panel arrangements. The IPA model includes some of the better features of a PPO in that physicians contract independently but are controlled as a panel with a defined patient population. The more members a physician has, the more capable the third party is able to analyze individual practitioners' practice patterns. This allows for comparative analyses between providers with respect to cost effectiveness. HMO programs also frequently employ gatekeepers as principal contact physicians for each patient who are responsible for assuring coordination of medical care. Pros and cons abound on this particular strategy, which is often viewed negatively by patients that are used to seeking widely open access to care (14).

5. Point of Service: POS programs have become increasingly popular in the past decade and present a hybrid between a fairly constrained closed panel of physicians in HMOs and the

more loosely controlled PPOs. In POS plans, members are usually directed by benefit (rather than fiat) to physicians within the third party payers' panel with lower deductibles, co-pays, or improved coverage benefits. Like managed indemnity, however, patients are able to see other physicians outside the panel. This is particularly attractive to members in an area that is largely fragmented or balkanized between competing health plans.

Thus, benefit design and network composition define the difference between the various third party plans currently available. Each is present along a continuum from higher to lower freedom of choice and cost for the individual payers of services. These represent only major categories along the continuum, however, and many variations exist. Thus, we may see gatekeepers in PPOs, open access HMOs, out of network coverage provisions of all types, etc.

Recent Developments

Recent developments in the organizational structure for the delivery of health care include the integrated delivery systems in which physicians combine with hospitals and risk managers to create a single package. Held out as the great answer to managed care, many of these integrated delivery systems failed to deliver the promise originally seen, in part due to organizational issues. The integration of a number of health care systems usually resulted in significant addition of management bureaucracy, without the anticipated significant reduction in health care delivery costs. The original thinking was that integrated delivery systems would reduce a large amount of the fat in the system, thus creating enough profit to support the bureaucratic systems and controls necessary to run them and allow premium reductions as a benefit (4). To date, these have only infrequently been demonstrated to do so.

Across the board, we see an increasing use of modern management systems to control the social structures of managed care systems. Multi-physician committees, quality oversight, credentialing protocols, and a variety of new methods designed to provide more uniform service levels and qualities for the members have developed simultaneously with the creation of new programs. Initial contracts for provider networks were fairly small, numbering as few as one or two pages in the past. Today, it is fairly typical for health plans to have 10 or even 30-page contracts for physician participation, specifying many aspects of behavior that are expected of the practitioners. The goal of the third party payer is also to maintain these organizational structures, while maintaining maximum benefit and access for the users who purchase these services.

In part, due to a growing national backlash against managed care, health plans are working to create programs that are more user friendly. Open access programs are becoming quite popular and allow patients wider latitude in seeing non-panel physicians. This often comes at the expense of higher co-pay and deductibles, higher premiums, or other underwriting methods to accommodate the accompanying higher health costs. Variations in employer financing are also being developed around more member choice. Employers, for example, are moving from defined benefit to defined contribution, cafeteria-style health care benefits to maintain health care cost exposure. As a consequence of moving more of the decision making to patients, the industry is gradually moving from wholesale (employer-purchased) to include a retail (employee-purchased) focus. Medical IRAs probably come under this heading, although efforts to develop this concept have not met with widespread public acceptance.

A number of other new developments are continuing to shape the rich texture of the problem and include:

- Significantly enlarging physician practices and their resultant willingness to accept insurance at risk for patient populations.
- Attempts by PHOs to work together.
- Development of several large national quality-oriented organizations.
- Pressure from a variety of sources to profile medical care down to the physician level.
- Involvement of various employer groups and coalitions in health care.
- Increased interest and involvement of payer coalitions.
- Expanded costs from leading edge pharmaceutical products, including new cell lines immunotherapies, and expensive new drugs.

ACTUARIAL AND COST CONTAINMENT CONSIDERATIONS RELEVANT TO PHYSICIANS

On the surface, health insurance is not too dissimilar from other types of risk management, including life insurance, liability insurance, auto/home insurance, etc. Basic health insurance is somewhat different, in that risk is managed based on a number of interfering influences. Particularly, employers, rather than individuals, by and large represent the purchasers of health insurance at the present time. This injects a very strong preference toward employed individuals (and secondarily, their families) and specific efforts to control costs. In the 1980s, a number of very large employers were concerned that the rate of health care cost inflation would erode corporate profitability and make them unfit to compete in a global marketplace. The creation and market influence of various labor coalitions in many cities resulted in the development of managed care organizations to address their cost concerns. In a number of states, the influence of large employers on the government was one of the many pressures to develop single payer nationalized health care and a variety of other initiatives. Health insurance is strongly influenced by the presence of organized labor, which is frequently mistrustful of the alliance between large businesses and insurance companies. It is very frequently the case that union negotiations focus around the level and the freedom of health care benefits, which are incorporated in labor contracts.

Health insurance differs from other insurance, in that group experience, rather than a community rating, frequently drive it. Experience rating applies when a specific purchaser seeks to have only their health care insurance costs reflected in the premiums. Community rating, on the other hand, distributes the health care costs from a large area among many purchasers of health care services. Many managed care organizations use experience rating, rather than community rating, for their products, resulting in significant alterations in the risk experience of a community. As an example, early in the development of managed care, managed care organizations sought to "cherry pick" low-risk individuals to whom they could charge appropriately lower health insurance premiums. Although this attracted healthy individuals, it had the secondary effect of concentrating sicker individuals in the standard indemnity pool, thus raising indemnity insurance prices. Because managed care organizations need only to be competitive with indemnity insurers, they were able to raise their premiums to "shadow price" the indemnity premiums,

while pocketing the difference in risk management as significant profit. This combination of cherry picking and shadow pricing has been theorized to paradoxically result in accelerated health care costs. It is important to consider the difference between rating, which calculates the actual exposure of a group of individuals and pricing, which sets the actual premium cost of a group of individuals. Large employers can minimize this effect by dealing with a single insurer who offers multiple programs—HMO, POS, and indemnity. By balancing the risk pool through individual pricing and cost sharing arrangements, the employer overall may continue to maintain low health insurance costs, while transferring high risks costs to employees in higher premium share, deductibles, and copayment.

The actual pricing of insurance programs is estimated from medical costs accumulated across the membership pool and retention, which is an additional portion of each premium added to account for unanticipated increased expenses in the following year, unpaid claims, and profit for the risk administrator. Large employers may hire third party administrators or enter into an administrative services only relationship with an insurer to minimize or control the profit included in the retention by the risk-taking entity. The use of multiple managers of this complex process may become very confusing to physicians and their patients trying to ascertain which benefits apply, how to appeal for services denied, etc. Composite strategies using different benefit administrators, claim payers, risk managers, and subcontracted management (e.g., for behavioral health) are common.

Third party pricing of health insurance has a number of objectives. The insurer must match prices to cover underlying medical costs and anticipated risks in the population being insured. Additionally, the insurer must be able to ride out cyclical changes in financial risk for the individuals being insured, in a way that both offers competitive premiums and insures overall continued financial viability of the program. This can principally be done only through insuring large numbers of individuals or through secondary re-insurance of a smaller groups' unexpected risk with a secondary insurer.

Overall, the cost of medical care runs between 70% and 90% of an insurance premium. Retention composes the remaining 10% to 30% and includes insurer's administrative cost, taxes (premium and federal income tax), investment income credits, profits (if the risk manager is a for-profit insurer), and risk charges.

The actual financial arrangements of a third party with a purchaser includes the rating methods, the levels of insurance desired, and funding methods. Rating methods include community or experience rated methods (described above) and occasionally are based on a certain class. Level of insurance may similarly be prospectively rated or retrospectively rated, and self-insured with stop-loss coverage or through pure self-insurance. Stop-loss coverage refers to secondary insurance for costs in excess of an amount that a self-insured entity would not be able to sustain losses. Typically, large or several employers will fund a risk pool on a monthly or quarterly basis and pay insurance claims from that pool. Significant exposure (e.g., transplants, critically ill newborns) tend to overshoot anticipated levels of insurance and result in tripping the stop-loss limits.

COST CONTROL MEASURES

Cost components often vary between managed care and indemnity programs. It is typically expected that managed care will reduce overall costs through a combination of benefits, such as benefits management, utilization savings, reduced trends, and more predictable retention rates. Significant alterations can occur through management of the risk pool. It is known, for example, that 5% of patients typically account for 50% of the cost, so careful selection of members, as with experience rating, can result in substantial differences in premium costs. Other managed care activities can result in monthly premium differences as much as $400 or $500 per member per month. Selection pressure for both commercial insurers, as well as Medicare and Medicare risk products is a very complex science but generally indicates that individuals move to various programs based on perceived benefit. This can have a substantial impact on the overall cost liability of a program.

Third parties use a variety of methods to reduce costs. These generally can be characterized by six processes (Fig. 20.2). Benefit design typically addresses what is and is not covered in an insurance plan. Measures to control cost include limitation on the number of visits or services

Cost Containment Measures

- *benefit design*
- *demand management*
- *depress supply*
- *reduce incentives for providers*
- *encourage competition*
- *management of the process.*

Figure 20.2 The six processes of cost containment measures.

available (e.g., psychiatric services, physical therapy), limitation on benefits that are considered experimental or investigational, and limitation on services that are considered non-essential (e.g., birth control pills). Demand management focuses on both under and over-utilization in the general population. Third party payers are most noted for concentrating on the over-utilization of services, particularly those that are unnecessary, such as an annual chest x-ray for someone who is concerned about the possible development of lung cancer. Third party payers are increasingly becoming sensitized to the long-term cost-effectiveness of preventive care and increasingly are covering vaccines, healthy patient visits, screening mammograms, and other types of medical care, encouraging members to seek these services as a method of long-term cost reduction. Depressing the supply of providers is a frequently used method for controlling over-utilization of services. Limiting the number of chiropractors or suppliers of alternative medicine and sharply restricting the numbers of over-utilized specialists are methods that have been attempted. Primary care physician scrutiny of specialists through the referral mechanism is a similar method of reducing access of patients to providers who might be tempted to provide services of marginal value. The reduction of incentives to providers is most typically characterized by the adoption of capitation as a method of payment to individual physicians. Other more subtle attempts to reduce provider incentive to perform unnecessary services include reducing fees to levels that eliminate a significant profit for providers, preventing self-referral for diagnostic lab or radiology tests, basing contract renewal on utilization records, etc. Encouragement of competition has recently emerged as a main strategy among business payers. Increasing physician populations in provider shortage areas or encouraging the development of competing HMOs has had a significant effect on reducing the prices in a number of areas. Similarly, business and consumer coalitions have worked to make information about different providers pub-

lic, encouraging consumer comparison of providers. Publication of individual provider mortality, or cost data, or publication of available provider options in a region have resulted in competition among providers for service delivery. Interestingly, this has had less of an impact on overall price than third party payers would prefer.

Current Utilization Review Tools

Scope

- Coordination and management of services and care delivery.
- Provider education.
- Supplement other network education efforts.
- Ensure PCP functions as gatekeeper.
- Assist PCPs in identifying appropriate specialists.
- Ensure medical necessity/appropriateness of services.
- 24 hour on call availability.

Function

- Pre-determination.
- Pre-certification.
- Admission review.
- Concurrent review.
- Retrospective review.
- Discharge Planning.
- Case management.
- Outpatient procedure review.
- Provider profiling.
- Referral management.
- Facility assessment/provider credentialing.
- Mental health option.
- Employer/employee education.
- Benefit design research.

Figure 20.3   Various utilization controls.

Hospital Illness Episode

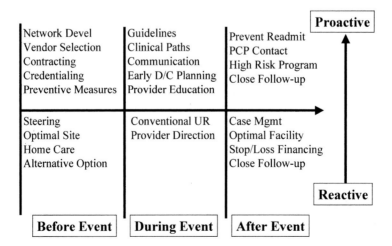

Figure 20.4   Shows process management, which begins before the patient enters the hospital and continues post-hospitalization.

Supplier Categories

- Hospital
- Rehab Facility
- Skilled Nursing Facility (SNF)
- Nursing Home
- Home Health Agency
- Pharmaceutical Benefit Management (PBM)
- Vendors
  - **Infusion Services**
  - **Durable Medical Equipment (DME)**
  - **Disease Management Companies**

Figure 20.5 Service supplier categories addressed by third party sources.

Third party administrators of various types also seek to manage the process of care delivery through various utilization controls as outlined in Figure 20.3. From the perspective of a payer of services, managing the process begins before the patient actually enters the hospital and continues post-hospitalization (Fig. 20.4). Surprisingly, most third party sources would prefer that physicians control their own activities and initially seek to interact with physicians in a collegial, non-confrontational way. Wide variation in practices results in inevitable conflict with physicians at the low end of the curve. It should be noted that the interaction of third parties with providers extends to a number of other suppliers of non-physician services. These include hospitals and a number of other ancillary service supplier categories also addressed by third party sources (Fig. 20.5).

MEDICAL POLICY

Third parties administer the essential elements of their program through the vehicle of their medical policy. The medical policy department is typically staffed by a physician who is asked to specifically input medical oversight into the development of benefits, utilization management, payment processes, etc. Medical policy, for the most part, has been fairly well worked out over the past three decades, as various medical services have been reviewed, priced, and placed into benefit programs. However, this area of administration is a dynamic one and frequently changes with employer and national needs. More recently, it is being overridden by local legislatures who seek, at the request of their constituents, to mandate minimum levels of medical coverage. In Pennsylvania, we have seen attempts to mandate cancer therapy, length of stay for deliveries, women's health issues, screening mammography, rectal exams, and a variety of other medical benefits. The medical policy process within managed care organizations tends to follow current medical literature and seeks consultation from professionals. Indeed, accreditation by both the Utilization Review Accreditation Commission (URAC) (34,35) and the National Committee for Quality Assurance (NCQA) mandates the involvement of physicians in this process. Physician reviewers often refer to the medical literature, state and national professional organizations, the Health Care Financing Administration, the Food and Drug Administration, and a variety of other sources. The medical policy review process is typically lengthy and thorough, but lags behind the state-of-the-art practice of medicine. It is at the cutting edge that the greatest likelihood of conflict arises.

Medical policy deals with a variety of topics, including benefit issues, defining ''medically necessary and appropriate,'' cataloging and review of experimental and investigational treatments, differentiating between cosmetic and reconstructive surgery, reimbursement issues for unusual or atypical situations, and other cost containment measures. Surgical physicians of all types at the cutting edge of medical care may experience problems with third party payers as medical policy forming bodies attempt to determine whether an investigational procedure is effective and should become a covered benefit. From an insurer or payers perspective, medical procedures are not reimbursed unless there is both a benefit listed and medical necessity. (Interestingly some contracts do not always have a medical necessity clause.) Defined benefits make it possible for actuaries to estimate what health insurance costs (and premiums) will be. All-inclusive benefits tend to be quite costly, so limitations on some benefits are used to maintain affordability. Thus, physicians may not understand why there is not an unlimited physical therapy or speech benefit for their patients when medical necessity is obvious. Benefit limitations exist in the policy to make the insurance affordable for the greatest number of individuals or at the level an employer can afford. Medical necessity is subtler and is often defined in volumes of medical policy designed to pay only for care that has been shown to have clear benefit. For the most part, as experimental techniques are proven, they rapidly move into the mainstream of covered medical services. Before that time, insurers are reluctant to pay for them, believing that other mechanisms (government or third party grants) are the appropriate source of funding for these endeavors. Indeed, all payers are now looking closely at the need, cost-benefit, and outcomes of new procedures. The burden of proof rests with the medical community to prove that procedures and treatments are worth the cost. Cost-effectiveness analysis is becoming increasingly important as health care demands and costs continue to rise (32, 33, 38). An excellent review of these issues has been outlined by Gold et al. (13). Although many physicians believe this is problematic in this era of rapid advances, the concept is not new (5).

PAYMENT FOR PROVIDER SERVICES

From an actuarial perspective, the calculation of per member per month costs can be developed from any one of a number of different provider payment strategies. The strategy that is selected depends on the individual market and the creativity of the contracting parties. Generally, large organizations seeking to manage risk prefer to shift some of that risk to providers of care. Capitation or per case payment systems generally are easier to administer, because the number of payments have become more predictable on a per member basis. Conversely, payments that bill individual services on a fee-for-service basis are both operationally complicated (each claim needs to be processed) and typically associated with higher levels of utilization and cost.

Payment schemes for individual providers are almost as numerous as the individuals making contracts and occur in a variety of arrangements, such as:

Group, practice, or enterprise global capitation
PHO or IDS capitation
"Contact capitation" of capitation designed for specific services
Specialty capitation
Individual physician or practice capitation
Relative value unit payment with Resource Based Relative Value Scale (RBRVS) system
Budget linked reimbursement (RBRVS multiplier inversely linked to costs)
Fee-for-service, with or without discounts or withholds

The opportunities for physicians vary from one region to the other, depending on how much over-utilization is in the system. For more efficient physicians, it is advantageous to seek capitation payment. The difference between their usual practice (which involves lower than average utilization) and the average for the region can simply be pocketed as profit with enough left over to allow for some discounting fees, as well. In areas of the country where capitation has substantially driven down costs, this represents less of an opportunity. The concern for an insurer, obviously, is that capitation arrangements tend to encourage under-utilization, the converse of fee-for-service payments that encourage over-utilization (12).

Whether or not capitation makes sense for an individual physician depends on the volume of patients under consideration. Specialty physicians should be particularly careful to make sure that the patient base is sufficiently large enough to allow balancing of risk from adverse selection. Expert help is often needed to avoid serious financial exposures. Typically, the amount of variation in health care costs begins to significantly diminish after a population of some 10,000 individual members is reached. Below the level of 500 to 1000 patients in a professional services contract, individual adverse selection may completely negate the averaging effect of capitation. It is the consideration of a large panel of patients as a portfolio of risks that capitation makes the most sense to individual providers. Physicians should shy away from capitation schemes, in which the number of patients under their control is small, because the effect of adverse selection can dramatically alter the profitability of the panel. An alternative approach to the small panel size problem is the purchase of stop-loss insurance or re-insurance, whereby unanticipated costs over a certain amount are insured with another entity. This clearly adds even further complexity to an already complicated system but is included as a part of the milieu in advanced managed care markets.

Hospital payments, although normally outside the sphere of relevance for a physician, are nevertheless important to understand, because hospital administrators are quite sensitive to payment measures in an era of decreasing reimbursement. Typically, hospitals may be reimbursed on a per case basis, in which hospitals are given a fixed amount of money for specific case class such as a Diagnosis Related Group (DRG) group. Hospitals may also be globally reimbursed for major surgical procedures, such as coronary artery bypass surgery, liver transplants, or other major cases transferring the risk of expensive case management back to individual hospitals. This process has been taken to an extreme with the development of for-profit specialty hospitals designed to perform a specific type of service. A third common method of reimbursing hospitals is per diem, which reimburses hospitals a fixed rate for each day that a patient stays, often with tiering for case severity level, etc. All methods may be found simultaneously in a geographic region, even from one managed care company source!

Clearly, the incentives for hospitals with each of these different types of reimbursement is quite different for everything from discharge planning and average lengths of stay to rates of transfer to step down units. For example, per case reimbursement of total hip fractures became popular with the introduction of DRG payments. Hospitals soon found that the length of stay for total hip patients could be dramatically reduced if patients were transferred shortly after surgery to step down skilled nursing facility units, which were reimbursed at a per diem rate. The institutions were essentially able to double bill for the intermediate period that had previously been covered within the DRG payment. This method of point-counterpoint reimbursement strategy between risk bearers and deliverers of services is maintained in a number of areas on a continuous basis. Although financial reimbursement schemes should not direct patient care, it is the foolish physician who does not pay attention to the financial pressures of distressed hospital organizations. How specialists, such as neurosurgeons, relate to acute patients moving into a rehab setting is clearly an important issue for administrators.

Of related interest, third party payers are capitated for services under Medicare risk contracts, in which the government provides a fixed rate reimbursement for each Medicare enrollee covered by the plan. A percentage (95% at this time) of the adjusted average per capita cost (AAPCC) becomes a single payment for the health plan to manage all medical costs for the members. Adjustments to the AAPCC are made by using a number of variables. These include age, gender, Medicare entitlement status, institutionalization, and Medicaid status (7). Third party payers must manage their provider networks to control costs within these limits. Problems with rates set by this method have recently resulted in the discontinuation of Medicare risk programs in a number of rural areas in this country.

MEDICAL MANAGEMENT

Reimbursement methodologies aside, third parties that were previously responsible only for calculating financial risk in member populations are increasingly becoming involved in medical management strategies designed to lower costs. Although most physicians see these strategies as a recent interference with their practices, the more appropriate view is to see various medical management controls in a state of evolution. As described above, from the early 1980s, medical management consisted of managing average lengths of stay determined by large actuarial houses processing claims for major employers. Patients who exceeded certain percentile cutoffs were usually targeted for case management and more intense scrutiny by medical management nursing staff and medical directors. This approach is predictably short-sighted in that patients who are extending into a high percentile cutoff range already may have underlying poor processes for discharge management. In the late 1980s and early 1990s, this inspection technology yielded to a more comprehensive approach to medical management that included early hospital discharge planning. Second surgical opinion programs often are met with similar fates. Early in their product life cycle, they appeared to reduce unnecessary surgeries and later appeared to only increase bureaucratic work for an additional surgeon. Thus, second surgical opinions, which are expensive, made way for the development of guidelines that surgical procedures would be compared. More recently, the use of surgical guidelines and clinical pathways has been criticized, because many patients do not fit into the standard category unless they are relatively young and without other co-existing comorbidities. It has also been problematic to enforce guidelines at the individual patient and physician level for a variety of reasons (17, 18, 20).

The 1990s have seen a move from the inspection technology demonstrated by the ''1-800-mother-may-I'' approach to one that is more in keeping with a statistical quality control orientation. In this latter approach, individual cases are not monitored, but overall statistics regarding a provider's approach to treating large numbers of patients are evaluated from a sophisticated statistical approach. The principle vehicle for administering this approach is the use of physician or group specific performance statistics, coupled with directed workplans to alter physician utilization behavior (25). The overall trend from an inspection approach in medical management to one that uses statistical quality control has been one of the most striking developments in medical management over the past decade. It has removed much of the micro management oversight over physicians, instead concentrating on overall performance of a physician management unit in the care of patients. This has resulted in increasing responsibility to the level of physician and has paralleled the overall approach to ensuring medical quality that emerged as a backlash to both imputed medical care problems, as well as concern over under-utilization, precipitated by managed care organizations (27).

Medical management activity going forward is moving from historical inspection methodologies aimed at individual case oversight of physicians to statistically driven approaches. Characteristics of modern medical management demonstrate that they have the following attributes (Fig. 20.6) (1).

Medical Management

- ◆ Information driven
- ◆ Population segmentation
- ◆ Risk stratification
- ◆ Targeted intervention
- ◆ Outcomes focused
- ◆ Continuous improvement strategies
- ◆ Modern analytic tools

Figure 20.6 Characteristics of modern medical management.

Information Driven

Health plans are increasingly using the large data warehouses that they have developed from claims payment information to assess potential sources of savings. This includes not only claims information but information obtained from provider credentialing activities, patient satisfaction surveys, public sources, and even credit card databases. The integration of all of these types of data into an information system has been the Holy Grail for health plan information officers over the past five years. The data collected through these various sources and the information it contains become the elements of the analysis that follows (1).

Population Segmentation

As health plans and health systems become larger, they are moving from the statistical analysis of an average member to a much more sophisticated, data driven analysis of various member segments. This movement parallels similar population segmentation initiatives in the general business community, which have yielded targeted marketing and improved sales techniques. Applied to the health of populations, it allows a more precise focusing of payer initiatives. Applied to provider populations, it allows the targeting of key physician members most responsible for outlier effects in cost, utilization, or practice styles.

Risk Stratification

Within population segments and across the health plan, risk stratification becomes important in an era where health plan management resources are highly scrutinized. Stratification of the population's sickest members is allowed by information driven processes and becomes the essential driver to disease management programs. As mentioned previously, approximately 5% of the population typically account for approximately 50% of the medical care costs. Twenty percent of the population typically accounts for 80% of the medical care costs. Stratifying the population to risk tiers allows precise focusing of medical management activities. (An example includes the development of congestive heart failure disease management programs that focus attention on the medical care of patients with New York Heart Association [NYHA] classifications of III or IV.) This allows for more appropriate use of resources and improved outcomes.

Targeted Intervention

Given the limitations in administrative resources, health plans are beginning to target the highest risk categories through the creation of disease state management or disease management programs. Thus, the plan's information systems will identify that the greatest impact and/or variance in medical costs comes from patients with congestive heart failure, diabetes, HIV, asthma, or other similar diseases. By targeting these subgroups of individuals for intensified medical management focus, significant benefit has been anticipated and is being demonstrated to accrue. Interestingly, there is a significant variation in the routine practice of medicine that has been well documented most famously in the Dartmouth Atlas studies (3). Through the effective application of evidence based medical guidelines, substantial reductions in overall medical costs can accrue to systems.

Outcomes Focused

Health plans have changed considerably from initial micro-management techniques to those that are population driven largely due to the recognition that individual traditional case management tools are ineffective in the outcomes they produce. Discharging patients from the hospital a day early only transfers cost to the outpatient arena. Micro-management of individuals results in considerable patient dissatisfaction. Accordingly, health plans are focusing on the production of medical and quality outcomes that demonstrate both increased medical cost savings and improved patient satisfaction. Thus, there is a movement to focus on major disease categories, patient satisfaction, case management for sicker members, and other initiatives that are calculated to achieve greater impact.

Continuous Improvement

The continuous quality improvement or total quality management revolution that effected businesses in the 1980s and 1990s came fairly late to the insurer and managed care communities. However, over the past four to six years, continuous quality improvement for both clinical and business operations has become de rigeur. The results are predictably quite measurable and impressive when implemented across large populations of individuals and sprawling bureaucratic companies. Continuous quality improvement methodologies have been widely embraced by hospital plans, insurers, and medical group practices, often at the coaching or insistence of traditional businesses who have found these methods effective in improving their product capabilities.

Modern Management Analytic Tools

One of the most striking changes in health care management over the past five years has been the widespread adoption of modern analytic tools. This may be secondary to the fact that many of the clinical staff within health plans are obtaining advanced business degrees, although it is also undoubtedly related to the widespread accessibility to these tools in common software packages. Analytic units that had previously analyzed things only at the level of gross number and simple averages are adopting spreadsheets, project planning software, and sophisticated techniques, such as scenario analysis, linear programming, and fuzzy systems. It is the combination of the above strategies that most characterizes the changing landscape of medical management activities. At the individual group practice level, the continuation of the strategies, supplemented by an epidemiologic approach to patient population management, is resulting in truly significant changes in the way that health care is delivered. Systems that are developed by third party payers are encouraged in individual medical practices. These sophisticated analytic tools are having significant impact on the medical management of large populations of patients at the payer and group medical practice level.

QUALITY MANAGEMENT

The introduction of continuous quality improvement methodologies at the level of the health plan has resulted in the progressive evolution of medical management strategies that address the quality of medical care. The evolution of quality measurement methodologies has, in many ways, corresponded to similar events within the business community. The evolution has progressed through a number of stages:

First Stage–Quality Assurance, Inspection

In the first stage of quality activities, health plans focused on event monitoring in a typical inspection mode. Activities included credentialing physicians and procedures, monitoring adverse outcomes, sentinel events, care delivery process, pharmacy usage patterns, case studies, and external accreditation. The typical feature of many of these methods was the descriptive statistic of things without the inclusion of systematic process analysis.

Second Stage–Process Analysis/Statistical Quality Control/Continuous Quality Improvement

During this period, which began in the mid-1980s, the focus moved from individual inspection of clinical practice to review at a more statistical level. Examples of items reviewed included diagnosis or DRG specific hospital admission variations, surgical procedure rates and results variation, ambulatory care pattern variation, preventive services standards, selected claims based variation analysis, and patient satisfaction instruments. During this stage in the evolution of analyses, we saw concern with variation across multiple examples of individual patient management. Physicians become less targeted for the occasional adverse outcome and more accountable for sources of variation within their population and the outcomes they achieve.

Third Stage–Outcomes

In this stage in the evolution of system measurement of quality, true outcomes became the target of analysis. Typical analysis items included clinical outcomes measures (a variety of measures have been described), disease specific patient perceptions of illness, linkages of initiatives to disability and absenteeism, life event risk interventions (e.g., smoking cessation, seat belts), and functional status evaluation analysis. During this period, we moved from focusing on variations in care or outcomes to truly what is important in the delivery of care, the functioning of individuals or populations of individuals. It is here where the goals of physicians and health plans coincide. Clearly, populations of individuals that maintain their health and get better quicker are significantly less expensive. Methods for increasing the numbers of these individuals in a population is of great interest to third party payers, because it is these individuals who fund the medical costs of the rest of the risk pool.

The current stage of quality analysis has become more fragmented but probably is most characterized by the application of large management systems and risk bearing agents in the overall process of care. It is also characterized by the development of breathtaking advances in the use of information systems. Additional measures of adjusting for the complexities of the system being analyzed must also be addressed. Typical elements that characterize this phase in the development improvement include integrated care management companies and cooperative ventures between PHOs; physicians, hospitals, and the community; larger networks that include laboratories (community health information networks); and others. Other issues center on the transfer of risk to group practices, the development of large data warehouses, severity adjustment systems for administrative data, the analysis of under-utilization, and new indicators for clinical outcomes (glycohemoglobin levels in diabetic populations).

Although the above changes are occurring at the level of the health plan, it is important to point out that because risk is often transferred to the level of individual group practices in some markets, individual group practices or physician hospital organizations face many of the same challenges. It has often been amusing to me as a medical director that many of the loudest opponents of the techniques used by the system are among the first to arrive at my door when risk is transferred to an organization in which they have financial interests.

Physician group profiling often includes all of the above activities, as well as specific items more focused at the individual physician or group practice operations, including attention to the ability to attract patients, attitude and professional identity, hours of practice contact time, hours of meeting attendants, time management skills, quality of medical services, patient complaints, loyalty to the group, malpractice problem rate, and accuracy and timeliness of service. Clearly, the next generation of medical groups and physicians will begin to think much more like epidemiologists rather than individual patient caregivers as they seek to improve their practice performance, both clinically and from an operational perspective. They will have familiarity with these complex clinical and management information systems that are now evolving and be able to use them at the local level.

One of the interesting side effects of the quality movement nationally is the development of several large organizations committed to evaluating the performance of health plans on their use of many of these tools. In many ways, comparable with the Joint Commission on Accreditation of Healthcare Organizations (JCAHO), these large, powerful national organizations have become central in the certification of third party payers in their use of the above tools. Although as problematic for third party payers as the JCAHO is for hospitals, the overall effect of these organizations has been to widely spread many of the above tools throughout organizations and to create the pressure for organizations to adopt these operational management tools. Most notable among these organizations is the NCQA and the URAC. Although the former initially focused on the use of continuous quality improvement and quality measures within health plans, and the latter focused more on traditional utilization management techniques, each organization has incorporated many of the standard attributes and standards of the other. Each has a web page that is worthwhile to review.

INFORMATICS AS AN EVOLVING THIRD PARTY TOOL

All of the key elements in the third party perspective outlined to date are becoming increasingly reliant on evolving information systems. It is widely believed that the payer/health plan that has the most advanced access to an understanding of information will best manage costs and control their market.

In the good old days, information systems were largely process oriented and focused as data processing in online transaction processing (OLTP). This environment was focused on daily operations, data entry, and simple tasks, such as collecting, processing, and paying claims. Within the past decade, we have seen health plans move to isolate the information previously contained in these OLTP environments to compile warehouses of data for research and analysis purposes. Data warehouses typically are focused mainly on reporting and may contain redundant data elements that are usually read only and allow widespread access across the enterprise to business information, both clinical and financial. It is the potential of the systems to allow intermixing of financial and clinical information that

is its greatest promise. The main limitation at this point to third party payers having almost omniscient knowledge is the fact that these information systems have developed slowly through a variety of legacy environments. Mainframe environments, data processing divisions, and processes focused on simple tasks, such as paying claims, resulted in the creation of systems that were not flexible for integrated health care delivery systems and their information needs. At the present time, health plans are rapidly moving to convert the information contained in largely financial databases to something usable at the senior management and analyst level.

The advent of managed care resulted in many challenges for third party payers. These included:

- Movement of focus from a financial service organization concentrating on claims processing to an integrated delivery systems focused on risk sharing and insurance analysis.
- Changing focus from simple payment of claims to healthcare outcomes analysis.
- Evolution of quality standards from simple inspection technology to widespread outcome measures.
- Evolution of organizational complexity in health plans.
- Presence of competition and need for increased marketing and actuarial insight.
- Demands by external creditors for defined information requirements.
- Increasingly empowered employer and customer coalitions and their requests.
- Cost of conversion and producing information.

Many of the challenges relate to the increasing complexity of the broad marketplace described above. Government reporting, accreditation needs, employer needs, marketplace demands, clinical knowledge requirements, and a variety of other forces are increasingly pressuring organizations to take the vast wealth of information that they have been compiling over the past decades and turn it into meaningful information that is useful in creating social change. Another problem owners of these data warehouses have is the relatively imperfect nature of data contained within them. Physicians and managed care organizations, however, are gradually coming to terms with the information and actions that can be obtained from them (11).

It had been the general impression of most physicians that large third party payers possess data warehouses, which are capable of producing sophisticated physician level analysis with a high degree of accuracy. Typically, data placed in large warehouses of third party payers has a number of imperfections, which makes this application less easy than one would anticipate. However, as data warehouses are completed, the data is cleaned and methodologies are developed to analyze it for this type of review. Large health systems will increasingly require unique patient identifiers, unique physician identifiers, and submission of electronic claims. This will increase homogeneity of the data at the front end and create fewer imperfections in the data warehouses. As standardization is created within the claims submission process, analysis of the material will become more reliable and sophisticated. The recommendation for physicians is not to attempt to retard this process but to carefully build their own practice information systems to complement and support it. Large information databases will increasingly be used to analyze individual physician performance; the proper submission of information to these systems will determine how fairly the resultant information analysis software treats one.

PHYSICIAN PROFILING

Many of the above arguments ultimately come down to the analysis of individual physician performance. The evolution of continuous quality improvement through the methods described above has increased pressure on informatics areas to analyze not only populations of individuals but also the performance of individual physicians. The reasoning and logic behind physician profiling is fairly important as health plans and third party payers identify the following goals of physician profiling:

- Improvement in the quality of care to members and reduced health care costs.
- Informing physicians about their practice pattern when compared with their peers.
- Identifying areas where opportunities exist for utilization, patient satisfaction, and quality of care change.
- Development of strategies to improve performance overall.
- Align provider incentives with third party

payer strategies and develop reimbursement methods.
- Maintain accreditation performance levels.
- Support strategies that eliminate reliance on inspection of micro-management techniques.

Profiling systems for physicians basically break down along two lines. Administratively based systems use existing claims databases to make determinations about the physicians at clinical performance. A number of products have been developed, including the systems 3M Health Information Systems, APR-DRGs, AVGs, and Quadramed. Clinically based systems incorporate actual clinical data and include Mediqual (Atlas, formerly MedisGroups System), ISIS (International Severity Information Systems), and Dyncorp. The administratively based systems generally are in favor at the present time, because they are less expensive to administer and do not require the additional collection of clinical information, which in the absence of the automated medical record is presently able to be performed with intensive chart extraction techniques. An excellent reference can be found in Iezzoni (15).

All of the physician profiling systems rely strongly on the accuracy of coded information input to the data warehouses. The important point for individual physicians is that how individual claims are coded becomes critical. Inappropriate coding and/or fraud can be easily detected by using these tools. More importantly, because clinical severity adjustment tools are developed by using the ICD-9 codes submitted individually and collectively on each claim, lack of attention by the clinician to these codes will result in miscalculation of the physician's overall patient severity and could result in inappropriate conclusions about his/her practice. Because of the complexities involved, specialist profiling at this time is often restricted to high volume specialties, high volume specialist procedures, or similar subsets of the physician population. Specialist profiling tools of necessity have evolved later than primary care physician tools, where patient volumes are higher and patient demographics are approximated by statistical processes. Specialist profiling adds the additional element of subspecialty specification and the wide clinical heterogeneity of patients being treated within specialist practices. Much of the current specialist profiling technology is focused on the economic and clinical performance of specialists in fairly homogenous patient treatment group categories. Specialists who have a fairly general practice and average patients will probably be favored over specialists who deal with unique or atypical patient categories (e.g., hand surgeons, pediatric ophthalmologists). For this reason, I anticipate that the focus on neurosurgery follow the focus on cardiologists, pulmonologists, gastroenterologists, orthopedists, and other specialties that are more widely known for significant variation in the way they practice medicine and relatively high procedural costs.

Physician response to profiling activities has been predictably angry as physicians detected early on that the data being used is imperfect and that patient severity, socioeconomic factors, and practice patient mix are not completely incorporated in the results. It should be quite clear, however, that the economic forces driving the profiling in the first place will not wait for the development of a perfect system. It is incumbent upon physicians to become actively involved in the analytic process and to understand how these analyses result in the interpretation of their practice performance. There is no longer any excuse for non-participation in the ongoing movement to lower health care costs and improve quality. Additional specialist profiling targets going forward will include patient satisfaction measures, which can be obtained fairly easily and quickly and focus in particular on the treatment of geriatric patients where cost increases are becoming increasingly critical for Medicare at-risk programs.

FUTURE DIRECTIONS

Given the rapid rate at which change has occurred in the field of medical management, the way that third party payers relate to physicians in the future remains uncertain. There are, however, a number of common themes that will clearly operate well into the 21st century and will drive much of the business relationship between physicians and the third party payers on whom they are becoming increasingly dependent. These will include some of the following:

- Breathtaking developments in information systems that will result in increasing sophistication in the ability to analyze the performance of individual physicians, medical groups, hospital organizations, and health plans.
- Increasing emphasis on outcomes over process

in the delivery of health care from both an operational and medical quality perspective.
- More, rather than less, rigorous accreditation standards.
- Every year, accreditation organizations, such as the NCQA, JCAHO, and URAQ up the ante by making accreditation standards increasingly complex and rigorous. Although there is a reasonable backlash to the bureaucracy that these organizations have introduced, it is quite clear that from a number of different perspectives, the demands on providers and third party payers alike will increase.
- An increasingly sharp focus will be brought to bear on individual providers beginning with primary care physicians followed by high volume, high variance specialties, such as cardiology, gastroenterology, orthopedics, and others.
- Involvement of the business community with the information produced by large health delivery systems will increase. Notable participation is already occurring with a number of business coalitions. An excellent reference to see the future of how this might evolve can be found at the web site for the Pacific Business Group on Health or the Washington Business Group on Health. These business coalitions are also driving the further development of quality organizations, such as the NCQA and the development of specific measurement systems, such as HEDIS and FAcct data sets.
- There is widespread expectation on the part of patient populations that they will have increased participation in the decision-making process. Direct marketing and pharmaceuticals not withstanding, patient participation in the review of physician performance statistics is anticipated as employers seek to involve their members in the selection of more cost-effective providers. Provider report cards at the individual physician level are already being produced, although in few areas. It is likely that this trend will continue.
- Confidentiality concerns will increase going forward, as owners of large data systems will find it increasingly difficult to maintain confidentiality at either the member or physician level. Significant government and public pressure exists to publish physician-specific information regarding their care cost and quality. Given the fact that these measurement tools are imperfect, it is likely that this will cause

considerable concern and anxiety on the part of physicians as this information is made public.

CONCLUSION

Generally, the best advice for physicians in any specialty is to keep alert and become actively involved in the development of these systems. Overall, I am optimistic that the application of intelligent management systems to what had been a fragmented, highly variable cottage industry will ultimately improve medical care. This will not occur without some stress and unfairness at the margins.

It is likely that neurosurgeons will need additional training in many of these techniques if they are to be prepared for coping with the exigencies of the 21st century (16). A rising senior population, increasing complexity of medical technology, and pressure to constrain health care costs will continue to prove an important challenge for the medical practitioners.

REFERENCES

1. Barish J, Breiner K, Fetterolf F, Heisler K, Moise J: The Highmark Pegasus Project Report. *Best Practices and Benchmarking in Healthcare*. 2:112, 1997.
2. Boland P: Special commentary: The challenge of documenting managed care cost savings and performance. *Managed Care Q* 1:36–40, 1993.
3. Center for Evaluative Clinical Sciences Dartmouth Medical School: The Dartmouth Atlas of Health Care. Chicago, American Hospital Association, 1998.
4. Coddington D: Making Integrated Health Care Work. Englewood, Colorado, Center for Research in Ambulatory Health Care Administration, 1996.
5. Cotter DJ, Renault P: Safety and clinical effectiveness of intracranial pressure monitors for purposes of Medicare coverage. *Med Instrum* 16:9–11, 1982.
6. Courtney H, Kirkland J, Viguerie P: Strategy Under Uncertainty. Harvard Business Review, 1997, Boston pp 67–79.
7. Dacso S, Dacso C: Managed Care Answer Book. New York, Aspen Publishers, 1999, ed 4, pp 6–45.
8. Doyle R: Healthcare Management Guidelines: Volume I–Inpatient and Surgical Care. Philadelphia, Milliman and Robertson, 1995.
9. Dunham N, Kindig D, Schulz R: The value of the physician executive role to organizational effectiveness and performance. *Health Care Manage Rev*, 19:56–63, 1994.
10. Ferguson J, Weinberger M: Case management programs in primary care. *J Gen Intern Med* 13:123–126, 1998.
11. Fetterolf D: The Use of Imperfect Data in Managed Care Organizations. Physician Executive, 1998, pp 42–46.
12. Fetterolf D: A framework for evaluating under-utilization of health care services. *Am J Med Quality* 14: 89–97, 1999.
13. Gold M, Siegel J, Russell L, Weinstein M: Cost-effectiveness in Health and Medicine: Report of the U.S. Public Health Service Panel on Cost-effectiveness in Health and Medicine. New York, Oxford University Press, 1996.
14. Halm E, Causino N: Is gatekeeping better than traditional care? *JAMA* 278:1677–1681, 1997.
15. Iezzoni L: Risk Adjustment for Measuring Healthcare Outcomes. Chicago, Health Administration Press, 1997, ed 2.
16. Jimenez D: Socioeconomic issues and education of neurologic surgery residents in the United States. *Surg Neurol* 50:179–81, 1998.
17. Khandker R, Manning W: The impact of utilization review on costs and utilization, in Zweifel P, Frech H (eds): Health Economics Worldwide. The Netherlands, Kluwer Academic Publishers, 1992, pp 47–62.
18. Kleinman L, Boyd E, Heritage J: Adherence to prescribed explicit criteria during utilization review. *JAMA* 278:497–501, 1997.
19. Kongstvedt P: The Managed Health Care Handbook. Gaithersburg, Aspen Publishers, 1996, pp 4–12.
20. Lomas J, Anderson G, Domnick-Pierre K, Vayda E, Enkin M, Hannah W: Do Practice Guidelines Guide Practice? *N Engl J Med* 321:1306–1311, 1989.
21. Martin M, Milstein A, Loveland D: Enhancing utilization review program results. *Health Cost Manage* 5: 10–16, 1988.
22. McClendon J, Politzer R, Christian E: Downsizing the physician workforce. *Public Health Reports* 112: 231–239, 1997.
23. Mills C: Case management programs improve patient outcomes but do not reduce costs. *ACP J Club* Sept/ Oct:53, 1998.
24. Muller C: Review of twenty years of research on medical care utilization: Part I. *Health Serv Res* 21: 130–144, 1986.
25. Nathanson P: Influencing physician practice patterns. *Top Health Care Finance* 20:16–25, 1994.
26. National Committee for Quality Assurance (NCQA). Standards for the Accreditation of Managed Care Organizations (MCOs). Washington, D. C., NCQA, 1997, 1998.
27. Payne S, Campbell D: New methods for evaluating utilization management programs. *QRB* October: 340–347, 1992.
28. Restuccia J: The effect of feedback in reducing inappropriate hospital utilization. *Med Care* 20:46–62, 1982.
29. Robinson J: Decline in hospital utilization and cost inflation under managed care in California. *JAMA* 276: 1060–1064, 1996.
30. Rosenberg S, Allen D, Handte M, et al: Effect of utilization review in a fee-for-service health insurance plan. *N Engl J Med* 333:1326–1354, 1995.
31. Santerre R, Neun S: Health Economics: Theories, Insights, and Industry Studies. Chicago, Irwin Publishers, 1996, pp 44–78.
32. Siegel J, Weinstein M: Recommendations for reporting cost-effectiveness analysis. *JAMA* 276:1339–1341, 1996.
33. Tarlov A: The medical outcomes study: An application of methods for monitoring the results of medical care. *JAMA* 262:925–930, 1989.
34. Utilization Review Accreditation Commission (URAC): National Utilization Review Standards. Washington, DC, URAC, April, 1994.

35. Utilization Review Accreditation Commission (URAC): Health Network Accreditation Standards Application Notebook. Washington, D. C., URAC, 1998.

36. Warren B, Puls T, Folgelstrom-DeZeeuw P: Cost-effectiveness of case management: Experiences of a university managed health care organization. *Am J Med Quality* 11:173–178, 1996.

37. Williamson J, Hudson J, Nevins M: Principles of Quality Assurance and Cost Containment in Healthcare. San Francisco, Josey Bass Publishers, 1982, pp 4–11.

38. Yates B: Analyzing Costs, Procedures, Processes, and Outcomes in Human Services: Applied Social Research Methods Series, Volume 42. London, Sage Publications, 1996.

CHAPTER 21

Understanding Standard Hospital Cost Indices

PAM ROSATO-LANGE, R.N., B.S., M.P.M.

With the passage and implementation of the Balanced Budget Act of 1997, the hospitals of the United States began facing the reality of declining revenues for several years into the future. The prospect of being paid less to provide the same, or potentially more, service has forced the industry to re-examine its use of resources and the way they are accounted for. A variety of new measures and cost indices has been developed in an attempt to maximize economic efficiency in patient care. Ms. Rosato-Lange provides us with an excellent account of the forces that have shaped these changes, an explanation of the hospital response, and an indication of the effect on the practicing physician.

Over the past 15 years, the health care system in the United States has undergone dynamic changes. The influx of managed care has placed a great demand on health care institutions to reduce price while maintaining quality. Historical methods of reimbursement by fee-for-service and full cost reimbursement have been replaced by restrictive pricing structures placing limits on remuneration for services provided. Recently, further limits have been imposed on these pricing mechanisms, minimizing the annual rate of payment increase to an amount less than the rate of inflation (8). Hospitals are under enormous pressure to implement strategies in response to declining patient revenues as a means for long-term survival.

This chapter discusses the common cost-indices experienced from the perspective of the health care institution. Methods of public and private third party hospital reimbursement are identified and discussed. The economic impact associated with the conversion from a fee-for-service to a capitated reimbursement environment is addressed. Information is presented that

relates to potential revenue retaining and enhancement strategies.

METHODS OF REIMBURSEMENT

Health care facilities are compensated for the service that they provide in a variety of diverse manners. Each third party reimbursement plan places a new set of requirements and responsibilities on the provider. Hospitals are compensated by these plans using variable or fixed payment rates, which expands the financial risk to the institution with the standardization of payment. The most common forms of recompense include fee-for-service payment, per diem payment, diagnosis related group (DRG) or fixed payment per discharge diagnosis, and global or capitated payment rates (1, 15).

Fee-for-service is a method by which payment is determined retrospectively from the providers itemized statement for services rendered to a patient during an inpatient or outpatient hospital encounter. Each service provided is matched with its corresponding fee and reimbursed accordingly. Currently, the majority of third party payers who employ this method compensate the health care facility a pre-negotiated percentage of total charges. This reimbursement process places the third party payer at risk for all service provided to its beneficiaries.

A per diem payment system compensates the provider for each day that care is provided within the health care institution. A flat per day rate is paid, regardless of the type of services that were performed during the beneficiary's admission. The third party payer may then retrospectively deny the admission or a certain portion of the patient's length of stay based on medical necessity or appropriateness of hospitalization.

The DRG method of payment reimburses the health care facility a pre-determined fixed dollar amount per hospital admission, which is determined by the patient's diagnosis. The DRG system classifies cases based on the primary diagnosis, secondary diagnoses, procedures performed, gender, age, and patient's discharge status (9). There are currently 496 DRGs in 25 major diagnostic categories (MDC), which generally refer to a particular organ system (for example, MDC 1, Diseases and Disorders of the Nervous System) (9). The prospective payment rate is calculated by multiplying each individual hospital's payment rate per case by an assigned DRG weight. The hospital specific payment rate is calculated using a labor rate (urban or rural) multiplied by the area wage index factor and adding a non-labor rate amount. This rate varies based on the geographic location and type of health care facility. The DRG weight calculation is reflective of the resources used to care for patients within a specific DRG category compared with the average resources used in all DRGs (9).

Global pricing combines the reimbursement for the physician, hospital, and ancillary components of care. A package price is determined based on these criteria for a specific diagnosis or procedure. This mode of compensation is often thought of as the precursor to capitated payment systems, providing limited risk sharing to the institution. Global pricing places the physician and health care institution at risk for increased lengths of stay and physician related costs (24).

Capitated payment plans reimburse the provider a fixed per member per month (PMPM) payment to provide medical care to a group of managed care plan members. The health care institution receives a pre-determined percentage of the PMPM premium dollar to provide care, whether or not it is utilized by the beneficiary. Acceptance of these PMPM fees places the health care institution at risk regardless of the number and nature of services needed to care for the capitated patient population.

Hospital care expenditures represented 371.1 billion of the 1 trillion dollars in national health care expenditures in 1997, with Medicare, Medicaid, commercial, and out of pocket payers comprising the bulk of third party hospital payers (11). The largest public providers of health care remuneration include Medicare and Medicaid, which reimbursed health care institutions 123.7 and 57.6 billion dollars in 1997, respectively (11). Administered by the Health Care Financing Administration (HCFA), Medicare is the largest public provider of health care insurance in the nation. Between 1965 and 1982, Medicare paid hospitals for service using the full cost reimbursement payment method. Hospitals were compensated retrospectively for all costs incurred during a patient's admission, including fees for operating costs, capital costs, and medical education pass-throughs in teaching institutions. In 1983, as part of the Social Security Amendments, the Medicare system drastically changed with the passage of Public Law 98-21, mandating the development of a prospective payment system under Medicare Part A (Hospital Insurance) (5). This prospective payment system currently reimburses hospitals a pre-determined DRG rate per patient admission.

The Balanced Budget Act of 1997 further curtailed payments to prospective payment system hospitals by establishing a ''0 percent increase for fiscal year 1998, a market basket index (MBI) minus 1.9 points for 1999, MBI minus 1.8 points for 2000, and a MBI minus 1.1 points for fiscal years 2001 and 2002'' (13). This law also placed restrictions on revenue available for capital improvements and medical education pass-throughs to teaching institutions. Consequently, it is anticipated that the increase in the Medicare inpatient hospital spending rate will decline to approximately 3% from an average of 8.2% per year in 1998 to 2000 (11, 38). Furthermore, these proposed curtailments in reimbursement are coupled by increases in regulation to limit Medicare fraud and abuse, necessitating an increase in expenditures for internal oversight programs to limit potential provider liability.

Title XIX of the Social Security Act established the Medicaid Program. Under this program, State agencies receive matched Federal funding to provide medical care for pregnant women, blind, disabled, families, and the aged. Since its inception, institutions have been paid by fee-for-service or by DRG payment for services rendered. Recently, states have been aggressively attempting to control their costs through a variety of managed care initiatives. In some states, beneficiary participation in a managed care plan is mandatory using a Health Maintenance Organization (HMO) or similar entity, which compensate health care providers using capitated payment rates. Medicaid capitated rates are calculated based on the fee-for-service per capita rates in a specific geographic region and are significantly lower than those rates acknowledged by commercial or Medicare insurers (7, 12). As reported by HCFA, Medicaid managed care enrollment rates have increased from 29.4% in 1995 to 53.6% in 1998 (10). This two-fold increase in the utilization of managed care contracting imposes a greater financial responsibility on the health care facility to provide care in an extremely prudent manner.

Commercial insurance contracts range from fee-for-service indemnity plans to capitated managed care payment plans. Payments for hospital care under these plans have risen from $36.5 billion in 1980 to $113 billion in 1997 (11). Many private insurance plans compensate health care facilities a certain percentage of charges over the Medicare base DRG payment for a given diagnosis. Employers that offer commercial insurance coverage to their workers encouraged the utilization of managed care plans to offset their employee benefit costs (19). Accordingly, managed care enrollment in the private sector has surpassed 85% in 1997 (38).

HOSPITAL COST INDICES AND THE RESPONSE TO REIMBURSEMENT CHANGES

To quantify the effect of the prospective payment system and managed care reimbursement on health care facilities, it is important to understand the common inpatient utilization indicators. Inpatient utilization is measured by a variety of different methods, including length of stay, inpatient days, cost per discharge, and hospital beds per 1000 persons. Inpatient length of stay encompasses the time elapsed in days from the date of admission to the acute care facility up to the date of discharge. Inpatient days are calculated based on the total number of days spent by all patients within the health care institution. This figure may be separated by specialty service and/or diagnosis to provide specific data related to service line volume. The total number of hospital or specialty inpatient days can be divided by the total number of patients within

those respective groups to determine an average length of stay for that specific population. The benchmark for the average length of stay in a neurosurgical patient population is approximately four days, with a slight increase for Medicare recipients' (27). The cost per discharge is determined by the addition of all costs incurred to the patient during a specific length of stay and may vary widely based on the geographic location and type of facility. Hospital beds per 1000 persons depict the total number of available beds in a certain geographic region. This figure is beneficial for determining global inpatient bed utilization and excess capacity.

Health care institutions initially responded to changes within the prospective payment system and an increase in the utilization of managed care plans through a reduction in inpatient length of stay. This is evident in the examination of MedPAR Neurosurgical DRG payment data from 1993 to 1997. During this period, length of stay declined nationally in short-term hospitals for DRG 001 (Craniotomy Age > 17 Except for Trauma), from 13.6 days to 9.43 days; for DRG 214 (Back and Neck Procedures with CC) from 8.4 days to 5.54 days; and for DRG 215 (Back and Neck Procedures without CC) from 4.70 days to 3.04 days (Table 21.1). A similar downward trend in length of stay is noted for most DRGs during this period, although the average reimbursement rate remained somewhat

TABLE 21.1
Health Care Financing Administration MedPAR Data for Short Stay Inpatient Hospitals, 1997

DRG	Year	Total Reimbursement ($)	Average Length of Stay	Average Payment ($)
001	1997	635,535,868	9.43	16,632
001	1996	606,602,452	10.1	16,347
001	1995	556,815,961	11.10	16,096
001	1994	521,793,702	12.40	15,829
001	1993	503,683,758	13.60	16,250
214	1997	539,623,399	5.54	9,043
214	1996	504,113,336	5.90	8,619
214	1995	466,514,537	6.40	8,453
214	1994	439,487,335	7.30	8,160
214	1993	411,649,054	8.40	8,150
215	1997	224,891,509	3.04	4,530
215	1996	199,787,277	3.30	4,375
215	1995	181,152,246	3.60	4,323
215	1994	178,493,700	4.10	4,294
215	1993	170,269,799	4.70	4,351

DRG = diagnosis related group.

stable. It is speculated that this occurred in part through the shifting of services from inpatient to outpatient care and through the increased utilization of alternate levels of care.

Since the inception of the Medicare prospective payment plan in 1983, inpatient rates have declined approximately 12% and outpatient utilization rates have risen 137%. As a result, outpatient reimbursement represents approximately 38% of the total revenue of an average health care institution (2, 10). This acceleration in outpatient utilization is a product of advances in medical technology, hospital based cost reduction stressors, and reimbursement incentives by third party payers (2, 25). The decline in inpatient utilization tends to be more significant in areas with an increase in managed care penetration. The greater the propensity of capitated managed care contracting within a certain geographic region further impacts inpatient utilization rates by decreasing the total number of acute care inpatient days. For example, in California, inpatient days and length of stay declined 29% and 19%, respectively, in markets with low managed care penetration and 44% and 20%, respectively, in areas with a higher managed care presence (35). The current rate of outpatient utilization is expected to slow in the future as a consequence of proposed provisions in the Balanced Budget Act of 1997, through the institution of a prospective payment plan for these services.

A wide variation in the cost of health care services is evident nationally (40). A variety of factors influences the cost per inpatient discharge within a health care facility. An overall reduction in hospital cost per discharge is evident in areas with a higher than average managed care presence. In the short-term, hospitals in competitive managed care environments were able to more effectively reduce cost and resource consumption (i.e., laboratory testing), resulting in a decline in the total cost per patient (43). The presence of positive cost drivers in a competitive market significantly influenced a reduction in price.

Hospital cost per discharge is inflated by the average age of the inpatient population, the number of secondary diagnoses per patient per admission, the number of paid hours per discharge, and an excess in the number of available beds per capita (6, 26). An increase in the number of employee paid hours per discharge, as well as a higher than average hospital wage index, contribute to a higher cost per discharge within the facility. An overabundance in the number of available beds per capita is also associated with an increase in the cost per discharge. Excess capacity and the expenses associated with maintaining it (labor, buildings, and equipment), generally represent fixed costs to the institution that cannot be reduced unless there is a consolidation or elimination of one or all of those components (26, 34). As length of stay, resource utilization, and the number of inpatient days decline, it is necessary to reduce simultaneously the number of health care facilities, poorly utilized beds, and their associated labor force. The inability to restrict capacity at the same rate as utilization can pose serious threats to the viability of the health care system.

To respond to the changing paradigm from fee-for-service reimbursement to capitated reimbursement plans, health care institutions must reanalyze administrative, fiscal, and patient care activities. As revenue streams begin to diminish, health care institutions must increase cost effectiveness and efficiency through the coordination and management of patient care. Activity-based costing, case management, clinical pathways, care mapping, and other revenue retaining strategies are methods by which health care institutions can continue to prepare for the shifting of financial burden (6, 26, 31).

It is imperative to recognize the actual costs incurred in providing patient care services. In general, hospital accounting systems are designed to maximize reimbursement and lack the sophistication necessary to determine these costs. Caution must be exercised not to confuse patient charges with the actual costs of care, because the two may differ widely. Activity-based costing is a method by which the actual costs of care may be identified and is defined as the "total cost of the service, including the cost to manufacture, deliver and service that product" (29). The product generated within the hospital is health care. The entire process of care must be carefully examined, assigning direct and indirect costs to each identified component (39). Direct costs are those costs easily traced to the product or service to be performed. Examples of direct costs include magnetic resonance imaging, drug, and supply costs. Indirect costs are much more difficult to realize, because they are not easily identified. Examples of indirect costs include administrative and overhead costs. Incertitude and improper allocation of indirect costs can lead to overpricing or underpricing of the health care product, thereby influencing the negotiation of managed care contracts resulting in poor fiscal decisions (29).

The use of internal proactive patient management systems is important for success in a managed care environment. Case management is a method by which all aspects of patient care are coordinated, integrated, and evaluated; thereby, influencing quality, cost, and access to care (4, 16). Through the facilitation of care, quality is increased by enhanced communication among patients/family members and all members of the health care team. Discharge planning begins within the first 24 hours of admission and extends throughout the continuum of care. These factors promote a reduction in length of stay, inpatient days, resource utilization, and readmissions to the acute care facility (4, 16). Case management activities vary from institution to institution; however, overall reductions in inpatient length of stay and resource utilization have been consistently realized.

Internal utilization management plays an important role in determining the continued financial solvency of the organization. The utilization review process coordinates the patient's insurance benefits with the written plan of care in the acute care setting. This method consists of four components: preadmission review, admission review, continued stay review, and discharge review. Criteria based on intensity of service, severity of illness, and readiness for discharge is utilized to determine the appropriateness of the admission or continued length of stay. Efficient patient management teams are easily able to identify those factors that limit or deny reimbursement based on these criteria.

Third party reimbursement to health care institutions is adversely effected by delays in the provision of service. An overall reduction in the number of avoidable days in service and denied days may be realized once the barriers to care are identified. Denied reimbursement from third party payers is directly correlated with system inefficiencies involving the hospital, the physician, and the patient (27). Hospital related barriers to care generally involve the inability to schedule or complete procedures within given time constraints. The failure to discharge a patient to an alternate level of care or to their home

in a timely manner represents the most commonly reported physician related delay. Patient issues generally involve the patient's refusal to be discharged to their home or an alternate level of care. The economic impact of these impediments to care may result in the denial of up to 30% of the total inpatient days within a health care institution (27).

The use of an appropriate alternate level of care setting is essential for the reduction in acute care length of stay and inpatient resource utilization. Some health care institutions have on-sight or established contracts with subacute, skilled (nursing home), and rehabilitation units. While decreasing the acute care length of stay, on-sight units afford the hospital with the opportunity to fill poorly utilized beds, cut costs, limit the avoidable days in acute-care service, and continue to receive compensation for service provided (17, 18). Medicare primarily reimburses these alternate levels of care under a fee-for-service payment method. The Balanced Budget Act of 1997 proposes the institution of a prospective reimbursement plan for skilled nursing care, home health, and rehabilitation care (13, 38). These proposed changes are expected to slow the growth of spending in these areas, mirroring the impact of the prospective payment plan in the acute care setting.

Another method of managing patient care utilization is the use of critical pathways or care maps. These tools provide standardization of best case scenarios to provide optimal patient care for a given diagnosis or procedure. They are generally used in conjunction with case management and should be formulated using a multidisciplinary team of clinicians and financial staff. The financial staff plays an integral role in providing physicians and clinical staff with information related to resource consumption and the costs that they are asked to control (6). When properly executed, clinical pathways can assist the health care facility to decrease their length of stay for a particular diagnosis or procedure, reduce redundancy of resources, and manage associated costs utilizing activity-based costing measures (24, 31, 39). Critical pathways should be continuously evaluated and variances in care documented. The differences between best case scenarios and actual practice should be carefully analyzed and shared with all members of the health care team.

With past and recently proposed changes in

the Medicare prospective payment system, optimization of reimbursement becomes a revenue retaining strategy within the health care organization. Medicare and some third party reimbursement rates continue to be reflective of hospital coding practices. An in-depth knowledge of Internal Classification of Diseases Coding (ICD-9) and its effect on DRG classification is crucial (8). Hospital staff must be aware of changes in regulation related to coding practices to maximize reimbursement, as well as reduce liability from external review compliance monitors.

At the onset of managed care growth and declining patient care revenues, health care institutions began to horizontally integrate. Hospitals bought, sold, collaborated with, and closed other health care institutions to reduce costs and gain market presence. This process enabled the institution to benefit from economies of scale while reducing administrative overhead (6, 43). This process evolved from horizontal integration with other hospitals to vertically integrated delivery systems. Integrated delivery systems provide the means to manage all aspects of care across the continuum, with a fundamental focus on health promotion and prevention of illness. These systems may provide hospital, physician, home care, skilled care, rehabilitation, and enterprise wide information systems. Advanced information system development is an essential component within these systems, availing pertinent patient related information at all levels of care. However, to be prosperous within a managed care environment, they must be proficient at providing high quality care within specified cost constraints (23). Successful integrated delivery systems demonstrate the ability to negotiate capitated contracts with managed care companies and/or directly with employers.

Once costs and utilization rates are driven to nationally equitable levels, the concept of total quality management and quality improvement will be the competitive force separating health care institutions. Mortality, morbidity, surgical complications, patient satisfaction, and physician credentialing will gain greater importance in contract negotiation. Physicians and facilities will be benchmarked against their peers for best practice scenarios and positive outcome indicators. Those facilities that can quantitatively demonstrate excellence in patient and financial management will gain bargaining power in negotiation with third party payers and employers.

CONCLUSION

The influx of managed care and changes within public insurance programs have placed additional financial responsibilities on hospitals. The challenge remains with creating a balance between a continued reduction in reimbursement and the maintenance of quality within health care institutions. Facilities must effectively coordinate and manage patient care and continue to investigate potential revenue enhancing and retaining strategies. It is abundantly clear that only those institutions that can incorporate cost, quality, and favorable patient outcomes will be the leaders in the highly competitive capitated markets of the future.

REFERENCES

1. Bodenheimer TS, Grumbach K: Reimbursing health care providers, in Understanding Health Policy. Connecticut, Appleton and Lange, 1995, pp 41–56.
2. Cleverley W: The Health Care Industry, in Evolution or Revolution? *J Health Care Finance* 25:2–14, 1999.
3. Coddington DC, Moore KD, Fischer EA: Integrating? Hang in there: The odds are in your favor. *Healthcare Forum J* Jan/Feb:72–75, 1995.
4. Cohen E, Cesta T: Nursing Case Management from Concept to Evaluation. St. Louis, Mosby, 1997.
5. Congress of the United States, Office of Technology Assessment: Predicted effects of Medicare's prospective payment system, in: Medicare's Prospective Payment System: Strategies for Evaluating Cost, Quality, and Medical Technology. Washington, D. C., U.S. Government Printing Office, 1985.
6. Conrad D, Wickizer T, Maynard C, et al: Managing care, incentives, and information: An exploratory look inside the "black box" of hospital efficiency. *HSR: Health Serv Res* 31:235–259, 1996.
7. Davidson H: Contracting for Medicaid Managed Care. *Healthcare Financial Manage* Nov:45–48, 1996.
8. Deatsch D: Revenue enhancement strategies. *Topics Health Care Finance* 17:21–29, 1991.
9. Department of Health and Human Services, Healthcare Financing Administration: Medicare program: Changes to the hospital inpatient prospective payment systems and fiscal year 1999 rates. *Federal Register* 63(89), May 8, 1998.
10. Department of Health and Human Services, Healthcare Financing Administration: Hospital admissions and outpatient visits. http://www.hcfa.gov/stats/indicatr/analysis.htm.
11. Department of Health and Human Services, Healthcare Financing Administration: Hospital care expenditures aggregate and per capita amounts and percent distribution, by Source of Funds: Selected Calendar Years 1960–1997. http://www.hcfa.gov/stats/stats.htm.
12. Department of Health and Human Services, Healthcare

Financing Administration: National summary of medicaid managed care programs and enrollment. June 30, 1998. http://www.hcfa.gov/medicaid/trends98.htm.

13. Department of Health and Human Services, Healthcare Financing Administration: Subtitle E: Provisions Relating to Part A only. http://www.hcfa.gov/regs/subt e.htm. pp 1–17.

14. Duncheon MA, Wolf DB: Key provisions strengthen hospital capitation contracts. *Healthcare Financial Manage* Nov:66–71, 1996.

15. Elliott SD: Taking control of managed care contracting. *Healthcare Financial Manage* Dec:40–45, 1996.

16. Etheridge P, Lamb G: Professional nursing management improves access, quality, and costs. *Nurs Manage* 20: 30–35, 1989.

17. Fogel LA: Financial advantages of operating a skilled nursing unit. *Healthcare Financial Manage* July: 50–55, 1994.

18. Fogel LA, Gossman-Kim K: Getting Started with Subacute Care. *Healthcare Financial Manage* Oct: 64–71, 1995.

19. Gaskin DJ, Hadley J: The impact of HMO penetration on the rate of hospital cost inflation: 1985–1993. *Inquiry* 34:205–216, 1997.

20. Goldsmith JC, Goran MJ, Nackel JG: Managed care comes of age. *Healthcare Forum J* Sept/Oct:14–24, 1995.

21. Herdman RC, Stevens RA: Proposals for funding graduate medical education. *Arch Gen Psychiatry* 55: 299–302, 1998.

22. Kauer RT, Silvers JB, Teplensky J: The effect of fixed payment on hospital costs. *J Health Polit Policy Law* 20:303–327, 1995.

23. Kaufman N: Competing in an integrated healthcare market: Four strategies for success. *Healthcare Executive* May/June:28–22, 1995.

24. Kelly MP: How global pricing works. *Healthcare Financial Manage* 18–19, 1995.

25. Lake T: Current trends in health plan payment methods for facility costs of outpatient care. *J Health Care Finance* 5:1–8, 1998.

26. Langabeer J: Competing on price: The economics of managed competition. *Acad Med* 71:1244–1246, 1996.

27. Lefton RB, Lefton RM: Expanding weekend and holiday clinical services: A financial perspective. *Healthcare Financial Manage* 37–40, 1998.

28. MacStravic S: Market and market segment portfolio assessment for hospitals. *Health Care Manage Rev* 14: 25–32, 1989.

29. Marrin CA, Johnson LC, Beggs VL, Batalden PB: Clinical process cost analysis. *Ann Thorac Surg* 64: 690–694, 1997.

30. Mechanic R, Coleman K, Dobson A: Teaching hospital costs. *JAMA* 280:1015–1019, 1998.

31. Meyer J, Feingold MG: Integrating financial modeling and patient care reengineering. *Healthcare Financial Manage* Feb:33–39, 1995.

32. Mulkerrin PF: What will create value in managed care? *Advest Healthcare Rev* Sept:5–9, 1995.

33. Reuter J, Gaskin D: Academic health centers in competitive markets. *Health Aff* 16:242–252, 1997.

34. Roberts R, Frutos P, Ciavarella G, et al: Distribution of variable versus fixed costs of hospital care. *JAMA* 281:644–649, 1999.

35. Robinson J: Decline in hospital utilization and cost inflation under managed care in California. *JAMA* 276: 1060–1064, 1996.

36. Schwartz M, Young DW, Seigrist R: The ratio of costs to charges: How good a basis for estimating costs? *Inquiry* 32:476–481, 1995/1996.

37. Skelton AG: The relationship among cost, quality and competition: An analysis of obstetrics services in Missouri hospitals. *J Health Care Finance* 24:30–44, 1997.

38. Smith S, Freeland M, Heffler S, McKusick D: Health expenditures projection team. The next ten years of health spending: What does the future hold? *Health Aff* 17:128–138, 1998.

39. Udpa S: Activity-based costing for hospitals. *Health Care Manage Rev* 21:83–96, 1996.

40. Weil TP: Competition versus regulation: Constraining hospital discharge costs. *J Health Care Finance* 2: 62–74, 1996.

41. Weil TP: The blending of competitive and regulatory strategies: A second opinion. *J Health Care Finance* 23:46–56, 1996.

42. Woolhander S, Himmelstein DU: Costs of care and administration at for-profit and other hospitals in the United States. *N Engl J Med* 336:769–773, 1997.

43. Zwanziger J, Melnick GA: Can managed care plans control health costs? *Health Aff* 15:186–199, 1996.

CHAPTER 22

Theory and Practice of Standard Billing Indices

GREGORY J. PRZYBYLSKI, M.D., AND WILLIAM MITCHELL, M.D.

The ability to correctly code medical services has become the single most important issue regarding the financial viability of medical practices in the United States. Cash flow is dependent upon timely payments by insurers, which require accurate coding of procedures and services. Equally as important is the avoidance of fraudulant billing practices incurred as a result of inaccurate coding. Many major academic medical centers have entered into settlements with The Healthcare Financing Agency (HCFA) over the issue of fraudulent and inaccurate billing. Many settlements are in the tens of millions of dollar range and require years of corporate compliance training and documentation. A large portion of the infractions sited resulted from inaccurate coding, insufficient documentation, or both. Drs. Przybylski & Mitchell provide us with an excellent chapter that outlines the origin of medical coding and its evolution into the structure that it has assumed today. The chapter provides a very good framework to help up understand the basis of this, oftentimes, very confusing issue.

Initially developed as a method of tracking diseases and physician services, medical coding systems have evolved into essential components of physicians' reimbursement. Yet, an understanding of coding systems was not a priority in physician practices until the last decade. A fee-for-service payment method based on customary, prevailing, and reasonable (CPR) charges was the cornerstone of third-party reimbursement until the 1980s. Because physician payment schedules were the basis for determining reimbursement, there was little motivation to understand the coding systems used to track services.

During the mid-1980s, total health care expenditures had reached $540 billion, representing an 11% share of the gross national product (GNP). In fact, proportional spending had more than doubled from the 5.6% of GNP in 1965

(11). Reimbursement for physician services by Medicare grew at a 15% compound rate between 1975 and 1987, nearly twice the 7.9% growth rate of the GNP (18). Along with other factors, observations of utilization of physician services suggested that excessive and unnecessary procedures further contributed to escalating costs (2, 4). The groundwork for dramatic reform of physician reimbursement methods had been established.

In 1986, Congress created the Physician Payment Review Commission (PPRC) to develop new methodologies for reimbursement under the Medicare system. The first recommendation of the commission was the development of a fee schedule (16). However, the payment schedule was initially based on CPR, which was felt to be a major contributor to spiraling health care expenditures. The pivotal reform recommended by the commission in 1988 was the creation of a fee schedule based on resource costs (17). Consequently, the resource-based relative value system (RBRVS) was developed, representing a dramatic change aimed at reducing the uninhibited growth pattern of health care expenditures of the previous decade. After the Health Care Finance Administration (HCFA) adopted the RBRVS for determining physician payment by Medicare, other third-party insurance companies adopted the system.

The dramatic reversal in compensation for medical services has prompted physicians to examine the coding and reimbursement systems that serve as the basis for these changes. Moreover, recent federal investigations into potentially fraudulent Medicare billing practices have demonstrated that an understanding of these methods is essential for the physician. The purpose of this chapter is to familiarize the neurosurgeon with the historical evolution of coding and billing systems. By understanding the underlying rationale of these methods, physicians should become more adept at applying these systems to develop successful billing practices. Initially, this chapter will examine the development of diagnostic coding methods. Although these may seem unrelated to reimbursement for services, procedural codes that identify services for payment require linked diagnostic codes. Moreover, assessment by the insurance industry of physician efficiency and cost in providing services is based on diagnostic coding. Secondly, the systems for coding physician services will be reviewed. Finally, the basis for the RBRVS will be examined with suggestions offered for application of this method to the physician's billing practice.

HISTORY OF DISEASE CLASSIFICATION

The basis for the current system of diagnostic coding was developed in 17th century England under the direction of John Graunt as a method for tracking mortality called the London Bills of Mortality. The following century, Francois Bossier de Lacroix first attempted to classify diseases systematically in a treatise entitled *Nosologia Methodica*. At the beginning of the 19th century, William Cullen developed the commonly employed disease classification system entitled *Synopsis Nosologiae Methodicae*. William Farr, the first medical statistician of the General Register Office of England and Wales, is credited with the adoption of a uniform classification that allowed for evolution of the system with advances in medicine.

The classification was evaluated annually by Farr until 1853, when the first International Statistical Congress asked Farr and his colleague, Marc d'Espine, to develop an international classification. Each recommended a different organization scheme. Whereas d'Espine classified disease by etiology, Farr organized disease into five broad categories comprising epidemic, general, anatomically local, developmental, and traumatic diseases. Although the compromise adopted by the Congress was never universally accepted, the system that was proposed by Farr served as the basis for the International List of Causes of Death. Subsequently, the International Statistical Institute asked a committee, chaired by Jacques Bertillon, to develop a classification system that represented a combination of English, German, and Swiss classification schemes and based on the organization recommended by Farr. The system, entitled the Bertillon Classification of Causes of Death, was adopted by the Institute with a plan to revise the classification each decade.

International Classification of Diseases

In 1946, the sixth revision of the Bertillon Classification of Causes of Death at the International Health Conference included causes of morbidity in the classification system. This conference is credited with the development of international cooperation in health statistics, linking national statistical institutions with the World Health Organization. The current classification, entitled the International Classification of Diseases, 9th revision, Clinical Modification (ICD-9-CM), represents the efforts of the World Health Organization in 1975 (10). Modifications included the creation of fifth digits to allow two additional levels of subclassification to the previous three-digit system, as well as an independent four-digit system to classify the histopathology of neoplasms. This internationally used classification scheme provides a uniform method for tracking morbidity data, as well as for preparing claims for reimbursement.

Current Procedural Terminology

Whereas the ICD-9 coding system helped the recording and tracking of disease and mortality, it failed to describe the treatment of disease. To standardize the description of procedures and to develop a method for compiling actuarial data, the American Medical Association (AMA) developed a listing of descriptive terms and associated numerical codes for reporting medical services that was published in 1966 as *Current Procedural Terminology* (CPT) (3). This first edition predominantly described surgical procedures with only limited reference to medical or radiological procedures. The second edition was published four years later and included an expanded description of medical services, as well as a five-digit coding system.

Two additional revisions to CPT were compiled later that decade. The fourth edition was completed in 1977 and contained substantial revisions to include improvements in medical technology. Although one of the intended applications of CPT was to facilitate communication between physicians and insurance agencies, HCFA did not adopt CPT as part of their Common Procedure Coding System (HCPCS) until 1983. Subsequently, HCFA mandated use of this system to report services for payment under Part B of the Medicare program. Three years later, HCFA also required Medicaid agencies to use the method.

The CPT system undergoes annual revision under the direction of the CPT Editorial Panel. A 16-member physician panel meets quarterly and is comprised predominantly of 11 physicians appointed by the AMA. The 11 AMA panelists serve four-year terms. Four of the seats rotate among specialists to allow a multi-disciplinary influence. The other members of the panel include the co-chairman of the Health Care Professionals Advisory Committee (HCPAC), a representative from HCFA, and appointees from the Blue Cross and Blue Shield Association, the Health Insurance Association of America, and the American Hospital Association. The CPT Editorial Panel is assisted by AMA staff with input from the CPT Advisory Committee, which is comprised predominantly of physicians selected by national medical specialty societies. The HCPAC was created by the Editorial Panel to facilitate participation of allied health professionals and limited license practitioners to participate in the process.

Despite a growing number of codes to describe medical services, the work included in many codes overlapped. The process of unbundling, which involves description of a larger procedure with several codes that contain overlapping work, resulted in significant increases in health care expenditures. On January 1, 1996, Medicare initiated the Correct Coding Initiative (CCI) to reduce unbundling and inappropriate reporting of CPT codes. HCFA contracted with Administar Federal, an Indiana Medicare carrier, to create and maintain a computer program to be used nationally. Despite the $700,000 development cost, Medicare reported savings of $700 million since the program's inception. In Version 5.1 of the CCI released on April 1, 1999, there were an estimated 120,000 coding edits (13). Most of the edits represented payment policies in which a comprehensive code would be paid while the component code would be disallowed, whereas a small percentage of edits identified mutually exclusive codes that would not be performed concurrently.

Although codes contained in CPT describe the procedures and services provided by physicians to patients, another national coding system was developed to describe non-physician services and supplies (12). For example, ambulance transportation and dental services, as well as various durable medical equipment and prosthetic devices are described by this system. These represent Level II HCPCS codes and are published and maintained by HCFA. In contrast to the five digit numeric codes of CPT, these are alphanumeric codes containing an initial letter (between A and V, excluding S) followed by four numbers. Moreover, modifiers can also append these codes but are comprised of either two letters (AA to VP) or alphanumeric symbols.

Finally, a third level of codes exists that is maintained by local Medicare carriers. These Level III codes describe new procedures and supplies not accounted for by the two sets of national codes. Similar to the Level II codes, these are alphanumeric codes containing an initial letter (between W and Z, including S) followed by four numbers. Although local Medicare carriers create these codes, prior approval by HCFA is required before implementation is permitted. Occasionally, one may encounter service or supply descriptions in two or all three coding levels. Whereas CPT takes priority over Level II codes with identical descriptors, the local Level III codes have the highest priority when overlap exists. However, Level II codes can supersede CPT when the descriptors are not identical and the Level II code is more specific than the CPT code.

RESOURCE-BASED RELATIVE VALUE SYSTEM

The greatest impact on the billing practices of physicians has occurred due to the development of the RBRVS. This payment system for physicians treating Medicare patients was fully implemented on January 1, 1996. The methodology was developed after years of coordinated efforts by physicians and HCFA to create a uniform way to account for physician work. This represented the first major change in determining how physicians were paid for their services since the inception of the Medicare program in 1965. To better understand this system, it would first be useful to review the historical development of RBRVS (19).

The impetus to revise the Medicare payment system arose from the rapidly increasing expenditures for payment of physician and hospital services by HCFA. Efforts to control costs of physician services followed implementation in 1983 of a prospective pricing system (PPS) for the hospital services reflected in Medicare Part A. Because hospital services accounted for more than two-thirds of Medicare expenditures, cost containment efforts were naturally directed at hospitals first. A diagnosis-related group (DRG) payment was developed for approximately 500 diseases based on the national average cost of hospital care for that particular illness. This method assumed that, over time, the cost for providing care for patients with a range of illness severity would equal the calculated DRG payment. Additional payments were also authorized to account for unusually severe illnesses requiring prolonged hospital stays. Because the payment was identical regardless of the hospital cost, the PPS provided a strong incentive for hospitals to improve cost-efficiency. As a result, the annual growth of Medicare expenditures was reduced by more than half between 1975 and 1990.

Several factors influenced the decision to develop an alternative method of physician payment, including dissatisfaction with the original payment scheme, growing Part B Medicare expenditures, and a reasonable proposal for a new method. The original method for determining the physician payment schedule was based on CPR charges. This resembled the usual, customary, and reasonable charge system utilized by private insurers to pay for physician's services based on their actual fees. To obtain some control over these costs, HCFA defined customary physician charges as the median of an individual physician's charges for a specific service within a specific time interval. In contrast, the prevailing charge was defined as the fee in the 90th percentile charged by specialty-specific physicians within a Medicare payment area. Finally, the reasonable charge reflected the lower of the customary and prevailing charges.

However, the wide variation in the amount that Medicare paid for physician services both among physician specialties and geographical regions caused dissatisfaction within the medical profession (1). Initially, costs were controlled by reducing the payment to the 75th percentile prevailing charge. Subsequently,

Medicare introduced a temporary price freeze on physician's services. This method of control was replaced in 1976 by relating increases in prevailing charges to the Medicare Economic Index (MEI), which measures the annual growth of physician practice costs based both on 1971 actual charges and overall economic trends. As a result, Medicare payments were based on prevailing charges in 1971 and remained nearly unchanged until 1992. However, compensation for procedures based on technological innovation continued to reflect high initial costs of development despite increasing availability and decline in costs over time. Additional dissatisfaction grew among physicians because of increasing disparity between the lower valuation of patient evaluation services and procedural services.

After a second freeze on payment levels in the 1980s and reduced payments for overpriced surgical procedures, several payment reform proposals were suggested by the government. Although additional modifications to CPR were considered, it seemed that this method evolved into a complex system that no longer reflected physician fee schedules. Consideration was given toward developing a DRG system similar to one developed for hospital payments under Medicare Part A (15). Another option was to create a managed care or capitation model of payment. Finally, a proposal was offered for replacing the CPR method with a payment schedule based on a relative value scale.

Only the CPR and the payment schedule represented fee-for-service methods. Many physicians voiced concern that a DRG or capitated system would threaten clinical judgment in patient-care decisions. Moreover, the AMA opposed policies which precluded physicians from charging patients the difference between their fee and the Medicare payment (i.e., balance billing). Because the courts supported congressional legislation to limit physicians' fees, development of a relative value system seemed to provide the best alternative to the CPR method.

The concept of a relative value system (RVS) was not new. In fact, the California Medical Association developed a RVS in 1956 that was regularly updated for nearly two decades. However, it was based on a median of charges reported by California Blue Shield in 1969, thereby still representing a CPR charge methodology. Physicians used this method to determine fee schedules, and government and private insurers alike used the system to establish payment rates. Subsequently, concerns raised by the Federal Trade Commission regarding the possibility of antitrust violations led the California Medical Association to discontinue updating the charge data collected.

Rather than continuing pursuit of a charge-based RVS as supported by most surgical subspecialty societies, a resource-based RVS was considered in which physician services were ranked based on the relative costs incurred in providing them. Most non-procedural specialty societies believed that wide variations among fee-for-service and geographical variations failed to adequately reflect costs incurred to provide the services. As a result, the AMA chose to support a RVS based on resource costs, provided that the payment system reflected geographical variations in practice costs and did not prevent physicians from balance billing. Although the AMA submitted a proposal to HCFA for development of a new RVS, continued antitrust concerns precluded direct physician involvement in their development. Consequently, the AMA accepted a proposal submitted by the Harvard University School of Public Health to perform a national study of resource-based relative value scales for physician services.

On July 1, 1986, the Consolidated Omnibus Budget Reconciliation Act mandated that the department of Health and Human Services develop a RBRVS to be submitted to Congress. In addition, the law created the Physician Payment Review Commission (PPRC) to study a variety of additional options for Medicare payment reform, including changing CPR, capitation, and physician DRG (16). The PPRC recommended development of a payment schedule linked to a RBRVS (17).

Concurrently, the Harvard study commenced in December of 1985 with funding from HCFA. The principal investigators, William Hsiao, Ph.D. and Peter Braun, M.D., had previously encountered limited success in a 1979 pilot study that attempted to rank 27 physician services from five specialties (8). Five years later, a follow-up study demonstrated more consistent results after estimates of work without the addition of complexity were considered. The first phase of the national study supported by HCFA developed a RBRVS for 12 physician specialties. In addition, independent funding was obtained for study of six additional specialties. Not only were

specialty-specific scales developed, but also a method for creating cross-specialty links allowed integration of a single cross-specialty RBRVS. The Omnibus Budget Reconciliation Act of 1986 provided a two-year extension for submission of RBRVS to Congress and mandated inclusion of 15 additional specialties during the second phase of the study (5, 6, 7, 9).

Although the AMA adopted in principle the results of the Harvard study, they also recommended that the new Medicare payment system include geographical differences in practice costs and professional liability, as well as a transition period to prevent disruptive changes between the CPR and RBRVS systems. The PPRC likewise endorsed the study and supported the AMA recommendations. However, the commission diverged from the AMA on two recommendations. Despite opposition to balance billing, the commission recommended placing limits on balance billing. In addition, expenditure targets for Medicare spending were recommended. Because RBRVS was still a variation of a fee-for-service payment system, PPRC believed that cost containment could only be achieved with expenditure targets.

In December of 1989, Congress enacted the Omnibus Budget Reconciliation Act (OBRA 89), which mandated a Medicare payment schedule based on RBRVS from the Harvard study with inclusion of physician work, practice expense, and professional liability costs. Geographical adjustments to all three components were included (Figure 22.1). The conversion factor for the calculated RVU was based on keeping the overall Medicare expenditure the same as the cost using the CPR system. A process was created to annually adjust the conver-

$$MFS = [RVUw \times GPCIw) + (RVUpe \times GPCIpe) + (RVUm \times GPCIm)] \times CF$$

Where,

    MFS = Medicare Fee Schedule
    RVU = Relative Value Unit
    GPCI = Geographical Practice Cost Index
      W = Work
     PE = Practice Expense
      M = Malpractice
     CF = Conversion Factor

Figure 22.1 Method for calculation of the RVU of a physician's service under RBRVS.

sion factor, maintaining a budget-neutral value, which limited increases in expenditures to $20 million annually. Additional reductions in limits on balance billing were included.

A five-year transition to the RBRVS Medicare payment system was to begin on January 1, 1992. Despite more than seven years of investigation in the Harvard study, relative value units (RVU) had not been assigned to all services listed in CPT by this date. At the direction of HCFA, regional carrier medical directors assigned RVU to the remaining codes until the third phase of the study was completed. The final comprehensive RBRVS for physician services was published in the November 25, 1992 Federal Register.

After implementation of the RBRVS fee schedule by HCFA for payments by Medicare, additional health insurers have gradually implemented an RVS, as well. Although RBRVS is the method most commonly used, an alternative RVS called St. Anthony's is also used in certain regions. This privately maintained system, formerly known as McGraw-Hill, utilizes relative value units based on the time, risk, and complexity of the physician service. In contrast, the RBRVS uses physician work, practice expense, and malpractice expense as the components for determining the relative value of a particular physician service. The physician work component comprises approximately 54% of the total relative value of the service, whereas practice expense comprises 41%. In addition, a geographic practice cost index is incorporated to adjust for geographical differences. Consequently, conversion factors between RBRVS and St. Anthony's RVS are different.

To coordinate changes in CPT with assignment of RVU by HCFA, the AMA/Specialty Relative Value Update Committee (RUC) was created in 1991. Twenty-three of the 28 members are appointed by major, national, medical specialty societies. The other five panelists include the RUC chair, the co-chair of HCPAC, and members of the AMA, American Osteopathic Association, and CPT Editorial Panel. A RUC Advisory Committee composed of members appointed by 94 specialty societies develop and suggest RVU for new codes to the RUC. Specialty society representatives are responsible for compiling physician survey data to determine the time spent in performing the medical service and ranking the service relative to exist-

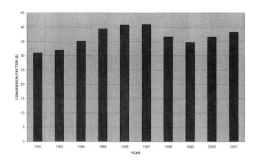

Figure 22.2 Variation in the Medicare surgical conversion factor over the past eight years.

ing services. Subsequently, consensus recommendations are forwarded to HCFA for annual consideration. During the five-year period ending in 1998, nearly 2300 relative value recommendations were made to HCFA with a recent acceptance rate of more than 90%.

An opportunity exists every five years to make significant adjustments in work values that were previously assigned. In 1995, representatives of the neurosurgical subspecialty societies requested changes in 77 surgical codes. Prior assignment of values by HCFA to some neurosurgical codes did not include certain components of the work involved, leading to an inappropriate reduction in value. All of the recommended changes were accepted by HCFA. However, the Balanced Budget Act required a budget neutral conclusion. Because the development of new CPT codes requires subsequent valuation, the new RVU assigned must come from previously valued codes to maintain budget neutrality. Typically, values are maintained within a family of codes, such as the musculoskeletal or neurosurgical sections of the CPT manual. Consequently, there is a disincentive to making significant changes in codes. Some allowance for new technology exists to account for innovations in medical care, thereby creating an opportunity for growth within a family of codes. The methods of maintaining budget neutrality have included reductions in practice expense and changes in the conversion factor. Beginning in 1996, HCFA decided that annual budget neutrality adjustments would be made to the physician fee schedule conversion factor (Figure 22.2).

PRACTICE EXPENSE DETERMINATION

Under RBRVS, work valuations were resource-based, whereas practice expense was based on the AMA's Socioeconomic Monitoring System 1989 Core Survey (SMS) of a representative sample of 4000 physicians in 34 specialties. Practice costs, including office rent, wages of non-physician personnel, equipment, and supplies were measured overall rather than specific to a given service. Moreover, practice expenses varied among specialties, representing 52.2% of family physicians' practice costs but only 38.9% of neurosurgeons' costs. The method enacted by OBRA 89 involved multiplying the specialty-specific practice expense factor by the average Medicare payment of the service in 1991. Similarly, professional liability was calculated based on the proportion of cost multiplied by the Medicare payment. The average, neurosurgical, professional liability component of practice cost was 7.6%, compared with a 3.9% proportion for the family physician. If the service was provided by more than one specialty, a weighted average of surveyed costs was utilized.

The Omnibus Budget Reconciliation Act of 1993 mandated reductions in the practice expense of over-valued services. Over a three-year period, the practice expense was reduced annually by 25% of the amount that the value exceeded the physician work RVU until it was no greater than 128% of the work component. However, concerns over the non-resource based OBRA 89 method of calculating practice expense, as well as a 1994 Social Security Act amendment mandating resource-based practice expense calculations prompted HCFA to contract with Abt Associates, Inc. to perform a national study of physician's practice expense. Fifteen Clinical Practice Expert Panels (CPEP) were formed from nominations by medical associations to develop a list of direct cost components of a selected group of reference codes. In addition, a national mail survey of 5000 practices was performed to obtain a sample of practice costs and service mix to validate the CPEP estimates. However, poor response rates from physicians led HCFA to abandon efforts at obtaining actual survey data. To meet the deadline of January 1998 set by Congress, HCFA planned to implement new practice expense values based on CPEP data. Lack of validation of the CPEP data with actual practice expense information, as well as failures to account for actual differences in practice cost among all specialties prompted the AMA to urge Congress to extend the deadline for implementation of new practice

expense values. As a result, Congress not only delayed implementation until 1999, but also directed the General Accounting Office (GAO) to review HCFA's methodology and make recommendations for a valid resource-based model. The GAO report supported the concerns raised by the AMA.

Beginning in January 1999, HCFA initiated a transition to a resource-based practice expense valuation that differs based on the site of the service. If a medical service can be performed either in an office or a hospital, then both a non-facility and facility practice expense value will be assigned. Whereas locations assigned non-facility practice expense include physician offices and independent imaging or laboratory centers, facility practice expense is attributed to hospitals, surgical centers, and nursing homes. The method for estimating practice costs is based on the AMA's SMS data. Because the SMS data came from small sample sizes with sufficient variability to introduce sampling bias, there continues to be concern regarding this methodology.

SUMMARY

There has been a dramatic change in the method of physician reimbursement that has occurred during the last two decades. Whereas reimbursement was previously based on charges, rapid escalation of spending for medical services resulted in the evolution of coding systems, originally intended to track diseases and services, to become a basis for reimbursement. The RBRVS represents a significant shift from a payment method based on charges to a system based on the costs for providing medical services. An understanding of the evolution of these systems is imperative in providing a foundation for developing a billing system that can lead to a successful neurosurgical practice.

REFERENCES

1. Burney IL, Schreiber GJ, Blaxall MO, Gabel JR: Geographic variation in physician's fees. *JAMA* 240: 1368–1371, 1978.
2. Chassin MR, Kosecoff J, Park RE, et al: Does inappropriate use explain geographic variations in the use of health care services? A study of three procedures. *JAMA* 258:2533–2537, 1987.
3. Gordon BL: Current Procedural Terminology. Chicago, American Medical Association, 1973.

4. Greenspan AM, Kay HR, Berger BC, Greenberg RM, Greenspon AJ, Gaughan MJS: Incidence of unwarranted implantation of permanent cardiac pacemakers in a large medical population. *N Engl J Med* 318: 158–163, 1988.

5. Hsiao WC, Braun P, Becker ER, Thomas SR: The resource based relative value scale. *JAMA* 258: 799–802, 1987.

6. Hsiao WC, Braun P, Dunn D, Becker ER: Resource based relative values: An overview. *JAMA* 260: 2347–2353, 1988.

7. Hsiao WC, Braun P, Dunn D, Becker ER: Results and policy implications of the resource based relative value study. *N Engl J Med* 319:881–888, 1988.

8. Hsiao WC, Stason WB: Toward developing a relative value scale for medical and surgical services. *Health Care Financing Rev* 1:23–29, 1979.

9. Hsiao WC, Braun P, Yntema D, Becker ER: Estimating physicians' work for a resource-based relative value scale. *N Engl J Med* 319:835–841, 1988.

10. International Classification of Diseases, Geneva, World Health Organization, 1977, pp 7–33.

11. Jacobs P: Behavior of supply, in The Economics of Health and Medical Care. Gaithersberg, Aspen Publishers, 1991, ed 3, pp 168–174.

12. Jones-Burns MK: St. Anthony's HCPCS Level II Code Book, Reston, St. Anthony's Publishing, 1997, pp 1–3.

13. Kirschner CG, Reyes D: An update on Medicare's correct coding initiative, in CPT Assistant. Chicago, American Medical Association, 1999, pp 7–9.

14. Medicode International Classification of Diseases, 9th Revision Clinical Modification, 1999, pp 1–2. Medicode Publications, Salt Lake City Utah.

15. Mitchell JB: Physician DRGs. *N Engl J Med* 313: 670–675, 1985.

16. Physician Payment Review Commission: Medicare physician payment: An agenda for reform, in Annual Report to Congress No. 68-227. Washington, D.C., U.S. Government Printing Office, 1987.

17. Physician Payment Review Commission: Medicare physician payment, in Annual Report to Congress. Washington, D.C., U.S. Government Printing Office, 1988.

18. Roper WL: Statement before Subcommittee on Health of the Committee on Ways and Means, U.S. House of Representatives. U.S. Department of Health and Human Services, Health Care Finance Administration, 1988.

19. Smith SL, Gallagher PE: Medicare RBRVS: The Physician's Guide. Chicago, American Medical Association, 1999, pp. 4–49.

CHAPTER 23

Cost Accounting and Cost Accounting Systems in Health Care Organizations

MARK E. TOSO, C.P.A.

As seen in Chapter 19 cost accounting has undergone a significant evolution in health care over the past few decades. This has been dictated by changes in reimbursement mechanisms, the regulatory environment, and falling revenue streams. The implementation of new accounting methods into a business is highly labor intensive, anxiety provoking, and expensive. The selection of appropriate methods and the systems to support them is of vital importance to the survival of any health care organization. Mr. Toso has contributed an excellent chapter that addresses these issues and discusses some of the solutions available today. It also provides one with an appreciation of the difficulty of applying cost-accounting principles to the delivery of medical care in the traditional sense.

HEALTH CARE INDUSTRY - COST ACCOUNTING OVERVIEW

The Health Care Environment during the 1990's has emphasized managed care principles where health care manager's efforts were directed to "reduce cost" and "maintain quality". The conflict created over cost reduction and quality improvement of health care services has created a greater need to know and understand the costs of the health care delivery system. This conflict has also created stress between government, employers, insurance companies (including HMO's), providers (including hospital, primary care physicians & specialty physicians) and ultimately patients. Each of these organizations has an interest in the cost and quality of the health care services being delivered, which has led to the increasing interest and development of cost accounting systems during the 1990's.

The driving force behind the development of cost accounting systems in health care organizations has been the change from fee for service and cost based reimbursement to prospective payment and capitation as a dominant form of payment to health care providers. Under the former reimbursement systems there was no incentive to reduce costs. If a provider performed a service they were paid a set fee or actual cost. The two major objectives under prospective payment and capitation are to control the growth of health care expenditures and manage the utilization of health care resources. Therefore, under these reimbursement systems cost management is integral to the success of the health care organization.

EVOLUTION OF COST ACCOUNTING

Departmental Costing

Historically, cost accounting has focused primarily on hospitals and hospital systems. This, in part, has determined the evolution of cost accounting. Initially, hospitals were interested in departmental costs, a department being defined as an organizational unit, which is responsible for a specific function, such as, laboratory, radiology etc. These departments could be responsible for strictly expenses or both expenses and revenues. Hospital's internal organizational structures, state cost reporting filings and the Medicare cost reimbursement filings have been set up based upon the departmental cost structure. Departmental costing would focus on the cost of producing a specific service (lab test, a radiology exam, etc). To the extent that different types of services were performed in a department the cost per unit might differentiate between the different types by assigning Relative Value Units ("RVU's) to each procedure. This is important to the management of the individual department.

Although departmental cost management is important to the management of the hospital it does not focus on the product being produced by the hospital, the care delivered to the patient. Diagnosis Related Groups (DRGs) represent one way of defining the product by patient by specialty. The ability to define the product is important prior to developing the cost accounting system in order to understand the required flow of cost information to provide the service. To paraphrase Yogi Berra, "If you don't know where you're going, you might end up somewhere else."

Product-Line Costing

Under the Prospective Payment System DRG's became the foundation for payment from Medicare and ultimately many other payers. The reimbursement for a specific DRG is a fixed amount. Under this type of reimbursement system the relationship between the product's price and cost is essential for understanding the financial impact different types of patients have on the health care organization. If the cost of DRG 1 (Craniotomy Age > 17) is substantially higher or lower than the revenue paid by the insurance companies, the health care managers need to know why. What is the impact on the organization if a service is added or dropped? What is the impact on the surgical service profitability if ambulatory surgical services have to be priced at the competitive rate of a local freestanding ambulatory surgery center? What is the lowest price the organization can charge to an HMO for a particular service or procedure? If they want to be able to able to answer these questions, it is imperative for management to have a product line costing system in place in order to manage effectively.

Process Costing, Job Order Costing and Standard Costing

Product line costing approaches to accumulating costs and assigning them to products or services are generally accomplished through some form of "job-order" or "process costing" system. Job order costing is used to directly assign

costs to patients that consume different amounts of resources. Process costing is used to allocate costs to patients that consume approximately the same amount of resources. Job order costing requires more detailed information to be retained and produces more accurate cost information. Process costing is less accurate than job order costing; however, it may generate costing data, which is reasonable for management purposes and is less expensive to obtain. Generally, most health care organizations use a combination of job order costing and process costing systems. No matter what product costing approach is chosen, there will invariably be some averaging of costs. Process costing averages costs over a large number of patients, whereas job order costing averages costs over a small number of patients.

In addition to developing actual incurred costs by patient, it is important to know how much it should have cost to treat the patient. Standard costs are predetermined estimates of what it should have cost to treat the patient for a specific illness. Standard costs are developed using actual costs, time-and-motion studies, etc. Several of the larger cost accounting systems build cost standards by cost types and cost categories. RVU's by cost type and category form the fundamental foundation for building cost standards. RVU's could represent minutes for the cost type variable labor but can represent any weighting scheme for all other cost types. The standard cost builders used in the more popular cost accounting systems utilize a variety of costs (fixed, semi-fixed, and variable) to derive a standard cost measure.

HEALTH CARE PRODUCTION PROCESS: INTERMEDIATE PRODUCTS AND PATIENTS

Typically the production process for health care product line costing is divided into two phases. Phase one converts hospital resources into intermediate products i.e. the cost of laboratory services, nursing services, operating room time, radiology services, etc. The second phase assigns the intermediate products to patients. The patients are identified as DRG's, ICD-9-CM's or any classification system deemed appropriate by the health care organization. The distinction between the two phases of the production process is important, in that, it reflects the difference in management control. The inter-

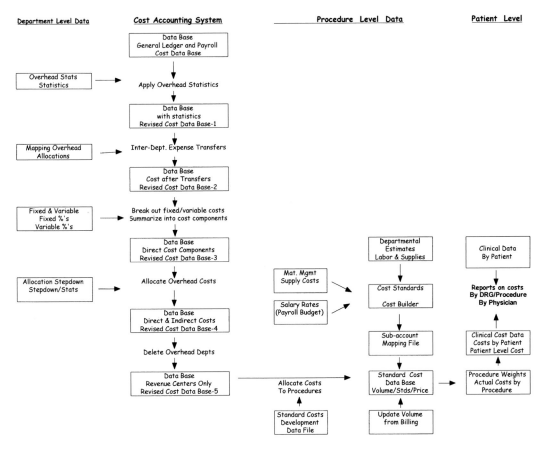

Figure 23.1 Product Line Costing Model.

mediate products are controlled in the departments and the efficient production of these products is the responsibility of the department managers. The utilization of these intermediate products is the responsibility of the physician; therefore, the amount and mix of intermediate products used by a patient will vary by physician. Both intermediate products and patient costs can have standard costs developed for management purposes. **Figure 1** outlines an example of the process used to develop a typical product line cost accounting model utilized by over 500 hospitals nationwide.

COST ACCOUNTING IN THE MILLENIUM–THE GROWTH OF ACTIVITY BASED COSTING

Traditional cost accounting, first developed by General Motors 70 years ago, postulates that

total cost is the sum of the costs of individual operations. Activity based costing shows us why traditional cost accounting has not worked for service (health care) companies. It is not because the techniques are wrong. It is because traditional cost accounting makes the wrong assumptions. Service (health care) companies cannot start with the cost of individual operations, as companies have done with traditional cost accounting. They must start with the assumption that there is only one cost: that of the total system.

The famous distinction between fixed and variable costs, on which traditional cost accounting is based, does not make much sense in services. Neither does the basic assumption of traditional cost accounting: that capital can be substituted for labor. In fact, in knowledge-based work especially, additional capital investment will likely require more, rather than less, labor. Organizations have found that: all costs are fixed over a given time period and that resources cannot be substituted for one another, so that the total operation has to be costed i.e. activity-based costing. Health care organizations are therefore beginning to shift from costing only what goes on inside their own organizations to costing the entire economic process, in which even the largest health care organizations are just one link. This is referred to as economic chain costing. In health care this move toward economic chain costing is the result of the shift from cost-led pricing to price-led costing. The advent of capitation and market pricing of services is forcing health care organizations along with insurers (HMO's) to look at the cost of the entire health care process. **Figure 2** outlines globally the various providers involved in the economic process.

Exhibit I summarizes the costs associated with providing care to patients over the contin-

uum of providers, the payers and the patient in the economic chain. By observation, the exhibit indicates that there must be areas of conflict between the various parties in the economic chain if there is a fixed budget. This conflict exists because managed care is forcing providers to deal with the fact that there is a fixed budget to be divided amongst the various providers and the HMO. There will also be conflicts between the providers and payers with the patient since the patient is ultimately responsible for paying the bill either in premiums or taxes. The following conflicts will make cost accounting for all of the various provider entities more important:

1. **The Providers, HMO's and the government (Medicare & Medicaid) and the Public will be in conflict** over the high cost of health care. The public will demand more services at the same or lower cost. The inclusion of prescription drugs for Medicare beneficia-

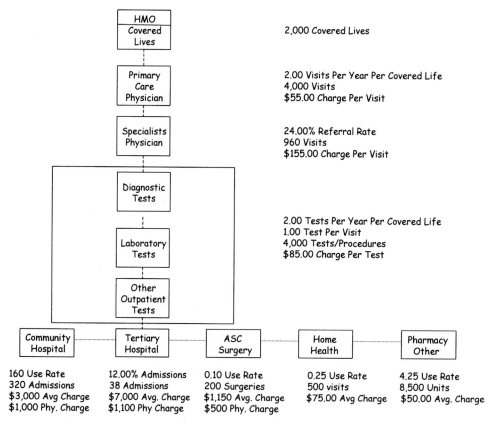

Figure 23.2 Activity Based Costing & Economic Chain Costing.

Healthcare Organization	Use Rate	Units	Cost or Price Per Unit	Total Cost or Price	Total Cost or Price PMPM	% Cost or Price PMPM
Subscriber Premium		2,000		$3,720,000	$155.00	100.00%
HMO / Insurer				**$631,500**	**$26.31**	**16.98%**
Medical Providers:						
Primary Care Physician	2 visits per member	4,000	$55.00	$220,000	$9.17	5.91%
Specialist Physician	24% Referral Rate	960	$155.00	148,800	6.20	4.00%
Outpatient Diagnostic/Other	2 Tests per member	4,000	$85.00	340,000	14.17	9.14%
Outpatient Surgery	.10 per member	200	$1,150.00	230,000	9.58	6.18%
Outpatient Surgery - Physician		200	$500.00	100,000	4.17	2.69%
Community Hospital	160 Admits/1,000	320	$3,000.00	960,000	40.00	25.81%
Community Hospital - Physician		320	$1,000.00	320,000	13.33	8.60%
Tertiary Hospital	12% of Admits	38	$7,000.00	268,800	11.20	7.23%
Tertiary Hospital - Physician		38	$1,000.00	38,400	1.60	1.03%
Home Health	.25 per member	500	$75.00	37,500	1.56	1.01%
Pharmacy/Other	4.25 per member	8,500	$50.00	425,000	17.71	11.42%
Total Medical Costs				$3,088,500	$128.69	83.02%
Panel Size		2,000				

Exhibit I   Activity Based Costing & Economic Chain Costing (Cost of the Entire Economic Process).

ries will be a critical debate during the next decade between the growing number of baby boomers and the ability of Medicare to fund the cost.

2. **Primary care physicians and specialty physicians will be in conflict with the hospital** over the distribution of the budget. Higher hospital payments per day will mean lower fees for physicians and vice versa.

3. **Primary care physicians and specialty physicians will be in conflict** over who has control of the patient. Physicians have been in debate over who should have control of the treatment for the patients and ultimately control the quality and cost of services that are provided.

4. **Managed care organizations and payers will be in conflict with the primary care physicians, specialty physicians, hospitals and other providers** on the cost and quality of services. They will also be in conflict over who has control of the premium dollar.

5. The government and providers will be in conflict over the amount of money the government will pay for Medicare, Medicaid and uncompensated care.

6. The academic medical centers and community hospitals will be competing for patients on the basis of cost and quality. Each has a distinct role; however, the payers and the government are pitting the various providers against each other in their quest to obtain a larger portion of the health care budget.

Exhibit I is an example of the distribution of the health care budget in the economic chain of a commercial health care product. The dollars are larger but similar for the Medicare health care budget. **Figure 3** shows the importance of cost accounting when there is a fixed budget for health care services.

The future does not look good from the standpoint of increased provider payments for health care services. The Medicare Balanced Budget

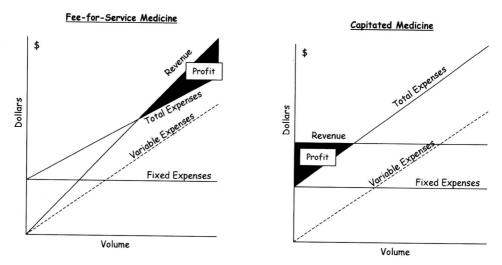

Figure 23.3 Evaluation of Capitated or Fixed Budgets.

Act of 1997 significantly reduced the reimbursement for Medicare services and yet a key component of the health care budget is still not provided as a benefit, prescription drugs. Over the next decade beneficiaries will demand more benefits, providers will want higher payments for the services they provide and the government will attempt to develop a revenue stream to pay for the added benefits and higher provider payments. Politically the baby boomers will have more and more political clout in order to increase the benefits provided to the elderly. Politically the government will have trouble increasing taxes to fund these benefit programs on a tax paying population, which will be smaller than it is today. Therefore, the providers will, in all probability, have to bear the brunt of the health care budget cuts. The implications are clear for hospitals, HMO's and other providers which represent a significant part of the health care budget: The hospitals, HMO's and other providers will have to figure out how to provide their health care services at a lower cost. This means that the importance of cost accounting will increase in the future. As good as a hospital or hospital system is in managing costs and maintaining quality, the health care organization will have to get better!

Despite the elegance of activity based costing, the economic as well as technical feasibility of implementing such a cost accounting system must be evaluated. That is, will the benefits derived from activity based costing system more than offset its costs of implementation and whether it is feasible to identify all of the activities that consume resources, in order to accumulate costs per type of activity. In the development of activity based costing systems, an activity analysis has to be conducted to identify activities that consume resources. This involves a detailed study of the entire organization's logistics and accounting information systems, and it is an expensive project in itself. It can be quite difficult and time consuming to identify and trace resource consumption to a specific activity because of the complexities involved. Therefore, it may be technically infeasible for some organizations to implement activity based costing.

II. DETERMINE WHEN COST ACCOUNTING SYSTEMS BE IMPLEMENTED

Goals and Objectives of a Cost Accounting System

Cost accounting systems generate information for a variety of purposes. Prior to implementing a cost accounting system management needs to determine the goals and objectives of the cost accounting system. The type of cost accounting system developed depends substantially on the type of information needed by management on a routine and on an ad-hoc basis. The managers within the organization must determine the provider organizations information needs. The installation of a cost accounting system often requires a major time commitment by all managers throughout the organization. If managers are not involved in the development and specification of the goals of the cost accounting systems it is unlikely they will support the efforts required to make the cost accounting system function effectively.

The development of the goals of the cost accounting system must find the link between the accuracy of the cost accounting system and the timeliness of the data and the cost of producing that data. When management has mastered the relationship between cost, accuracy and timeliness, they will be able to make decisions on whether increased levels of accuracy or timeliness are worth the cost.

An example of some goals and objectives of the provider organization are as follows:

Organizational Goals (Management Costing and Product Costing):

- Implementation of detailed cost management capabilities
- Evaluation of service line profitability and the financial impact of the promotion of specific product lines
- Assessment of strategic initiatives
- Negotiation of contracts with third parties based upon fixed and variable costs
- Facilitate performance measurement through cost variance analysis
- Support systems of utilization management and efficiencies
- Assist in long term planning and capital acquisition
- Improve the budget process

Departmental Goals:

- Supplement analytical tools available to department managers enabling them to further understand and manage their areas of responsibility
- Quantify resources required to perform patient services on a procedural level
- Identify the interrelationship between departments in providing total patient care
- Provide cost based input in establishing prices
- Allow department managers to better identify areas of economy and efficiency

Reporting Goals:

- To be able to report costs at a number of different levels:
  - Procedure Charge Code
  - Department
  - Patient
  - Physician
  - Payer or Financial Class
  - CPT-4 Code
  - ICD-9-CM diagnosis or procedure
  - DRG or MDC
  - Product Line
- To be able to break down the components of cost:
  - Direct fixed salary
  - Direct variable salary
  - Direct fixed nonsalary
  - Direct variable nonsalary
  - Direct capital
  - Indirect capital
  - Indirect other

There are additional considerations in designing and implementing a cost accounting system. When is the information needed and at what level of detail. There are trade-offs in system responsiveness and the level of detail which management would like to see.

Information should never be collected if the cost of the data collection exceeds the benefit from the improved decisions made based on the availability of that information.

Cost accounting systems are very complex by their nature. In order to mitigate the potential problems arising from this complexity it is important to consider several factors in the design of the cost accounting system;

- Development of Ad-Hoc and Exception Reporting in order to minimize the impact of information overload
- Establish Quality Control procedures to maintain the reliability of the system
  - Test the cost accounting system frequently
  - Verify data input
  - Validate the system
- Cost accounting system should be flexible and accommodate a variety of users
- Cost accounting system should be dynamic, not static. The cost accounting system should be able to respond to changes in the environment.
- Individuals throughout the organization should be able to access and use the system. The successful operation of the system should not depend on one person!

Who Will Use the Cost Accounting System

A survey of healthcare financial managers by the National Healthcare Financial Managers Association found that the most important management information system application for the next five years will be cost accounting. This survey was prepared in the early 1990's and is still valid today. The primary users of the cost accounting information have been identified as:

- Outside third parties such as:
  - HMO's
  - American Hospital Association
  - Internal Revenue Service
  - Medicare and Medicaid
  - Other third parties
  - Community
  - Politicians
- Executive Management
- Operational Managers
- Physicians

III. WHAT IS THE PROCESS AND THE COSTS TO IMPLEMENT A COST ACCOUNTING SYSTEM?

The evolution of cost accounting systems is dynamic and will continue to change over the next decade. In the future management information systems will be collecting claims data by patient in order to capture the total cost of treating a particular patient. Technological change will allow health care managers to deal with this level of detail in an efficient manner. The process to implement a cost accounting system and the costs of implementing a cost accounting system will also change as the health care system changes. However, there are certain steps in the process of implementing a cost accounting system, which should not change significantly. Additionally, the cost of a cost accounting system will vary based upon a number of factors. The following steps are generally followed in the installation of a cost accounting system:

1. Establish goals and objectives of a cost accounting system
2. Plan and design the cost accounting system
3. Evaluate and select the cost accounting system
   - Determine the cost of the cost accounting system
     - Cost of Software

- Cost of Hardware
- Cost of Installation
- Cost of Maintenance
- Cost of Service and Support
  - Cost of software updates
4. Determine how costs are going to be measured
   - Product line costs
   - Management costs
   - Process & Job order costs
   - Standard costs
   - Industry Relative Value Units
   - Provider defined standards
   - Engineered Standards(time and motion studies)
5. Evaluate the reliability of the outcomes of the system

Establish Goals and Objectives of a Cost Accounting System

Section II identified in detail the goals and objectives, which need to be, determined prior to implementing a cost accounting system. Prior proper planning will limit the mistakes many providers have made when implementing a cost accounting system. As indicated before, there is a relationship between the accuracy of the system, the timeliness of the system and the cost of the system. Increasing the accuracy without lengthening the time to get a report may increase the cost of the system. Increasing the frequency of the reports without lowering the accuracy increases the cost of the system. Reducing the cost of the system will eventually mean sacrificing the accuracy and timeliness of the system.

Management must then decide if the major goal is to determine product costs or develop a management costing system. Product costs are designed to determine the cost of delivering the hospital's services to patients. Management costing systems are more elaborate and focus mainly on properly modeling the cost behavior of service producing departments. Management costing focuses on internal control and is similar to a flexible budgeting system.

Plan and Design the Cost Accounting System

Planning and designing a health care cost accounting system has a number of distinct, yet interrelated requirements. Hospital managers at all levels of the organization will require concise, meaningful, and timely cost information to understand and control the costs for which they are responsible. Cost information must be organized to support management decision making throughout the organization. The cost accounting system must have the flexibility and adaptive structure to meet the specific and varying needs of strategic analysis and planning. Patient services must appropriately and consistently costed on a timely basis by DRG or other appropriate product line classification. To the extent possible, the hospital cost accounting system should be integrated with existing financial systems to ensure cost-effective operation.

The following factors should be considered as much as possible in the design of the cost accounting system because they are inherent in providing patient care services:

- Each patient's treatment is uniquely defined and modified to meet the patient's specific needs and the varying conditions of that patient
- Patient treatment and care can be defined as a number of service units, which are similar to component parts. The total treatment of a patient can be defined as a list of service units provided, that is, a bill of services.
- The individual service units provided are fairly uniform in nature and for the purpose of costing can be defined in terms of standard cost units.
- Identify the level of detail and number of areas to be costed.

Evaluate and Select the Cost Accounting System

The provider organization has primarily two options in developing a cost accounting system. Management can develop the cost accounting system internally or they can purchase the software from a management information systems vendor. The vast majority of healthcare institutions have opted for the latter choice i.e. purchase the system from an MIS vendor. The cost of cost accounting system include the following:

- **Cost of Software**
  How often does the software get updated, if at all? What is the cost of the updated software?
- **Cost of Hardware**
  Is the hardware compatible with the institutions existing hardware? Hardware estimates will vary depending upon whether microcomputers, mini computers or main frame computers are used.

- **Cost of Installation**
  Many organizations require assistance in installing the software. Sometimes installation services are packaged in with a software sale, and sometimes they are sold separately. A separate part of the installation process is the actual development of the cost standards and design of the cost accounting system. This may require a consulting study costing in excess of $100,000.
- **Cost of Maintenance(Hardware & Software Licenses)**
  The cost of maintenance includes the software, hardware, cost accounting design and internal staff training. The cost of the software many times is the least expensive part of an accounting system. If the software is inexpensive but the cost accounting system is expensive to maintain and install, then management may have a problem.
- **Cost of Service and Support**
  The vendor support for the product will be very important. Generally, only one or two individuals within the organization will have an in-depth knowledge of the cost accounting system. If either one or both of these individuals leave the investment in the system will be at risk. One solution to mitigate this risk is to have a vendor who can support the system while other staff are trained to operate the cost accounting system.

The estimated total cost of the system will vary depending on many of the factors previously discussed, however, the cost of a cost accounting system can easily approach $1,000,000 to get the system operational. In addition, the on-going costs could approach $250,000 annually with the internal staff support that is required. HBOc, SMS, Transition Systems Ins. (TSI), Kreg Corp. and HCM are some of the larger vendors offering complete cost accounting systems. There are a significant number of specialty cost accounting vendors for specific areas within the hospital.

The following criteria should be evaluated when selecting a vendor to implement a cost accounting system:

- **Vendor Experience** - How many clients does the vendor have locally and nationally. How many clients have they lost and why? It is important to make several visits to clients who use the system well and discuss the pros and cons of the system without the vendor present.

- **Service and Support Network** - What service organization is in place locally? What importance does the vendor place on service support nationally? What is the ratio of service support staff to clients? What level of service exists as part of the licensing agreement and what service is charged on an hourly basis?
- **System Functionality** - What is the flexibility of the vendors system? Does the vendors system meet the goals and objectives established by management? Is the provider's cost accounting design consistent with the vendor's specifications.
- **Cost Types and Cost Elements** - Does the vendor support the cost types and cost elements identified by management of the provider unit? Does the increase in detailed cost types and cost elements reduce the functionality of the system?
- **Integration with Provider Financial and Clinical Systems** - Has the vendor successfully integrated its cost accounting system with the provider's financial and clinical management information systems? Poor integration will result in more costly installation and will likely result in higher maintenance costs.
- **System Speed and Updating Process** - The speed of the system to produce reports and the ability to update or change the cost accounting should be carefully ascertained. A slow system many be unacceptable and not being able to add new procedures will limit the usefulness of the system.
- **Ownership and Price** - Does the hospital own the software license or is it leased? Can the software be installed at multiple sites? Finally, the price of the system given all of the above considerations needs to be determined.

Determine How Costs are going to be Measured

The measurement of costs is usually the most expensive part of the cost accounting system after maintenance of the system. The purpose of this process is to translate the costs from the general ledger to the individual procedures. The general ledger costs cannot be directly assigned to the procedures, first they have to be mapped to the cost elements. In other words, individual salary accounts have to be mapped to either fixed or variable salary or some other cost elements. Several methods exist for this mapping,

and they can be broken down into four general categories, from least costly to most costly.

Direct Assignment

This method requires the manager to directly assign the costs to a cost component. The salary accounts are identified as fixed or variable as are the nonsalary and overhead costs of each department. This may seem overly simplistic, however, it is the most cost effective and is used frequently.

Direct Inspection

The assignment of costs are based upon reading contracts and other items which directly assign costs to a specific function.

Direct Observation

Observational techniques include work sampling, time studies, regression analysis, and many others. The technique requires going in and observing the services being performed and is used largely for measuring direct labor inputs.

Engineered Studies

These are the most expensive techniques and should be reserved for areas of highly repetitive work or for areas that have a high potential for staff reduction. A hospital will use a combination of direct assignment, direct inspection, direct observation and engineered studies for tracing costs to products. The technique chosen will be based upon the item to be costed.

Evaluate the Reliability of the Outcomes of the System

Once the cost accounting system is operational it needs to be tested. The department managers should verify the cost data and routine reports should be generated and tested for accuracy. The credibility of the system with internal management and physicians will depend on their input and the accuracy of the data. To minimize the testing phase will totally undermine the usefulness of the system. Once the system has been tested and found to be working effectively the system can be used for its intended purpose.

The most expensive part of a cost accounting system is continually maintaining the system each year. Part of the maintenance is related to updating the product costing as the production process changes. Switching to a unit dose in pharmacy or primary nursing on a nursing unit requires changing the cost accounting data. The second part of maintaining the system is the education of sufficient internal staff to make the system work effectively. As indicated previously, at least two people need to know how the system works in order to have the appropriate backup.

FUTURE FOR COST ACCOUNTING

The use of cost accounting by healthcare providers has gained tremendous momentum in the 1990's as the result of the implementation of prospective payment. The acceptance of capitation and fixed budgets for healthcare organizations as a means of payment and the continued pressure to reduce Medicare costs will make cost accounting more important in the future. Information must be available on what costs are for each health care organization product or product line, with the product typically being identified as the patient, but detailed information is also desired concerning the intermediate products required to treat each type of patient.

CHAPTER 24

Cost Principles of Practice Management

CHARLES A. PECK, M.D., F.A.C.P.

The immense change that has occurred in the health care profession over the past thirty years has resulted in a highly complex business environment for medical practices. The dramatic changes in reimbursement (both financially and administratively), along with a consistent increase of regulatory requirements have made it essential that physicians understand and control practice expense to ensure financial survival. Dr. Peck and Mr. Heacox have contributed a timely chapter that is dedicated to understanding practice costs and their management. Such information has become of vital importance to the practicing physician, whether in solo practice or as part of the largest multi-specialty clinic.

Health care inflation over the past three decades has resulted in enormous changes to the regulatory and reimbursement environment in which physicians operate. The practice of medicine has increasingly become a business, as well as a profession. Neurosurgical practice has been impacted along with other specialty surgical services. As with any business, one's practice must be run in an efficient manner to be profitable, and the practice can be greatly impacted by changes in the health care marketplace. This means that the neurosurgeon, in addition to practicing medicine, must develop skills in office and practice management and continuously be updated with new business skills and knowledge as the market evolves.

THE BASICS OF PRACTICE MANAGEMENT

Practice cost management has become increasingly important to maintain practice viability. In other words, the market sets the price (or reimbursement) and the physician determines

the profit (or compensation) required and then manages the expenses of the practice to meet his or her desired income level. The basics of practice management can be demonstrated with the following formula:

Revenue (reimbursement) − Expense (cost)

= Income (compensation)

It becomes evident that in an environment of flat or declining reimbursement, practices can remain viable only if they are able to control costs. This becomes particularly difficult in an era of increasing regulatory obligations. Although one may reduce costs without a change in reimbursement, it is evident that changes in reimbursement drive changes in expense management to maintain income. Figure 24.1b depicts a five-year (1993–1997) trend in neurosurgical practice reimbursement, expenses, and income. The graph demonstrates that there have been minimal changes in each of the practice variables for neurosurgeons. In other words, over this five-year period, neither revenue nor physician compensation changed dramatically overall. However, when each variable is viewed as year over year percentage change (Fig. 24.1a) it becomes clearer that reimbursement is tending downward while expenses are trending upward. This results in reduced physician income, a trend expected to continue or accelerate over the next several years.

WHAT DO WE MEAN BY COST?

To manage costs, one must understand the different components of practice expense. (Editor's note: For a more detailed discussion of practice

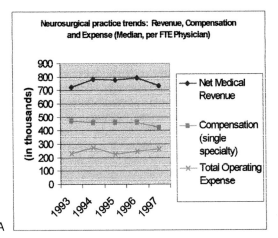

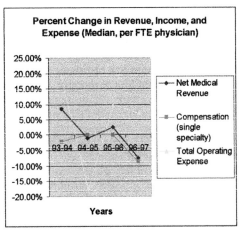

A   B

Figure 24.1   Practice revenue, operating expenses, and physician compensation trends for neurosurgery on an absolute (*A*) and percentage change (*B*) basis. Source: MGMA Physician Compensation and Production Survey and MGMA Cost Survey.

TABLE 24.1
Practice Cost Comparisons for Three Specialities

	Neuro-surgery	Family Practice	Anesthesiology
Operating Cost to Total Cost	35.4%	58.1%	12.1%
Provider Cost to Total Cost	64.6%	41.9%	87.9%
Total Operating Cost	$263,039	$230,880	$58,436
Physician Compensation	$420,625	$127,753	$265,000

Source: MGMA Cost Survey and Physician Compensation and Production Survey—1998, based on 1997 data.

costs, see Chapter 19.) Practice expense is traditionally broken into two major categories, direct and indirect costs. Direct costs are costs associated with the delivery of medical care (e.g., physician's time, medical supplies used during procedures, pharmaceuticals). Indirect costs, sometimes referred to as overhead, are costs incurred for maintaining the practice (e.g., billing, scheduling, rent, support staff, printing) but not associated with the delivery of medical care. In addition, both direct and indirect costs can be further defined as fixed (i.e., costs that remain stable over time, such as rent) or variable (i.e., costs that change based on usage).

Table 24.1 compares the practice costs of neurosurgery with family practice (primarily an office-based specialty) and anesthesiology (a hos-

pital-based specialty). These data show that nearly two-thirds of the costs associated with a typical neurosurgical practice (n = 18) are attributable to the physician. Operating costs account for only one-third of total costs, which is consistent with the fact that few office procedures are preformed in neurosurgery. Besides spending a significant portion of time in the inpatient setting, a neurosurgeon's compensation is relatively high when compared with other subspecialties. Table 24.1 demonstrates that the median compensation for a neurosurgeon ($421,000) is three times that of their primary care counterparts ($128,000). This difference in salary is due both to a smaller revenue stream generated by family practice, as well as higher operating costs due to the heavy dependency on the office setting. In comparison, another specialty that spends significant time in the inpatient setting but has a lesser median salary, anesthesiology, has an operating cost to total cost ratio of approximately 12%.

The distribution of practice costs (operating or provider) becomes more important when practices are faced with declining reimbursement. For specialties in which operating costs make up a small percentage of total costs the impact of reduced reimbursements are more directly borne on the provider's costs, and ultimately, income. Neurosurgeons are less susceptible to this phenomenon than anesthesiologists because of higher operating costs, and thus, op-

an activity-based accounting system, reliable and timely data, and accessibility to the latest evidence-based clinical guidelines (Editor's note: See Chapter 19). Data must be collected and turned into meaningful information, such as dashboards, physician profiles, and other physician-friendly reporting tools.

Typical areas of overhead cost savings opportunities include the following:

- Reduction of staffing overtime
- Revaluation of current staffing mix
- Volume discounts
- Negotiation with vendors for equipment and supplies
- Evaluation of facility costs

Typical areas of focus for managing the cost of patients in a capitated environment include the following:

- Variances in clinical practice by and among physicians
- Duplication of procedures for a patient throughout the continuum
- Misalignment of incentives
- Current utilization and payment model does not support significant enough bonus distribution to change physician behavior
- Lack of information or current information systems must be able to support measurements and monthly reporting
- Lack of fully implemented disease management programs, practice management guidelines, and quality measurements

GAINSHARING

In addition to cost management specific to a practice setting, many health systems are partnering with physicians in a gainsharing program to reduce cost in the hospital. Gainsharing is a customized program that is (a) designed to share hospital clinical savings with physicians, and (b) built on a foundation of objective measurements of clinical improvement, quality outcomes, and cost savings. An operationally successful program of physician gainsharing must be grounded in the following:

- Must be focused on improving clinical practice
- Must be focused on maintaining or enhancing clinical outcomes
- Must be centered around clinical improvement

and may use strategies, such as case management, clinical pathways, and guidelines
- Must involve physicians and hospitals as partners with no barriers to change
- Must never be designed to withhold necessary care
- Must incorporate timely measurement of cost and outcomes

Physician gainsharing programs are carefully crafted incentive arrangements to motivate physicians to take the lead in developing new systems and protocols for more effective care management by sharing the resulting savings with them. An effective physician gainsharing program provides the following benefits:

- Can systematically decrease costs within key, high volume, high dollar clinical service lines
- Creates a "win/win" alignment strategy between physicians and hospitals around a critical mass of established business
- May be accomplished without changes in structure or legal entity
- Can be a catalyst to the development of a system that measures and improves quality
- Creates a solid clinical foundation as a precursor to risk-based managed care contracting

If gainsharing incentives are structured appropriately, a program can be developed that is in full compliance with federal law. It is important to avoid making compensation systems overly complicated. The compensation model should be as straightforward as possible, yet flexible enough to reward physicians adequately for positive health outcomes achieved in the most cost-effective manner feasible.

WHAT ABOUT VALUE AND SATISFACTION?

The specialist must try to ensure satisfaction for both the patient and the physician referral source. This includes patient access, providing information to referral sources and the patient, and of course, quality clinical care. Arthur Andersen LLP (Atlanta, GA) recently conducted a benchmarking study of ambulatory surgery that included responses from 120 health care companies. The report generated from the Arthur Andersen Global Best Practices (AA GBP) study includes data from the patient satisfaction and physician relations sub-processes. The patient

satisfaction process included all activities related to monitoring patient satisfaction and responding to customer needs. Among the areas
in this process were method and frequency of
obtaining customer feedback, measurement of
satisfaction, responsiveness of comments, and
establishment of performance goals.

The best practices that were addressed in patient satisfaction include the following: (a) use
of formal techniques to monitor patient satisfaction and response to comments in a timely manner; and (b) establish performance goals for
monitoring and improving patient satisfaction.
An effective formal technique for monitoring results is a standard questionnaire format that allows for consistent compilation of satisfaction
results. The results can then be trended from
time period to time period. Examples of survey
questions found in the study include the following:

- Quality of physician interaction with the pa-
  tient
- Efficiency of the pre-registration process
- Efficiency of the registration process
- Diagnostic testing services available on-site
- Patient waiting time
- Quality of discharge teaching, education, and
  follow-up
- Accessibility/convenience of practice sites
- Quality of nursing care delivered

Once the questionnaire is established, the
practice must monitor and act on feedback that
indicates a need to improve patient satisfaction.
This means that the practice reacts to both positive and negative feedback in an expedient manner. In the best practice study, one facility's
feedback indicated that their patients were receiving too many contacts before surgery. Consequently, the organization redesigned the entire
pre-surgical process and eventually eliminated
all pre-registration activities.

One of the questions posed in the best practice
study was, "Do you know your physicians' concerns?" The AA GBP study results indicated
that although the majority of those surveyed
value the importance of customer satisfaction,
fewer than half could assess the level of physician satisfaction. The physician satisfaction process includes all activities related to monitoring
physician satisfaction and responding to their
concerns. Among the areas included are method
and frequency of obtaining customer feedback,

measurement of satisfaction, responsiveness to
comments, and involvement of physicians in decision-making to establish goals and influence
change.

The best practices that were addressed within
physician satisfaction were the following: (a) development of team alliances with physicians to
communicate cost management and to develop
patient responsiveness strategies; (b) use appropriate measurement techniques to obtain physicians' feedback and proactively respond to their
concerns; and (c) active involvement of the medical director in open communication and participation in decision making with physicians to establish focused goals and influence change
management.

Developing team alliances can apply to the
primary care referral relationship, as well as internal physician relationships. The AA GBP
study showed that best performers:

- Fostered and sustained good physician relationships, enabling them to react quicker to
  changing reimbursement methodologies, increased managed care, and increased competition;
- Involved providers in the demonstration of the
  value of cost management and its direct benefit
  to attracting more managed care organizations,
  resulting in increased patient volume;
- Educated physicians in the patient screening
  process enabling them to match the types of
  patients with established clinical protocols.

The best performers (a) surveyed their physicians; (b) were proactive in discussing issues
with their physicians; and (c) promptly reacted
to their comments. Important issues to physicians that were identified in the survey included
cost of services for patients, quality of services,
and atmosphere and quality of nursing care.
Common issues important to physicians who
provide outpatient surgery care included extended operating reduced turnaround times;
more reliable start times; better conditions of
waiting/holding area room hours; and better
scheduling.

FUTURE ISSUES FOR
NEUROSURGICAL PRACTICE

The future for neurosurgical practice is filled
with opportunity. Gamma knife surgery, stereotactic abilities, and other non-invasive tech-

niques will make practices more cost-efficient and higher quality. As with other specialties, more demands will be placed on neurosurgical practice management. These demands include decreased reimbursement, increased administrative costs, patient and customer service issues, and competition from neurosurgical practice management companies.

The Health Care Finance Administration (HCFA) is impacting medical practices by potentially reducing reimbursement and increasing regulation. The new Medicare fee schedule is expected to decrease neurosurgical income when the new system is implemented in 2002. Although the exact impact has not been finalized, sources have cited anywhere from 10% to 35% reductions in fees paid to neurosurgical specialties. It should be noted that this impact would also impact commercial payers who reimburse based on the Medicare fee schedule.

In addition to decreasing reimbursement, HCFA (as well as private payers) will continue to audit a practice's documentation and coding procedures to lessen possible Medicare fraud and overpayments to providers. This may lead to additional administrative costs for internal audits, coding education, and utilization management. In addition, some practices may develop compliance plans while others may face fines and continued hassle practices.

If capitation continues to grow in neurosurgical practice, information systems must be able to support measurements and monthly reporting that in many cases will include clinical outcomes. Employers, patients, and payers will increasingly demand value for services delivered that are defined as low cost and high quality. Quality will be measured quantitatively through mortality rates, return to work timeframes, and patient satisfaction. These measurements will be published publicly and an informed population will direct referrals to those practitioners whose ratings appear superior. Qualitative measures like communication, patient wait times, and accessibility will also become more important. Neurosurgical practice will have to adapt to these new health care marketplace demands.

SUGGESTED READINGS

1. Arthur Andersen LLP: Ambulatory Surgery Global Best Practices Study, 1997.
2. Baum MD, Zablocki N, Zablocki E: Take Charge of Your Medical Practice. . .Before Someone Else Does It for You. Gaithersburg, Aspen Publishers Inc., 1996.
3. Benedict GS: The Development and Management of Medical Groups. Chicago, Medical Group Management Association and American Medical Association, 1996.
4. Burns L: Multispecialty group practice. *J Ambulatory Care Manage* 19:77–86, Gaithersburg, Aspen Publishers Inc., 1996.
5. Green B: Understanding the forces driving medical group practice activities. *J Ambulatory Care Manage* 19: 87–95, 1996.
6. Jaklevic MC: S.D. Hospital, Docs Battle Over Patients. *Modern Healthcare* Jan 18, 1999.
7. Micklitsch N, Ryan-Mitlyng C, Ryan-Mitlyng TA: Physician Performance Management: Tools for Survival and Success. Englewood, CO, Medical Group Management Association, 1996.
8. Powell M: Neurosurgery: Recent advances. *BMJ* 318: 35–38, 1999.
9. Ryan JV: Hospital Cost Accounting and Cost Management: The Expense Absorption Method of Cost Accounting. Mobile, James V. Ryan, 1994.

CHAPTER 25

Neurosurgical Education: Cost and Workforce Issues

KRISTEN UPCHURCH, M.D., AND PETE MCLAREN BLACK, M.D., PH.D.

The education of medical school graduates in their chosen specialty has been a primary mission of academic medical centers. Traditionally, funded directly by Medicare payments and indirectly by clinical revenues, the reductions in both of these revenue streams represents a significant threat to the future of resident education. Recent legislation in the form of the Balanced Budget Act of 1997 will have profound impacts on the number and types of residents educated. Drs. Upchurch and Black present an excellent discussion of the present state of funding for graduate medical education, changes caused by the Balanced Budget Act of 1997, initiatives for future changes, and issues concerning the size and future requirements of the neurosurgical workforce.

In the new competitive medical marketplace, teaching hospitals are struggling to survive financially while at the same time uphold their special missions of teaching and research (14). One of the most important academic missions of teaching hospitals is graduate medical education (GME), the training of new physicians in their specialties of choice. Because it is a public good, GME has historically been financed in large part by federal programs, with Medicare as the greatest single source of funding (18, 35).

As part of the drive to control expansionary health care costs (17) and due to the perception that a physician surplus exists (8, 9), recent legislation in the form of the Balanced Budget Act of 1997 (BBA 97) has drastically reduced Medicare funding of GME. These funding reductions have created incentives for teaching hospitals to reduce the size of their residency training programs and, in particular, to decrease the number of specialist positions. These changes in funding impact the ability of teaching hospitals to train all physicians, both generalists and specialists, but affect most profoundly the viability of residency training for specialists, such as neurosurgeons.

FINANCING OF GRADUATE MEDICAL EDUCATION

Residency training has historically been financed from several sources, including Medicare, Medicaid, private insurers, faculty practice plans, and other cross-subsidies. Before the Medicare program was enacted in 1965, GME was funded directly by teaching hospitals, which provided to their residents a small cash stipend, room, board, laundry, and other services. The hospitals recovered these costs directly or indirectly from insurance payments (6). Since 1965, Medicare, the federal insurance program for the elderly administered by the Health Care Finance Administration (HFCA), has become the largest source of funding for graduate medical education (35, 9).

Medicare financing of GME consists of two funding streams: direct medical education (DME) payments and indirect medical education (IME) adjustment. Direct payments cover part of the costs that can be attributed directly to resident training, such as salaries and benefits for residents (55% of DME total dollars), compensation to faculty for teaching (26%), administrative expenses, and other overhead (19%). Annual DME payments have been determined by the following formula:

$$\text{DME payment} = (\text{Hospital-specific base-year direct cost per resident}) \times (\text{Inflation adjuster}) \times (\text{number of residents}) \times (\text{Medicare inpatient days} / \text{Total inpatient days})$$

This formula reveals that two key variables for determining DME payments are the number of residents and the percentage of the teaching hospital's inpatients represented by Medicare patients (34). Note also that the inflation adjuster has been reduced for residents in non-primary care specialties (6).

IME payments cover part of the costs to teaching hospitals that are indirectly incurred by the operating inefficiencies associated with resident training, such as longer inpatient stays and perhaps the ordering of greater numbers of diagnostic tests. They also cover expenses that are not educational but are related to the role of teaching hospitals as institutions burdened by higher severity of patients' illnesses, the use of more complex technical procedures, and a larger proportion of uninsured and underinsured in their payer mix (1, 5, 24). Because these indirect costs cannot be calculated using cost-accounting techniques, Medicare developed a complex adjustment factor that takes into account the relationship between teaching hospitals' costs, the number of residents, and the number of beds the hospitals operate. The resulting IME payment is calculated by applying this adjustment factor to each hospital's diagnostic reference group (DRG) revenues to generate the following IME formula (as it was before the BBA 97) (34):

IME adjustment = 1.89 ((1 + number of

house staff/number of available beds)

0.405 − 1) × Total DRG revenues

It is extremely difficult to calculate accurately these higher patient care costs of teaching hospitals. As one health-policy expert has written, "The adjustment for indirect medical education is only a proxy to account for a number of factors which may legitimately increase costs in teaching hospitals" (18).

Before 1997, increasing the number of residents in a teaching hospital's residency program led directly to an increase in GME Medicare payments. When the teaching hospital added residents to a program, the only increase in costs that it incurred to itself was the additional residents' salaries and benefits. At the same time, it received increases in both DME and IME funds, which covered these costs. Of note, IME payments to teaching hospitals have always been much greater than DME payments; for example, between 1990 and 1994, IME reimbursement ac-

counted for approximately 70% of total Medicare GME payments (6). Due to this fact, the teaching hospital that increased its number of residents gained extra monies, even after subtracting the salaries and benefits of the new residents from the Medicare payments received. That is, DME payments covered salaries and benefits, leaving IME payments as a net gain (34).

This Medicare payment system for GME created an obvious financial incentive for teaching hospitals to increase the number of residents in their training programs. From 1984 through 1995, the period during which this funding system was in place, the total number of residents in the United States increased by 42%, from 72,400 in 1984 to 102,600 in 1995. As explained above, the increase in the number of residents resulted in significant growth in the amount of GME payments made by the Medicare program to teaching hospitals (34).

This system of Medicare GME financing was altered by the BBA 97 (Public Law 105-83) (35). In this Act, Congress reduced Medicare payments to teaching hospitals for GME and also created incentives for decreasing resident numbers. These changes were thought necessary for two reasons, the impending insolvency of the Medicare Hospital Insurance Trust Fund and a presumed surplus of physicians.

Many economic analysts, including the trustees for Medicare, predict that the Medicare Trust Fund will be insolvent within the next 15 years. The expenses of the Medicare Trust Fund are outstripping its income because of increased spending for beneficiaries and an increase in the number of persons eligible for Medicare. Medicare spending for beneficiaries increased from $21.5 billion in 1977 to $214.6 billion in 1997, that is, by a factor of 10 over the past 20 years. The number of persons eligible for Medicare (those over age 65, the permanently disabled of all ages, and those with end-stage renal disease) has grown from 26 million to 38.6 million (18, 32).

According to public opinion polls, most Americans support the safety net that Medicare provides to the elderly and disabled (3). Because Medicare is so popular with the public, politicians take great risks when they attempt changes within the program, as seen with President Clinton's 1996 re-election. In 1995, the newly elected Republican Congressional majority attempted to reduce Medicare expenses in part by increasing the annual premiums paid by elderly beneficiaries, and Clinton's veto of their plan led to increased support from the elderly, who helped vote him to a second term (18).

Despite the political risks involved in tampering with this popular program, Congress has been forced by the impending insolvency of the Medicare Hospital Insurance Trust Fund to cut Medicare expenses via the BBA 97. Through this legislation, these expenses have been drastically reduced. Although the Medicare program accounts for only 12% of all federal spending, the BBA 97 extracts 56.5% of all savings to the government that it contains solely from reductions in Medicare's estimated future expenditures (18).

In shaping the BBA 97, the Senate and the House took different stances regarding how best to reduce Medicare expenses. The Senators, whose six-year terms make it unnecessary for them to run constant re-election campaigns, wanted to lower Medicare expenses in part by asking beneficiaries to pay for more of their health-care costs. They voted to raise the age of initial eligibility for Medicare from 65 to 67 years, to adjust a beneficiary's premium on the basis of his or her income, and to require co-payments for home health services. The House members, whose two-year terms make them more immediately accountable to voters, rejected all three of the Senate's proposals. Instead, the House voted to lower Medicare expenses by reducing payments to health care providers. In the BBA 97, most of the savings to the Medicare program, $116.6 billion from 1998 to 2002, are extracted from future payments to health care providers (18). Because the American public holds the view that "doctors and hospitals overcharge Medicare," Congress has taken no political risks with the voting public at large (3).

The Balanced Budget Act of 1997

The BBA 97 represents the most far-reaching reform in the 34-year history of Medicare, in the form of some 300 new provisions (18). The BBA 97 has reduced both direct and indirect Medicare payments for GME. Specifically, the BBA 97 altered DME resident-counting methods, IME resident-counting methods, components of the formula used to calculate the IME adjustment, and treatment of GME payments in the calcula-

tion of rates for Medicare managed care contractors (34).

Under the BBA 97 regulations, a teaching hospital cannot count more residents for DME or for IME than were counted in Fiscal Year 1996. That is, if a hospital adds more residents to its training programs, the hospital will not receive Medicare funding for those residents (34). In addition, the BBA 97 bases the house staff count used for both DME and IME on a three-year rolling average. Under this regulation, if a teaching hospital reduces the number of its residents over time, the smaller more recent total is averaged in with the larger past totals (e.g., 90 house staff in 1997, 85 in 1998, and 80 in 1999, for an average of 85). The hospital benefits financially by reducing the number of its residents from 90 to 80, because it will receive a DME payment for 85 residents in 1999 even though it is paying the salaries of only 80 residents. This same financial benefit for the teaching hospital also holds for the IME adjustment. In this way, the BBA 97 imposes significant financial penalties on teaching hospitals that increase their resident numbers and bestows financial rewards on those that actively cut the number of available positions (1).

The BBA 97 also requires changes in the IME adjustment formula, specifically that the coefficient in the IME adjustment formula be decreased over time, with the obvious result that the IME adjustment itself is reduced. The decrease in the multiplier for the formula used to calculate the actual IME adjustment is as follows: 1.89 in 1997, 1.72 in 1998, 1.60 in 1999, 1.47 in 2000, and 1.35 in 2001 and after. In other words, the IME adjustment in 1997 represented a payment to each hospital of an additional 7.7% of its total annual DRG payment for each 0.1 in the ratio of house staff to beds. This will be reduced in the following manner to 7.0% in 1998, 6.5% in 1990, 6.0% in 2000, and to 5.5% in 2001 and thereafter. At the end of the five-year phase-in period, the result will be a 29% reduction in IME funding to teaching hospitals (1).

The impact of the funding cuts mandated by the BBA 97 on the fate of teaching hospitals and on the fate of residency training programs cannot be overestimated. Prior to the implementation of the BBA 97's regulations in 1997 total direct and indirect GME-related costs paid by Medicare to U.S. teaching hospitals were between $18.1 billion and $22.8 billion (24). The Association of

Education Trust Fund legislation: Washington Highlights. *Association of American Medical Colleges* 1999:10(4):5–6.

5. Bajaj A: Commission reviewing GME funding disbands without a proposal. *JAMA* 281:1556b, 1999.

6. Bajaj A: How Medicare calculates GME payments: Part I. *JAMA* 281:1958a, 1999.

7. Council on Graduate Medical Education: Summary of Sixth Report: Managed health care–Implications for the physician workforce and medical education. COGME website. September 1995.

8. Council on Graduate Medical Education: Summary of Eighth Report: Patient care physician supply and requirements–Testing COGME recommendations. COGME website. November 1996.

9. Council on Graduate Medical Education: Summary of Ninth Report: Graduate medical education consortia–Changing the governance of graduate medical education to achieve physician workforce objectives. COGME website. June 1997.

10. Council on Graduate Medical Education: Summary of Fourteenth Report: COGME physician workforce policies–Recent developments and remaining challenges in meeting national goals. COGME website. March 1999.

11. Flannery AM: Pediatric neurosurgery work force: A pilot study. *Pediatr Neurosurg* 29:114–116, 1998.

12. Friedlich DL, Feustel PJ, Popp AJ: Workforce demand for neurosurgeons in the United States of America: A 13-year retrospective study. *J Neurosurg* 90:993–997, 1999.

13. GME Study Group: GME study group discusses workforce issues: Washington Highlights. *Association of American Medical Colleges* 1998:9.

14. Goldberg C: Teaching hospitals battling cutbacks in Medicare money. *New York Times*. May 6, 1999; sect A:1.

15. Greene J: States scramble for ways to fund medical education. *American Medical News* 1999:42(16):??–??.

16. Harrington TR: Neurosurgical manpower needs: Achieving a balance. *Surg Neurol* 47:316–325, 1997.

17. Hoff JT, Polinsky MN, Bean JR: Health-care reform and neurosurgery training, in Bean JR: Neurosurgery in Transition: The Socioeconomic Transformation of Neurological Surgery. Baltimore, Williams & Wilkins, 1998.

18. Iglehart JK: The American health care system: Medicare. *N Engl J Med* 340:327–332, 1999.

19. Jacoby I, Meyer GS: Creating an effective physician workforce marketplace. *JAMA* 280:822–824, 1998.

20. Landers SJ: Congress to consider new options for GME funding. *American Medical News* 1999:42(16):??–??.

21. Landers SJ: Senate panel weighs Medicare options. *American Medical News* 1999:42(19):5–6.

22. Laws ER, Friedman WA, Orrico KO: Letter stating the official position of the AANS and CNS, addressed to Murray Ross, Ph.D. of the Medicare Payment Advisory Committee. CNS website. March 31, 1998.

23. McClendon BJ, Politzer RM, Christian E, Fernandez ES: Downsizing the physician workforce. *Public Health Rep* 112:231–239, 1997.

24. Mechanic R, Coleman K, Dobson A: Teaching hospital costs: Implications for academic missions in a competitive market. *JAMA* 280:1015–1019, 1998.

25. Miller RS, Dunn MR, Richter TH, Whitcomb ME: Employment-seeking experiences of resident physicians completing training during 1996. *JAMA* 280:777–783, 1998.

26. Miller RS, Dunn MR, Whitcomb ME: Initial employment status of resident physicians completing training in 1995. *JAMA* 277:1699–1704, 1997.

27. Miller RS, Jonas HS, Whitcomb ME: The initial employment status of physicians completing training in 1994. *JAMA* 275:708–712, 1996.

28. Patterson RH Jr: How many residents should we train? The USA experience. *Acta Neurochir Suppl (Wien)* 69:30–32, 1997.

29. Popp AJ: The neurosurgical workforce: Market effects, public policy, and professional constraints, in Bean JR: Neurosurgery in Transition: The Socioeconomic Transformation of Neurological Surgery. Baltimore, Williams & Wilkins, 1998.

30. Popp AJ, Toselli R: Work force requirements for neurosurgery. *Surg Neurol* 46:181–185, 1996.

31. Seifer SD, Troupin B, Rubenfeld GD: Changes in marketplace demand for physicians. *JAMA* 276:695–699, 1996.

32. Travis RL, Orrico KO: Neurosurgery and politics, in Bean JR: Neurosurgery in Transition: The Socioeconomic Transformation of Neurological Surgery. Baltimore, Williams & Wilkins, 1998.

33. Weiner JP: Forecasting the effects of health reform on U.S. physician workforce requirements. *JAMA* 272:222–230, 1994.

34. Wray JL, Sadowski SM: Defining teaching hospitals' GME strategy in response to new financial and market challenges. *Acad Med* 73:370–379, 1998.

35. Young JQ, Coffman JM: Overview of graduate medical education: Funding streams, policy problems, and options for reform. *West J Med* 168:428–436, 1998.

Glossary

A

Act Phase: Fourth stage of the **Plan-Do-Check-Act (PDCA) cycle** during which decisions are made regarding adopting changes that were tested, proposing new changes, or continuing through the cycle.

Action plan: an explicit identification of the tasks, responsibilities, and timetable required to implement the **strategic plan**. Typically, action plans are prepared on an annual basis and ideally are linked to the annual operating and capital budget so that resources required for implementation can be identified and committed.

Activity-Based Costing (ABC): A method of cost accounting that identifies activities that drive costs for any given activity.

Activity Network Diagram: Also known as an **arrow diagram**, a tool used to plan the most appropriate path and schedule for the completion of any complex task.

Affinity Diagram: A planning tool that groups spoken thoughts (language data) such as ideas, options, or issues according to their natural relationships. The emphasis is on a pre-rational, gut-feel sort of grouping, often done by the members of the group with little or no talking. Also known as the KJ method after its creator, Kawakita Jiro.

Arrow Diagram: Also known as an **activity network diagram**, a tool used to plan the most appropriate path and schedule for the completion of any complex task.

Attribute Data: Data that result from counting the number of occurrences or items in a single category of similar items or occurrences. The alternative to attributes data is **variables data**, which is data that is measured on a continuous and infinite scale such as temperature or distance. Charts that use attribute data include **bar charts, pie charts**, **Pareto charts** and some **control charts**.

B

Balanced Scorecard: Graphics data used to document important process outcomes over time. Reporting is balanced between outcomes for cost, patient satisfaction, and clinical indicators. This balanced approach insures that cost cutting measures do not negatively impact upon patient satisfaction or clinical outcomes.

Baseline Data: Data from a stable process that are used to determine the effectiveness of process changes by serving as an initial reference point for subsequent comparison.

Basic Graphic Tools: Charting & graphing procedures commonly use for process description or to depict process performance. They can visually identify areas for improvement as well as the effects of any process changes (i.e. PDCA cycle). Common graphic tools include **flow charts, check sheets, cause and effect diagrams, Pareto charts, control charts, run charts, histograms**, and **scatter diagrams**.

Benchmarking: In quality terms, a strategic and analytic process of continuously measuring an organization's products, services, and practices against a recognized leader in the studied area. Also a management technique designed to conserve time, effort, & resources by identifying an organization who excels at a given process and then initially stabilizing your organization's analogous process based on their model. Benchmarking eliminates the need to begin process improvement at ''ground zero'' and the need to ''re-invent the wheel'' for processes that are common to multiple organizations. However, since every **extended system** is unique, the benchmarked process will need to be optimized for any given organization through **continuous process improvement** (continuous **PDCA cycles**). (see also **best practice analysis**)

Best Practice: Guidelines that result from clinical trials as the currently accepted best way to prevent, detect, or treat a medical condition; guidelines that insurance plans or managed care organizations may require physicians to follow in order to be part of their panel; provide specific treatment options or steps to follow when a provider sees a patient with a particular set of clinical symptoms or lab data.

Best practice analysis: (see **benchmarking**) Determining recognized leaders in a particular product, service, or process and studying these leaders' approaches to provide a foundation for an organization's own improvement efforts.

Bias: In statistical terms, bias is the degree to which the mean value of a sample approximates the distribution parameter. In descriptive scientific terms, bias is an un-accounted or uncontrolled influence on a data set causing the objective measurement resulting from that data set to skew either positively or negatively from the value that would have been apparent if that influence were not present.

Big Hairy Audacious Goals (BHAG's): the term created by Collins and Porras in their widely acclaimed book *Built to Last* to characterize the 10–30 year goals that are part of an organization's **vision** and establish targets that stretch it beyond current capabilities to provide a compelling focal point for future effort; eg. NASA's target to put a man on the moon by the end of the sixties articulated by President Kennedy in 1961.

Boundary: Something that delineates a limit or extent. Boundaries may be spatial, temporal or organizational and can be established by agreement or by definition.

Brainstorming: An idea-generating technique used by teams to generate many ideas in a short period of time. Ideas are solicited in a non-judgmental manner from all team members until all ideas are exhausted. No discussion, evaluation, or criticism of ideas is allowed until the brainstorming session is complete. Hearing each other's ideas usually triggers many more ideas than would have been solicited individually from team members.

Bureaucratic Hierarchy: A traditional form of organization and management characterized by specialization of functions, adherence to fixed rules, and a hierarchy of authority. On an organizational flow chart, it tends to have a vertical organization with information flow proceeding up and down the organizational columns (see **silo effect**).

Buy-in: agreement by the key **stakeholders** in an organization with the direction established by the **strategic plan**.

C

c-Chart: A type of attributes **control chart** that plots the number of defects for samples of a constant size.

Capable Process: A process that is stable (running within statistical control limits) *and* meets customer needs.

Capitation: A payment system in which a provider is paid a flat amount for each covered individual on a monthly basis.

Case Mix Adjustment: Methodology used to modify anticipated health outcomes based on the severity of illness of patients being treated by a given provider or healthcare organization.

Causal System: The combination of influences or sources of variation that determine the nature of an output characteristic.

Cause and Effect Diagram: A graphic representation that organizes potential causes of process variation into general categories. A tool used to analyze all factors (causes) that contribute to a given situation or occurrence (effect) by breaking down main causes into smaller and smaller sub-causes. Typically these categories include methods, material, machines, people, and environment. Also called a **fishbone diagram** or an **Ishikawa diagram** (after its developer).

Chain Reaction: A graphic demonstration of Deming's theory that relates quality to a series of beneficial results. The theory states that as you improve quality, you also improve productivity, capture markets with better quality and lower price, stay and business and provide jobs.

Charter: A written document that describes the boundaries, expected results, and resources to be used by a quality improvement team. A charter should go through a process of validation by the accepting team prior to attempting implementation.

Check Phase: The third phase of the **Plan-Do-Check-Act (PDCA) cycle** in which the effects of the "**Do**" phase are assessed. Sometimes referred to as the "study" phase if the alternative "Plan-Do-Study-Act (PDSA) cycle" terminology is used.

Check Sheet: An organized form designed for the efficient collection, organization, and analysis of data.

Clinical Outcomes: A subset of **Outcomes Data** focusing on the morbidity and mortality with treatment (e.g. complications of surgery, treatment failure, etc.) or without treatment (natural history).

Clinical Pathway: Is a documented interdisciplinary plan of care that describes current best management of a specific disease, condition, or procedure. It is designed to reduce unwanted variation in clinical care where adequate data exists to support standardization, and to improve patient outcomes. Components include **discharge outcomes, daily-anticipated outcomes**, and daily orders and interventions. The pathway defines the expected length of hospital stay.

Common Causes: Those causes of variation that are inherent in the process over time and affect all outputs of the process. Since they are inherent in the process, they are not within the power of individuals participating in the process to change, and can only be altered by actually changing the process.

Complexity: Unnecessary or redundant steps within a process. During **standardization** of a process, complexity should be identified and minimized (see **process improvement**).

Consensus: Consensus means, literally, shared thought. A decision by a group that is acceptable to all members and that all members can publicly and privately support. A feeling that all members of a group have been heard, and all can live with the decision of the group. One of the most important and fundamental concepts of total quality management, achieving consensus is hard work and often occupies a large portion of a quality management team's time and energy. It does not imply universal agreement on every aspect of the decision by all group members and is not arrived at by a vote. It should never be confused with "leadership by democracy", majority rule, political compromise, unanimous agreement or **"group think"**.

Constancy of Purpose: A leadership obligation to establish and demonstrate unwavering commitment to the long-term purpose of the organization. This purpose is usually formally codified within a **strategic framework** with a formal organizational **mission statement**, and **vision statement**, as well as an organizational statement of **guiding principles**.

Continuous Improvement: see **continuous process improvement**.

Continuous Process Improvement: The continuous (regular and frequent) endeavor to learn about the causal system of a process and to use this knowledge to change the process by reducing variation and complexity as well as improving customer satisfaction. At minimum, continuous process improvement requires (1) process definition & stabilization (see **stable process**), (2) regular and frequent **customer feedback**, and (3) continuous **PDCA cycles**. Also known as **continuous quality improvement (CQI), continuous improvement,** and **process improvement.**

Continuous Quality Improvement (CQI):   see **continuous process improvement**.

Control Charts: A statistical process control tool used to distinguish between process variation due to common cause and variation due to special causes. A chart that indicates upper and lower statistical control limits, and an average line, for samples or subgroups of a given process. If all points on the control chart are within the limits, variation may be ascribed to common causes and the process is deemed to be ''in control.'' If points fall outside the limits, it is an indication that special causes of variation are occurring, and the process is said to be ''out of control.'' The type of control chart necessary depends on the characteristics of the data collected.

Control Limit: A line on a control chart, calculated from process data, that represents the limits of the common cause system of the process.

Core competencies: the basic capabilities that define an organization and distinguish it from its competitors.

Core ideology: the enduring and unchanging character of an organization. In the model of Collins and Poras presented in *Built to Last,* core ideology consists of two parts: **core values** and **core purpose**.

Core purpose: **mission**.

Core strategies: the specific approaches through which an organization plans to address its opportunities and overcome its competitive disadvantages. Core strategies provide the basic framework of a **strategic plan**.

Core values: the guiding principles and tenets of an organization.

Correlation: A statistical measure of the degree and nature of relation between variables.

Cost: The amount of resources consumed for a given purpose or to perform a given task.

Cost Driver: Represents the measurement unit (in **ABC** accounting) of demand for the activity required to produce goods and services.

Cost-Effectiveness Analysis: A type of decision analysis where resource utilization required (e.g. dollars spent) to achieve a quantified benefit (e.g. 20 **Quality Adjusted Life Years**) is the result of the analysis.

Critical Mass: A state in which a sufficient number of people with position, knowledge, and **leadership** have the necessary knowledge to effect, and are sufficiently committed to, transformation, so that **organizational transformation** becomes self-sustaining without need for external pressure or energy.

Critical Paths: 1. The longest sequential series of tasks in a project. 2. Minimum necessary tasks to accomplish an objective or meet a goal. 3. In health care, a treatment protocol, based on a consensus of clinicians, that includes only those few vital components or items proved to affect patient outcomes, either by the omission or commission of the treatment or the timing of the intervention.

Critical Process: A stage within a **significant process** that is deemed most important for improvement (see **process**).

Cross-Functional Team: A team with members from more than one organizational function that each have responsibility for some portion of an identified **process.**

Customer: The person or group who establishes the requirements of a process and receives or uses the **output** of that process. Also known as an **end user**. Customers can be either **internal customers** or **external customers**.

Customer Feedback System: A system used by production organizations or groups for obtaining information from **customers** about relevant quality characteristics of products and services.

Customer Satisfaction: The degree to which a customer perceives that a product or service meets expectations.

Cycle for Improving Performance: A well-known performance improvement method developed by the Joint Commission on Accreditation of Healthcare Organizations that integrates a number of different approaches to performance improvement.

D

Daily Outcomes: represent the expected condition on each day or phase of hospital stay on a **clinical pathway**. Outcomes are the result of providing clinical care. For example, on post-operative day 1 a patient should be taking food by mouth, ambulating 50 feet, and have their pain adequately controlled on oral medication.

Dashboard: the key measures of performance that monitor an organization's progress toward achieving its strategic goals and provide feedback that supports necessary modification to plans over time.

Data Collection Plan: A plan that provides guidance for gathering information establishing the why, who, what, how, where, and when of data collection.

Data Synthesis Studies: Studies employing statistical methodologies for combining the results of individual studies.

Deadly Diseases, 7:   Deming's list of seven roadblocks to institutionalizing the quality transformation that are inherent in most organizations in the western world. Their cure requires a complete change in management style.

Decision Analysis: Methodology in which competing therapeutic strategies are specified and assigned probabilities of achieving various clinical outcomes based on results published in the medical literature. This methodology is used to determine the most beneficial treatment for an individual patient or to assess the value of various treatment strategies for a cohort of patients.

Defect: A nonconformity to **customer** requirements.

Defective: An item or service that contains one or more **defects**.

Diagnosis Related Group (DRG) Method: A payment method in which a provider is paid a predetermined amount for each admission determined by the patient's diagnosis.

Direct Costs: Resources that are clearly and directly consumed for a given purpose or by a given cost-object.

Direct Medical Education (DME) Payments: Payments by Medicare to hospitals to cover the direct cost of resident training such as salaries and benefits.

Disability: The loss of personal activity or function as measured at the level of the individual.

Discharge Outcomes: represent the overall condition the patient should achieve on a **clinical pathway** to allow safe discharge from the hospital. These criteria help communicate to all caregivers when a patient is ready for discharge. For example, for some conditions, a patient may be discharged when afebrile and ambulating independently, with pain controlled with oral medication only.

Discounting: The process of adjusting future costs and benefits to present value terms.

Dispersion: see **variation**.

Distribution: A graphic representation of the **dispersion**, location, and density of measured values.

Do Phase: The second phase of the **Plan-Do-Check-Act (PDCA) cycle** in which the **plan** is executed.

Dreadful Diseases, 10:   Deming's list of ten management practice roadblocks to institutionalizing the **quality transformation** that are harmful but curable through application of the **14 "obligations" of management.**

E

Effectiveness: The degree to which actions achieve desired effects.

Efficiency: The ratio of useful **output** to the total **input** in a system.

Empowerment: Delegation of *authority* as well as the necessary *means* to improve a process or achieve a specified end.

End User: see **customer**.

End of Stay Insert Day: Is an **insert day** added when a patient stayed in the hospital longer than was outlined in the **clinical pathway** and includes the reason for the extension.

Environment: Circumstances and conditions external to organizational boundaries that interact with, and affect, an organization. These may be economic, political, cultural, regulatory, or physical factors.

Envisioned future: in the construct presented by Collins and Porras in *Built to Last,* the combination of **"Big Hairy Audacious Goals" (BHAG's)** and vivid descriptions of what the future will be like if these goals are achieved.

Executive Steering Committee (ESC):   A permanent team of guiding members of an organization who comprise the highest level quality improvement team in the organization. This team is comprised of all major organizational leaders as well as the responsible members for each of the organization's **significant processes**. This team is responsible for organizational **strategic planning** as well as providing the **charters** for each permanent organizational **quality management board (QMB)**.

Extended System: A system that extends beyond the boundaries of the producing organization to include the **suppliers** the **customers**, and the environmental **stakeholders** of the organization. Interaction among the components are managed by the producing organization using the principles of system **optimization**. Processes internal to the producing organization that link the customer to the supplier are regarded as **significant processes.**

External Customer: An individual or group outside the **boundaries** of the producing organization who receives or uses the **output** of a process.

External Supplier: An individual or group outside the **boundaries** of the receiving organization who provides **input** to the receiving organization.

F

Fee-for-Service: A reimbursement method in which each service provided is paid for, usually at a pre-determined rate.

Fishbone Diagram: See **cause-and-effect diagram**.

Flow Chart: A schematic diagram that uses various graphic symbols to depict the nature and flow of the steps in a process. "Deployment" and **opportunity flow charts** are the two types most commonly used. Flow charts can be drawn to represent different detail and complexity, reflecting different levels of analysis (e.g. macro, mini, & micro).

FOCUS-PDCA: A variation on the classic Shewhart **Plan-Do-Check-Act (PDCA) cycle** developed by the Hospital Corporation of America and (now part of Columbia Health Care Corporation) adopted by many healthcare organizations. It Stands for: **F**ind a process improvement opportunity, **O**rganize a team that understands the process, **C**larify the current knowledge of the process, **U**ncover the **root cause** of **variation**, **S**tart the **PDCA cycle**. It's advantage is that multiple quality improvement efforts can begin immediately (albeit ad hoc) throughout the organization. However, since these efforts are not planned or managed at an organizational level, they run the risk of contributing to **suboptimization** (see **managed participation, strategic planning** and **optimization**).

Force Field Analysis: A tool, developed by social psychologist Kurt Lewin, which is used to analyze the opposing forces involved in causing/resisting any change. It is shown in balance sheet format with forces that will help (driving forces) listed on the left and forces that hinder (restraining forces) listed on the right.

Forming: The first stage of team psychological evolution. In this stage, the team members are just getting to know one another's personalities, position within the organization, and area and degree of subject matter expertise. During this stage, members cautiously explore the boundaries of acceptable group behavior and often test the leader's guidance both formally and informally. Personal insecurity is still present, so member's are cautious in offering input into group activities and discussions, and personal interactions may be overly courteous (see **team evolutionary stages**). Teams may reform during their life.

Functional Outcomes: A subset of **Outcomes Data** focusing on the functional capabilities of patients with or without treatment. Generic and disease specific functional outcomes instruments are available for quantifying functional health status.

G

Gainsharing: A program designed to share savings between hospitals and physicians using objective measurements of clinical improvement, quality outcomes and cost savings.

Gantt Chart: A diagram used to plan and manage work in relation to time. A bar chart that shows planned work and finished work in relation to time. Each task in a list has a bar corresponding to it. The length of the bar is used to indicate the expected or actual duration of the task.

Gap: In the context of **strategic planning**, a gap is the difference between what an organization is doing today to accomplish its mission and what it needs to do to achieve its vision of the future organization.

Global Pricing: A method of payment that combines the reimbursement for the physician, hospital, and all ancillary services into a single payment.

Government Performance and Results Act (GPRA):   Public law 103-62 enacted by the 103rd U.S. Congress. It establishes the requirement for **strategic planning** and performance measurement in Federal Executive Agencies.

Group Think: Groupthink is the term, borrowed from George Orwell's classic book, *1984*, to describe the tendency of people in a group to be afraid to think outside of the group's perceptual boundaries. A negative potential result of group psychology where, due to unwillingness to disrupt group harmony, all members agree to a decision that no member individually supports. A mode of thinking that people engage in when they are deeply involved in a cohesive in-group, when members' striving for unanimity overrides their motivation to realistically appraise alternative courses of action.

Guiding Principles: A set of principles generated by the guiding members of the organization intended to guide the behavior of all the members of the organization towards each other as well as their **customers** and **suppliers**. These statements are based on an agreed-upon set of **organizational values** sometimes referred to as "core values".

H

Histogram: A vertical bar graph depicting the distribution of a set of continuous data. A specialized bar chart showing the distribution of measurement data. It will pictorially reveal the amount and type of variation within a process.

Hoshin Planning: A planning and management technique with seven specific tools designed to help an organization target one or two breakthrough goals, rather than trying to accomplish too many things at once.

I

Impairment: The loss or abnormality of psychological, physiological, or anatomic structure or function at the organ level.

Implementation Plan: A plan for starting **total quality management** in an organization with the aim of establishing **critical mass** and beginning the practice of **process management**.

Incremental Cost-Effectiveness Analysis: A comparison of the cost and effects of one treatment strategy with the next most expensive or invasive treatment.

Indirect Costs: Resources used in the ultimate production of a good or service that cannot be directly linked to a particular activity in their production.

Indirect Medical Education (IME) Payments: Payments by Medicare to hospitals to cover the **indirect cost** of resident training represented in operating inefficiencies.

Innovation: The application of knowledge leading to the development of new processes, products, or services in response to anticipated customer requirements.

Inputs: Materials or information used to produce a product or service.

Insert Day: A defined set of orders and interventions that are added to a **clinical pathway** because a patient's **length of stay** has been extended. This document states the reason stay has been extended at any given point in the **clinical pathway.**

Internal Customer: An individual or group inside the boundaries of the producing organization who receives r uses output from a previous stage of a process **(internal supplier)** to contribute to the production of the final product or service.

Internal Supplier: An individual or group within the boundaries of an organization who provides input to another individual or group within the organization **(internal customer)** for use in a subsequent stage of a process leading to the production of the final product or service

International Classification of Diseases (ICD): Classification scheme used to provide an internationally consistent method of tracking morbidity data.

Ishikawa Diagram: See **cause-and-effect diagram**.

ISO 9000: A generic term for the series of standards sponsored by the International Organization for Standardization (ISO); the intent is to establish, document, and maintain a system for ensuring output quality for manufacturing and service firms.

J

Job-Order Costing: A process used to directly assign costs to patients that consume different amounts of resources.

Just-In-Time: The concept of supplying inputs only when they are immediately needed for use. Examples of commonly planned just-in-time inputs include inventory, personnel, and personnel training. A strategy to maximize efficiency within an organization.

Just in time Training: Providing training and resources for people on a topic at a time when they have an immediate need and will quickly apply their new learning to their own situation.

K

Kurtosis: The kurtosis of a frequency distribution is a measure of its flatness or pointiness. A standard normal distribution has zero kurtosis. Mont Blanc is pointier than a normal distribution, and has negative kurtosis.

L

Leadership: The process of motivating others to take action towards a common goal (contrast with **management**).

Length of Stay: The number of days of hospitalization calculated by subtracting the admission date from the discharge date.

Lesional Outcomes: A subset of **Outcomes Data** bearing on the effectiveness of treatment in correcting a physiological (e.g. hypertension) or structural (e.g. carotid artery stenosis) abnormality. Radiological imaging, physiological monitoring, laboratory evaluation, or other means of determining the effects of treatment are needed.

Linking Pin: A member of the **executive steering committee (ESC)** or **quality management board (QMB)** who is assigned to work with a subordinate **QMB** or **process action team (PAT)** in order to help them interpret their team charter, and provide guidance and support for the team's activities. The linking pin serves both as a "down link" from the authorizing team, and as an "up link" from the subordinate team for purposes of communication and maintaining focus on organizational **optimization**. The linking pin is a non-voting member of the subordinate team.

M

Managed Indemnity: A payment system in which claims are paid by the insurer as they are received often after the treatment has been approved by some method.

Management: The exercise of either formal or informal authority to direct and coordinate the work of others (contrast with **leadership**).

Management by Objective: Manaement by objective is a process that specifies that superiors and subordinates will jointly set goals for a specified time period and then meet again to evaluate the subordinate's performance in terms of the previously established goals.

Management of Participation: The boundaries, limits, and controls placed upon participatory management. In **total quality management (TQM)**, individual participation in **quality management boards (QMB's)** and **process action teams (PAT's)** is authorized by organizational leadership, is planned to compliment organizational priorities, and is coordinated to contribute to organizational **optimization**.

Marginal Cost-Effectiveness Analysis: The additional cost and effect obtained from the use of one additional unit of treatment.

Matrix Diagram: A graphic tool that shows the relationships and the perceived subjective strength of relationship between two or more qualitative variables.

Mean: A summary indicator of central tendency or location on a measurement scale obtained by summing the values in a set of data and dividing by the number of values in the set.

Median: A summary indicator of central tendency or location on a measurement scale which is the point on the scale above and below which 50% of the measurements fall.

Meta-Analysis: Statistical methodology used to combine compatible results from smaller prospective randomized studies into a larger database in order to gain additional statistical power for analysis.

Mission: the fundamental reason for an organization's existence; **core purpose** that is unchanging, timeless, and provides the organization's foundation.

Mission Statement: A written document that defines the fundamental and unique purpose that sets one organization apart from others and identifies the scope of operations. It literally and concretely describes what the organization does, who it does it for, and how it does it. It is written primarily for internal consumption within the organization as part of leadership's obligation to maintain **constancy of purpose**. It should never contain exhortations to the work force, and should not be designed for advertising or public promotion purposes.

Mode: A summary indicator of central tendency or location on a measurement scale which is the most frequently occurring value in the measurement set.

Moving Range: The absolute value of the difference between two successive observations. Used as a measure of the variability of a process.

Multi-voting: A repetitive process used by a team to conduct a straw poll to select the most important or popular items from a large list of items generated by the team. The process is purposefully conducted with limited discussion to minimize peer influence.

N

National Performance Review (NPR):   An executive initiative aimed at reducing cost and improving productivity in public sector organizations.

Neurosurgical Report Card: A brief outcomes reporting instrument for monitoring clinical outcomes data and resource utilization for neurosurgical procedures developed by the Outcomes Committee of the American Association of Neurological Surgeons and the Congress of Neurological Surgeons.

Nominal Group Technique (NGT):   A weighted ranking technique that allows a team to generate and prioritize a large number of issues without creating ''winners'' and ''losers'' among the team members. Technique used to encourage creative thinking and new ideas, but is more controlled than **brainstorming**. Each member of a group writes down his or her ideas and then contributes one to the group pool. All contributed ideas are then discussed and prioritized.

Norming: The second stage of team psychological evolution. In this stage, the team members are beginning to take pride in group identity and responsibility. However, the good feelings arising from coordinated group effort and accomplishment can lead to hesitancy to risk group harmony by offering dissenting or conflicting ideas or points of view. While this maintains overall group harmony, it means that the team is deprived of potentially valuable individual input (see **team evolutionary stages**). Teams may cycle through this stage several times.

Notetaker: The notetaker records key topics, main points raised during discussions, decisions made, action items, and items to be discussed at future meetings. These minutes are the permanent record of the team's work in meetings.

np-Chart: A type of attributes **control chart** that plots the number of defective units for samples of a constant size.

O

Objectives: Specific, measurable, mid-term and short-term performance targets necessary for achieving long-term goals.

Objectives Matrix: A technique used to combine different measures of performance into a summary index that allows for meaningful comparisons of performance.

"Obligations" of management, 14:   A different title for the 14 points that emphasizes management's obligation.

Operational Definition: A definition that gives communicable meaning to a concept by specifying how the concept is measured and applied within a particular set of circumstances. It is composed of three elements: criterion, test, and decision. Operational definitions change according to their application and the given set of operational circumstances.

Opportunities: possibilities provided by the internal and external environment to improve an organization's competitive position and move toward its vision. Identifying opportunities is the "O" in **SWOT analysis**.

Opportunity Costs: A measure of the benefit forgone by using resources for an alternative purpose.

Opportunity Flow Chart: A graphic technique that differentiates process activities that add value from those that only add cost. During **standardization** of a process, complexity should be minimized by eliminating unnecessary and costly activities while retaining all **value added activities**.

Optimization: Organizing and orchestrating the combined efforts of all components of a system toward achievement of the same stated aims. A major responsibility of organizational **leadership** (see **suboptimization**).

Organizational Culture: A collection of basic assumptions, invented, discovered, or developed by a given group, as it learns to cope with its problems of external adaptation and internal integration, that has worked well enough to be considered valid and, therefore is taught to new members as the correct way to perceive, think, and feel in relation to those problems.

Organizational Transformation: The end result of instituting fundamental changes in the strategies, design, management, and leadership of an organization.

Organizational Values: Enduring beliefs and assumptions about modes of conduct or states of existence that are deemed worthwhile or desirable within the organization.

Outcome: The way customers respond to products or services.

Outcomes Analysis: An umbrella term used to describe various methodologies for evaluating the effectiveness of medical care.

Outcomes Data: Outcome endpoints used in **Outcomes Analysis**. Outcomes data include **Clinical Outcomes, Lesional Outcomes, Functional Outcomes,** and **Patient Satisfaction.**

Output: The products or services produced by a process

Overadjustment: One form of **tampering.**

P

p-Chart or **percent control chart:**   A types of attributes control chart that plots the proportion of defective units for samples of varying sizes.

Paradigm: A set of rules based on an explicit or implicit set of assumptions that explains how thing work or ought to work.

Paradigm Shift: A change in the way one perceives the way things work or ought to work.

Pareto Chart: A vertical bar graph that displays categories of items in decreasing order of frequency or magnitude from left to right which is used to prioritize items for attention.

Pareto Principle: The principle that one's impact for change can be maximized by focusing one's energy on a few priority causes that account for the majority of effects within a system. From the Italian economist Vilfredo Pareto in 1897, who note that the vast majority of wealth in his society was held by a remarkably small percentage of the population. Sometimes paraphrased as ''the vital few and the trivial many'', or ''the 80/20 rule'', it postulates that ~20% of the total causes within a system usually account for ~80% of the effects within that system.

Participative Management: A management approach in which supervisors and their subordinates interact in defining and structuring how work is done.

Patient Level Analysis: A subset of **Outcomes Analysis** with the focus of data collection being the individual patient.

Patient Satisfaction: A subset of **Outcomes Data** focussing on patient's degree of satisfaction with their care. Patient satisfaction is strongly influenced by timeliness, convenience, and cost, and often does not correlate with other more clinically-oriented **Outcomes Data** endpoints.

Per diem Payment System: A system in which the provider is paid a flat day rate for each day a patient is cared for in their institution.

Performance Measure: Performance Measures (also known as indicators) are quantitative tools that provide an indication of an organization's performance in relation to a specified process or outcome. Typically, data on the numerator event of interest and on the denominator population at risk are reported in the form of indicator rates or ratios.

Performing: The fourth and final stage of team psychological evolution. In this stage, the team members have come to know and respect each of their fellow team members. They are secure in their own position within the team and have learned how to resolve conflict within the group with without negative effects. All members are contributing to the group effort and all ideas and points of view are brought forth for discussion (see **team evolutionary stages**). Team members have discovered and accepted each other's strengths and weaknesses, and learned what their roles are. The team is now an effective, cohesive unit. Teams may cycle through the performing stage several times.

Personality Types: Descriptions of the primary tendencies individuals possess that describe how they behave and feel. Personality types are not necessarily good or bad.

Physician Profiling: The process of evaluating a physician's performance with regard to **clinical outcomes** and cost-effectiveness of treatments, usually by a third party payer.

Plan-Do-Check-Act (PDCA) Cycle: Also known as the Shewhart or Deming cycle or the ''Plan-Do-Study-Act (PDSA) cycle, it is an application of the scientific method useful for gaining knowledge about, and improving, **processes**.

Plan Phase: The first phase of the **Plan-Do-Check-Act (PDCA) cycle**. A plan based upon a prediction is developed in this phase. The plan identifies what needs to be improved, how it is to be implemented, and how the results are to be evaluated.

Planning Assumption: A belief, based upon past knowledge and experiences, about how current and future events, both internal and external to the organization, are likely to effect the achievement of desired results.

Points, 14: Deming's guidance for application of his theory of management for improvement of Quality, productivity, and competitive position.

Prioritization Matrix: A graphic tool used to prioritize tasks. Issues, or possible options based on known, weighted, criteria.

Process: A set of causes and conditions that repeatedly come together to transform **inputs** into **outputs** (see **significant process** and **critical process**).

Process Action Team (PAT): A temporary cross functional quality management team chartered by the **executive steering committee (ESC)** or a **quality management board (QMB)** composed of individuals actually working within a process for the purpose of gathering process data and/or improving a particular stage of the process (usually a **critical process**).

Process Capability: The predictable distribution of performance of a **stable process**.

Process Costing: A method used to assign costs to a group of patients that use approximately the same amount of resources.

Process Decision Program Chart (PDPC): A graphic tool that maps out conceivable negative events and contingencies that can occur in the execution of a plan and appropriate counter measures.

Process Improvement: see **continuous process improvement**.

Process Management: Actions taken by a quality management team to identify **critical processes** within a **significant process**, stabilize them, and then continually improve them.

Process Owner: Coordinates the various functions and work activities at all levels of a process, has the authority to make changes in the process as required, and manages the process end-to-end so as to ensure optimal overall performance.

Producible Quality Characteristic: Those quality characteristics identified by a **stakeholder** that a providing organization can produce.

Profound Knowledge: Deming's term to describe the system of knowledge required to achieve **organizational transformation** and system **optimization**. It consists of four equally-important and interdependent parts or disciplines: appreciation for a **system**, knowledge about **variation**, **psychology**, and the **theory of knowledge**. In general, it is more important to have a broad understanding of how the components interact than to have in-depth knowledge of any individual part of the system.

Psychology: One of the four disciplines of Deming's theory of **profound knowledge**. In quality terms, it involves the understanding of individual character types, values, motivations and learning styles, as well as group interpersonal dynamics and **team evolutionary stages**. Without an understanding of human psychology, **leadership** is not possible.

Q

Quality: The extent to which a product or service meets or exceeds customer requirements and expectations.

Quality Adjusted Life Years (QALYs): A widely used term for quantifying the benefit obtained from a medical or surgical intervention. One year of life in perfect health equals 1.0 QALY. Ten years of life with a disability assigned a utility value of 0.8 equals 8.0 QALYs.

Quality Advisor: A support person within an organization trained in **total quality management** theory, methods, and tools, who assists **quality management boards (QMB's)** or **process action teams (PAT's)** in data collection, analysis, and interpretation, provides **just-in-time** training for the team in the use of quality methods and tools for process improvement, and assists the team leader in interpreting and optimizing group dynamics.

Quality Characteristic: A property or attribute of a product or service that is considered important to a **stakeholder**.

Quality Circle: A small group that voluntarily performs quality improvement activities within the workplace, carrying out its work continuously as a part of quality control, self-development, mutual education, flow control, and improvement within the workplace.

Quality Function Deployment: A system for designing products or services based on customer requirements and involving all necessary functions of the producing organization.

Quality Improvement Teams: Any team that has been established to improve quality through the improvement of an organization's processes. They may be voluntary and informal such as **quality circles**, or they may be formally **chartered** and assigned through organizational **participative management**. In the Department of the Navy, these teams include the permanent **executive steering committee (ESC)** and **quality management boards (QMB's)**, as well as temporary **process action teams (PAT's)**.

Quality Leadership: The practice of Deming's 14 points by any person having formal authority within an organization.

Quality Loss Function: see **Taguchi loss function**.

Quality Management Board (QMB): A permanent cross functional team, **chartered** by the **executive steering committee (ESC)**, composed of managers, usually at the same organizational level within a **bureaucratic hierarchy,** who are jointly responsible for a process, system, product, or service. Separate QMB's are usually established for each of an organization's significant processes and membership includes all **process owners**.

Quality Philosophy: An enduring, value-based, set of interrelated statements created by an organization's guiding members that reflect the quality principles, concepts, and methods that address what the organization stands for and how it conducts its business.

R

Radar chart: A chart used to plot performance along several axes, which makes it easy to see areas of relative strength and weakness.

Random: Having no pattern

Random Sample: A sample selected in such a way that all potential candidates have an equal chance of being selected.

Range: A representation of the extent of **dispersion** in a set of data. It is determined by calculating the difference between the largest and smallest values in the data set.

Range chart: **Control chart** in which the range of the subgroup is used to track the instantaneous variation within a process, i.e. the variation in the process at any one time, when many input factors would not have time to vary enough to make a detectable difference. Range charts are usually paired with average charts for complete analysis.

Rational Subgrouping: A method for dividing data into subgroups based on some rational hypothesis in order to answer specific questions.

Rational Subgroup: A criterion for the **X-bar & R control chart** that requires samples (groups of observations used to plot points on the chart) to have the following characteristics:
- observations within the sample likely to be similar
- samples likely to differ from one another

Reengineering: The fundamental rethinking and radical redesign of business processes to bring a dramatic improvements in performance. Also known as "business process reengineering".

Reliability: A quality of measurement characterized by the same data being collected each time in repeated observations of the same phenomenon. In relation to performance measures, it is the ability of the indicator to consistently identify the events it was designed to identify across multiple health care settings.

Report Card: Publicly released reports on the actual performance of health care organizations (e.g. health plans or hospitals) on specific measures/indicators. The reports cards are frequently intended to help inform consumer or purchaser selection of providers and/or to foster competition on the basis of quality.

Representative Sample: A sample created with the intention of limiting **bias** and therefore increasing the validity of the study results.

Resource-Based Relative Value System (RBRVS): A methodology used for reimbursement calculations that considers physician work, practice expense, and malpractice expense to determine the relative value of a particular physician service.

Rice Bowl: The collection of all resources perceived to be within one's span of control.

Risk Adjustment: Methodology used to adjust anticipated health outcomes to compensate for the severity of illness in the patients treated.

Risk Stratification: After various factors are considered that may influence anticipated health outcomes (**Risk Adjustment**), patients can be grouped into appropriate risk categories.

Roadblock: An impediment, either internal or external to an organization, that hinders progress toward a goal.

Root Cause: Original reason for non-conformance within a process. When the root cause is removed or corrected, the non-conformance will be eliminated.

Root Cause Analysis: A process for identifying the basic or causal factor(s) that underlie variation in performance including the occurrence or possible occurrence of a **sentinel event**.

Run Chart: A line graph depicting data values over time which is used to assess and achieve process stability. A chart that plots data over time, allowing you to identify trends and anomalies.

Run Tests: see **zone tests.**

S

Sample: Data taken from a subset of potentially measurable subjects.

Sampling Plan: see **data collection plan**.

Scatter Diagram: A graph depicting the strength ad shape of the relationship between to variables.

Scorecard: the key measures of performance that monitor an organization's progress toward achieving its strategic goals and provide feedback that supports necessary modification to plans over time.

Scribe: During a meeting, the scribe posts ideas on a flipchart or whiteboard as the discussion unfolds so that everyone can see them. Posting the ideas prevents the "team memory" from changing as the dialogue or discussion unfolds and to keep team members focused on the topic or task.

Selection Grid: A grid (or **prioritization matrix**) designed to help a team select one option out of several possibilities. It involves deciding which criteria are important and using them as a basis for reaching a decision acceptable to the group.

Sensitivity Analysis: A method used to test the impact of variations of individual assumptions on the overall analysis outcome.

Sentinel Event: An unexpected occurrence involving death or serious physical or psychological injury, or the risk thereof. Such events are called "sentinel" because they signal the need for immediate investigation and response.

Significant Process: a **process** producing **outputs** that address external customer requirements, that can be traced back through the producing organization to organizational **inputs**. Improving this process will affect customer outcomes.

Silo Effect: A negative result of vertically-oriented **bureaucratic hierarchies** where horizontal, cross-functional, cooperation is limited by the absence of horizontal flow of necessary information within an organization, as well as conflicts of jurisdiction & authority between figures in vertically-oriented columns.

Small Area Analysis: An analysis used to determine population-based rates of medical care usage by patients, hospitals, and health care providers.

Special Cause: Causes that are not in the process all the time or do not affect every product or service, but arise because of specific circumstances. These sources of variation are unpredictable and unstable. Causes of variation in a process that are not inherent in the process itself but originate from circumstances that are out of the ordinary. Special causes are indicated by points that fall outside the limits of a **control chart**.

Specification Limits: A range of values, based on customer requirements, used to judge the acceptability of a product or service.

Stability: A state in which a process has displayed a certain degree of consistency in the past and is expected to continue to do so in the future.

Stable Process: A process in which **variation** in **outputs** arises only from **common cause**. A process that is stable and predictable.

Stages of Team Growth: As a team works together and matures, members gradually learn to cope with the emotional and group pressure they face together. As a result, the team goes through fairly predictable stages: **forming, storming, norming** and **performing**.

Stakeholder: The groups and individuals inside or outside the organization who affect and are affected by the achievement of the organization's mission, goals and strategy.

Standard Gamble: A method used to measure the utility of **clinical outcomes** obtained by asking patients to compare a variety of given health states obtained with certainty or attempt to obtain perfect health by assuming a gamble, the loss of which results in death.

Standardization: A method used to achieve uniform practice within a process, i.e., that all workers are following a standard operating procedure.

Statistical Control: The condition describing a **process** from which all **special causes** have been eliminated and only **common causes** remain; evidenced on a **control chart** by the absence of points beyond the **control limits** and by the absence of nonrandom patterns or trends within the control limits (see **stable process**).

Statistical Process Control: The application of statistical methods for the purpose of reducing process **variation**.

Statistical Quality Control: The application of statistical methods to improve the quality of products. The emphasis is on acceptance sampling of the product rather than the process that produced the product.

Storming: The third stage of team psychological evolution. The stage of team growth in which team members begin to realize that the task is different and more difficult than they imagined. In this stage, the team members tend to disagree with one another's ideas and viewpoints and begin to assert themselves to assess their degree of support among the others in the group, as well as establish their position in the group social "pecking order" (see **team evolutionary stages**). Team members struggle for power and influence, become impatient about the lack of progress, and resist collaborating with other team members. This is often the most difficult stage for the team. Teams may experience several phases of storming during their life.

Storyboarding: Originally, the process used by cartoonists to rough out the story line of a new television program. Quick sketches would be drawn, and pasted up on a common bulletin board, to make it easy for a group to plan together. This technique has grown now to include idea generation techniques using cards or sticky notes, and the rather different ideas of the graphical display of project achievements.

Strategic Framework: The combination of an organization's **mission statement, vision statement**, and **guiding principles** which serves as a context for practicing **strategic management**.

Strategic Goal: A long-range target that guides an organization's efforts in moving toward a desired future state.

Strategic Intent: A driving force compelling leadership toward its vision.

Strategic Management: A process that links **strategic planning** and **strategic intent** with day-to-day operational management in a single management process.

Strategic Plan: A document that describes an organization's **mission, vision, guiding principles, strategic goals, strategies,** and **objectives.**

Strategic Planning: The process by which the guiding members of an organization develop a **strategic plan**.

Strategy: A means for achieving a long-range strategic goal.

Strengths: the particular capabilities that distinguish an organization relative to others and provide competitive advantage. Determining an organization's strengths is the "S" in **SWOT analysis**, the basic approach to strategic assessment.

Suboptimization: A negative condition for an organization that occurs when the component of a system component has a net negative effect on the aim of the total system. In this situation the performance of the component is improved at the expense of the other components of the system as well as the system as a whole.

Suppliers: The person or group who provides an input to a process. Suppliers can be either **internal** or **external suppliers**.

Supporting Plans: Operating plans developed at lower levels of the organization that support the organization's **strategic plan** and contribute to organizational **optimization**.

SWOT Analysis: a succinct and honest evaluation of an organization's competitive position—its **strengths** (S), **weaknesses** (W), **opportunities** (O), and **threats** (T).

System: A network of interdependent components that work together to try to accomplish the aim of the system. Components of the system include management style, employees, customers, environmental constraints, stakeholders, training, and recruitment, among others.

System Optimization: see **optimization**.

T

Taguchi Loss Function: The concept that there is an increasing economic loss as product **quality characteristics** deviate from their target value even if these characteristics remain within absolute **specification limits**.

Tampering: Inappropriate action taken because process variation is erroneously ascribed to a **special cause** when, in fact, the cause is part of the **common cause** system. Tampering wastes time and resources, is harmful to morale, often increases overall process variation, and can lead to increased complexity within a process.

Team: A group of individuals organized to work together to accomplish an aim.

Team Evolutionary Stages: The concept that a group of individuals must sequentially work through four psychological stages before emerging as an effective team. These four stages are known as the **"forming"**, **"norming"**, **"storming"**, and "**performing"** stages.

Team Facilitator (or Coach): Someone who helps keep the team on track and provides **Just in Time Training** as needed. A facilitator usually focuses more on how the team gets its work done than on the content or subject of the team's work. They usually have extensive technical skills in problem solving, process improvement methodologies, data collection and analysis. They also are experienced in communication, group dynamics, and running meetings. The facilitator may attend meetings, but is neither the team leader nor a team member.

Team Leader: A member of a team responsible for leading the team in the accomplishment of the aim. The leader is responsible for setting and keeping to meeting agendas, publication of meeting minutes, ensuring meeting attendance, motivating team members, working with the **quality advisor** to manage group dynamics, and communicating with the authorizing quality management team through the **link pin**.

Theory of Knowledge: Deming's theory that **process** knowledge is acquired and advanced through a slow, continuous stream of empirical tests and experiments. While occasional "breakthroughs" do occur bringing rapid advances in knowledge, he believed that the majority of advances are made through slow incremental growth based on experimentation and guided by theory.

Threats: challenges to an organization's current and future competitive position. Identifying threats is the "T" in **SWOT analysis**.

Time Trade-Off: A method used to measure the utility of **clinical outcomes** by asking patients to exchange years of life for optimal health.

Timekeeper: The timekeeper helps the group keep track of time during the meeting. This person is responsible for alerting the team when the time allocated for an item is almost up so the team can decide whether to continue the discussion or cut it short.

Total Quality: An extension of the total quality concept to include improvement of all the **quality characteristics** that influence customer-perceived quality. This includes sources of **variation** from incoming supplies, all of the **significant processes** within an organization, and all those that can influence customer satisfaction, needs, or expectations when the product or service has left the organization.

Total Quality Management: The application of quantitative methods and the knowledge of people to assess and improve: materials and services supplied to the organization; all **significant processes** within the organization; and meeting the needs of the **end-user**, now and in the future.

Tree Diagram: A graphic tool for mapping the full range of tasks needed to achieve the end goal, purpose, or objective. A chart used to break any task, goal, or category into increasingly detailed levels of information. Family trees are the classic example of a tree diagram.

U

u-Chart: A type of attributes **control chart** that plots the number of defects per unit (defect rate) for samples of varying sizes.

Under-adjustment: Not taking action on a process when action is needed.

"Unknowable" Costs: Costs that result from poor quality which cannot be readily quantified in financial terms. For example, the cost to an organization of a dissatisfied customer, or of employees who are afraid to make suggestions or take risks that might lead to better quality.

Unmanaged Indemnity: A payment system in which claims are paid by the insurer as they are received.

Unstable Process: A **process** in which **variation** is a result of both **common** and **special causes**.

Utilitarianism: An economic philosophy that is concerned with the strength of an individual's preference for certain circumstances and outcomes.

Utilization Research: Clinical studies evaluating the rate of use of various medical and surgical interventions. Most commonly this methodology has been used to determine the rate of surgical procedures or rate of hospitalization among geographic areas or healthcare organizations.

V

Validity: The extent to which a measure accurately reflects the concept or *construct* that it is intended to measure. For performance measurement in health care, it is the ability of an indicator to measure processes or outcomes reflective of the quality of health care services provided. This can be determined by assessing a measure's ability to identify opportunities to improve the quality of care.

Value-Added Activity: Activities or steps within a **process** that actually contribute value, as defined by the **customer**, to the **output** of the process.

Values: the guiding principles and tenets of an organization; also referred to as "**core values**."

Variables Data: Values resulting from measurement of a continuous variable rather than discreet units or yes/no options. Variables data is used to create **histograms**, some **control charts**, and sometimes **run charts**.

Variation: The observed differences in output characteristics produced by a **process**. Causes of variation can be separated into **common** and **special causes**.

Vision: the combination of "**core ideology**" and "**envisioned future**" that articulates an organization's future direction for a period of time. Unlike "**mission**", which is timeless, "vision" changes over time as an organization achieves major goals and pursues new opportunities created by changes in the external environment and its own resources and capacity.

Vision Statement: An idealized view of a desirable and potentially achievable future state for the organization.

Voice of the Customer: The **quality characteristics** of a product or service that customers define as important to meet their needs.

Voice of the Process: The actual performance of the process.

W

Weaknesses: organizational characteristics that limit its performance, create competitive disadvantages, and must be improved if it is to be successful in achieving its vision. Identifying an organization's weaknesses is the ''W'' in **SWOT analysis**.

White Space: The space represented on an organizational flow chart between adjacent functions (vertical columns) that must be managed and improved by owners of those functions to achieve system **optimization**.

X

X & MR Chart: A type of variables control chart that plots individual measurements and **moving ranges**. This chart is commonly used in service industries.

X-bar & R Chart: A type of variables control chart that plots sample means and sample **ranges**.

X-bar & S Chart: A type of variables control chart that plots sample means and sample standard deviations.

Y

Z

Zero Defects: A situation that exists when all quality characteristics are produced within design specifications. This concept is reflected in the attitude that defects can be prevented, especially if more attention is given to the task at hand. The theme that embodies this concept is ''do it right the first time''. A quality philosophy attributed to Philip B. Crosby.

Zone Tests: Criteria applied to three or more consecutive points on a **control chart** to detect unnatural patterns that would indicate **special cause variation** even if the data points on the **control chart** lie within the **control limits**. Also called **run tests**.

Index

Page numbers followed by letters *f* and *t* denote figures and tables, respectively.